INTRODUCTION TO
Orthotics

INTRODUCTION TO
Orthotics

A Clinical Reasoning & Problem-Solving Approach

FOURTH EDITION

BRENDA M. COPPARD, PhD, OTR/L, FAOTA

Professor, Associate Dean for Assessment
Special Assistant to the Provost
Department of Occupational Therapy
Creighton University
Omaha, Nebraska

HELENE LOHMAN, MA, OTD, OTR/L, FAOTA

Professor
Department of Occupational Therapy
Creighton University
Omaha, Nebraska

ELSEVIER
MOSBY

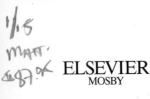

ELSEVIER
MOSBY

3251 Riverport Lane
St. Louis, Missouri 63043

INTRODUCTION TO ORTHOTICS: A CLINICAL REASONING
AND PROBLEM-SOLVING APPROACH, FOURTH EDITION

ISBN: 978-0-323-09101-5

Notices

Knowledge and best practice in this field are constantly changing. As new research and experience broaden our understanding, changes in research methods, professional practices, or medical treatment may become necessary.

Practitioners and researchers must always rely on their own experience and knowledge in evaluating and using any information, methods, compounds, or experiments described herein. In using such information or methods they should be mindful of their own safety and the safety of others, including parties for whom they have a professional responsibility.

With respect to any drug or pharmaceutical products identified, readers are advised to check the most current information provided (i) on procedures featured or (ii) by the manufacturer of each product to be administered, to verify the recommended dose or formula, the method and duration of administration, and contraindications. It is the responsibility of practitioners, relying on their own experience and knowledge of their patients, to make diagnoses, to determine dosages and the best treatment for each individual patient, and to take all appropriate safety precautions.

To the fullest extent of the law, neither the Publisher nor the authors, contributors, or editors, assume any liability for any injury and/or damage to persons or property as a matter of products liability, negligence or otherwise, or from any use or operation of any methods, products, instructions, or ideas contained in the material herein.

ISBN: 978-0-323-09101-5

Content Strategy Director: Penny Rudolph
Content Development Manager: Jolynn Gower
Publishing Services Manager: Julie Eddy
Senior Project Manager: Marquita Parker
Designer: Paula Catalano

Printed in the United States of America

Last digit is the print number: 9 8 7 6 5 4 3 2 1

*This work is dedicated to the late Roman Renner, my beloved father,
my family, and the Creighton community.*
Brenda M. Coppard

*This book is dedicated to my parents, Mira Lee and
Henry Goldstein, who instilled in me the love of learning,
and to my students who continue to inspire me.*
Helene Lohman

CONTRIBUTORS

Debbie Amini, EdD, OTR/L, CHT
Assistant Professor
Department of Occupational Therapy
East Carolina University
Greenville, North Carolina

Omar Aragón, OTD, OTR/L
Assistant Clinical Professor
Department of Occupational Therapy
Creighton University
Omaha, Nebraska

Janet Bailey, OTR/L, CHT
Hand and Arm Therapy Specialists
Columbus, Ohio

Shirley Blanchard, PhD, OTR/L, ABDA, FAOTA
Associate Professor
Department of Occupational Therapy
Creighton University
Omaha, Nebraska

Salvador L. Bondoc, OTD, OTR/L, FAOTA
Associate Professor and Chairperson of Occupational
    Therapy
Quinnipiac University
Hamden, Connecticut

Cynthia Cooper, MFA, MA, OTR/L, CHT
Director of Hand Therapy
Arizona VibrantCare Rehabilitation
Phoenix, Arizona

Brenda M. Coppard, PhD, OTR/L, FAOTA
Professor, Associate Dean for Assessment
Special Assistant to the Provost
Department of Occupational Therapy
Creighton University
Omaha, Nebraska

Lisa Deshaies, OTR/L, CHT
Adjunct Instructor
Department of Occupational Science & Occupational
    Therapy
University of Southern California
Los Angeles, California
Occupational Therapy Clinical Specialist
Occupational Therapy Department
Rancho Los Amigos National Rehabilitation Center
Downey, California

Stefania Fatone, PhD
Associate Professor
Physical Medicine and Rehabilitation
Northwestern University
Chicago, Illinois

Deanna J. Fish, MS, CPO
Chief Clinical Officer
Clinical Operations
Linkia, LLC
Bethesda, Maryland

Sharon Flinn, PhD, OTR/L, CHT
Assistant Professor
Division of Occupational Therapy
The Ohio State University
Columbus, Ohio

Linda S. Gabriel, PhD, OTR/L
Assistant Professor
Department of Occupational Therapy
Creighton University
Omaha, Nebraska

Amy Marie Haddad, PhD
Director, Center for Health Policy and Ethics
Dr. C.C. and Mabel L. Criss Endowed Chair
    in the Health Sciences
Creighton University
Omaha, Nebraska

Karyn Kessler, OTR/L
Vice President, Clinical Operations
Linkia, LLC
Bethesda, Maryland

Dulcey G. Lima, OTR/L, CO
Clinical Education Manager
Orthomerica Products, Inc.
Orlando, Florida

Helene Lohman, MA, OTD, OTR/L, FAOTA
Professor
Department of Occupational Therapy
Creighton University
Omaha, Nebraska

Michael Lohman, MEd, OTR/L, CO
Adjunct Clinical Professor
Department of Occupational Therapy
Creighton University
Director of Clinical Education
Lifestyles Orthotics and Prosthetics
Omaha, Nebraska

Ann McKie, OTR/L
Owner of McKie Splints, LLC
Duluth, Minnesota

Deborah A. Rider, OTR/L, CHT
Occupational Therapist
Fieldwork Coordinator
Therapy Department
Hand Surgery and Rehabilitation
Marlton, New Jersey

Marlene A. Riley, MMS, OTR/L, CHT
Clinical Associate Professor
Department of Occupational Therapy and
    Occupational Science
Towson University
Owner Occupational Therapy Associates of Towson
Towson, Maryland

Christopher Robinson, MBA
Assistant Professor
Physical Medicine and Rehabilitation
Northwestern University
Chicago, Illinois

Linda S. Scheirton, PhD
Associate Professor
Department of Occupational Therapy
Associate in the Center for Health Policy and Ethics
Creighton University
Omaha, Nebraska

Deborah A. Schwartz, OTD, OTR/L, CHT
Product and Educational Specialist
Orfit Industries America
Leonia, New Jersey

Brittany Bennett Stryker, OTD, OTR/L, CO
Practice Manager
Orthopedic Motion, Inc.
Las Vegas, Nevada

Kris M. Vacek, OTD, OTR/L
Chairperson and Associate Professor
Department of Occupational Therapy
Rockhurst University
Kansas City, Missouri

Jean Wilwerding-Peck, OTR/L, CHT
Clinical Coordinator
Creighton University Medical Center
Omaha, Nebraska

Aviva Wolff, OTR/L, CHT
Section Manager
Hand Therapy Department of Rehabilitation
    Hospital for Special Surgery
New York, New York

STUDENT CONTRIBUTORS
Martha Earney, OTS, Creighton University
Bob Gillmore, OTS, Creighton University
Nicole Cortes, OTS, Creighton University
Alexandria Neville, OTS, Creighton University
Jenny Junker, OTS, Creighton University
Mackenzie Raber, OTS, Creighton University

As instructors in a professional occupational therapy program who were unable to find an introductory orthotic textbook that addressed the development of orthotic theory and skills, we wrote the first edition and subsequent editions of *Introduction to Splinting: A Clinical Reasoning and Problem-Solving Approach*. Entry-level occupational therapy practitioners are expected to have fundamental skills in orthotic theory, design, and fabrication. It is unrealistic to think that students gain these skills through observation and limited experience in didactic course work or fieldwork. With the growing emphasis in the health care environment on accountability, productivity, and efficacy, educators must determine the skills students need to apply theory to practice.

Several features are improved in this fourth edition. Evidence-based orthotic provision is emphasized throughout the chapters, both in narrative and chart formats. A focus on occupation-based orthosis is present, including a chapter dedicated to the topic. The Occupational Therapy Practice Framework terminology is incorporated throughout the book. The use of the term *orthosis* and its derivatives are used throughout the text. An emphasis on safety is present in each chapter.

The fourth edition of *Introduction to Orthotics: A Clinical Reasoning and Problem-Solving Approach* was again designed with a pedagogy to facilitate the process of applying theory to practice in relationship to orthotic provision. This text is primarily designed for entry-level occupational therapy students, occupational therapy practitioners and interdisciplinary practitioners who need development in orthotic provision, therapists re-entering the field, and students on fieldwork. In past editions, students found the book beneficial because it facilitated the mastery of basic theory and the principles and techniques of orthotics that entry-level clinicians need for clinical competence. Instructors enthusiastically welcomed the text because the text was targeted for novice occupational therapy students. Novice practitioners also reported that the book enhanced the development of knowledge and skills related to orthotics.

The pedagogy employed within the book facilitates learning to meet the unique needs of students' preferred learning styles. Resources for students and educators on the EVOLVE website are expanded. Students have access to more video clips, learning activities, and additional case studies to create a personalized approach to learning. Educators have access to PowerPoint lecture slides, image collections, and a test bank.

The website provides visual and auditory instructions on orthotic provision. Additional case studies stimulate clinical reasoning and problem-solving skills. Self-quizzes and review questions with answers provide the reader with excellent tools to test immediate recall of basic information. Readers are guided through orthotic fabrication in the laboratory with more illustrations and photographs than in the previous editions. The forms provided in the book present opportunities to promote reflection and to assist students' development of their self-assessment skills. Case studies, orthotic analyses, and documentation exercises are examples of learning activities designed to stimulate authentic problem solving. The learning exercises and laboratory experiences provide opportunities to test clinical reasoning and the technical skills of orthotic pattern design and fabrication.

A cadre of expert contributors revised and expanded chapters that reflect current practice. This edition of *Introduction to Orthotics* contains 19 chapters. The first 5 chapters consist of foundations of orthotics; occupation-based orthotic provision; orthotic tools, processes, and techniques; anatomic and biomechanical principles; and assessment related to orthotic provision. These chapters provide fundamental information, which undergirds content in the remaining chapters.

Chapter 6 addresses thorough clinical reasoning processes used in making decisions about practice involving orthotic design and construction. The material presented in this chapter relates to answering questions of case studies presented in subsequent chapters.

Chapters 7 through 11 present the theory, design, and fabrication process of common orthoses used in general clinical practice. Orthoses acting on the wrist, hand, thumb, elbow, and fingers are addressed.

The remaining chapters in the book are geared toward more specialized topics and to intermediate-to-advanced orthotic provision. Topics include mobilization orthoses, orthotic provision for nerve injuries, antispasticity orthoses, orthotics for elders and children, orthoses for the lower extremity, prosthetics, and ethical issues related to orthotic provision.

A glossary of terms used throughout the book follows Chapter 19. This book contains 3 appendixes. Appendix A provides answers to quizzes, laboratory exercises, and case studies. Appendix B and C contain listings of web resources.

Although many therapists reviewed this book, each experienced therapist and physician may have a personal view on orthotic provision and therapeutic approaches and techniques. This book represents the authors' perspectives and is not intended to present the only correct approach. Thus, therapists employ their clinical reasoning skills in practice.

We hope this fourth edition of the book complements your professional development and continued competence!

**Brenda M. Coppard, PhD, OTR/L, FAOTA and
Helene Lohman, MA, OTD, OTR/L, FAOTA**

The completion of this fourth edition was made possible through the efforts of many individuals. We are grateful to Cynthia Cooper, MFA, MA, OTR/L, CHT, for the peer-reviewing of the manuscripts. Additionally, we appreciate the talent and expertise of the following contributor authors to the current and previous editions: Debbie Amini, EdD, OTR/L, CHT; Omar Aragon, OTD, OTR/L; Janet Bailey OTR/L, CHT; Serena M. Berger, MA, OTR; Shirley Blanchard, PhD, OTR/L, ABDA, FAOTA; Salvador Bondoc, OTD, OTR/L, FAOTA, Maureen T. Cavanaugh, MS, OTR; Cynthia Cooper, MFA, MA, OTR/L, CHT; Lisa Deshaies, OTR/L, CHT; Beverly Duvall-Riley, MS, BSOT; Stefania Fatone, PhD; Deanna J. Fish, MS, CPO; Sharon Flynn, PhD, OTR/L, CHUT; Linda Gabriel, PhD, OTR/L; Amy Marie Haddad, PhD; Karyn Kessler, OTR/L; Dulcey G. Lima, OTR/L, CO; Michael Lohman, MEd, OTR/L, CO; Peggy Lynn, OTR, CHT; Ann McKie, OTR/L; Debra A. Monnin, OTR/L; Sally E. Poole, MA, OT, CHT; Debbie Rider, OTR/L, CHT; Marlene A. Riley, MMS, OTR, CHT; Christopher Robinson, MBA: Susan Salzberg, MOT, OTR/L; Linda Scheirton, PhD; Deborah A. Schwartz, OTD, OTR/L, CHT; Lauren Sivula, OTS; Brittany Bennett Stryker, OTD, OTR/L, CO; Joan L. Sullivan, MA, OTR, CHT; Kris Vacek, OTD, OTR; Jean Wilwerding-Peck, OTR/L, CHT; and Aviva Wolff, OTR/L, CHT.

Preparing the artwork and filming for this book was time and labor intensive. We are grateful for the skills of Rik Cannon and the staff of Redline Production and Alexandra Kobrin, OTS, for assistance with videotaping.

The staff at Elsevier has given steadfast support (and patience) for this book. We are grateful for the guidance and assistance from Kathy Falk, Jolynn Gower, Penny Rudolph, and Marquita Parker.

We thank our families and friends for their continual support, encouragement, and patience. We also thank our students for enabling us to learn from them.

BMC
HL

CONTENTS

Orthotic Foundations

CHAPTER 1

Foundations of Orthotics

Brenda M. Coppard, PhD, OTR/L, FAOTA

Key Terms
dorsal
evidence-based practice
immobilization
mobilization
orthosis
splint
torque transmission
volar

Chapter Objectives
1. Define the terms *splint* and *orthosis*.
2. Identify the health professionals who may provide orthotic services.
3. Appreciate the historical development of orthotics as a therapeutic intervention.
4. Apply the Occupational Therapy Practice Framework (OTPF) to optimize evaluation and intervention for a client.
5. Describe how frame-of-reference approaches are applied to provision of orthoses.
6. Familiarize yourself with orthotic nomenclature of past and present.
7. List the purposes of immobilization (static) orthoses.
8. List the purposes of mobilization (dynamic) orthoses.
9. Describe the six orthotic designs.
10. Define *evidence-based practice*.
11. Describe the steps involved in evidence-based practice.
12. Cite the hierarchy of evidence for critical appraisals of research.

Chrystal is a student who is enrolled in an orthotics course. She is a bit anxious, but is looking forward to gaining the knowledge and skills to be competent in orthotic provision.

Note: This chapter includes content from previous contributions from Peggy Lynn, OTR, CHT.

The instructor told Chrystal and her classmates that it takes time to build skills, and much practice is necessary.

Determining orthotic design and fabricating hand orthoses are extremely important aspects in providing optimal care for persons with upper extremity injuries and functional deficits. Fabrication of orthoses is a combination of science and art. Therapists must apply knowledge of occupation, pathology, physiology, kinesiology, anatomy, psychology, payment systems, and biomechanics to best design orthoses for persons. In addition, therapists must consider and appreciate the aesthetic value of orthoses. People who are novices at making orthoses should be aware that each person is different, requiring a customized approach to orthoses. The use of occupation-based and evidence-based approaches to orthoses guides a therapist to consider a person's valued occupations. As a result, those occupations are used as both a means (e.g., as a medium for therapy) and an end to outcomes (e.g., intervention goals).[1]

Therapists must also develop and use clinical reasoning skills to effectively evaluate and treat clients with upper extremity conditions who may need orthotic interventions. This book emphasizes and fosters such skills for people who are learning how to make orthoses in general practice areas. After therapists are knowledgeable in the science of orthotic design and fabrication (including instructing clients on their use and on precautions regarding them, checking for proper fit, and making revisions as deemed appropriate), practical experience is essential for them to become comfortable and competent.

Definition of Splint and Orthosis

According to the American Society of Hand Therapists (ASHT) a **splint** "refers to casts and strapping used for reductions of fractures and dislocations. *Splinting* is a term that should not be used by therapists [who] are fabricating and issuing...orthoses. [Splinting] is used by physician offices for applying a cast. There are Current Procedural Terminology (CPT) codes for splinting that are used when billing for this purpose."[2] An **orthosis** is defined by ASHT as a single device that is rigid or semi-rigid. Orthoses are used to support a weak or deformed body part, or restrict or eliminate motion of a body part. Orthoses can be custom made or prefabricated. The terms *splint* and *orthosis* are often used synonymously. However, for payment purposes, therapists must use the proper term.

Historical Synopsis of Orthotic Intervention

Reports of primitive orthoses date back to ancient Egypt.[3] Decades ago, blacksmiths and carpenters constructed the first orthoses. Materials used to make the orthoses were limited to cloth, wood, leather, and metal.[4] Hand orthoses became an important intervention in physical rehabilitation during World War II. Survival rates of injured troops dramatically increased because of medical, pharmacologic (e.g., the use of penicillin), and technological advances. During this period, occupational and physical therapists collaborated with orthotic technicians and physicians to provide orthoses to clients: "Sterling Bunnell, MD, was designated to organize and to oversee hand services at nine army hospitals in the United States."[5] In the mid 1940s, under the guidance of Dr. Bunnell many orthoses were made and sold commercially. During the 1950s, many children and adults needed orthoses to assist them in carrying out activities of daily living (ADLs) secondary to poliomyelitis.[5] During this time, orthoses were made of high-temperature plastics. With the advent of low-temperature thermoplastic materials in the 1960s, hand orthoses became a common intervention for clients.

Today, some therapists and clinics specialize in hand therapy. Hand therapy evolved from a group of therapists in the 1970s who were interested in researching and rehabilitating clients with hand injuries.[6] In 1977, this group of therapy specialists established the ASHT. In 1991, the first certification examination in hand therapy was administered. Those therapists who pass the certification examination are credentialed as certified hand therapists (CHTs).

Specialized organizations (e.g., American Society for Surgery of the Hand and ASHT) influence the practice, research, and education of upper extremity orthoses.[7] For example, the ASHT Splint Classification System offered a uniform nomenclature in the area of orthotics.[8]

Professionals Who Make Orthoses

A variety of health care professionals design and fabricate orthoses. Occupational therapists (OTs) constitute a large group of health care providers whose services include orthotic design and fabrication. Certified occupational therapy assistants (COTAs) also provide orthotic services. Along with OTs and COTAs, physical therapists (PTs) specializing in hand rehabilitation often fabricate orthoses for their clients who have hand injuries. PTs are also frequently involved in providing orthoses for the lower extremities. In addition, certified orthotists (COs) are trained and skilled in the design, construction, and fitting of braces and orthoses prescribed by physicians. Dentists often fabricate orthoses to address selective dental problems. Occasionally, nurses who have had special training fabricate orthoses.

Orthotic design must be based on scientific principles. A given diagnosis does not specify the orthosis that the practitioner will make. Orthotic fabrication often requires creative problem solving. Such factors as a client's occupational needs and interests influence orthotic design, even among clients who have common diagnoses. Health care professionals who make orthoses must allow themselves to be creative and take calculated risks. Making orthoses requires practice for one to be at ease with the design and fabrication process. Students or therapists beginning to design and fabricate orthoses should be aware of personal expectations and realize that their skills will likely evolve with practice. Therapists with experience in orthotics tend to be more efficient with time and materials than novice students and therapists.

Occupational Therapy Theories, Models, and Frame-of-Reference Approaches for Orthotic Intervention

The Occupational Therapy Practice Framework (OTPF) outlines the occupational therapy process of evaluation and intervention and highlights the emphasis on the use of occupation.[9] Performance areas of occupation as specified in the framework include the following: ADLs, instrumental activities of daily living (IADLs), education, work, play, leisure, and social participation. Performance areas of occupation place demands on a person's performance skills (i.e., motor skills, process skills, and communication/interaction skills). Therapists must consider the influence of performance patterns on occupation. Such patterns include habits, routines, and roles. Contexts affect occupational participation. Contexts include cultural, physical, social, personal, spiritual, temporal, and virtual dimensions. The engagement in an occupation involves activity demands placed on the individual. Activity demands include objects used and their properties, space demands, social demands, sequencing and timing, and required actions, body functions, and body structures. Client factors relate to a person's body functions and body structures. Table 1-1 provides examples of how the framework assists one in thinking about orthotic provision to a client.

The practice of occupational therapy is guided by conceptual systems.[10] One such conceptual system is the Occupational Performance Model, which consists of performance areas, components, and contexts. A therapist using the Occupational Performance Model may influence a client's performance area or component while considering the context in which the person lives, works and plays. The therapist is guided by several approaches in providing assessment and intervention. The therapist may use the biomechanical,

Table 1-1   Examples* of the Occupational Therapy Practice Framework and Orthotic Provision

CATEGORY	QUESTIONS
Performance in Areas of Occupation	
Activities of daily living (ADLs)	What ADLs will a person need to perform while wearing an orthosis? Will ADLs need to be modified because of orthotic provision?
Instrumental activities of daily living (IADLs)	What types of IADLs will the person wearing an orthosis have to carry out (e.g., child care, shopping, pet care)? Will IADLs need to be modified because of orthotic provision?
Education	Can the person who just received an orthosis read the brochure that explains the home program? What type of client education must be provided for optimum care?
Work	What paid or volunteer work does the client want or need to perform while wearing the orthosis? Will work activities need to be modified because of orthotic provision?
Play	Can a child who wears an orthosis interact with toys?
Leisure	Can the person who wears an orthosis engage in leisure activities? Do modifications in leisure equipment or activities need to be made for full participation?
Social participation	Will the orthosis provided cause an adolescent to withdraw from particular social situations because the orthosis draws unwanted attention?
Performance Skills	
Motor skills	Does the person have the coordination and strength to don and doff his new resting hand orthosis?
Process skills	Can the person who has developmental delays correctly complete the steps and sequence to don and doff an orthosis?
Communication/ interaction skills	Will the person who communicates via sign language be hindered in wearing an orthosis? Will the person feel like she can engage in sexual activity while wearing her orthosis?
Performance Patterns	
Habits	How will the therapist enable a habit for the person to take care of his orthosis?
Routines	How might ADL routines be interrupted because the orthosis interferes with established sequences?
Roles	What roles does the person fulfill, and will any related behaviors be affected by wearing an orthosis?
Contexts	
Cultural	What if the person does not believe the orthosis will help his condition?
Physical	Does the client have accessibility to transportation to the clinic for follow-up visits?
Social	How might a caregiver be affected if the person receiving care is provided an orthosis?
Personal	What happens when a client needs an orthosis but has no means of paying for it?
Spiritual	How can the therapist tap into a client's motivation system to improve her outlook on the outcome of wearing an orthosis and receiving treatment?
Temporal	Should the client who has a 6-month life prognosis be issued an orthosis?
Virtual	Will the person who wears an orthosis be able to access his email?
Activity Demands	
Objects used and their properties	Will the teenager who is on the high school chess team be able to manipulate the chess pieces while wearing bilateral orthoses?
Space demands	Will wearing the orthosis impede a client's work tasks due to space restrictions?
Social demands	Will the teacher help the child don and doff an orthosis for participation in particular activities?
Sequencing and timing	Will the intensive care unit nursing staff be able to don and doff a client's orthosis according to the specified schedule?
Required actions	Can the client with arthritis thread the orthotic strap through the D-ring?
Required body functions	Does the client have the strength to lift her arm to dress while wearing an elbow orthosis?
Required body structures	How will the client with one arm amputated don and doff his orthosis?
Client Factors	
Body functions	Does the client have sensation to determine if a dynamic orthosis is exerting too much force on joints?

*Examples are inclusive, not exclusive.

sensorimotor, and rehabilitative approaches. The biomechanical approach uses biomechanical principles of kinetics and forces acting on the body. Sensorimotor approaches are used to inhibit or facilitate normal motor responses in persons whose central nervous systems have been damaged. The rehabilitation approach focuses on abilities rather than disabilities and facilitates returning persons to maximal function using their capabilities.[10] (See Self-Quiz 1-1.)

Each approach can incorporate orthoses as an intervention, depending on the rationale for orthotic provision. For example, if a person wears a tenodesis orthosis to recreate grasp and release to maximize function in ADLs, the therapist is using the rehabilitation approach.[11] If the therapist is using the biomechanical approach, a dynamic (mobilization) hand orthosis may be chosen to apply kinetic forces to the person's body. If the therapist chooses a sensorimotor approach, an antispasticity orthosis may be used to inhibit or reduce tone.

Pierce's notions[12] of contextual and subjective dimensions of occupation are powerful concepts for therapists who appropriately incorporate orthotics into a client's care plan. Understanding how an orthosis affects a client's occupational engagement and participation are salient in terms of meeting the client's needs and goals, which may result in increased adherence. Contextual dimensions include spatial, temporal, and sociocultural contexts.[12] Subjective dimensions include restoration, pleasure, and productivity. Box 1-1 explicates both contextual and subjective dimensions of occupation. Pierce's framework is used to structure questions for a client interview.

Categorization of Orthotics

According to the ASHT,[13] there are six orthotic classification divisions (Figure 1-1):
- Identification of articular or nonarticular
- Location
- Direction
- Purpose

Box 1-1 Contextual and Subjective Dimensions of Occupation

Contextual Dimensions	Subjective Dimensions
• Temporal	• Restoration
• Circadian rhythms	• Eating
• Social schedules	• Sleeping
• Time (clocks)	• Self-care
• Patterns of occupations	• Hobbies
• Spatial	• Spirituality
• Physical body	• Pleasure
• Environmental conditions	• Play
• Object use	• Leisure
• Symbolic meanings of space	• Humor
• Sociocultural	• Ritual
• Identity	• Productivity
• Cultural diversity	• Challenge to avoid boredom
• Genders	• Worth ethic
• Health care cultures	• Work identity
• Relationships	• Stress

- Type
- Total number of joints

Identification of Articular or Nonarticular

The first element of the ASHT classification indicates whether or not an orthosis affects articular structures. Articular orthoses use three-point pressure systems "to affect a joint or joints by immobilizing, mobilizing, restricting, or transmitting torque."[7] Most orthoses are articular, and the term *articular* is often not specified in the technical name of the orthosis.

Nonarticular orthoses use a two-point pressure force to stabilize or immobilize a body segment.[7] Thus, the term *nonarticular* should always be included in the name of the orthosis. Examples of nonarticular orthoses include those that affect the long bones of the body (e.g., humerus).

SELF-QUIZ 1-1*

Match the approach used in each of the following scenarios.

a. Biomechanical approach
b. Sensorimotor approach
c. Rehabilitation approach

1. _____ This approach is used on a child who has cerebral palsy. The goal of the orthosis is to decrease the amount of tone present.
2. _____ This approach allows a person who had a stroke to grasp the walker by using orthoses that are adapted to assist with grasp.
3. _____ This approach helps a person who had a tendon repair that resulted in flexor contractures of the metacarpophalangeal (MCP) joint regain full range of motion.

---

*See Appendix A for the answer key.

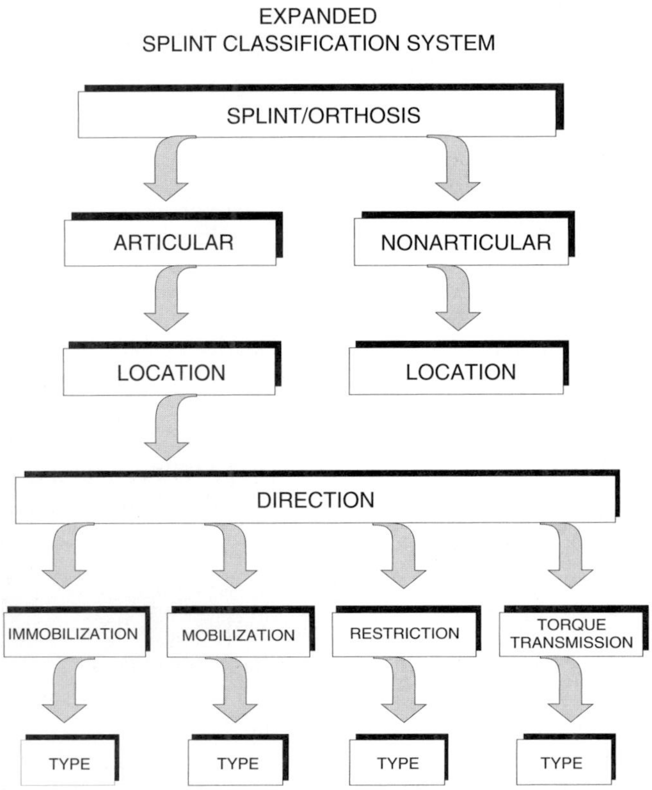

**EXPANDED
SPLINT CLASSIFICATION SYSTEM**

Figure 1-1 Expanded orthotic classification system division. (From Fess EE, Gettle KS, Philips CA, et al: *Hand and upper extremity splinting: principles and methods,* ed 3, St Louis, 2005, Elsevier Mosby.)

Location

Orthoses, whether articular or nonarticular, are classified further according to the location of primary anatomic parts included in the orthosis. For example, articular orthoses will include a joint name in the orthosis (e.g., elbow, thumb metacarpal [MP], index finger proximal interphalangeal [PIP]). Nonarticular orthoses are associated with one of the long bones (e.g., ulna, humerus, radius).

Direction

Direction classifications are applicable to articular orthoses only. Because all nonarticular orthoses work in the same manner, the direction does not need to be specified. Direction is the primary kinematic function of orthoses. Such terms as *flexion, extension,* and *opposition* are used to classify orthoses according to direction. For example, an orthosis designed to flex the PIP joints of index, middle, ring, and small fingers would be named an *index–small-finger PIP flexion orthosis.*

Purpose

The fourth element in the ASHT classification system is purpose. There are four purposes of orthoses: (1) mobilization, (2) immobilization, (3) restriction, and (4) torque

transmission. The purpose of the orthosis indicates how the orthosis works. Examples include the following:

- Mobilization: Wrist/finger-MP extension mobilization orthosis
- Immobilization: Elbow immobilization orthosis
- Restriction: Elbow extension restriction orthosis
- Torque transmission: Finger PIP extension torque transmission orthosis, type 1 (2) (The number in parentheses indicates the total number of joints incorporated into the orthosis.)

Mobilization orthoses are designed to move or mobilize primary and secondary joints. **Immobilization** orthoses are designed to immobilize primary and secondary joints. Restrictive orthoses "limit a specific aspect of joint range of motion for the primary joints."[13] **Torque transmission** orthoses' purposes are to "(1) create motion of primary joints situated beyond the boundaries of the orthosis itself or (2) harness secondary 'driver' joint(s) to create motion of primary joints that may be situated longitudinally or transversely to the 'driver' joint(s)."[7] Torque transmission orthoses, illustrated in Figure 1-2, are also referred to as *exercise orthoses.*

Type

The classification of orthosis type specifies the secondary joints included in the orthosis. Secondary joints are often incorporated into the orthotic design to affect joints that are proximal, distal, or adjacent to the primary joint. There are ten joint levels that comprise the upper extremity: shoulder, elbow, forearm, wrist, finger MP, finger PIP, finger distal interphalangeal (DIP), thumb carpometacarpal (CMC), thumb metacarpophalangeal (MCP), and thumb interphalangeal (IP) levels. Only joint levels are counted, not the number of individual joints. For example, if the wrist joint and multiple finger PIP joints are included as secondary joints in an orthosis, the type is defined as 2. (PIP joints account for one level and the wrist joint accounts for another level, thus totalling two secondary joint levels.) The technical name for an orthosis that flexes the MCP joints of the index, middle, ring, and small fingers and incorporates the wrist and PIP joints is an *index–small-finger MCP flexion mobilization orthosis, type 2.* If no secondary joints are included in the orthotic design, the joint level is type 0.

Total Number of Joints

The final ASHT classification level is the total number of individual joints incorporated into the orthotic design. The number of total joints incorporated in the orthosis follows the type indication. For example, if an elbow orthosis includes the wrist and MCPs as secondary joints, the orthosis would be called an *elbow flexion immobilization orthosis, type 2 (3).* The number in parentheses indicates the total number of individual joints incorporated into the orthosis.

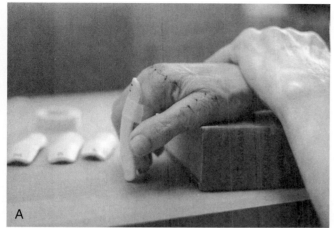

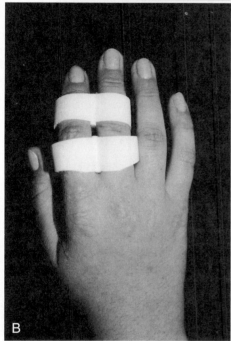

Figure 1-2 Torque transmission orthoses may create motion of primary joints situated longitudinally **(A)** or transversely **(B)** according to secondary joints. (From Fess EE, Gettle KS, Philips CA, et al: *Hand and upper extremity splinting: principles and methods,* ed 3, St Louis, 2005, Elsevier Mosby.)

Orthotic Designs

In the past, orthoses were categorized as static or dynamic. This classification system has its problems and controversies. In some clinics, ASHT orthotic terminology is not often used. Therefore, therapists must be familiar with the ASHT classification system and other commonly used nomenclature. Static orthoses have no movable parts.[14] In addition, static orthoses place tissues in a stress-free position to enhance healing and to minimize friction.[15] Dynamic orthoses have one or more movable parts[16] and are synonymous with orthoses that employ elastics, springs, and wire, as well as with multipart orthoses.

The purpose of an orthosis as a therapeutic intervention assists the therapist in determining its design. Orthotic design classifications include[15]:

- Static
- Serial static
- Dropout
- Dynamic
- Static-progressive

A static or immobilization orthosis (Figure 1-3) can maintain a position to hold anatomical structures at the end of available range of motion, thus exerting a mobilizing effect on a joint.[15] For example, a therapist fabricates an orthosis to position the wrist in maximum tolerated extension to increase extension of a stiff wrist. Because the orthosis positions the shortened wrist flexors at maximum length and holds them there, the tissue remodels in a lengthened form.[15]

Serial static orthoses (Figure 1-4) require the remolding of a static orthosis. The serial static orthosis holds the joint or series of joints at the limit of tolerable range, thus promoting tissue remodeling. As the tissue remodels, the joint gains range and the practitioner remolds the orthosis to once again place the joint at end range comfortably.

A dropout orthosis (Figure 1-5) allows motion in one direction while blocking motion in another.[13] This type of orthosis may help a person regain lost range of motion while preventing poor posture. For example, an orthosis may be designed to enhance wrist extension while blocking wrist flexion.[15]

Elastic tension dynamic (mobilization) orthoses (Figure 1-6) have self-adjusting or elastic components, which may include wire, rubber bands, or springs.[17] An orthosis that applies an elastic tension force to straighten an index finger PIP flexion contracture exemplifies an elastic tension/traction dynamic (mobilization) orthosis.

Static progressive orthoses (Figure 1-7) are types of dynamic (mobilization) orthoses. They incorporate the use of inelastic components, such as hook-and-loop tapes, outrigger line, progressive hinges, turnbuckles, and screws. The orthotic design incorporates the use of inelastic components to allow the client to adjust the amount of tension so as to prevent overstressing of tissue.[15] Chapter 12 more thoroughly addresses mobilization and torque transmission (dynamic) orthoses.

Many possibilities exist for orthotic design and fabrication. A therapist's creativity and skills are necessary for determining the best orthotic design. Therapists must stay updated on orthotic techniques and materials, which change rapidly. Reading professional literature and manufacturers' technical information helps therapists maintain knowledge about materials and techniques. A personal collection of reference books is also beneficial, and continuing-education courses and professional conferences provide ongoing updates on the latest theories and techniques.

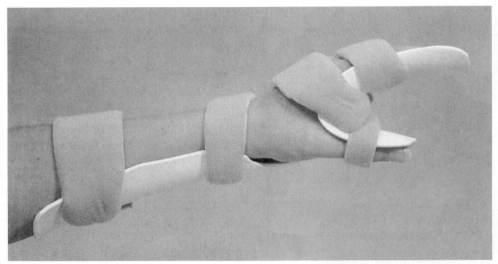

Figure 1-3 **Static immobilization orthosis.** This static orthosis immobilizes the thumb, fingers, and wrist.

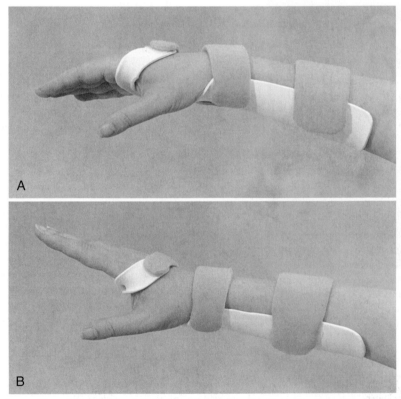

A

B

Figure 1-4 Serial static orthoses (**A** and **B**). The therapist intermittently remolds the orthosis as the client gains wrist extension motion.

Evidence-Based Practice and Orthotic Provision

Calls for **evidence-based practice** have stemmed from medicine but have affected all health care delivery, including orthoses.[18] Sackett and colleagues[19] defined evidence-based practice as "the conscientious, explicit, and judicious use of current best evidence in making decisions about the care of individual clients. The practice of evidence-based medicine

means integrating individual clinical expertise with the best available external clinical evidence from systematic research."

The aim of applying evidence-based practice is to "ensure that the interventions used are the most effective and the safest options."[20] Additionally, the American health care system increasingly emphasizes effectiveness and cost-efficiency and less credibility of provider preferences.[21] Essentially, therapists apply the research process during practice. This process includes (1) formulating a clear question based on

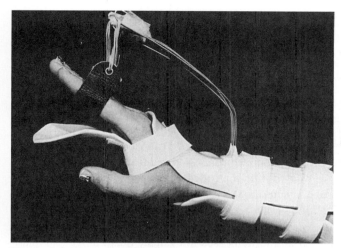

Figure 1-5 Dropout orthosis. A dorsal–forearm-based dynamic extension orthosis immobilizes the wrist and rests all fingers in a neutral position. A volar block permits only the predetermined metacarpophalangeal (MCP) joint flexion. (From Evans RB, Burkhalter WE: A study of the dynamic anatomy of extensor tendons and implications for treatment, *J Hand Surg* 11A:774, 1986.)

a client's problem, (2) searching the literature for pertinent research articles, (3) critically appraising the evidence for its validity and usefulness, and (4) implementing useful findings to the client case. Evidence-based practice is not about finding articles to support what a therapist does. Rather, it is reviewing a body of literature to guide the therapist in selecting the most appropriate assessment or intervention for an individual client.

Sackett and colleagues[19] and Law[22] outlined several myths of evidence-based practice and described the reality of each myth (Table 1-2). A misconception exists that evidence-based practice is impossible to implement or that it already exists. Although we know that keeping current on all health care literature is impossible, practitioners should consistently review research findings related to their specific practice, and even consider collecting their own data for evidence. Unfortunately, some practitioners rely primarily on their training or clinical experience to guide decision making. Novel clinical situations present a need for evidence-based practice.

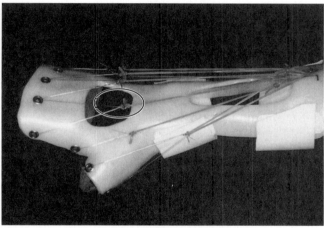

Figure 1-6 Elastic tension orthosis. This orthosis for radial nerve palsy has elastic rubber bands and inelastic filament traction. (Courtesy of Dominique Thomas, RPT, MCMK, Saint Martin Duriage, France; from Fess EE, Gettle KS, Philips CA, et al: *Hand and upper extremity splinting: principles and methods,* ed 3, St Louis, 2005, Mosby.)

Table 1-2 Evidence-Based Practice Myths and Realities

MYTH	REALITY
Evidence-based practice exists.	Practitioners spend too little time examining current research findings.
Evidence-based practice is difficult to integrate into practice.	Evidence-based practice can be implemented by busy practitioners.
Evidence-based practice is a "cookie cutter" approach.	Evidence-based practice requires extensive clinical experience.
Evidence-based practice is focused on decreasing costs.	Evidence-based practice emphasizes the best clinical evidence for individual clients.

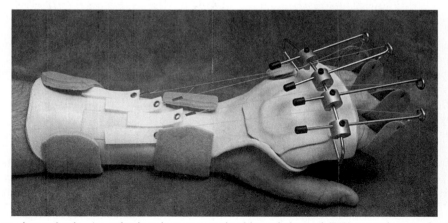

Figure 1-7 Static progressive orthosis. An orthosis to increase proximal interphalangeal (PIP) extension uses hook-and-loop mechanisms for adjustable tension.

Some argue that evidence-based practice leads to a "cookie cutter" approach to clinical care. Evidence-based practice involves a critical appraisal of relevant research findings. It is not a top-down approach. Rather, it adopts a bottom-up approach that integrates external evidence with one's clinical experience and client choice. After reviewing the findings, practitioners must use clinical judgment to determine if, why, and how they will apply findings to an individual client case. Thus, evidence-based practice is not a one-size-fits-all approach because all client cases are different.

Evidence-based practice is not intended to be a mechanism whereby all clinical decisions must be backed by a random controlled trial. Rather, the intent is to address efficacy and safety using the best current evidence to guide intervention for a client in the safest way possible. It is important to realize that efficacy and safety do not always result in a cost decrease.

Important to evidence-based practice is the ability of practitioners to appraise the quality of the evidence available. A hierarchy of evidence is based on the certainty of causation and the need to control bias (Figure 1-8).[23] The highest quality (gold standard) of evidence is the meta-analysis of randomized controlled studies. Next in the hierarchy are randomized controlled trials (RCTs). A well-designed cohort study is next in the hierarchy, followed by case-controlled studies and case reports. Last in the hierarchy is expert opinion or editorials. Box 1-2 presents a list of appraisal questions used to evaluate quantitative and qualitative research results.

Throughout this book, the authors made an explicit effort to present the research relevant to each chapter topic. Note that the evidence is limited to the timing of this publication. Students and practitioners should review literature to determine applicability of contemporary publications. The Cochrane Library, Cumulative Index of Nursing and Allied Health Literature (CINAHL), EBSCOHost, EMB Reviews, MEDLINE, EMBASE (comprehensive pharmacological and biomedical database), OT Search, OTCATS, OTseeker, Google Scholar, Health and Psychosocial Instruments (HAPI), Applied Social Sciences Index of Abstracts (ASSIA), and HealthStar are useful databases to access during searches for research.

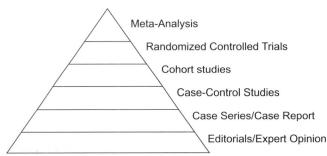

Figure 1-8 Evidence-based levels of evidence. (Adapted from: http://ebp.lib.uic.edu/nursing/node/2?q=node/12 and Feree N, Kreider CM: Defining and applying strategies to find and critically assess the evidence, Presentation at AOTA conference, April 16, 2011.)

Box 1-2   Appraisal Questions Used to Evaluate Quantitative and Qualitative Research

Evaluating Quantitative Research
- Was the assignment of clients to treatments randomized?
- Were all subjects properly accounted for and attributed at the study's conclusion?
- Were subjects, health workers, and research personnel blinded to treatment?
- Were the groups similar to each other at the beginning of the trial?
- Aside from experimental intervention, were the groups treated equally?
- How large was the treatment effect?
- How precise was the treatment effect?
- Can the results be applied to my client care?
- Were all clinically important outcomes considered?
- Are the likely benefits worth the potential harms/costs?

Evaluating Qualitative Research
- Are the results trustworthy?
- Was the research question clearly articulated?
- Was the setting in which the research took place described?
- Were the sampling measures clearly described?
- Were methods to ensure the credibility of research used?
- Did the researchers address issues of confirmability and dependability?
- Was the collection of data prolonged and varied?
- Is there evidence of reflexivity?
- Was the research process subjected to internal or external audits?
- Were any steps taken to triangulate the outcomes?
- Where were the primary findings?
- Were the results of the research kept separate from the conclusions drawn?
- If quantitative methods were appropriate as a supplement, were they used?
- Will the results help me care for my clients?

Data from Gray JAM: *Evidence-based healthcare*, Edinburgh, 1997, Churchill Livingstone; Krefting L: Rigour in qualitative research: the assessment of trustworthiness, *Am J Occup Ther* 45:214-222, 1990; Rosenberg W, Donald A: Evidence-based medicine: an approach to clinical problem-solving, *BMJ* 310:1122-1126, 1995.

Review Questions

1. What health care professionals provide orthotic services to persons?
2. What are the three therapeutic approaches used in physical dysfunction? Give an example of how orthoses could be used as an intervention for each of the three approaches.
3. How might the OTPF[9] assist a therapist in orthotic provision?
4. What are the six divisions of the ASHT orthosis classification system?
5. For what purposes might an orthosis be used as part of an intervention plan?
6. What is evidence-based practice? How can it be applied to orthotic intervention?
7. In evidence-based practice, what is the hierarchy of evidence?

References

1. Gray JM: Putting occupation into practice: occupation as ends, occupation as means, *Am J Occup Ther* 52(5):354–364, 1998.
2. American Society of Hand Therapists. http://www.asht.org/practic emgmt/codingreimb.cfm
3. Fess EE: A history of splinting: to understand the present, view the past, *J Hand Ther* 15(2):97–132, 2002.
4. War Department: *Bandaging and splinting*, Washington, D.C, 1944, United States Government Printing Office.
5. Rossi J: Concepts and current trends in hand splinting, *Occup Ther Health Care* 4(3-4):53–68, 1988.
6. Daus C: Helping hands: a look at the progression of hand therapy over the past 20 years, *Rehab Manag* 64–68, 1998.
7. Fess EE, Gettle KS, Philips CA, et al.: A history of splinting. In Fess EE, Gettle KS, Philips CA, et al.: *Hand and upper extremity splinting: principles and methods*, St Louis, 2005, Elsevier Mosby, pp 3–43.
8. Bailey J, Cannon N, Colditz J, et al.: *Splint classification system*, Chicago, 1992, American Society of Hand Therapists.
9. American Occupational Therapy Association: Occupational therapy practice framework: Doman and process, ed 3, *Am J Occup Ther* 68(Suppl):S1–S48, 2014.
10. Pedretti LW: Occupational performance: a model for practice in physical dysfunction. In Pedretti LW, editor: *Occupational therapy: practice skills for physical dysfunction*, ed 4, St Louis, 1996, Mosby, pp 3–12.
11. Hill J, Presperin J: Deformity control. In Intagliata S, editor: *Spinal cord injury: a guide to functional outcomes in occupational therapy*, Rockville, MD, 1986, Aspen Publishers, pp 49–81.
12. Pierce DE: *Occupation by design: building therapeutic power*, Philadelphia, 2003, FA Davis.
13. American Society of Hand Therapists: *Splint classification system*, Garner, NC, 1992, The American Society of Hand Therapists.
14. Cailliet R: *Hand pain and impairment*, ed 4, Philadelphia, 1994, FA Davis.
15. Schultz-Johnson K: Splinting the wrist: mobilization and protection, *J Hand Ther* 9(2):165–177, 1996.
16. Malick MH: *Manual on dynamic hand splinting with thermoplastic material*, ed 2, Pittsburgh, 1982, Harmarville Rehabilitation Center.
17. Fess EE, Philips CA: *Hand splinting principles and methods*, ed 2, St Louis, 1987, Mosby.
18. Jansen CW: Outcomes, treatment effectiveness, efficacy, and evidence-based practice: examples from the world of splinting, *J Hand Ther* 15(2):136–143, 2002.
19. Sackett DL, Rosenberg WM, Gray JA, et al.: Evidence-based medicine: what it is and what it isn't, *BMJ* 312(7023):71–72, 1996.
20. Taylor MC: What is evidenced-based practice? *Br J Occup Ther* 60:470–474, 1997.
21. American Occupational Therapy Association (April 2010). AOTA's evidence-based practice resources, using evidence to inform occupational therapy practice. http://www.aota.org/Educate/Research/2011-EBP-Resources.aspx?FT=.pdf
22. Law M: Introduction to evidence based practice. In Law M, editor: *Evidence-based rehabilitation*, Thorofare, NJ, 2002, Slack, pp 3–12.
23. Lloyd-Smith W: Evidence-based practice and occupational therapy, *Br J Occup Ther* 60:474–478, 1997.

APPENDIX 1-1   CASE STUDY

Case Study 1-1

Read the following scenario, and answer the questions based on information in this chapter.

Simon is a new therapist working in an outpatient care setting. He has an order to make a wrist immobilization orthosis for a person with a diagnosis of carpal tunnel syndrome who needs an orthosis to provide rest and protection.

1. According to the American Society of Hand Therapists (ASHT) orthotic terminology, which name appropriately indicates the orthosis indicated in Figure 1-9?
   a. Forearm neutral mobilization, type 1 (2)
   b. Wrist neutral immobilization, type 1 (1)
   c. Wrist neutral immobilization, type 0 (1)
2. If Simon focuses on the person's ability to perform activities of daily living (ADLs) with the orthosis, what is the guiding approach?
   a. Rehabilitation
   b. Biomechanical
   c. Sensorimotor
3. Listed below are several types of evidence. Rank the studies in descending order (1 = highest level, 3 = lowest level).
   ___ a.   Talking to a certified hand therapist (CHT) about the protocol she believes is best for a particular client
   ___ b.   A randomized control trial with one group of clients serving as the control group and another group of clients receiving a new type of treatment
   ___ c.   A case study describing the treatment of an individual client

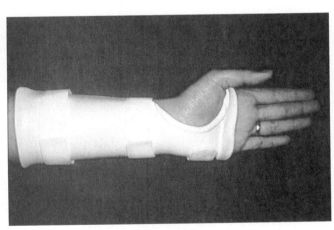

Figure 1-9

CHAPTER 2

Occupation-Based Orthotic Intervention

Debbie Amini, EdD, OTR/L, CHT, C/NDT

Key Terms

client-centered intervention
context
occupational deprivation
occupational disruption
occupational profile
occupation-based orthotic intervention
treatment protocol

Chapter Objectives

1. Define *occupation-based treatment* as it relates to orthotic design and fabrication.
2. Describe the influence of a client's occupational needs on orthotic design and selection.
3. Review evidence to support preservation of occupational engagement through orthotic intervention.
4. Describe how to utilize an occupation-based approach to orthotic intervention.
5. Review specific hand pathologies that create the potential for occupational dysfunction.
6. Describe orthotic design options to promote occupational engagement while ensuring safety of body structures and functions.
7. Apply knowledge of application of occupation-based practice to a case study.

Jacob is a 37-year-old self-employed builder who fell from a second story rooftop approximately 5 months ago. His injuries included a fractured femur of his left leg, fractured metatarsals of his right foot, a compression fracture of his distal right dominant radius, and a volarly angulated fracture of his left nondominant radius. As a result of these injuries, Jacob was unable to engage in his work activities while he was immobilized in bilateral lower extremity casts, a cast on his left wrist, and an external fixator on his right wrist.

One month following injury, Jacob began outpatient occupational therapy. He expressed a desire to return to his vocation as soon as possible due to the financial difficulty that he was experiencing from being unemployed and having no disability insurance. His occupational therapist helped him implement strategies to revive his company while addressing his client factor difficulties surrounding bilateral hand function. Jacob returned to work when his fractures were fully consolidated.

Unfortunately, through constant use of his left upper extremity, Jacob began to experience chronic wrist pain and painful snapping of his forearm with rotational movements. He was diagnosed with ulnocarpal impingement syndrome due to positive ulnar variance in addition to a TFCC tear. Surgery was suggested, but it was expected to take him out of work for an additional 2 to 3 months. This was not acceptable to Jacob who consulted with his occupational therapist in hopes of finding an alternate strategy that would allow him to work without pain until surgery became a feasible option. The occupational therapist and Jacob designed a custom forearm-based wrist orthosis that immobilized his wrist and allowed him to work without pain. Jacob plans to undergo a corrective surgery in approximately 1 year.

As stated eloquently by Mary Reilly, "Man, through the use of his hands as they are energized by mind and will, can influence the state of his own health."[23] This phrase reminds us that the hand, as directed by the mind and spirit, is integral to function. **Occupation-based orthotic intervention** is an approach that promotes the ability of the individual with hand dysfunction to engage in desired life tasks and occupations. Occupation-based orthotic intervention is defined as "attention to the occupational desires and needs of the individual, paired with the knowledge of the effects (or potential effect) of pathological conditions of the hand, and managed through client-centered orthotic design and provision."[2]

Prior to starting the orthotic process, the therapist must adopt a personal philosophy that supports occupation-based and client-centered practice. Multiple models of practice exist that adopt this paradigm, including the Canadian Occupational Performance Measure (COPM); Person, Environment, Occupation Model; and the Model of Human Occupation and Occupational Adaptation. In addition, the occupational therapist (OT) should understand the tenets of the Occupational Therapy Practice Framework (OTPF) that provides a foundation for OT practice within the US and its relationship to the International Classification of Functioning (ICF), Disability and Health.

The profession of occupational therapy adopted the use of orthoses, an ancient technique of immobilization and mobilization, in the mid part of the twentieth century.[10] According to Fess, the most frequently recorded reasons for orthotic intervention include increasing function, preventing deformity, correcting deformity, protecting healing structures, restricting movement, and allowing tissue growth or remodeling.[11] Such reasons for orthotic intervention relate to changing the condition of the neuromusculoskeletal and movement-related functions and body structures within the client factors category of the OTPF. However, body functions and structures comprise only a part of the overall occupational behavior of the client; and despite the importance of assisting the healing or mobility of the hand, the occupational therapy practitioner must immediately and concurrently tend to the needs of the client that transcend movement and strength of the body.

This chapter provides definitions of client-centered and occupation-based practice. The process of combining both approaches to orthotic intervention is presented, as are suggested assessment tools and additional intervention models that are compatible. Orthotic options that promote occupational functioning are described.

Client-Centered versus Occupation-Based Approaches with Orthotic Intervention

Client-centered and occupation-based practice are compatible, but a distinction is made between the two.[22] **Client-centered** practice is defined as "an approach to service which embraces a philosophy of respect for, and partnership with, people receiving services."[17] Law[15] outlined concepts and actions of client-centered practice that articulate the assumptions for shaping assessment and intervention with the client (Box 2-1).

Occupation-based practice is "the degree to which occupation is used with reflective insight into how it is experienced by the individual, how it is used in natural contexts for that individual, and how much the resulting changes in occupational patterns are valued by the client."[12] Methods of employing empathy, reflection, interview, observation, and rigorous qualitative inquiry assist in understanding

---

Box 2-1   Concepts and Actions of Client-Centered Practice
• Respect for clients and their families and choices they make
• Clients' and families' right to make decisions about daily occupations and therapy services
• A communication style that is focused on the person and includes provision of information, physical comfort, and emotional support
• Encourage client participation in all aspects of therapy service
• Individualized occupational therapy service delivery
• Enabling clients to solve occupational performance issues
• Attention to the person-environment-occupation relationship

---

Box 2-2   Description of Contexts
• Cultural: The ethnicity, family values, attitudes, and beliefs of the individual
• Physical: The physical environment in all respects
• Social: Relationships the individual has with other individuals, groups, organizations, or systems
• Personal: Features of the person specific to them (age, gender, socioeconomic status, and so on)
• Temporal: Stages of life, time of day, time of year
• Virtual: Realistic simulation of an environment and the ability to communicate in cyberspace

From American Occupational Therapy Association (2008). Occupational therapy practice framework: Domain and process. American Journal of Occupational Therapy. 62,625–683

---

the occupations of others.[22] Christiansen and Townsend[6] described occupation-based occupational therapy as an approach to treatment that serves to facilitate engagement or participation in recognizable life endeavors. Pierce[22] described occupation-based treatment as including two conditions: (1) the occupation as viewed from the client's perspective and (2) the occupation occurring within a relevant context. According to the OTPF, context and environment relate "to a variety of interrelated conditions within and surrounding the client that influence performance."[1] **Contexts** include cultural, physical, social, personal, temporal, and virtual aspects.[1] Thus, therapists should consider both input from the client, (views and perspective) and external conditions. Box 2-2 describes the contexts and environments as set forth in the OTPF.

Occupation-Based Orthotic Design and Fabrication

Occupation-based orthotic intervention is a treatment approach that supports the goals of the intervention plan to promote the ability of clients to engage in meaningful and relevant life endeavors. Unlike a more traditional biomechanical model of orthotic intervention that may initially focus on body structures and functions, occupation-based orthotic intervention incorporates the client's occupational needs and desires, cognitive abilities, and motivation. When using occupation-based orthotic intervention, the therapist recognizes that the client is an active participant in the treatment and decision-making process. Orthoses as occupation-based and client-centered intervention focuses on meeting client goals as opposed to therapist-designed or protocol-driven goals. Body structure healing is not the main priority. It is a priority equal to that of preservation of occupational engagement.

Occupation-based orthotic intervention can be viewed as part of a top-down versus bottom-up approach to occupational therapy intervention. According to Weinstock-Zlotnick and Hinojosa,[27] the therapist who engages in a top-down approach always begins treatment by examining a client's occupational performance and grounds treatment in a client-centered frame of reference. A therapist who uses a bottom-up approach first evaluates the pathology and then attempts to connect the body deficiencies to performance difficulties. To be truly holistic, one must never rely solely on one method or frame of reference for intervention. A practitioner may choose one primary model to guide selection of assessments and interventions and then choose one or more additional secondary models that further inform assessment and intervention choices.[14] Treating a client's various needs using the most appropriate and holistic approach(es) is the first and foremost priority.

Occupation-Based Orthotic Intervention: Contexts and Environments

According to the OTPF, occupational therapy is an approach that facilitates the individual's ability to participate in meaningful engagements within specific areas of occupation and varied contexts of living.[1] The areas of occupation are one part of the domain of occupational therapy and include activities of daily living (ADLs), instrumental activities of daily living (IADLs), leisure, play, work, education, social participation and rest and sleep.[1] Context and environment are also a part of the domain of occupational therapy and include all levels of the occupational therapy process including evaluation, intervention (including treatment planning), and outcomes. The contexts described in the OTPF include cultural, physical, social, personal, temporal, and virtual contexts.

An often overlooked issue surrounding orthotic intervention is attention to the client's cultural needs. Unfortunately, to ignore culture is to potentially limit the involvement of clients in their orthotic programs. For example, there are cultures whereby the need to rely on an orthosis is viewed as an admission of vulnerability or as a weakness in character. Such feelings can exist due to large group beliefs or within smaller family dynamic units. Orthotic intervention within

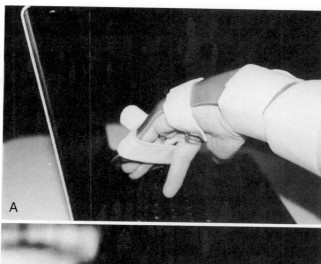
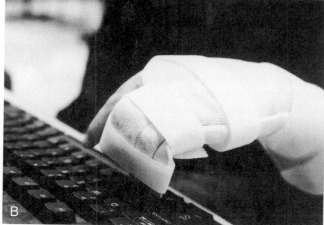

Figure 2-1 A, Excessive pronation required to accurately press keys while using standard dorsal blocking orthosis. **B,** Improved ability to work on computer using modified volar-based protective orthosis.

this context must involve a great deal of client education and possibly education of family members. Issuing small, unobtrusive orthoses that allow as much function as possible may diminish embarrassment and a sense of personal weakness.

Knowledge of physical environments may contribute to an understanding of the need for orthotic provision. Physical environments may also hamper consistent use if clients are unable to engage in required or desired activities. For example, if a client needs to drive to work and is unable to drive while wearing an orthosis, he might remove it despite the potential for reinjury. Figure 2-1, *A,* depicts a young woman wearing an orthosis because she sustained a flexor digitorum profundus injury. She found that typing at her workplace while wearing the orthosis was creating shoulder discomfort. She asked the therapist if she could remove her orthosis for work, and with physician approval the therapist created a modified protective orthosis (see Figure 2-1, *B*). The newly modified orthosis allowed improved function and protected the healing tendon.

Social contexts pertain to the ability of clients to meet the demands of their specific group or family. Social contexts are taken into consideration with orthotic provision. For example, a new mother is recently diagnosed with de

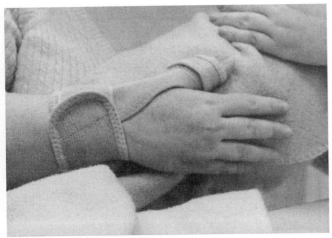

Figure 2-2 Prefabricated thumb immobilization orthosis. It improves comfort while holding the infant.

Quervain tenosynovitis and is issued a thumb orthosis. The mother feels inadequate as a mother when she cannot cuddle and feed the infant without contacting the infant with a rigid orthosis. In such a case, a softer prefabricated orthosis or alternative wearing schedule is suggested to maximize compliance with the orthotic program (Figure 2-2).

Personal context involves attention to issues, such as age, gender, and educational and socioeconomic status. When clinicians who employ occupation-based orthotic intervention fabricate orthoses for older adults or children, they consider specific guidelines (see Chapters 15 and 16). The choices in material selection and color may be different based on age and gender. For example, a child may prefer a bright-colored orthosis, whereas an adult executive may prefer a neutral-colored orthosis. Concerns may arise about the role educational level plays in orthotic design and provision. For clients who have difficulty understanding new and unfamiliar concepts, it is important to have an orthosis that is simple in design and can be donned and doffed easily. Precautions and instructions should be given in a clear manner.

Temporal concerns are addressed through attention to issues, such as comfort of the orthosis during hot summer months or the use of devices during holidays or special events such as proms or weddings. An example is the case of a bride-to-be who was 2 weeks postoperative for a flexor tendon repair of the index finger. The young woman asked repeatedly if she could take off her orthosis for 1 hour during her wedding. A compromise reached between the therapist and the client ensured that her hand would be safe during the ceremony. A shiny new orthosis was made specifically for her wedding day to immobilize the injured finger and wrist (modified Duran protocol). The therapist discarded the rubber-band/finger-hook component (modified Kleinert protocol). This change made the orthosis smaller and less obvious. The client was a happy bride and her finger was well protected. Virtual context addresses the ability to access and use electronic devices. The ability to access devices (e.g., computers, iPads, radios, PDAs, MP3 players, cell phones)

plays an important role in lives of many people in the twenty-first century. Fine motor control is paramount when using these devices and should be preserved as much as possible to maximize electronic contact with the outside world for social participation, education, and work-related occupations. Attention to orthosis size and immobilizing only those joints required can facilitate the ability to manipulate small buttons and dials required to use such devices. For an orthosis to be accepted as a legitimate holistic device, it must work for clients within their context(s) and environments. Since contextual concerns are not always apparent to the practitioner, all clients should be asked if their orthoses are in any way inhibiting their ability to engage in any life experience. Most orthoses affect a person's ability to perform activities. Orthoses might perpetuate dysfunction and may prolong the return to meaningful life engagement. Thus, it is important to pay attention to the specifics of lifestyle and geographic context. The impact is a matter of degree, and consideration needs to be given to the trade-off between how an orthosis enables clients (if only in the future) and how the orthosis presently disables them. Therapists must be aware of the balance between enablement and disablement. Therapists must do their best to appropriately modify the orthosis or the wearing schedule to facilitate clients' occupational engagement. To ignore the interconnection of function is to practice a reductionist form of intervention, because it only emphasizes isolated skills and body structures without regard to engagement in selected activities.

Occupation-Based Orthotics and Intervention Levels

The OTPF[1] describes three types of activities and occupations used as occupational therapy interventions: preparatory methods, purposeful activities, and occupations-based interventions. Preparatory methods prepare clients for purposeful activity, and they do not imply activity or occupation. Examples include exercise, inhibition or facilitation techniques, and positioning devices that are used in preparation for purposeful or occupation-based interventions. Enabling activities that are part of preparatory methods simulate purposeful activity. For example, simulated activities (e.g., driving simulators) begin to prepare the client for participation in actually driving a vehicle. Purposeful activities are goal directed and have an inherent purpose to the client; they are readily understood by others in the pragmatic sense. In the case of driving, when a client gets into a vehicle and drives, the intervention level is considered purposeful activity. Occupation is the highest level of intervention. Clients participate in occupations within their natural context and affix personal meaning to the experience. The ability to complete one's morning routine and drive to his or her place of employment is considered an occupation.

At first blush, orthoses could appear to be less than occupation oriented, because it is not an activity; it is initiated prior to occupational engagement and discontinued when hand function resumes. However, from an occupation-based orthotic perspective, an orthotic intervention is not only a technique used in preparation for occupation. For appropriate clients, orthoses are an integral part of ongoing intervention to support occupational engagement at all levels of intervention: preparatory, purposeful, and occupation-based. For example, some clients may receive an orthosis to decrease pain while simultaneously being allowed engagement in work and leisure pursuits that would otherwise not be possible.

Orthotic Intervention as a Therapeutic Approach

The OTPF[1] intervention approaches are defined as "specific strategies selected to direct the process of intervention that are based on the client's desired outcome, evaluation data, and evidence."[1] These intervention approaches include processes to[1]:

- Create or promote health
- Establish or restore a skill or ability
- Maintain performance capabilities
- Modify context or activity demands through compensation and adaptation
- Prevent disability

From an occupation-based perspective, when orthoses enable occupation, they are elevated to the status of an integral part of function versus relegated to being a preparatory method only. Custom fitted orthoses within the context of clients' occupational experience can promote health, remediate dysfunction, substitute for lost function, and prevent disability. When teamed with a full occupational analysis and knowledge of the appropriate use of orthoses for specific pathologies (supported by evidence of effectiveness), orthotic options are selected to produce the outcomes that reach the goals collaboratively set by the client and the practitioner.

Orthotic Intervention as a Facilitator of Therapeutic Outcomes

Within the context of occupation-based practice, orthotic intervention is a therapeutic approach interwoven through all levels of intervention. Orthotic intervention is a facilitator of purposeful and occupation-based activities. The OTPF[1] describes specific therapeutic outcomes expected from intervention. Outcomes are occupational performance, participation, role competence, adaptation, health and wellness, prevention, quality of life, self-advocacy, and occupational justice.[1] Positive outcomes in occupational performance are the effect of successful intervention. Such outcomes are demonstrated either by improved performance within the presence of continued deficits resulting from injury or disease or the enhancement of function when disease is not currently present.

Orthotic intervention addresses both types of occupational performance outcomes (improvement and enhancement).

Orthoses that improve function in a person with pathology result in an "increased independence and function in an ADL, IADL, education, work, play, leisure, or social participation."[1] For example, a wrist immobilization orthosis is prescribed for a person who has carpal tunnel syndrome. The orthosis positions the wrist to rest the inflamed anatomical structures and maximize the carpal tunnel space, thus decreasing pain and paresthesias and improving work performance. Orthoses that enhance function without specific pathology result in improved occupational performance from one's current status or prevention of potential problems. For example, some orthoses position the hands to prevent overuse syndromes resulting from hand-intensive repetitive or resistive tasks.

Role competence is the ability to satisfactorily complete desired roles (e.g., worker, parent, spouse, friend, and team member). Roles are maintained through orthotic intervention by minimizing the effects of pathology and facilitating upper extremity performance for role-specific activities. For example, a mother who wears an orthosis for carpal tunnel syndrome should be able to hold her child's hand without extreme pain. Holding the child's hand makes her feel like she is fulfilling her role as a mother.

Orthoses created to enhance adaptation to overcome occupational dysfunction address the dynamics of the challenges and the client's expected ability to overcome it. An example orthotic intervention to improve adaptation might involve a client who experiences carpal ligament sprain but must continue working or risk losing employment. In this case, a wrist immobilization orthosis that allows for digital movements may enable continued hand functions while resting the involved ligament.

Health and wellness are collectively described as the absence of infirmity and a "state of physical, mental, and social well-being."[1] Orthoses promote health and wellness of clients by minimizing the effects of physical disruption through protection and substitution. Enabling a healthy lifestyle that allows clients to experience a sense of wellness facilitates motivation and engagement in all desired occupations.

Prevention in the context of the OTPF involves the promotion of a healthy lifestyle at a policy creation, organizational, societal, or individual level.[1] When an external circumstance (e.g., environment, job requirement, and so on) exists with the potential for interference in occupational engagement, an orthotic program may be a solution to prevent the ill effects of the situation. If it is not feasible to modify the job demands, clients may benefit from the use of orthoses in a preventative role. For example, a wrist immobilization orthosis and an elbow strap are fitted to prevent lateral epicondylitis of the elbow for a client who works in a job that involves repetitive and resistive lifting of the wrist with a clenched fist. In addition, the worker is educated on modifying motions and posture that contribute to the condition.

One of the most difficult concepts to define is the concept of quality of life. Despite this, most individuals from

Western cultures have a tacit understanding of its meaning and typically know it to be a condition that includes general health, physical, emotional, cognitive, role and social function with an absence of signs and symptoms of pathology. Quality of life entails one's appraisal of abilities to engage in specific tasks that beneficially affect life and allows self-expressions that are socially valued.[9] One's state of being is determined by the ability of the client to be satisfied, engage in occupations, adapt to novel situations, and maintain health and wellness. Ultimately, orthotic intervention focused on therapeutic outcomes improves the quality of life through facilitating engagement in meaningful life occupations.

Self-advocacy refers to the ability of the individual to advocate for oneself to obtain necessary and desired goods, services, and financial assistance. When an individual understands the needs and rights to service and has the physical functions necessary, he/she is able to tap into available resources. Occupational therapy practitioners educate clients and facilitate functional abilities that enable them to interface with appropriate organizations and agencies. Orthoses that enhance function with regard to communication, community integration and mobility, social participation, and work pursuits can assist clients to gain requisite skills and abilities needed as they advocate for training, funding, housing, and transportation assistance.

Occupational justice refers to the rights of people to be included in desired life pursuits including education and movement within the community. When provided with orthoses that enable function, individuals who are at a disadvantage and cannot participate fully within society without a device may become empowered and able to take full advantage of all that society has to offer. For example, an individual who is not able to access a computer in the public library due to significant hand contractures may be able to search the Internet in this publically-funded facility if an orthosis is provided that isolates the index finger of the dominant hand for one-finger typing.

The Influence of Occupational Desires on Orthotic Design and Selection

The **occupational profile** phase of the evaluation process described in the OTPF involves learning about clients from a contextual and performance viewpoint.[1] For example, what are the interests and motivations of clients? Where do they work, live, and recreate? Tools (i.e., COPM; Disabilities of the Arm, Shoulder, and Hand [DASH]; Patient-Rated Wrist Hand Evaluation [PRWHE]; and the Manual Ability Measure-36 [MAM-36]) that offer clients the opportunity to discuss their injuries in the context of their daily lives lend insight into the needs that must be addressed. Table 2-1 lists such tools. When used in conjunction with traditional methods of hand and upper extremity assessment (e.g., goniometers, dynamometers, and volumeters), they help therapists

learn about the specific clients they treat and assist in orthotic selection and design.

The assessment tools listed in Table 2-1 emphasize client occupations and functions as the focus of intervention. Information obtained from such assessments supports the goal of occupation-based orthotic intervention, which is to improve the client's quality of life through the client's continued engagement in desired occupations.

An orthosis that focuses on client factors alone does not always treat the functional deficit. For example, a static orthosis to support the weak elbow of a client who has lost innervation of the biceps muscle protects the muscle yet allows only one angle of function of that joint. A dynamic flexion orthosis protects the muscle from end-range stretch yet allows the client the ability to change the arm angle through active extension and passive flexion. Assessment tools that measure physical client factors exclusively (e.g., goniometry, grip strength, volumeter, and so on) must remain as adjuncts to determine orthotic design, because physical functioning is an adjunct to occupational engagement.

Canadian Occupational Performance Measure

The COPM is an interview-based assessment tool for use in a client-centered approach.[16] The COPM assists the therapist in identifying problems in performance areas, such as those described by the OTPF. In addition, clients' perceptions of their ability to perform the identified problem area and their satisfaction with their abilities are determined when using the COPM.[16] Therapists can use the COPM with clients from all age groups and with any type of disability. Parents or family members can serve as proxies if the client is unable to take part in the interview process (e.g., if the client has dementia). When the COPM is re-administered, objective documentation of the functional effects of orthotic intervention through comparison of pre- and post-intervention scores is made.

When using the COPM, contextual issues arise during the client interview about satisfaction with function. Clients may indicate why certain activities create personal dissatisfaction despite their ability to perform them. An example is the case of a woman who resides in an assisted living setting. During administration of the COPM, she identifies that she is able to don her orthosis by using her teeth to tighten and loosen the straps. She needs to remove the orthosis to use utensils during meals. However, she is embarrassed to do this in front of other residents while at the dining table. The use of the COPM uncovers issues that are pertinent to individual clients and must be considered by the therapist.

Disabilities of the Arm, Shoulder, and Hand

The DASH is a condition-specific tool that measures a client's perception of how current upper extremity disability has

Table 2-1 Client-Centered Assessments

TOOL	GENERAL DESCRIPTION	CONTACT INFORMATION
Manual Ability Measure-36 (MAM-36)	A 36-item self-report questionnaire. Tool consists of two parts: (1) a client demographic sheet, and (2) a self-report task list consisting of items that clients rate on a four-point scale based upon their perceived ability to complete tasks. It also includes a visual analog pain scale and column for indicating if skill can be completed with the noninvolved hand.	*Archives of Physical Medicine and Rehabilitation*, 91(3), p. 414-420
Canadian Occupational Performance Measure (COPM)[16]	The COPM is a client-centered approach to assessment of perceived functional abilities, interest, and satisfaction with occupations. This interview-based valid and reliable tool is scored and can be used to measure outcomes of treatment.	The COPM can be purchased through the Canadian Association of Occupational Therapists (CAOT) at http://www.caot.ca. Visit the DASH/QuickDASH website at http://www.dash.iwh.on.ca.
Disabilities of the Arm, Shoulder, and Hand (DASH) assessment[13]	DASH is a condition-specific tool. The DASH consists of 30 predetermined questions addressing function within performance areas. Clients are asked to rate their recent ability to complete skills on a scale of 1 (no difficulty) to 5 (unable). The DASH assists with the development of the occupational profile through its valid and reliable measure of clients' functional abilities.	
Patient-Rated Wrist Hand Evaluation (PRWHE)[19]	The PRWHE is a condition-specific tool through which the client rates pain and function in 15 preselected items.	MacDermid JC, Tottenham V. (2004). Responsiveness of the disability of the arm, shoulder, and hand (DASH) and patient-rated wrist/hand evaluation (PRWHE) in evaluating change after hand therapy. Journal of Hand Therapy 17:18-23.

impacted function.[8] The DASH consists of 30 predetermined questions that explore function within performance areas. The client is asked to rate on a scale of 1 (no difficulty) to 5 (unable) his or her current ability to complete particular skills, such as opening a jar or turning a key. The DASH assists the therapist in gathering data for an occupational profile of functional abilities. The focus of the assessment is not on body structures or on the signs and symptoms of a particular diagnostic condition. Rather, the merit of the DASH is the information obtained is about the client's functional abilities.

An interview, although not mandated by the DASH, should become part of the process to enhance the therapist's understanding of the identified problems. The therapist must also determine why a functional problem exists and how it may be affecting quality of life. The DASH is an objective means of measuring client outcomes when re-administered following orthosis provision or other treatment interventions.

When selecting the DASH as a measure of occupational performance, the therapist may consider several additional facts. For example, the performance areas measured are predetermined in the questionnaire and may limit the client's responses. In addition, the DASH does not specifically address contextual issues or client satisfaction or provide insight into the emotional state of the client. Additional information can be obtained through interview to gain insight needed for proper orthotic design and selection.

Patient-Rated Wrist Hand Evaluation

The PRWHE is a condition-specific tool through which clients rate their pain and functional abilities in 15 preselected areas.[19] PRWHE assists with the development of the occupational profile through obtaining information about clients' functional abilities. The functional areas identified in the PRWHE are generally much broader than those in the DASH. Similar to the DASH, the PRWHE's questions to elicit such information are not open-ended questions as in the COPM. Information about pain levels during activity and client satisfaction of the aesthetics of the upper limb are gathered during the PRWHE assessment.

The PRWHE does not specifically require an inquiry into the details of function, but such information would certainly assist the therapist and make the assessment process more occupation based. The PRWHE does not include questions related to context. Therefore, the therapist should include such questions in treatment planning discussions.

The Manual Ability Measure-36

The MAM-36 was developed by OTs[3] and can be used with both musculoskeletal- and neurological-based hand function deficits. The tool was originally described in 2005 in the *Journal of Hand Surgery* (British and European Volume) as the Manual Ability Measure-16. The tool consists of two parts: (1) a client demographic sheet, (2) and a self-report task list consisting of items that clients rate on a four-point scale based upon their perceived ability to complete the task. The rating scale ranges from 1, "cannot do," to 4, "easy." The 0 (zero) option indicates "almost never do (even prior to condition)." The tool also includes a visual analog pain scale and a column to indicate if a task is being completed with the opposite hand. The MAM-36 takes a positive wellness stance and addresses function versus dysfunction. The client scores higher when higher levels of function are present. Research has supported the validity and reliability of the MAM-36.[3]

Analysis Phase

Following the data collection part of the evaluation process, the analysis of occupational performance occurs. If a therapist uses one of the aforementioned tools, analysis of the performance process has been initiated. Further questions will be asked based on the answers of previous questions. The therapist continues to gain specific insight into how orthotic intervention can be used to remediate the reported dysfunction.

During the analysis phase, the therapist may actually want to see the client perform several functions to gain additional insight into how activity affects, or is impacted by, the diagnosis or pathology. For example, a client states that he cannot write because of thumb carpometacarpal (CMC) joint pain. Therefore, the therapist asks the client to show how he is able to hold the pen while describing the type of discomfort experienced with writing. The therapist begins orthotic design analysis by holding the client's thumb in a supported position to simulate the effect of a hand-based orthosis. The client actively participates in the process by giving feedback to the therapist during orthotic design and fabrication.

After a client-centered occupation-based profile and analysis is completed, an occupation-based orthotic intervention plan is developed. Measuring only physical factors to create a client profile results in a therapist seeing only the upper extremity and not the client. The upper extremity does not dictate the quality of life. Rather, the mind, spirit, and body do so collectively! (See Self-Quiz 2-1.)

Evidence to Support Preservation of Occupational Engagement and Participation

Fundamental to occupational therapy treatment is the belief that individuals must retain their ability to engage in meaningful occupations or risk further detriment to their subjective experience of quality of life. If humans behaved as automatons (completing activities without drive, interest, or attention), correcting deficits would become reductionist and mechanical. A reductionistic approach could guarantee that an adaptive device or exercise could correct any problem and immediately lead to the continuation of the required task (much like replacing a spark plug to allow a car to start). Fortunately, humans are not automatons, and occupational therapy exists to support the ability of the individual to engage in and maintain participation in desired occupations.

The literature supports the premise that any temporary or permanent disruption in the ability to engage in meaningful occupations can be detrimental. For example, with a flexor tendon repair therapists must follow protocols to facilitate appropriate tissue healing. Such protocols typically restrict the hand from performing functional pursuits for a minimum of 6 to 8 weeks. However, occupational dysfunction must be effectively minimized as soon as possible to maintain quality of life.[20]

Evidence to Support Occupational Engagement

Supported by research, in addition to anecdotal experiences and reports of therapists, is the importance of multidimensional engagement in meaningful occupations. Described by Wilcock,[29] the term **occupational deprivation** is a state wherein clients are unable to engage in chosen meaningful life occupations due to factors outside their control. Disability, incarceration, and geographic isolation are but a few circumstances that create occupational deprivation. Depression, isolation, difficulty with social interaction, inactivity, and boredom leading to a diminished sense of self can result from occupational deprivation.[6] **Occupational disruption** is a temporary and less severe condition that is also caused by an unexpected change in the ability to engage in meaningful activities.[6] Additional studies conducted by behavioral

SELF-QUIZ 2-1

Answer the following questions.

1. Consider an orthotic intervention plan with a client of a different culture than yourself. What factors of orthotic design and provision may need special attention to ensure acceptance, compliance, and understanding? _____

2. When designing orthoses to match the occupational needs of a young child, what performance areas and personal contextual factors will you be interested in addressing? _____

scientists interested in how individual differences, personality, and lifestyle factors influence well-being have shown that engagement in occupations can influence happiness and life satisfaction.[5]

Ecological models of adaptation suggest that people thrive when their personalities and needs are matched with environments or situations that enable them to remain engaged, interested, and challenged.[4] Walters and Moore[26] found that among the unemployed, involvement in meaningful leisure activities (not simply busy-work activities) decreased the sense of occupational deprivation.

Palmadottir[21] completed a qualitative study that explored clients' perspectives on their occupational therapy experience. Positive outcomes of therapy were experienced by clients when treatment was client-centered and held purpose and meaning for them. Thus, when a client who has an upper extremity functional deficit receives an orthosis, the orthosis should meet the immediate needs of the injury while meeting the client's desire for occupational engagement.

According to Clark and colleagues,[7] older adults from federally subsidized housing complexes realized positive outcomes in life satisfaction, role functioning, and physical and emotional health after receiving lifestyle interventions. These interventions include education for safety, time use and cultural awareness, goal setting, and activities for social participation. The ability to engage in this program and the occupations targeted can be facilitated through orthoses that prevent or correct occupational dysfunction resulting from upper extremity changes associated with aging (e.g., joint changes, pain, weakness) or pathological conditions (e.g., arthritis, fractures, carpal tunnel syndrome).

Research offers evidence that orthoses of all types and for all purposes are indeed effective in reaching the goals of improved function.[24,25,18,28] Refer to the chapters throughout this book for current evidence related to specific orthoses. Three examples are presented to demonstrate such evidence of client-centered and occupation-based orthotic intervention. One study was conducted on the effects of orthotic intervention of the CMC joint of individuals with basal joint osteoarthritis. Two orthoses were provided to determine client preference and effects of custom versus prefabricated orthoses. Both orthoses demonstrated modest improvements in hand function. The prefabricated orthosis was the preferred orthosis, although the custom-made orthosis decreased pain slightly more. According to the authors, this reinforces the client-centered approach to orthotic intervention in that clients can be given a choice in orthotic design knowing that both types are effective in enhancing occupational engagement.[24]

Thiele and colleagues[25] found that individuals using wrist immobilization orthoses for pain control during functional activities did have positive results in pain reduction, occupational performance, and strength. In addition, it was found that customized leather orthoses were preferred to commercially-available fabric orthoses.

A nocturnal wrist extension orthosis was found to be effective in reducing the symptoms of carpal tunnel syndrome experienced by Midwestern auto assembly plant workers.[28] This evidence leads us to conclude that orthotic intervention with attention to occupational needs can and should be used to preserve quality of life.

Utilizing an Occupation-Based Approach to Orthotic Intervention

With guiding philosophies in place, the therapist using an occupation-based approach to orthotic intervention begins the following problem-solving process of orthotic design and fabrication.

Step 1: Referral

The clinical decision-making process begins with the referral. Some orthotic referrals come from physicians who specialize in hand conditions. A referral may contain details about the diagnosis or requested orthosis. However, some orders may be from physicians who do not specialize in the treatment of the hand. If this is the case, the physician may depend on the expertise of the therapist and may simply order an orthosis without detailing specifics. An orthotic intervention order for a client with a condition may also rely on the knowledge and creativity of the therapist. At this step, the therapist must begin to consider the diagnosis, the contextual issues of the client, and the type of orthosis that must be fabricated.

Step 2: Client-Centered Occupation-Based Evaluation

Therapists use assessments (such as, the COPM, DASH, MAM-36, or PRWHE) to learn which occupations clients desire to complete during orthotic wear, which occupations orthoses can support, and which occupations the orthoses will eventually help accomplish. The therapist and the client use this information for goal prioritization and orthotic design in Step 4.

Step 3: Understand/Assess the Condition and Consider Intervention Options

Review biology, cause, course, and traditional interventions of the person's condition, including protocols and healing timeframes. Assess the client's physical status. Research orthotic options, and determine possible modifications to result in increased occupational engagement without sacrificing orthotic effectiveness. When an orthosis is ordered to prevent an injury, the therapist must analyze any activities that may be impacted by wearing the orthosis and determining how it may affect occupational performance.

Step 4: Analyze Assessment Findings for Orthotic Design

Analyze information about pathology and protocols to reconcile needs of tissue healing and function (occupational engagement). Consider whether the condition is acute or chronic. Acute injuries are those that have occurred recently and are expected to heal within a relatively brief time period. Acute conditions may require orthoses to preserve and protect healing structures. Examples include tendon or nerve repair, fractures, carpal tunnel release, de Quervain release, Dupuytren release, or other immediate post-surgical conditions requiring mobilization or immobilization through orthotic intervention.

If the condition is acute, orthotic intervention adheres to protocols and knowledge of client occupational status and desires. Determine if the client is able to engage in desired occupations within the orthosis. If the client can engage in occupations while wearing the orthosis, continue with a custom occupation-based treatment plan in addition to orthotic intervention.

Step 5: Determining Orthotic Design

If the client is unable to complete desired activities and functions within the orthosis, the therapist must determine modifications or alternative orthotic designs to facilitate function. Environmental modifications or adaptations may be needed to accommodate lack of function if no further changes can be made to the orthosis.

Figure 2-3, *A,* is an example of a hand-based trigger finger orthosis that allows unrestricted ability of the client to engage in a craft activity. Compare the orthosis shown in Figure 2-3, *B,* to the orthosis shown in Figure 2-3, *C,* that was previously issued and limited mobility of the ulnar side of the hand and diminished comfort and activity satisfaction.

To ensure that an occupation-based approach to orthotic intervention has been undertaken, the occupation-based orthotic intervention checklist can be used (Form 2-1). This checklist focuses the therapist's attention on client-centered occupation-based practice. Using the checklist helps ensure that the client does not experience occupational deprivation or disruption.

Orthotic Design Options to Promote Occupational Engagement and Participation

The characteristics of an orthosis have an influence on a client's ability to function. The therapist faces the challenge of trying to help restore or protect the client's involved anatomic structure while preserving the client's performance. To achieve optimal occupational outcomes, specific designs and materials must be used to fabricate orthoses that are user friendly. The therapist must employ clinical reasoning that considers the impact on the injured tissue and the desires of the client. Such consideration

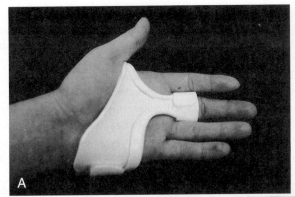

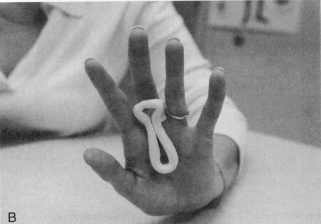

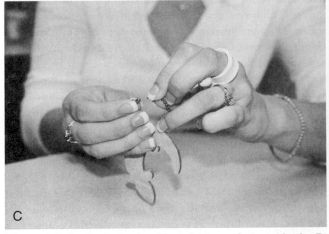

Figure 2-3 A, Confining hand-based trigger finger orthosis. **B,** Finger-based metacarpophalangeal (MCP) blocking trigger finger orthosis. **C,** Functional ability while using finger-based trigger finger orthosis.

results in an orthosis that best protects the anatomic structure at the same time it preserves the contextual and functional needs of the client.

Summary

Engagement in relevant life activities to enhance and maintain quality of life is a concept to be considered with orthotic provision. The premise that orthotic intervention of the hand and upper extremity can improve the overall function of the hand is supported in the literature. Hence, orthotic intervention that includes attention to the functional desires of the client is a valid occupation-based treatment approach that enhances life satisfaction and facilitates therapeutic outcomes.

Review Questions

1. According to this chapter, what is the definition of *occupation-based orthotic intervention?*
2. What is occupational deprivation, and how is it impacted by occupation-based orthotic intervention?
3. What are the reasons therapists provide orthoses to clients who have upper extremity pathology?
4. Why is it important for the client to be an active participant in the orthotic process?
5. Why is attention to the context of the client integral to occupation-based orthotic intervention?
6. What could occur if concern for patient safety is not present when selecting orthoses used for individuals with acute conditions of the hand or upper extremity?
7. Why should a therapist be knowledgeable about tissue healing and treatment protocols despite the fact that such factors do not imply occupation-based treatment?

References

1. American Occupational Therapy Association: Occupational therapy practice framework: domain and process, *Am J Occup Ther* 68(Suppl):S1–S48, 2014.
2. Amini D: The occupational basis for splinting, *Adv Occup Ther Pract* 21:11, 2005.
3. Chen CC, Bode RK: Psychometric validation of the Manual Ability Measure-36 (MAM-36) in patients with neurologic and musculoskeletal disorders, *Arch Phys Med Rehabil* 91(3):414–420, 2010.
4. Christiansen C: Three perspectives on balance in occupation. In Zemke R, Clark F, editors: *Occupational science: the evolving discipline*, Philadelphia, 1996, FA Davis, pp 431–451.
5. Christiansen CH, Backman C, Little BR, et al.: Occupations and subjective well-being: a study of personal projects, *Am J Occup Ther* 53(1):91–100, 1999.
6. Christiansen C, Townsend E: In *Introduction to occupation: the art and science of living*, ed 2, Upper Saddle River, NJ, 2009, Pearson Education.
7. Clark F, Jackson J, Carlson M, et al.: Effectiveness of a lifestyle intervention in promoting the well-being of independently living older people: results of the Well Elderly 2 Randomized Controlled Trial, *J Epidemiol Community Health* 66(9):782–790, 2012.
8. Institute for Work & Health: *The DASH outcome measure* (website). Accessed www.dash.iwh.on.ca, February 4, 2014.
9. Fayers P, Machin D: *Quality of life: the assessment, analysis and interpretation of patient reported outcomes*, ed 2, West Sussex, 2007, John Wiley & Sons Ltd.
10. Fess EE: A history of splinting: to understand the present, view the past, *J Hand Ther* 15(2):97–132, 2002.
11. Fess EE, Gettle KS, Philips CA, et al.: *Hand and upper extremity splinting: principles and methods*, ed 3, St Louis, 2005, Elsevier Mosby.
12. Goldstein-Lohman H, Kratz A, Pierce D: A study of occupation-based practice. In Pierce D, editor: *Occupation by design: building therapeutic power*, Philadelphia, 2003, FA Davis, pp 239–261.
13. Hudak et al. 1996 [Need full ref]
14. Ikiugu MN, Smallfield S, Condit C: A framework for combining theoretical conceptual practice models in occupational therapy practice, *Can J Occup Ther* 76(3):162–170, 2009.
15. Law M, editor: *Client-centered occupational therapy*, Thorofare, NJ, 1998, Slack.
16. Law M, Baptiste S, Carswell A, et al.: *Canadian occupational performance measure*, Ottawa, ON, 2005, CAOT.
17. Law M, Baptiste S, Mills J: Client-centered practice: what does it mean and does it make a difference? *Can J Occup Ther* 62(5):250–257, 1995.
18. Li-Tsang et al. 2002 [Need full ref]
19. MacDermid JC, Tottenham V: Responsiveness of the disability of the arm, shoulder, and hand (DASH) and patient-rated wrist/hand evaluation (PRWHE) in evaluating change after hand therapy, *J Hand Ther* 17(1):18–23, 2004.
20. McKee P, Rivard A: Orthoses as enablers of occupation: client-centered splinting for better outcomes, *Can J Occup Ther* 71(5):306–314, 2004.
21. Palmadottir G: Client perspectives on occupational therapy in rehabilitation services, *Scand J Occup Ther* 10:157–166, 2003.
22. Pierce D: *Occupation by design: building therapeutic power*, Philadelphia, 2003, FA Davis.
23. Reilly M: Occupational therapy can be one of the great ideas of 20th century medicine, *Am J Occup Ther* 16:1–9, 1962.
24. Sillem H, Backman CL, Miller WC, et al.: Comparison of two carpometacarpal stabilizing splints for individuals with thumb osteoarthritis, *J Hand Ther* 24(3):216–226, 2011.
25. Thiele J, Nimmo R, Rowell W, et al.: A randomized single blind crossover trial comparing leather and commercial wrist splints for treating chronic wrist pain in adults, *BMC Musculoskelet Disord* 10:129, 2009.
26. Walters L, Moore K: Reducing latent deprivation during unemployment: the role of meaningful leisure activity, *J Occup Organ Psychol* 75:15–18, 2002.
27. Weinstock-Zlotnick G, Hinojosa J: Bottom-up or top-down evaluation: is one better than the other? *Am J Occup Ther* 58(5):594–599, 2004.
28. Werner R, Franzblau A, Gell N: Randomized controlled trial of nocturnal splinting for active workers with symptoms of carpal tunnel syndrome, *Arch Phys Med Rehabil* 86(1):1–7, 2005.
29. Wilcock A: *An occupational perspective of health*, ed 2, Thorofare, NJ, 2006, Slack.

APPENDIX 2-1   CASE STUDIES

CASE STUDY 2-1

Read the following scenario, and use your clinical reasoning skills to answer the questions based on information in this chapter.

Natasha is a 68-year-old woman who is legally blind. Natasha underwent a metacarpophalangeal (MCP) joint silicone arthroplasty procedure for long, ring, and small fingers of her left hand due to severe rheumatoid arthritis 3 days ago. You received an order to fabricate "forearm-based dynamic extension orthosis to hold the fingers in neutral alignment but allow flexion and extension of the MCPs throughout the day." Natasha attends her first therapy appointment accompanied by her husband , who is now her primary caregiver.

1. During the initial session, you attempt to conduct an interview using the Canadian Occupational Performance Measure (COPM) with Natasha. Her answers seem unrealistic and you suspect that she is not providing accurate information. What steps can you take to verify that the information you obtained is reflective of her current level of function?

   _____

   _____

2. How will you be certain that Natasha is able to read and comprehend the printed orthosis care sheet?

   _____

   _____

3. How will you be certain that Natasha is able to follow the home exercise program pamphlet?

   _____

   _____

4. You design a creative way to allow safe range of motion exercises while maintaining neutral alignment of the digits. How will you ensure that the orthosis modification is appropriate and will not cause harm?

   _____

   _____

APPENDIX 2-2   FORM

Form 2-1 Occupation-based orthotic intervention checklist

1. Orthosis meets requirements of protocol for specific pathology; ensuring attention to bodily functions and structures.   Yes ○   No ○   NA ○

2. If indicated, orthotic design is approved with referring physician.   Yes ○   No ○   NA ○

3. Orthosis allows client to engage in all desired occupation-based tasks through support of activity demands.   Yes ○   No ○   NA ○

4. Orthosis supports client habits, roles, and routines.   Yes ○   No ○   NA ○

5. Orthotic design fits client's cultural needs.   Yes ○   No ○   NA ○

6. Orthotic design fits with temporal needs, including season, age of client, and duration of use.   Yes ○   No ○   NA ○

7. Orthotic design takes into consideration the client's physical environment.   Yes ○   No ○   NA ○

8. Orthotic design supports the client's social pursuits.   Yes ○   No ○   NA ○

9. Client's personal needs are addressed through orthotic design.   Yes ○   No ○   NA ○

10. Client is able to engage in the virtual world (e.g., cellular phone, PDA, computer use).   Yes ○   No ○   NA ○

11. Orthosis is comfortable.   Yes ○   No ○   NA ○

12. Client verbalizes understanding of orthosis use, care, precautions, and rationale for use.   Yes ○   No ○   NA ○

13. Client demonstrates the ability to don and doff orthosis.   Yes ○   No ○   NA ○

14. Adaptations to the physical environment are made to ensure function in desired occupations.   Yes ○   No ○   NA ○

15. Client indicates satisfaction with orthotic design and functionality within orthosis.   Yes ○   No ○   NA ○

CASE STUDY 2-2

Read the following scenario, and use your clinical reasoning skills to answer the questions based on information in this chapter.

Graysen is a 29-year-old man with a 2-year status post multiple trauma, which was secondary to an improvised explosive device (IED) blast in Kabul, Afghanistan. Graysen was referred to occupational therapy by his current orthopaedic physician for treatment of residual hand and upper extremity dysfunction and difficulty participating in desired occupations. An occupational therapist (OT) evaluated him using goniometry, dynamometry, the nine-hole peg test, and the Canadian Occupational Performance Measure (COPM). The results of the range of motion measurements indicate full passive motion in flexion and extension with 75% impairment of active flexion of all digits and full active extension of all digits of both hands. Thumbs are functional yet lack 10% of passive and active motion. Grip strength testing indicated 15 pounds of force bilaterally with 5 pounds of lateral pinch strength. The nine-hole peg test indicated impaired fine motor coordination (FMC) with a score of 60 seconds on the left nondominant hand and 72 seconds on the right hand using lateral pinch only.

Graysen indicated three areas of functional concern while completing the COPM. These include the inability to (1) complete independent bill paying, (2) use the computer to communicate with friends and family on social network sites, and (3) prepare his plate for independent eating. Graysen has scored his ability and satisfaction with these skills as follows (10 = high; 1 = low).

- Bill paying:
  - Performance: 2
  - Satisfaction: 3
- Computer use and social communication:
  - Performance: 2
  - Satisfaction: 1
- Eating/plate preparation:
  - Performance: 3
  - Satisfaction: 4
- Average scores:
  - Performance: 8/3, 2.6
  - Satisfaction: 7/3, 2.3

1. According to the information presented previously, what areas should be addressed first to assist Graysen with occupational satisfaction? Why?

   _____

   _____

2. What approach to treatment facilitates the most expedient return to function? Why?

   _____

   _____

3. What components of this assessment indicate a concern for the occupational participation and context of the client?

   _____

   _____

4. What occupational areas would you need to consider for Graysen's orthotic design?

   _____

   _____

CHAPTER 3

Orthotic Processes, Tools, and Techniques

Brenda M. Coppard, PhD, OTR/L, FAOTA
Shirley Blanchard, PhD, OTR/L, FAOTA

Key Terms
conduction
convection
handling characteristics
hard end feel
heat gun
memory
performance characteristics
physical agent modality (PAM)
soft end feel
superficial agents
thermoplastic material

Chapter Objectives
1. Categorize orthotic materials according to their properties.
2. Recognize tools commonly used to make orthoses.
3. Identify various methods to optimally prepare a client for orthotic intervention.
4. Explain the process of cutting and molding an orthosis.
5. List common items that should be available to a therapist for making orthoses.
6. List the advantages and disadvantages of using prefabricated orthoses.
7. Explain the reasons for selecting a soft orthosis over a prefabricated orthosis.
8. Explain three ways to adjust a static progressive force on prefabricated orthoses.
9. Relate an example of how a person's occupational performance might influence prefabricated orthosis selection.
10. Summarize the American Occupational Therapy Association's (AOTA's) position on occupational therapists' use of physical agent modalities (PAMs).
11. Define *conduction* and *convection*.
12. Describe the indications, contraindications, and safety precautions for the use of PAMs in preparation for making orthoses.

Lola is a new therapist beginning her first week of practice in an outpatient clinic. She receives her first referral for a client who needs evaluation and intervention, including the provision of an orthosis. Lola's heart beats quickly and for a few seconds, she panics! Then she calms down and remembers her education whereby she gained foundational knowledge and skills required for orthotic intervention. With a clear head, she rises up to the challenge.

Therapists who engage in orthotic intervention must have competency in a variety of processes, tools, and techniques. This chapter presents commonly used processes, tools, and techniques related to making orthoses. Orthoses and their purposes needed to address a variety of clients who require custom-made or prefabricated orthoses are discussed. Physical agent modalities (PAMs) are briefly addressed in relationship to how they can be used to prepare a client for optimal positioning during the orthosis-making process.

Thermoplastic Materials

Low-temperature thermoplastic (LTT) materials are most commonly used to fabricate orthoses. The materials are considered "low temperature" because they soften in water heated between 135° F and 180° F,[19] and the therapist can usually safely place them directly against a person's skin while the plastic is still moldable. These compare to high-temperature thermoplastics that become soft when warmed to greater than 250° F[27] and cannot touch a person's skin while moldable without causing a thermal injury. When LTT is heated, it becomes pliable and then hardens to its original rigidity after cooling. The first commonly-available LTT material was Orthoplast. Currently, many types of thermoplastic materials are available from several companies. Types of materials used in clinics vary on the basis of patient population, diagnoses, therapists' preferences, and availability.

In addition to orthotic use, LTT material is commonly used to adapt devices for improving function. For example, thermoplastic material may be heated and wrapped around pens, handles, utensils, and other tools to build up the circumference and decrease the required range of motion needed to use such items.

Therapists select the best type of **thermoplastic material** to use for orthotic fabrication. Decisions are based on such factors as cost, properties of the thermoplastic material, familiarity with orthotic materials, and therapeutic goals. One type of thermoplastic material is not the best choice for every type or size of orthosis. If a therapist has not had experience with a particular type of thermoplastic material, it is beneficial to read the manufacturer's technical literature describing the material's content and properties. Therapists should practice using new materials before fabricating orthoses on clients.

Thermoplastic Material Content and Properties

Thermoplastic materials are elastic, plastic, a combination of plastic and rubberlike, and rubberlike.[18] Thermoplastic materials that are elastic-based have some amount of memory. (Memory is addressed later in this section.) Typically, elastic thermoplastic material has a coating to prevent the material from adhering to itself. (Most thermoplastic materials have a nonstick coating, but there are a few that specify that they do not.) Elastic materials have a longer working time than other types of materials and tend to shrink during the cooling phase.

Thermoplastic materials with a high plastic content tend to be drapable and have a low resistance to stretch. Plastic-based materials are often used because they result in a highly conforming orthosis. Such plastic requires great skill in handling the material (e.g., avoiding fingerprints and stretch) during heating, cutting, moving, positioning, draping, and molding. Thus, for novice practitioners positioning the client in a gravity-assisted position is best to prevent overstretching of the material.

Thermoplastic materials that are described as rubbery or rubberlike tend to be more resistant to stretching and fingerprinting. These materials are less conforming than their more drapable plastic counterparts. Therapists should not confuse resistance to stretch during the molding process with the rigidity of the orthosis upon completion. Materials that are quite drapable become extremely rigid when cooled and set, and the opposite is also true. In addition, the more contours that an orthosis has, the more rigid it will be.

Some LTT materials are engineered to include an antimicrobial protection. Orthoses can create a moist surface on the skin where mold and mildew can form.[20] When skin cells and perspiration remain in a relatively oxygen-free environment for hours at a time, it is conducive to microbe growth and results in odor. Daily isopropyl alcohol cleansing of the inside surface of the orthosis effectively combats this problem. Thermoplastic materials containing the antimicrobial protection offer a defense against microorganisms. The antimicrobial protection does not wash or peel off.

Each type of thermoplastic material has unique properties,[13] which are categorized by handling and performance characteristics. **Handling characteristics** refer to the thermoplastic material properties when heated and softened, and **performance characteristics** refer to the thermoplastic material properties after the material has cooled and hardened.

Handling Characteristics

Memory

Memory is a property that describes a material's ability to return to its preheated (original) shape, size, and thickness when reheated. The property ranges from 100% to little or no memory capabilities.[17] Materials with 100% memory return to their original size and thickness when reheated. Materials with little to no memory do not recover their original thickness and size when reheated or stretched.

Most materials with memory turn translucent (clear) during heating. Using the translucent quality as an indicator, the therapist can easily determine that the material is adequately heated and can prevent over- or under-heating. The ability to see through the material also assists the therapist to properly position and contour the material on the client.

Memory allows therapists to reheat and reshape orthoses several times without the material stretching excessively. Materials with memory must be constantly molded throughout the cooling process to sustain maximal conformability to persons. Novice or inexperienced therapists who wish to correct errors in a poorly-molded orthosis frequently use materials with memory. Materials with memory accommodate the need to redo or revise an orthosis multiple times while using the same piece of material over and over. LTT material with memory is often used to make orthoses for clients who have high tone or stiff joints, because the memory allows therapists to serially adjust a joint(s) into a different position. Clinicians use a serial adjustment approach when they intermittently remold to a person's limb to accommodate changes in range of motion.

Materials with memory may pose problems when a therapist is attempting to make fine adjustments. For example, spot heating a small portion may inadvertently change the entire orthosis because of shrinkage. Therapists must carefully control duration of heat exposure. It may be best in these situations to either reimmerse the entire orthosis in water and repeat the molding process, or prevent the problem and select a different type of LTT material.

Drapability

Drapability is the degree of ease with which a material conforms to the underlying shape without manual assistance. The degree of drapability varies among different types of material. The duration of heating is important. The longer the material heats, the softer it becomes, and the more vulnerable it becomes to gravity and stretch. When a material with drapability is placed on a surface, gravity assists the material in draping and contouring to the underlying surface. Material exhibiting drapability must be handled with care after heating. A therapist should avoid holding the plastic in a manner in which gravity affects the plastic and results in a stretched, thin piece of plastic. Therefore, this type of plastic is best positioned on a clean countertop during cutting. Material with high drapability is difficult to use for large orthoses and is most successful on a cooperative person who can place the body part in a gravity-assisted position.

Thermoplastic materials with high drapability may be more difficult for beginning practitioners because the materials must be handled gently, and often the material is handled too aggressively. Successful molding requires therapists to refrain from pushing the material during shaping. Instead, the material should be lightly stroked into place. Light touch and constant movement of therapists' hands result in orthoses that are cosmetically appealing. Materials with low drapability require firm pressure during the molding process. Therefore, persons with painful joints or soft-tissue damage have better tolerance for materials with high drapability.

Elasticity

Elasticity is a material's resistance to stretch and its tendency to return to its original shape after stretch. Materials with memory have a slight tendency to rebound to their original shapes during molding. Materials with a high resistance to stretch can be worked more aggressively than materials that stretch easily. As a result, resistance to stretch is a helpful property when one is working with uncooperative persons, those with high tone, or when one orthosis includes multiple areas (i.e., forearm, wrist, ulnar border of hand, and thumb in one orthosis). Materials with little elasticity stretch easily and become thin. Therefore, light touch must be used.

Bonding

Self-bonding or self-adherence is the degree to which material sticks to itself when properly heated. Some materials are coated; others are not. Coated materials always require surface preparation with a bonding agent or solvent. Self-bonding (uncoated) materials may not require surface preparation, but some thermoplastic materials have a coating that must be removed for bonding to occur.

Coated materials tack at the edges, because the coating covers only the surface and not the edges. Often, the tacked edges can be pried apart after the material is completely cool. If a coated material is stretched, it becomes tackier and is more likely to bond. When heating self-bonding material, the therapist must take care that the material does not overlap on itself during the heating or draping process. If the material overlaps, it sticks to itself. Noncoated materials may adhere to paper towels, towels, bandages, and even the hair on a client's extremity! Thus, it may be necessary to apply an oil-based lotion to the client's extremity. To facilitate the

therapist's handling of the material, wetting the hands and scissors with water or lotion can prevent sticking.

All thermoplastic material, whether coated or uncoated, forms stronger bonds when surfaces are prepared with a solvent or bonding agent (which removes the coating from the material). A bonding agent or solvent is a chemical that can be brushed onto both pieces of the softened plastic to be bonded. In some cases, therapists roughen the two surfaces that will have contact with each other. This procedure, called *scoring*, can be carefully done with the end of a scissors, an awl, or a utility knife. After surfaces have been scored, they are softened, brushed with a bonding agent, and adhered together. Self-adherence is an important characteristic for mobilization orthoses when a therapist must secure outriggers to bases of the orthoses (see Chapter 12) and when the plastic must attach to itself to provide support—for example, when wrapping around the thumb as in a thumb spica orthosis (see Chapter 8).

Self-Finishing Edges

A self-finishing edge is a handling characteristic that allows any cut edge to seal and leave a smooth rounded surface if the material is cut when warm. This handling characteristic saves time for therapists, because they do not have to manually roll or smooth the edges.

Other Considerations

Other handling characteristics to be considered are heating time, working time, and shrinkage. The time required to heat thermoplastic materials to a working temperature should be monitored closely, because material left too long in hot water may become excessively soft and stretchy. Therapists should be cognizant of the temperature the material holds before applying it to a person's skin to prevent a burn or discomfort. After material that is ⅛ inch thick is sufficiently heated, it is usually pliable for approximately 3 to 5 minutes.[4] Some materials will allow up to 4 to 6 minutes of working time. Materials thinner than ⅛ inch and those that are perforated heat and cool more quickly.[18]

Shrinkage is an important consideration when therapists are properly fitting any orthosis, but particularly with a circumferential design. Plastics shrink slightly as they cool. During the molding and cooling time, precautions should be taken to avoid a shrinkage-induced problem, such as difficulty removing a thumb or finger from a circumferential component of an orthosis.

Performance Characteristics

Conformability

Conformability is a performance characteristic that refers to the ability of thermoplastic material to fit intimately into contoured areas. Material that is easily draped and has a high degree of conformability can pick up fingerprints and crease marks (as well as therapists' fingerprints). Orthoses that are intimately conformed to persons are more comfortable, because they distribute pressure best and reduce the likelihood of the orthosis migrating on the extremity.

Flexibility

A thermoplastic material with a high degree of flexibility can take stresses repeatedly. Flexibility is an important characteristic for circumferential orthoses, because these orthoses must be pulled open for each application and removal.

Durability

Durability is the length of time thermoplastic material will last. Rubber-based materials are more likely to become brittle with age.

Rigidity

Materials that have a high degree of rigidity are strong and resistant to repeated stress. Rigidity is especially important when therapists make medium to large orthoses (such as orthoses for elbows or forearms). Large orthoses require rigid material to support the weight at larger joints. In smaller orthoses, rigidity is important if the plastic must stabilize a joint. Rigidity can be enhanced by contouring an orthosis intimately to the underlying body shape.[33] Most LTT materials cannot tolerate the repeated forces involved in weight bearing on an orthosis, such as in foot orthoses. Most foot orthoses have fatigue cracks within a few weeks.[14]

Perforations

Theoretically, perforations in material allow for air exchange to the underlying skin. Various perforation patterns are available (e.g., mini-, maxi-, and micro-perforated).[20] Perforated materials are also designed to reduce the weight of orthoses. Several precautions must be taken if one is working with perforated materials.[33] Perforated material should not be stretched, because stretching enlarges the holes in the plastic and thereby decreases its strength and pressure distribution. When cutting a pattern out of perforated material, therapists should attempt to cut between the perforations to prevent uneven or sharp edges. If this cannot be avoided, the edges of the orthosis should be smoothed.

Finish, Color, and Thickness

Finish refers to the texture of the end product. Some thermoplastics have a smooth finish, whereas others have a grainy texture. Generally, coated materials are easier to keep clean because the coating resists soiling.[14]

The color of the thermoplastic material may affect a person's acceptance and satisfaction with the orthosis and compliance with the wearing schedule. Darker-colored orthoses tend to show less soiling and appear cleaner than white orthoses. Brightly-colored orthoses tend to be popular with children and youth. Colored materials may be used to help a person with unilateral neglect call attention to one side of the body.[14] In addition, colored orthoses are easily seen and therefore useful in preventing loss in institutional settings. For example, it is easier to see a blue orthosis in white bed linen than to see a white orthosis in white bed linen.

A common thickness for thermoplastic material is ⅛ inch. However, if the weight of the entire orthosis is a concern, a thinner plastic may be used—reducing the bulkiness of the orthosis and possibly increasing the person's comfort and improving compliance with the wearing schedule. Some thermoplastic materials are available in thicknesses of ¹⁄₁₆, ³⁄₃₂, and ³⁄₁₆ inch. Thinner thermoplastic materials are commonly used for small orthoses, arthritic joints, and pediatric orthoses. The ³⁄₁₆-inch thickness is commonly used for lower extremity orthoses and fracture braces.[15,20] Therapists should keep in mind those plastics thinner than ⅛ inch soften and harden more quickly than thicker materials. Therefore, therapists who are novices in orthotic intervention may find it easier to use ⅛-inch-thick materials than thinner materials.[14] Table 3-1 lists property guidelines for thermoplastic materials. (See also Laboratory Exercise 3-1.)

Process: Making the Orthosis

Orthotic Patterns

Making a good pattern for an orthosis is necessary for success. Giving time and attention to the making of a well-fitting pattern saves the practitioner's time and the materials involved in making adjustments for an entirely new orthosis. A pattern should be made for each person who needs an orthosis. Generic patterns rarely fit persons correctly without adjustments. Having several sizes of generic patterns cut out of aluminum foil for trial fittings may speed up the pattern process. A standard pattern can be reduced on a copy machine for pediatric sizes.

To make a custom pattern, the therapist traces the outline of the person's hand (or corresponding body part) on a paper towel (or foil), making certain that the hand is flat and in a neutral position. If the person's hand is unable to flatten on the paper, the contralateral hand may be used to draw the pattern and fit the pattern. If the contralateral hand cannot be used, the therapist may hold the paper in a manner so as to contour to the hand position. The therapist marks on the paper any anatomical landmarks needed for the pattern before the hand is removed. The therapist then draws the pattern over the outline of the hand, cuts out the pattern with scissors, and completes final sizing.

Fitting the Pattern to the Client

As shown in Figure 3-1, moistening the paper and applying it to the person's hand helps the therapist determine which adjustments are required. Patterns made from aluminium foil work well to contour the pattern to the extremity. If the pattern is too large in areas, the therapist can make adjustments by marking the pattern with a pen and cutting or folding the paper. Sometimes it is necessary to make a new pattern or to retrace a pattern that is too small or that requires major

Table 3-1 Thermoplastic Property Guidelines*

THERMOPLASTIC NAME	DEGREE OF HEATING TEMPERATURE (F)	THERMOPLASTIC NAME	DEGREE OF HEATING TEMPERATURE (F)
Memory		Polyflex II	150-160
Aquaplast-T	160-170	Polyflex Light	150-160
Colours	150-160	Orfit NS (non-stick)	150
NCM Encore	160	Orfit Natural NS (non-stick)	150
FiberForm Soft	150-160	Orfit Soft-Fit NS (non-stick)	150
FiberForm Stiff	150-160	Orthoplast II	150-160
Watercolors	160-170	Encore	140-160
Aquaplast Resilient T	160-170	NCM Clinic D	160
Aquaplast ProDrape-T	160-170	Omega Max	140-160
Encore	140-160	Orfit	135
NCM Spectrum	140-145	Watercolors	160-170
NCM Prism	160		
Omega Max	140-160	**Moderate Drapability**	
Omega Plus	140-160	Aquaplast-T	160-170
Orfibrace	150	NCM Clinic	160
Orfilight	150	NCM Prism	160
Orfit NS (non-stick)	150	NCM Spectrum	160
Orfit Natural NS (non-stick)	150	NCM Vanilla	160
Orfit Soft-Fit NS (non-stick)	150	Ezeform	160-170
Orfit Stiff	135	Ezeform Light	150-160
Prism	140-160	Orfilight	150
Rebound	150-160	Orfibrace	150
		Solaris	160
Rigidity		NCM Clinic	160
NCM Clinic	160	NCM Preferred	160
Colours	150-160	NCM Spectrum	140-145
Excel	150-160	Prism	140-160
Ezeform	160-170	Watercolors	160-170
FiberForm Soft	150-160		
FiberForm Stiff	150-160	**Resistance to Drape**	
Infinity	150-160	Aquaplast Resilient T	160-170
Marque-Easy	150-160	Caraform	140-145
NCM Clinic	160	Colours	150-160
NCM Clinic D	160	FiberForm Soft	150-160
NCM Preferred	160	FiberForm Stiff	150-160
NCM Spectrum	160	Rebound	150-160
NCM Vanilla	160	Synergy	160-170
Omega Max	140-160	Omega Plus	140-160
Omega Plus	140-160		
Orfibrace	150	**Resistance to Stretch**	
Polyform	150-160	Aquaplast Original Resilient	160-170
Solaris	160	Aquaplast Resilient T	160-170
		Colours	150-160
Conformability, Drapability		Excel	150-160
Aquaplast ProDrape-T	160-170	Ezeform	160-170
Contour Form	140-145	FiberForm Soft	150-160
NCM Encore	160	FiberForm Stiff	150-160
NCM Clinic	160	Infinity	150-160
NCM Spectrum	160	NCM Prism	160
Excel	150-160	NCM Spectrum	160
Ezeform	160-170	NCM Vanilla	160
Infinity	150-160	Rebound	150-160
Marque-Easy	150-160	Solaris	160
Polyform	150-160	Synergy	160-170
Polyform Light	150-160	San-splint	160-175

Continued

Table 3-1 Thermoplastic Property Guidelines*—cont'd

THERMOPLASTIC NAME	DEGREE OF HEATING TEMPERATURE (F)	THERMOPLASTIC NAME	DEGREE OF HEATING TEMPERATURE (F)
Omega Max	140-160	Prism	140-160
Omega Plus	140-160	Rebound	150-160
Orfibrace	150	Solaris	160
		Spectrum	160
Self-Adherence		Synergy	160-170
Aquaplast Original	160-170		
NCM Clinic (with dry heat)	160	**Antimicrobial Defense**	
NCM Vanilla (with dry heat)	160	Polyform with antimicrobial built in	150-160
Contour Colors	140-145	Aquaplast ProDrape-T with antimicrobial built in	160-170
Contour Form	140-145		
Encore	140-160	Polyflex II with antimicrobial built in	150-160
Ezeform	160-170		
Marque-Easy	150-160	Aquaplast-T with antimicrobial built in	160-170
NCM Spectrum	140-145		
Omega Max	140-160	TaylorSplint with antimicrobial built in	150-160
Orfilight (with dry heat)	150		
Orfit Soft	135		
Orfit Stiff	135		

NCM, North Coast Medical, Inc.
*Not all-inclusive.
Courtesy of Serena Berger, Smith & Nephew Rolyan, Inc., Germantown, Wisconsin, and North Coast Medical, Inc., San Jose, California.

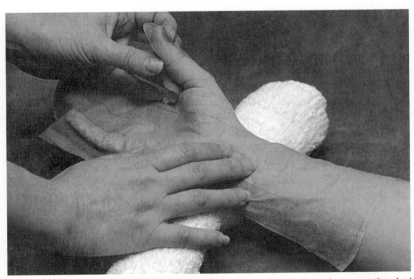

Figure 3-1 To make pattern adjustments, moisten the paper and apply it to the extremity during fitting.

adjustments. The therapist ensures that the pattern fits the person before tracing it onto and cutting it out of the thermoplastic material. It is well worth the time to make an accurate pattern because any ill-fitting pattern directly affects the finished product.

Throughout this book, detailed instructions are provided for making different orthotic patterns. Keep in mind that therapists with experience and competency may find it unnecessary to identify all landmarks as indicated by the detailed instructions. Form 3-1 lists suggestions helpful to a beginning practitioner when drawing and fitting patterns.

Building the Orthosis from the Pattern

After making and fitting the pattern to the client, the therapist places it on the sheet of thermoplastic material in such a way as to conserve material and then traces the pattern on the thermoplastic material with a pencil. (Conserving materials ultimately saves expenses for the clinic or hospital.) Pencil

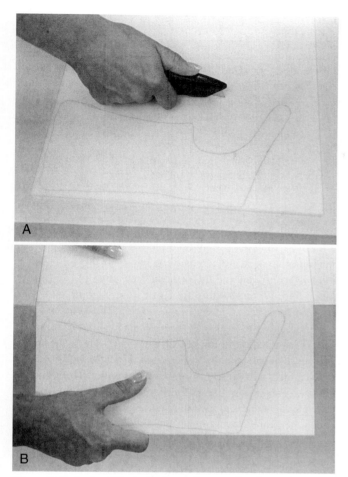

Figure 3-2 **A,** A utility knife is used to cut the sheet of material with the pattern outline on it in such a way that the thermoplastic material fits in the hydrocollator or fry pan. **B,** The score from the utility knife is pressed against a countertop.

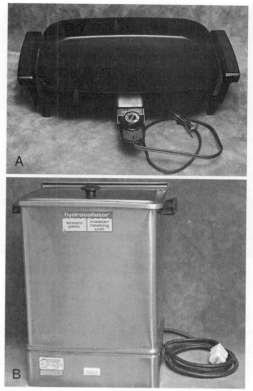

Figure 3-3 Soften thermoplastic material in **(A)** an electric fry pan or **(B)** a hydrocollator.

lines do not show up on all plastics. Using an awl to "scratch" the pattern outline on the plastic works well. Another option is to use grease pencils or china pencils. Caution should be taken when a therapist uses an ink pen, because the ink may smear onto the plastic. On occasions, the ink might be removed with chlorine.

Once the pattern is outlined on a sheet of material, a rectangle slightly larger than the pattern is cut with a utility knife (Figure 3-2). After the cut is made, the material is folded over the edge of a countertop. If unbroken, the material can be turned over to the other side and folded over the countertop's edge. Any unbroken line can then be cut with a utility knife or scissors.

Heating the Thermoplastic Material

Thermoplastic material is softened in an electric fry pan, commercially-available orthotic pan, or hydrocollator filled with water heated to approximately 135° F to 180° F (Figure 3-3). (Some materials can be heated in a microwave oven or in a fry pan without water.) To ensure temperature consistency, the temperature dial should be marked to indicate the correct setting of 160° F by using a hook-and-loop (Velcro)

dot or piece of tape. When softening materials vertically in a hydrocollator, the therapist must realize the potential for problems associated with material stretching due to gravity's effects. If a fry pan is used, the water height in the pan should be a minimum of three-fourths full (approximately 2 inches deep).

Adequate water height allows a therapist to submerge portions of the orthosis later when making adjustments. If the thermoplastic material is larger than the fry pan, a portion of the material should be heated. When soft, place the material on a wet paper towel. The remaining hard material is placed in the fry pan for softening. A nonstick mesh may be placed in the bottom of a fry pan to prevent the plastic from sticking to any materials or particles. However, it can create a mesh imprint on some plastics. When the thermoplastic piece is large (and especially when it is a high-stretch material), it is a great advantage to lift the thermoplastic material out of the pan on the mesh or a hefty paper towel or with two spatulas. This keeps the plastic flat and minimizes stretch.

Cutting the Thermoplastic Material

After removing the thermoplastic material from the water with a spatula or on the mesh, the therapist cuts the material with either round- or flat-edged scissors (Figure 3-4). The therapist uses sharp scissors and cuts with long blade strokes (as opposed to using only the tips of the scissors). Scissors should be sharpened at least once each year and possibly more often, depending on use. Dedicating scissors for specific materials

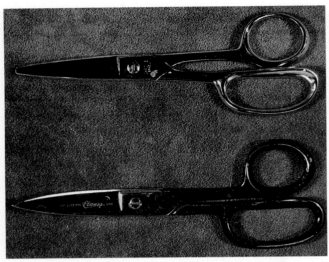

Figure 3-4 Sharp round- or flat-edged scissors work well for cutting thermoplastic.

prolongs the edge of the blade. For example, one pair of scissors should be used to cut plastic, another for paper, another for adhesive-backed products, and so on. Solvent or adhesive removers remove adhesive that builds up on scissor blades. Sharp scissors in a variety of sizes (e.g., fingernail scissors) are helpful for intricate contoured cutting and trimming.

Reheating the Thermoplastic Material

After the pattern is cut from the material, it is reheated. During reheating, the therapist positions the person to the desired joint position(s). If the therapist anticipates positioning challenges and needs to spend time solving problems, positioning should be done before the material is reheated to prevent the material from overheating.[24] During this time frame, the therapist explains that the material will be warm, and if it is too intolerable, the client should notify the therapist. The therapist completes any pre-padding of bony prominences and covers dressings and padding prior to the molding process. (The LTT sticks to the dressings and padding if not covered with stockinette.)

Positioning the Client

Several client positioning options exist. The client is placed in a position that is comfortable, especially for the shoulder and elbow. A therapist may use a gravity-assisted position for hand orthoses by having the person rest the dorsal wrist area on a towel roll while the forearm is in supination to maintain proper wrist positioning. Alternatively, a therapist may ask the person to rest the elbow on a table and work with the hand while it is in a vertical position. This position allows for taking joint measurements, but the material may stretch with the effects from gravity.

For persons with stiffness, a warm water soak or whirlpool, ultrasound, paraffin dip, or hot pack can be used before positioning the client for the orthotic-making process. Orthotic making is easiest when persons take their pain medication 30 to 60 minutes before the session. For persons with hypertonicity, it may be effective to use a hot pack on the joint that needs to be positioned in the orthosis. Then the joint is positioned and the orthosis is applied in a submaximal range. When the orthotic fabrication is completed after warming or after an intervention session, the joints are usually more mobile. However, the orthosis may not be tolerated after the preconditioning effect wears off. Thus, the therapist must find a balance to complete a gentle warm-up and avoid aggressive preconditioning treatments.[24] Goniometers are used, when possible, to measure joint angles for optimal therapeutic positioning. With experience, joint angles can be "eyeballed" and a goniometer may not be needed.

Molding the Orthosis to the Client

Once positioning is accomplished, the therapist retrieves the softened thermoplastic material (Box 3-1). Any hot water is wiped off on a paper towel, a fabric towel, or a pillow that has a dark-colored pillowcase on it. (The dark-colored pillowcase helps identify any small scraps or snips of material from previous orthotic intervention activities that may adhere to the thermoplastic material.) The therapist checks the temperature of the softened plastic and finally applies the thermoplastic material to the person's extremity. The thermoplastic material may be extremely warm, and thus the therapist uses caution to prevent skin burn or discomfort. For persons with fragile skin who are at risk of burns, the extremity may be covered with stockinette before the thermoplastic material is applied. Some thermoplastic materials stick to hair on the person's skin, but this situation can be avoided by using a stockinette or applying lotion on the skin before application of the thermoplastic material. Care must be taken not to use lotions on open wounds.

Therapists may choose to hasten the cooling process to maintain joint position and the orthoses' shape. Several options exist. First, a therapist can use an environmental friendly cold spray. Cold spray is an agent that serves as a surface coolant. Cold spray should not be used near persons who have severe allergies or who have respiratory problems.

Because the spray is flammable, it should be properly stored. A second option is to dip the person's extremity with the orthosis into a tub of cold water. This must be done

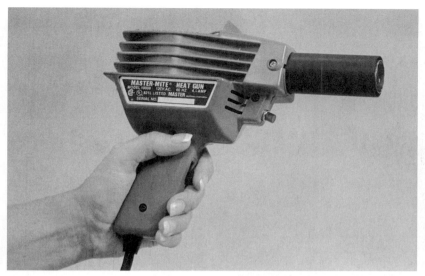

Figure 3-5 A heat gun is used for spot heating.

cautiously with persons who have hypertonicity, because the cold temperature could cause a rapid increase in the amount of tone, thus altering joint position. Similar to using a tub of cold water, the therapist may carefully walk the person wearing the orthosis to a sink and run cold water over the orthosis. Third, a therapist can use frozen Theraband and wrap it around the orthosis to hasten cooling. An Ace bandage immersed in ice water and then wrapped around the orthosis may also speed cooling.[33] However, Ace bandages often leave their imprints on the thermoplastic material.

Making Adjustments

Adjustments can be made to an orthosis by using a variety of techniques and equipment. While the thermoplastic material is still warm, therapists can make adjustments to orthoses—such as, marking a trim line with their fingernails or a pencil or stretching small areas of the orthosis. The amount of allowable stretch depends on the property of the material and the cooling time that has elapsed. If the plastic is too cool to cut with scissors, the therapist can quickly dip the area in hot water. A professional-grade metal turkey baster or ladle assists in directly applying hot water to modify a small or difficult-to-immerse area of the orthosis.

A **heat gun** (Figure 3-5) may also be used to make adjustments. A heat gun has a switch for off, cool, and hot. After using a heat gun, before turning it to the off position, the therapist sets the switch to the cool setting. This allows the motor to cool down and protects the motor from overheating. When a heat gun is on the hot setting, caution must be used to avoid burning materials surrounding it and reaching over the flow of the hot air.

Heat guns must be used with care. Because heat guns warm unevenly, therapists should not use them for major heating and trimming. Use of heat guns to soften a large area on an orthosis may result in a buckle or a hot/cold line. A hot/cold line develops when a portion of plastic is heated and its adjacent line or area is cool. A buckle can form where the hot area stretched and the cooled material did not. Heat guns are helpful for warming small focused areas for finishing touches. When using a heat gun, it is best to continually move the heat gun's air projection on the area of the orthosis to be softened. In addition, the area to be softened should be heated on both sides of the plastic. Attachments for the heat gun's nozzle are available to focus the direction of hot air flow. Small heat guns are available and may assist in spot heating thinner plastics and areas of the orthosis that have attachments that cannot be exposed to heat (i.e., orthosis line).[24,25]

Strapping

After achieving a correct fit, the therapist uses strapping materials to secure the orthosis onto the person's extremity. Many strapping materials are available commercially. Velcro hook and loop, with or without an adhesive backing, is commonly used for portions of the strapping mechanism. Velcro is available in a variety of colors and widths. Therapists trim Velcro to a desired width or shape. For cutting self-adhesive Velcro, sharp scissors other than those used to cut thermoplastic material should be used. The adhesive backing from strapping materials often accumulates on the scissor blades and makes the scissors a poor cutting tool. The adhesive can be removed with solvent. When a self-adhesive Velcro hook is used, the corners should be rounded. Rounded corners decrease the chance of corners peeling off the orthosis. Pre-cut self-adhesive Velcro hook dots can be purchased and save therapists' time not only in cutting and rounding corners but in keeping adhesive off scissors. A clinic may have an aide or volunteer cut self-adhesive Velcro hook pieces that have rounded corners to save therapists' time. Briefly heating the adhesive backing and the site of attachment on the orthosis with a heat gun increases the bond of the hook or loop to the thermoplastic material.

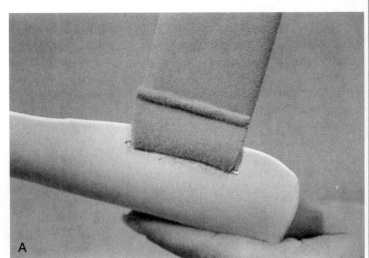
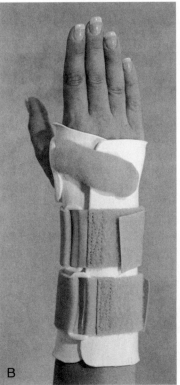

Figure 3-6　A, Strap is threaded through a slit in forearm trough. The strap is overlapped upon itself and securely sewn. **B,** D-ring strapping mechanism.

Alternative pressure-sensitive straps, which attach to the Velcro hook, are available. Strapping materials are often padded to add comfort, but these tend to be less durable than Velcro loop. Some padded strapping materials, when cut, have a self-sealing or more finished look than others. Soft straps without self-sealing edges tend to tear apart with use over time. The therapist may cut extra straps and give them to the client to take home if necessary. Commercially sold orthotic strapping packs provide all the straps needed for a forearm-based orthosis in one convenient package.

Spiral or continuous strapping can be employed to evenly distribute pressure along the orthosis. A spiral or continuous strap is a piece of soft strapping that is spiralled around the forearm portion of an orthosis. Rather than several pieces of Velcro hook being cut to attach to selected sites on the orthosis, both sides of the forearm trough can be the sites for placement of a long strip of Velcro hook. The spiral or continuous strap attaches to the Velcro hook. Spiral or continuous straps can be used in conjunction with compression gloves for persons who have edematous hands. The spiral strapping and glove prevent the trapping of distal edema.

To prevent the person wearing the orthosis from losing straps, the therapist may attach one end of the strap to the orthosis with a rivet or strong adhesive glue. Another helpful technique is to heat the end of a metal butter knife with a heat gun and push it through the thermoplastic material to make a slit. The area is cooled and the knife is removed. The therapist threads the strap through the slit, folds the strap end over itself, and sews the strap together (Figure 3-6, *A*). D-ring straps are available commercially. This type of strapping material affords the greatest control over strap tension and distal migration of the orthosis (see Figure 3-6, *B*).

Strap placement is critical to a proper fit. Many therapists fail to place the straps strategically for joint control and render the orthosis useless.[24] Schultz-Johnson particularly stresses wrist strap placement at the wrist, rather than proximal to the wrist.

Padding and Avoiding Pressure Areas

Therapists attempt to remediate portions of orthoses that may potentially cause pressure areas or irritations. The therapist can use a heat gun to push out areas of the thermoplastic material that may irritate bony prominences. Any bony prominences should be padded before the orthosis is formed. Padding should not be added as an afterthought. Padding over these areas or lining of an entire orthosis may also be considered to prevent irritation. Sufficient space must be made available for the thickness of the padding. Otherwise, the pressure may actually increase over the area.

Use of a self-adhesive gel disk (other paddings work as well) is helpful in cushioning bony prominences, such as the ulnar head. To use gel disks, the therapist adheres the disk to the person's skin and then forms the orthosis over the gel disk. Upon cooling of the orthosis, the gel disk is removed from the person and adhered to the corresponding area inside

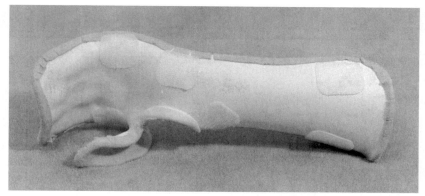

Figure 3-7 Moleskin overlaps the orthosis' edges.

the orthosis. To bubble out or dome areas over bony prominences, a therapist can place elastomer putty over the prominence before applying the warm thermoplastic material.

If an entire orthosis is to be lined with padding, the therapist can use the pattern to cut out the padding needed. The therapist can trace the pattern ¼ to ½ inch larger on the padding if the intention is to overlap the self-adhesive padding onto the orthosis' edges, as shown in Figure 3-7.

Gel lining is often used within the interior of the orthosis to assist in managing scars. Two types of gel lining are available: silicone gel and polymer gel. Silicone gel sheets, which are flexible and washable, can be cut with scissors into any shape. The silicone gel sheets are often positioned in conjunction with pressure garments or orthoses, or they are positioned with Coban. Persons using silicone gel sheets must be monitored for the development of rashes, skin irritations, and maceration. Polymer gel sheets are filled with mineral oil, which is released into the skin to soften "normal," hypertrophic, or keloid scars. Polymer gel sheets adhere to the skin and can be used with pressure garments or orthoses.

Various padding systems are commercially available in a variety of densities, durabilities, cell structures, and surface textures.[17] A self-adhesive backing is available with some types of padding, which saves the therapist time and materials, because glue does not have to be used to adhere the padding to an orthosis. Some cushioning and padding materials have an adhesive backing for easy application. Other types of padding are applied to any flat sheet of thermoplastic material and put in a heavyweight sealable plastic bag before immersion in hot water. The padding and thermoplastic material are adhered prior to molding the orthosis on the client. Putting the plastic with the padding adhered to it in a plastic bag prevents the padding from getting wet and can save the therapist time. Table 3-2 outlines available padding products.

Padding has either closed or open cells. Closed-cell padding resists absorption of odors and perspiration, and it can easily be wiped clean. Open-cell padding allows for absorption. Because of low durability and soiling, padding used in an orthosis may require periodic replacement. Some types of padding are virtually impossible to remove from

an orthosis. Thus, when padding needs replacement so does the orthosis.

Edge Finishing

Edges of an orthosis should be smooth and rolled or flared to prevent pressure areas on the person's extremity. The therapist may use a heat gun or heated water in a fry pan or hydrocollator to heat, soften, and smooth edges. Fingertips moistened with water or lotion help avoid finger imprints on the plastic. Most of the newer thermoplastic materials have self-finishing edges. When the warm plastic is cut, it does not require detailed finishing other than that necessary to flare the edges slightly.

Reinforcement

Strength of an orthosis increases when the plastic is curved. Thus, a plastic that has curves is stronger than a flat piece of thermoplastic material. When the thermoplastic material has been stretched too thin or is too flexible to provide adequate support to an area such as the wrist, it must be reinforced. If an area of an orthosis requires reinforcement, an additional piece of material bonded to the outside of the orthosis increases the strength. A ridge molded in the reinforcement piece provides additional strength (Figure 3-8).

Prefabricated Orthoses

In addition to making a custom-made orthosis, therapists have options to use prefabricated orthoses. The manufacturing of commercially-available prefabricated orthoses is market driven. Therefore, changes in style or materials may appear from year to year. Styles and materials are also affected by the manufacturing processes. Manufacturers are slow to change materials and design even when the market requests it. When a material, cut, or style of a prefabricated orthosis does not sell well, it may be discontinued or replaced with a different design. Vendors often attempt to manufacture prefabricated orthoses for broad populations. Based on research evidence, custom-made orthoses are preferred for some diagnostic conditions.

Table 3-2 Padding Categorization Guidelines

PADDING NAME	DENSITY	DURABILITY	SURFACE TEXTURE	SELF-ADHESIVE
BioPad	Thin	Short	Soft	Yes
Contour foam	Semi-dense	Medium	Textured	Yes
Elasto-gel splint pads	Dense	Medium	Semi-soft	Yes
Firm foam padding	Dense	Long	Semi-soft	Yes
Hapla padding	Semi-dense	Long	Textured	Yes
Luxafoam	Semi-dense	Medium	Soft	Yes
Microtape	Thin	Medium	Soft	Yes
Moleskin	Thin	Long	Soft	Yes
Orthopedic adhesive	Dense	Long	Semi-soft	Yes
Orthopedic felt	Dense	Long	Semi-soft	No
Plastizote padding	Semi-dense	Medium	Semi-soft	No
Reston foam padding	Thin	Short	Semi-soft	Yes
Silopad pressure	Dense	Long	Semi-soft	Yes
Slo-Foam padding	Semi-dense	Medium	Textured	No
Splint cushion	Semi-dense	Medium	Semi-soft	Yes
Splint pad	Semi-dense	Long	Textured	Yes
Soft splint padding	Thin	Medium	Soft	Yes
Sorbothane	Dense	Medium	Semi-soft	No
Terry cushion	Thin	Long	Textured	Yes

From North Coast Medical: *Hand therapy catalog,* San Jose, CA, 2012-2013, NCM.

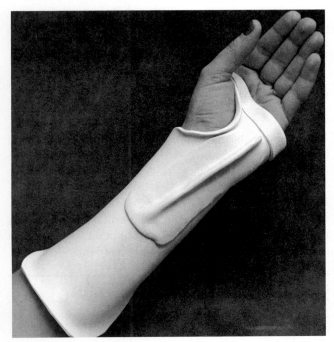

Figure 3-8 **Orthosis reinforcement.** This ridge on the reinforcement piece adds strength.

Manufacturing for a specific population is often costly and not financially rewarding unless that "specific population" has a large market. Improvements in the quality of prefabricated orthoses are affected by market economics, which stimulate companies to manufacture better products in terms of comfort, durability, and therapeutics. Current catalogs serve as the ultimate reference to what is available.

Vendors selling prefabricated orthoses are listed at the end of this chapter.

In addition to market economics, the proliferation of various styles of prefabricated orthoses can be attributed to two factors. First, the proliferation of prefabricated orthoses is influenced by the third-party payers' willingness to reimburse for orthoses. For example, the variety of soft hand and wrist orthoses for the elderly is an outgrowth of Medicare reimbursement policies during the 1980s and early 1990s. In contrast, because pediatric orthoses are typically not well reimbursed (except for orthopedic injuries), the market is small. Pediatric orthoses marketed for orthopedic needs tend to be smaller versions of adult-size orthoses.

Another reason for the proliferation of prefabricated orthoses involves the conceptual advances in design and the recognition that a need for these types of orthoses exists. For example, the refinement of wrist and thumb prefabricated orthoses has been influenced by the advancement of ergonomic knowledge and the public's awareness of the incidence and effects of cumulative trauma disorders.

Prefabricated orthoses are available from numerous vendors in a variety of styles, materials, and sizes. Prefabricated orthoses are available for the head, neck, joints of the upper and lower extremities, and trunk. Typically, prefabricated orthoses are ordered by size—and in some cases for right or left extremities. Some orthoses have a universal size, meaning that one orthosis fits the right or left hand. Before deciding to provide a prefabricated orthosis for a client, the therapist must be aware of the advantages and disadvantages of prefabricated orthoses.

Box 3-2 Advantages and Disadvantages of Using Soft and Prefabricated Orthoses

Advantages

- May save time and effort (if the orthosis fits the person well)
- Immediate feedback from client in terms of satisfaction and therapeutic fit
- Variety of material choices
- Some clients prefer the sports-brace appearance

Disadvantages

- Unique fit is often compromised
- Little control over therapeutic positioning of joints
- Expensive to stock a variety of sizes and designs
- Prefabricated and soft splints usually made for a few target populations (cannot address all conditions requiring unique or creative splint designs)

Advantages and Disadvantages of Prefabricated Orthoses

The advantages and disadvantages of using prefabricated orthoses are listed in Box 3-2.

Advantages

An obvious advantage of using a prefabricated orthosis is saving of the therapist's time and effort. The time required designing a pattern, tracing and cutting the pattern from plastic, and molding the orthosis to the person is saved when a prefabricated orthosis is used. However, keep in mind the time and expense involved in ordering and paying for the prefabricated orthoses. The costs and wage-hours involved in processing an order through a large facility are considerable. Maintaining inventory takes time and space.

If a prefabricated orthosis is in a clinic's inventory, the ability to immediately assess the orthosis in terms of therapeutics and customer satisfaction is an advantage. After orthosis application, the client is readily able to see and feel the orthosis. When fabricating a custom orthosis, the therapist may find that it does not meet the client's expectations or needs. When this occurs, a considerable amount of time and effort is expended in modifying the current orthosis or in designing and fabricating an entirely new orthosis. With prefabricated orthoses, an educated trial-and-error process can be used to find the best orthosis to meet the client's goals and therapeutic needs.

A third advantage is the variety of materials used to make prefabricated orthoses. Many prefabricated orthotic materials offer sophisticated technology that cannot be duplicated in the clinic. For example, a prefabricated orthosis made from high-temperature thermoplastic material is often more durable than a counterpart made of LTT material. Softer materials (combinations of fabric and foam) may be more acceptable to persons, especially those with rheumatoid arthritis.

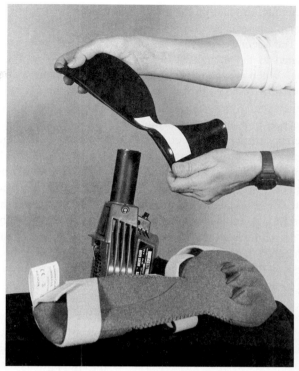

Figure 3-9 Adjustments can be made to commercial low-temperature thermoplastic (LTT) orthoses with the use of a heat gun. (Courtesy of Medical Media Service, Veterans Administration Medical Center, Durham, North Carolina.)

Soft orthoses can be more comfortable than the LTT ones usually used for custom orthoses. In a study comparing soft versus hard resting hand orthoses in 39 persons with rheumatoid arthritis, Callinan and Mathiowetz[6] found that compliance with wearing the orthosis was significantly better with the soft orthosis (82%) than with the hard orthosis (67%). However, therapists must realize that a person who needs rigid immobilization for comfort will not prefer a soft orthosis, because soft orthoses allow some mobility to occur. Some clients may think that the sports-brace appearance of a prefabricated orthosis is more aesthetically pleasing than the medical appearance of a custom-fabricated orthosis. For these clients, wearing compliance may increase.

Disadvantages

Several disadvantages must be noted with regard to prefabricated orthoses. A major disadvantage of using a prefabricated orthosis is that a custom, unique fit is often compromised. Soft prefabricated orthoses vary in how much they can be adjusted. If a high degree of conformity or a specialized design or position is needed, a prefabricated orthosis will usually not meet the person's needs. LTT prefabricated orthoses can be spot heated and adjusted somewhat (Figure 3-9), but they will never conform like a custom-made orthosis of the same material. Some prefabricated orthoses require adjustments. For example, thumb orthoses may require adjustment of the palmar bar to prevent chafing in the thumb web space.

Other preformed orthoses must be adjusted by trimming the forearm troughs for proper strap application.

The second disadvantage of prefabricated orthoses is related to the therapist's lack of control over customization. When using prefabricated orthoses, therapists often have little or no control over joint angle positioning. Often a therapeutic protocol or specific client need prescribes a specific joint angle for positioning. In such instances, the therapist must select a prefabricated orthosis that is designed with the appropriate joint angle(s) or choose one that can be adjusted to the correct angle. If unavailable, a custom orthosis is warranted. For example, therapists must use prefabricated orthoses cautiously with persons who have fluctuating edema. The orthosis and its strapping system must be able to accommodate the extremity's changing size. In addition, when conditions require therapists to create unique orthotic designs the desired prefabricated orthoses may not always be commercially available.

A third disadvantage of using a prefabricated orthosis is that the orthosis may not be stocked in the clinic and may have to be ordered. Many clinics cannot afford to stock a wide variety of prefabricated orthoses because of cost and storage restrictions. When an orthosis must be applied immediately and the prefabricated orthosis is not in the clinic's stock, a time delay for ordering it is unacceptable. A custom-made orthosis should be fabricated instead of waiting for the prefabricated orthosis to arrive.

Once the advantages and disadvantages have been weighed, a decision must be made regarding whether to use a prefabricated or a custom-made orthosis. The therapist engages in a clinical reasoning process to select the most appropriate orthosis.

Selecting an Orthosis

Therapists rarely use custom or prefabricated orthoses for 100% of their clientele. The therapist uses clinical reasoning based on a frame of reference to select the most appropriate orthosis. Outcome research is beginning to surface that addresses custom versus prefabricated orthosis usage. To determine whether to use a prefabricated or a custom-made orthosis, the therapist must know the specific orthotic needs of the person and determine how best to accomplish them. Some questions to ask are:

- Would a soft material or an LTT best meet the person's needs?
- How would the function and fit of a prefabricated orthosis compare with that of a custom-made orthosis?
- To properly evaluate whether a prefabricated orthosis or a custom-made orthosis would best meet a person's needs, the factors and questions discussed in the following sections must be considered and answered.

Diagnosis

Therapists should provide orthoses to people, not diagnoses. However, one must be well-versed in clinical conditions that often require orthotic intervention. Questions about orthotic intervention and diagnoses include:

- Is a prefabricated orthosis available for the diagnosis?
- Which orthotic design meets the therapeutic goals?
- Is there a match between the therapeutic goals and the design of a prefabricated or soft orthosis?
- What evidence exists to indicate a particular orthotic design for a particular diagnostic category?

For example, if a therapist must provide an orthosis to immobilize a wrist joint in neutral position, a prefabricated orthosis must have the ability to position and immobilize the wrist in the required neutral position.

Age of the Person

Thinking about age-related issues that impact orthotic intervention includes asking questions such as:

- Is the client at an age where he or she may have an opinion about the orthotic cosmesis?
- What special considerations are there for an older adult or a young child? (See Chapters 15 and 16.)
- What are the age-related activities that the person completes?

For example, an adolescent who is self-conscious may be unwilling to wear a custom-made elastic tension radial nerve orthosis at school because of its appearance. However, the adolescent might agree to wear a prefabricated wrist orthosis because of its less conspicuous sports-brace appearance.

Medical Complications

Medical complications can impact making orthoses. Questions to consider include:

- Does the person have compromised skin integrity, vascular supply, or sensation?
- Is the person experiencing pain, edema, or contractures?

Medical conditions must be considered because they may influence orthotic design. For example, the therapist may choose an orthosis with wide elastic straps to accommodate the change in the extremity's circumference for a person who has fluctuating edema.

Goals

Clients often have goals—things they wish to accomplish and symptoms they want to eliminate. Therapists should consider the following questions:

- What are the client's goals?
- What are the therapeutic goals?

The therapist determines the client's priorities and goals from an interview. The therapist can facilitate clients' compliance by understanding each person's capabilities and expectations.

Orthotic Design

Choosing an orthotic design should be individualized for each client. Questions to consider include:

- Which joints must be immobilized or mobilized?

- What are the therapeutic goals?
- Will the orthosis achieve the desired therapeutic goals?

It is important to avoid immobilizing unnecessary joints. Any orthosis that limits active range of motion may result in joint stiffness and muscle weakness. For example, if only the hand is involved, use a hand-based orthosis to avoid limiting wrist motion.

Occupational Performance

Clients lead lives that are filled with participation in meaningful activities and occupations. Participation in such activities is important to keep in mind. The therapist should reflect on the following questions:

- Does the orthosis affect the client's occupational performance?
- Does the orthosis maintain, improve, or eliminate occupational performance?
- Does wearing the orthosis interfere with participation in valued activities?

Occupational performance should be considered, regardless of the age of the client. Stern and colleagues[30] studied 42 persons with rheumatoid arthritis and reported that the "major use of wrist orthoses occurs during instrumental activities of daily living where greater stresses are placed on the wrist."[30] Therapists should observe or ask the client about his or her occupational participation while wearing the orthosis. Functional problems that occur while the orthosis is being worn require clinical reasoning. Resolution of functional problems may lead to a modification of performance technique, an adjustment in the wearing schedule, or a change in the orthotic design.

Person's or Caregiver's Ability to Adhere to Orthotic Instructions

Many clients and caregivers need to be educated on issues related to orthotic intervention. One should consider the following questions:

- Is the person or caregiver capable of following written and verbal instruction?
- Is the person motivated to comply with the wearing schedule? Are there any factors that may influence compliance?
- What is the client's health literacy level?

Forgetfulness, fear, cultural beliefs, values, therapeutic priorities, and confusion about the orthosis' purpose and schedule may influence adherence to a therapeutic plan. A therapist should consider a person's motivation, cognitive functioning, and physical ability when determining an orthotic design and schedule.

Adherence tends to increase with proper education.[1] For example, persons receiving education often have a better outcome if instructions are presented in verbal and written formats.[22] Therapists often explain to clients that long-term gains are usually worth short-term inconveniences. When adherence is a problem, the orthotic intervention may require modification.

Independence with Orthotic Regimen

A client's follow-through with a therapeutic intervention is important to achieve optimal outcomes. If there is no caregiver, can the client independently apply and remove the orthosis? Can the person monitor for precautions, such as the development of numbness, reddened areas, pressure sores, rash, and so on? For example, Fred (an 80-year-old man) is in need of bilateral resting hand orthoses to reduce pain from an exacerbation of rheumatoid arthritis. His 79-year-old wife is forgetful. Fred's therapist designs a wearing schedule so that Fred can elicit assistance from his wife. The therapist recommends putting the orthoses on the bed so that Fred can remind his wife to assist him in donning the orthoses before bedtime.

Comfort

If an orthosis is uncomfortable to the client, chances are it will not be worn. Therapists should ask questions related to comfort including:

- Does the person report that the orthosis is comfortable?
- Does the person have any condition, such as rheumatoid arthritis, that may warrant special attention to comfort?
- Are there insensate areas that may be at risk when wearing the orthosis?

Therapists should monitor the comfort of an orthosis on each client. If the orthosis is not comfortable, a person is not likely to wear it. In studying three prefabricated wrist supports for persons with rheumatoid arthritis, Stern and colleagues[31] concluded that "satisfaction appears to be based not only on therapeutic effect, but also the comfort and ease of its use."

Environment

Where people live, work, and recreate has an impact on orthotic intervention. Therapists must consider the following:

- In what type of environment will the person be wearing the orthosis?
- How might the environment affect orthotic wear and care?

Industrial Settings

Industrial settings may warrant orthoses made of more durable materials, such as leather, high-temperature thermoplastics, or metal. For example, orthoses may need extra cushioning to buffer vibration from machinery or tools that often aggravate cumulative trauma disorders.

Long-Term Care Settings

Therapists providing prefabricated orthoses to residents in long-term care settings must consider the influence of multiple caretakers and the fragile skin of many older adults. The following suggestions may assist in dealing with multiple caretakers and older adults' fragile skin. Orthoses should be labeled with the person's name. To avoid strap loss, consider attaching them to the orthosis or choose a prefabricated orthosis with attached straps. Select orthotic materials that are durable and easy to keep clean. Orthoses made from colored, thermoplastic material provide a contrast and may be more easily identified and distinguished from white or neutral-colored backgrounds.

School Settings

Several factors relating to pediatric orthoses must be considered by the therapist. Pediatric prefabricated orthoses should be made of materials that are easy to clean. Orthoses for children should be durable. Consider attaching straps to the orthosis or choose a prefabricated orthosis with attached straps. Because multiple caretakers (parents and school personnel) are typically involved in the application and wear schedule, instructions for wear and care should be clear and easy to follow. When the child is old enough, personal preferences and parental preferences should be considered during orthotic selection. If the orthosis is for long-term use, the therapist must remember that the child will grow. If possible, the therapist should select an orthosis that can be adjusted to avoid the expense of purchasing a new orthosis. In addition, orthoses with components that may scratch or be swallowed by the child should be avoided.

Education Format

Educating the client and/or caregiver on the orthotic intervention plan is linked to outcomes. The therapist must consider:

- What education do the client and caregiver need to adhere to the orthotic-wearing schedule?
- What is the learning style of the person and caregiver?
- How can the therapist adjust educational format to match the person's and caregiver's learning styles?

Educating clients and caregivers in methods consistent with their preferred learning style may increase compliance. Learning styles include kinesthetic, visual, and auditory.[8]

Written instructions should include the orthosis' purpose, wearing schedule, care, precautions, and emergency contact information. Because correct use of an orthosis affects intervention outcomes, the client should demonstrate an understanding of instructions in the presence of the therapist. A therapist may complete a follow-up phone call at a suitable interval to detect any problems encountered by the client or caregiver in regard to the orthosis (see Chapter 6).[21]

Fitting and Making Adjustments

If a decision is made to use a prefabricated orthosis and a selection is made, the therapist must evaluate the orthosis for size, fit, and function. Just as with custom orthoses, a particular prefabricated orthotic design does not work for every client. As professionals who provide orthoses to clients, therapists have an obligation and duty to fit the orthosis to the client rather than fitting the client to the orthosis! The implications of this duty suggest that clinics should stock a variety of commercial orthotic designs. Although a large clinic's overhead is expensive, limiting choices may result in poor client compliance.[31] When a variety of orthotic designs are available, a trial-and-error approach can be used with commercial orthoses, because most clients are able to report their preference for an orthosis after a few minutes of wear. When fitting a client with a commercial orthosis, the therapist should ask the following questions[31]:

- Does the orthosis feel secure on your extremity?
- Does the orthosis or its straps rub or irritate you anywhere?
- When wearing the orthosis, does your skin feel too hot?
- What activities will you be doing while wearing your orthosis?
- When you move your extremity while wearing the orthosis, do you experience any pain?
- Does the orthosis feel comfortable after wearing it for 20 to 30 minutes?

In addition to fit and size, therapists must evaluate the prefabricated orthosis' effect on function. Stern and colleagues[30] investigated three commercial wrist orthoses for their effect on finger dexterity and hand function. Dexterity was reduced similarly across the three orthoses. In addition, dexterity was significantly affected when the orthoses were used during tasks that required maximum dexterity. In such cases, therapists and clients should decide whether dexterity reduction outweighs the known benefits of orthotic intervention.

Jansen and colleagues'[11] research indicated that grip strength decreased when clients wore wrist orthoses. However, for women with rheumatoid, arthritis grip strength increased during orthotic wear.[16] A reduction in grip strength occurs because wrist orthoses prevent the amount of wrist extension required to generate maximal grip strength in the "normal" population. Those with rheumatoid arthritis have poor wrist stability. Thus, the orthoses allow them to generate improved grip strength because of improved stability. Prefabricated orthoses often require adjustments to appropriately fit the person and condition.

Technical Tips for Custom Adjustments to Prefabricated Orthoses

The following points describe common adjustments made to commercial low-temperature thermoplastic orthoses. High-temperature thermoplastic orthoses cannot be adjusted using equipment, such as heat guns and hydrocollators. The provider must be competent to make adjustments to high-temperature thermoplastic orthoses as is a certified orthotist/prosthetist.

1. Therapists should ensure that orthoses do not irritate soft tissue, reduce circulation, or cause paresthesias.[31] Adjustments may include flaring ends, bubbling out pressure areas, or addition of padding.
2. Although soft orthoses are intended to be used as is, minor modifications to customize the fit to a person can be accomplished. Some soft orthoses can be trimmed

with scissors to customize fit. If a soft orthosis has stitching to hold layers together, it will need to be resewn. (Note that it is beneficial to have a sewing machine in the clinic.)

3. Modification methods for preformed orthoses include heating, cutting, or reshaping portions of the LTT orthosis. Minor modifications can be made with the use of a heat gun, fry pan, or hydrocollator to soften LTT preformed orthoses for trimming or slight stretching.

   - Some elastic traction/tension prefabricated orthoses may be adjusted by bending and repositioning portions of wire, metal, or foam orthotic components. Occasionally, technical literature accompanying the orthosis describes how to make adjustments in the amount of traction. Often traction can be adjusted with the use of an Allen wrench on the rotating wheels on a hinge joint, as shown in Figure 3-10. When there are no instructions describing how to make adjustments on prefabricated orthoses, the therapist must use creative problem-solving skills to accomplish the desired changes.

   - When a static prefabricated orthosis is used and serial adjustments are required to accommodate increases in passive range of motion (PROM), the orthosis must be reheated and remolded to the client. It is advantageous to select a prefabricated orthosis made of material that has memory properties to allow for the serial adjustments.

   - The amount of force provided by some static-progressive orthoses is made through mechanical adjustment of the force-generating device. Force may be adjusted by manipulating the orthotic turnbuckle, bolt, or hinge.

   - The force exerted by elastic traction components of a prefabricated orthosis is also made through adjustments of the force-generating device. Therapists can adjust the forces by changing elastic component length by gradually moving the placement of the neoprene or rubber band–like straps on an orthosis throughout the day, as shown in Figure 3-11.

   - Adding components to prefabricated orthoses can be helpful. For example, putty-elastomer inserts that serve as finger separators can be used in a resting hand orthosis. Finger separators add contour in the hand area to maintain the arches. A therapist may choose to add other components, such as wicking lining or padding.

   - Prefabricated orthoses can be modified by replacing parts of them with more adjustable materials. For example, if a wrist orthosis has a metal stay, replacing it with an LTT stay results in a custom fit with the correct therapeutic position.

   - It is often necessary to customize strapping mechanisms for prefabricated orthoses. The number and placement of straps are adjusted to best secure the orthosis on the person. Straps must be secured properly, but not so tightly as to restrict circulation. Straps coursing through web spaces must not irritate soft tissue. The research by Stern and colleagues[31] on commercial wrist orthoses indicates that clients with stiff joints experienced difficulty threading straps through D-rings. Clients reported having to use their teeth to manipulate straps. Straps that are too long also appear to be troublesome because they catch on clothing.[31]

   - Stern and colleagues[29] showed that although commercial orthoses are often critiqued for being too short, some persons prefer shorter forearm troughs. Shorter orthoses seem to be preferred by clients when wrist support, not immobilization, is needed.

After the necessary adjustments are completed and a proper fit is accomplished, a therapist determines wearing schedule.

Wearing Schedule

Although there are no easy answers about wearing protocols, experienced therapists have several guidelines for decision making as they tailor wearing schedules to each client.[23]

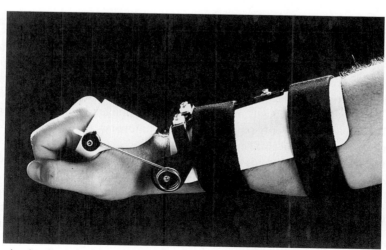

Figure 3-10 Tension is adjusted with an Allen wrench on the rotating wheels on the hinge joint of this orthosis.

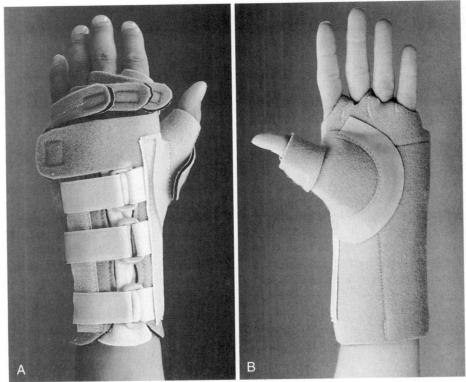

Figure 3-11 A, The Rolyan In-Line orthosis with thumb support can be adjusted by loosening or tightening the neoprene straps. **B,** Volar view of the Rolyan In-Line orthosis with thumb support. (Courtesy of Rehabilitation Division of Smith & Nephew, Germantown, Wisconsin.)

Evidence from the literature may also provide information on wearing schedules.

- For orthoses designed to increase PROM, light tension exerted by an orthosis over a long period of time is preferable to high tension for short periods of time.
- For joints with **hard end feels** (i.e., an abrupt, hard stop to movement when bone contacts bone during PROM) and PROM limitations, more hours of orthotic wear are warranted than for joints with **soft end feels** (i.e., a soft compression of tissue is felt when two body surfaces approximate each other).
- Persons tolerate static orthoses (including serial and static-progressive orthoses) better than dynamic orthoses during sleep.
- When treatment goals are being considered, wearing schedules should allow for facilitation of active motion and functional use of joints when appropriate.

As with any orthotic provision, the orthotic-wearing schedule should be given in verbal and written formats to the person and caregiver(s). The wearing schedule depends on the person's condition and dysfunction and the severity (chronic or acute) of the problem. The wearing schedule also depends on the therapeutic goal of the orthosis, the demands of the environment, and the ability of the person and caregiver(s).

Care of Prefabricated Orthoses

Always check the manufacturer's instructions for cleaning the orthosis. Give the client the manufacturer's instructions on orthotic care. If a client is visually impaired, make an enlarged copy of the instructions. For soft orthoses, the manufacturer usually recommends hand washing and air drying, because the agitation and heat of some washers and dryers can ruin soft orthoses. Because air drying of soft orthoses takes time, occasionally two of the same orthosis are provided so that the person can alternate wear during cleaning and drying. The inside of LTT orthoses should be wiped out with rubbing alcohol. The outside of LTT orthoses can be cleaned with toothpaste or nonabrasive cleaning agents and rinsed with tepid water. Clients and caregivers should be reminded that LTT orthoses soften in extreme heat, as in a car interior or on a windowsill or radiator.

Precautions for Patient Safety

In addition to selecting, fitting, and scheduling the wear of a prefabricated orthosis, the therapist must educate the client or caregiver about any precautions and how to monitor for them. There are several precautions to be aware of with the use of commercial orthoses. These are discussed in the section following.

Dermatological Issues Related to Orthotic Wear
Latex Sensitivity
Some prefabricated orthoses contain latex. More latex-sensitive people, including clients and medical professionals, are being identified.[10,19] Therapists should request a list of both latex and latex-free products from the suppliers of commercial orthoses used.

Allergic Contact Dermatitis

Recently, dermatologic issues related to neoprene orthoses have come to therapists' attention. Allergic contact dermatitis (ACD) and miliaria rubra (prickly heat) are associated in some persons with the wearing of neoprene (also known as *polychloroprene*) orthoses.[28] ACD symptoms include itching, skin eruptions, swelling, and skin hemorrhages. Miliaria rubra presents with small, red, elevated, inflamed papules and a tingling and burning sensation. Before using commercial or custom neoprene orthoses, therapists should question clients about dermatologic reactions and allergies. If a person reacts to a neoprene orthosis, wear should be discontinued, and the therapist should notify the manufacturer. An interface, such as polypropylene stockinette, may also serve to resolve the problem.

Clients need to be instructed not only in proper orthotic care but in hygiene of the body part included in the orthosis. Intermittent removal of the orthosis to wash the body part, the application of cornstarch, or the provision of wicking liners may help minimize dermatologic problems. Time of year and ambient temperatures need to be considered by the therapist. For example, neoprene may provide desired warmth to stiff joints and increase comfort while improving active and passive range of motion. However, during extreme summer temperatures, the neoprene orthosis may cause more perspiration and increase the risk of skin maceration if inappropriately monitored.

Ordering Commercial Orthoses

A variety of vendors sell prefabricated orthoses. Companies may sell similar orthotic designs, but the item names can be quite different. To keep abreast of the newest commercial orthoses, therapists should browse through vendor catalogs, communicate with vendor sales representatives, and seek out vendor exhibits during meetings and conferences for the ideal "hands-on" experience.

It is most beneficial to the therapist and the client when a clinic has a variety of commercial orthotic designs and sizes for right and left extremities. Keeping a large stock in a clinic can be expensive. To cover the overhead expense of stocking and storing prefabricated orthoses, a percentage mark-up of the prefabricated orthosis is often charged in addition to the therapist's time and materials used for adjustments.

Orthotic Workroom or Cart

Having a well-organized and stocked orthotic area benefits the therapist who must make decisions about the orthotic design and construct the orthosis in a timely manner. Clients who need orthotic intervention also benefit from a well-stocked orthotic supply inventory. Readily available materials and tools expedite the orthotic-making process.

Clinics should consider the services commonly rendered and stock their materials accordingly. In addition to a stocked orthotic inventory, therapists may find it useful to have a cart organized for orthotic provision in a client's

room or in another portion of the health care setting. The cart can assist the therapist in readily transporting orthotic supplies to the client, rather than a client coming to the therapist. For therapists who travel from clinic to clinic, orthotic supply suitcases on rollers are ideal. Orthotic carts or cases should contain such items as the following:

- Paper towels
- Pencils/awl
- Masking tape
- Thermoplastic material
- Fry pan
- Scissors (various sizes)
- Strapping materials, including Ace bandages
- Padding materials
- Heat gun
- Spatula, metal turkey baster
- Thermometer
- Pliers
- Revolving hole punch
- Glue
- Goniometer
- Solvent or bonding agent
- Other specialized supplies as needed (e.g., finger loops, outrigger wire, outrigger line, springs, turnbuckles, rubber bands, and so on)

Documentation and Reassessment

Orthotic provision must be well documented. Documentation assists in third-party reimbursement, communication to other health care providers, and demonstration of efficacy of the intervention. Documentation should include several elements, such as the type, purpose, and anatomic location of the orthosis. Therapists should document that they have communicated in oral and written formats with the person receiving the orthosis. Topics addressed with each person include the wearing schedule, orthotic care, precautions, and any home program activities.

In follow-up visits, documentation should include any changes in the orthotic design and wearing schedule. In addition, the therapist should note whether problems with compliance are apparent. The therapist should determine whether the range of motion is increasing with orthotic wearing time and draw conclusions about orthotic efficacy or compliance with the program. Function in and out of the orthosis should be documented. For example, the therapist determines whether the person can independently perform some type of function as a result of wearing the orthosis. The therapist must listen to the client's reports of functional problems and solve problems to remediate or compensate for the functional deficit. If function or range of motion is not increased, the therapist needs to consider orthotic revision or redesign or counseling the client on the importance of wearing the orthosis.

The therapist should perform reassessments regularly until the person is weaned from the orthosis or discharged from services. Facilities use different methods of documentation, and the therapist should be familiar with the routine method of the facility. (Refer to the documentation portion of Chapter 6 for more information.)

Physical Agent Modalities

Physical agent modalities (PAMs) are defined as those modalities that produce a biophysiologic response through the use of light, water, temperature, sound, electricity, or mechanical devices.[2] The AOTA's PAM position paper indicates that PAMs "may be used by occupational therapy practitioners as an adjunct to or in preparation for intervention that ultimately enhances engagement in occupation; physical agents may only be applied by occupational therapists who have documented evidence of possessing the theoretical background for safe and competent integration into the therapy treatment plan."[2] Therapists must comply with their respective state's scope of practice requirements regarding the use of PAMs as preparation for orthotic intervention.

Experienced therapists often use PAMs as an adjunctive method to effect a change in musculoskeletal tissue. Select PAMs may be used before, during, or after orthotic provision for management of pain, to increase soft-tissue extensibility, reduce edema, increase tendon excursion, promote wound healing, and decrease scar tissue. Occasionally, PAMs are used to prepare the upper extremity for optimal positioning for orthotic intervention. Prior to using any PAM, the therapist must develop and use clinical reasoning skills to effectively select and evaluate the appropriate modality; identify safety precautions, indications, and contraindications; and facilitate individualized treatment outcomes.

The type of PAM selected and the parameter setting(s) affects the neuromuscular system and tissue response. Changes in tissue response depend on how sensory information is processed to produce a motor response. Thermotherapy (heat) and cryotherapy (cold) have a significant effect on the peripheral nervous system and on neuromuscular control, and may enhance sensory and motor function when applied as an adjunctive method.

Therapists who use PAMs to effect a change in soft tissue, joint structure, tendons and ligaments, sensation, and pain level must consider the agent's effects on superficial structures within the skin (i.e., epidermis, dermis, and hypodermis). Because orthoses are usually applied to an extremity (e.g., hand or foot), therapists must consider which sensory structures are stimulated and which motor responses are expected when applying a PAM prior to orthotic intervention. PAMs can be generally categorized in numerous ways. An overview of superficial agents commonly used to position the client for orthotic intervention follows.

Superficial Agents

Superficial agents penetrate the skin to a depth of 1 to 2 cm.[7] These heating agents or thermotherapy agents include moist hot packs, fluidotherapy, paraffin wax therapy, and cryotherapy. Table 3-3 lists superficial agents and their physiologic responses, indications, contraindications, and precautions.

Heat Agents

Heat is transferred to the skin and subcutaneous tissue by conduction or by convection. **Conduction** transfers heat from one object to another. Heat is conducted from the higher-temperature object to the lower-temperature material (such as moist heat packs or paraffin). Table 3-4 lists the temperature ranges for heat application.

Hot Packs

Superficial heat may be used for the relief of pain with non-inflammatory conditions, general relaxation, and to stretch contractures and improve range of motion prior to orthotic intervention. For example, a client fractures her wrist and upon removal of the cast demonstrates limited wrist extension. The therapist intends to gain wrist extension by applying a moist hot pack to her wrist to increase the extensibility of the soft tissue. After application of the heat, the therapist is able to range the wrist into 10 degrees of wrist extension (an improvement from neutral). The client is positioned in slight wrist extension. A serial static orthotic approach is used to gain a functional level of wrist extension.

Heat may be used to decrease muscle spasms by increasing nerve conduction velocity. According to Cameron, "Nerve conduction velocity has been reported to increase by approximately 2 meters/second for every 1° C (1.8° F) increase in temperature."[7] Elevation of muscle tissue to 42° C (108° F) has been shown to decrease firing rate of the alpha motor neurons resulting in decreased muscle spasm.[7] Thus, in some cases heat is applied to reduce muscle spasms with a client who needs an orthosis.

Fluidotherapy

Convection transfers heat between a surface and a moving medium or agent. Examples of convection include fluidotherapy and whirlpool (hydrotherapy). Fluidotherapy is a form of dry heat consisting of ground cellulose particles made from corn husks. Circulated air heated from 100° F to 118° F suspends the particles,[7] creating agitation that functions much like a whirlpool turbine. Fluidotherapy is frequently used for pain control and desensitization and sensory stimulation. It is also used to increase soft tissue extensibility and joint range of motion and to reduce adhesions. Fluidotherapy is often used prior to applying static and dynamic hand orthoses for increasing soft-tissue extensibility. Fluidotherapy can increase edema due to the heat and dependent positioning of the upper extremity. Caution must be taken when using fluidotherapy on those who have asthma or when using fluidotherapy around those near the machine who have respiratory conditions, because particles can trigger a respiratory attack.

Table 3-3 Superficial Agents

TYPE OF PAM	PHYSIOLOGIC RESPONSE	INDICATIONS	CONTRAINDICATIONS	PRECAUTIONS
Hot packs (conduction)	• Increased collagen extensibility • Increased activity of thermoreceptors • Increased blood flow increases nutrients to the area and facilitates removal of prostaglandin, bradykinin, and histamine • Changes muscle spindle firing rate • Increased sensory nerve conduction velocity	• Clients with subacute and chronic conditions who experience stiffness and/or pain that interferes with positioning needed for making an orthosis	• Do not use with clients who have absent sensation or decreased circulation	• Use tongs to who have absent sensation. • Clients should not lie on top of heat packs. • Do not use in presence of severe edema. • Be careful with clients who have decreased sensation.
Fluidotherapy (convection)	• Increased collagen extensibility • Increased activity of thermoreceptors • Increased blood flow increases nutrients to the area and facilitates removal of prostaglandin, bradykinin, and histamine • Changes muscle spindle firing rate • Increased sensory nerve conduction velocity	• Clients with subacute and chronic conditions who experience stiffness and/or pain that interferes with positioning needed for making an orthosis	• Do not use with clients who have open wounds or draining wounds	• Be cautious with clients who have decreased sensation and circulation. • Caution needed when used with persons who have asthma or respiratory problems.
Paraffin (conduction)	• Increased collagen extensibility • Increased activity of thermoreceptors • Increased blood flow increases nutrients to the area and facilitates removal of prostaglandin, bradykinin, and histamine • Changes muscle spindle firing rate • Increased sensory nerve conduction velocity	• Clients with subacute and chronic conditions who experience stiffness and/or pain that interferes with positioning needed for making an orthosis	• Do not use with clients who have open wounds, infections or absent sensation	• Check the thermostat on the machine. • Keep a CO_2 fire extinguisher available. • Be careful with clients who have decreased sensation or circulation.
Cold cryotherapy • Ice packs • Ice towels • Vapo-coolant sprays	• Vasoconstriction • Decreased velocity of nerve conduction • Decreased metabolism • Increased pain threshold • Reduced spasticity due to decreased muscle spindle activity	• Decreased pain, edema, and spasticity	• Cardiac dysfunction • Chronic or deep open wounds, arterial insufficiency • Hypersensitivity to cold • Impaired sensation • Regenerating peripheral nerves • Older adults who have decreased tolerance to cold	

PAM, Physical agent modality.

Table 3-4	Temperature Ranges for Heat Application	
TEMPERATURE RANGE	**°F**	**°C**
Normal temperature	98.6	37
Mild heating	98.6-104	37-40
Vigorous heating	104-110	40-43
Tissue damage	>110	>43

Data from Bracciano A: *Physical agent modalities: theory and application for the occupational therapist*, Thorofare, NJ, 2002, Slack.

Paraffin Wax Therapy

Heated paraffin wax is another source of superficial warmth that transfers heat by conduction. The melting point of paraffin wax is 54.5° C (131° F).[7] Administration includes dipping the clean hand in the wax for ten consecutive immersions. The hand is then wrapped in a plastic bag and covered with a towel. Clients with open wounds, infections, or absent sensation should not receive paraffin therapy. Clients with chronic conditions, such as rheumatoid arthritis, may benefit from paraffin therapy to reduce stiffness prior to orthotic intervention.

Cryotherapy

Cryotherapy is defined as the therapeutic use of cold modalities. Cold is considered a superficial modality that penetrates to a depth of 1 to 2 cm[7] and produces a decrease in tissue temperature. Cold is transferred to the skin and subcutaneous tissue by conduction. Examples of cold modalities include cold packs, ice packs, ice towels, ice massage, and vapo sprays. Cold packs are usually stored at −5° C (23° F) and treatment time is 10 to 15 minutes.[7] The effectiveness of the cold modality used depends on intensity, duration, and frequency of application.

There are four sensations of cold associated with reduced pain and inflammation: cold, burning, aching, and numbness. Hayes[9] suggested that cold modalities used to reduce swelling and slow metabolism must be mild. To block pain, cold must be very cold. Duration of cold application depends on the targeted tissue. Deeper tissues must be cooled for longer periods of time. The colder the medium the shorter the duration. Cryotherapy may be used in the treatment of acute injury or to control bleeding associated with recent wounds. Other therapeutic benefits of cold include increased vasoconstriction, decreased metabolic response (reduces oxygen and thus decreases inflammation), decreased nerve conduction velocity, increased pain threshold, decreased muscle spindle activity, and reduced spasticity.

Cryotherapy is contraindicated for clients with cardiac dysfunction, chronic or deep open wounds, arterial insufficiency, hypersensitivity to cold, impaired sensation, and regenerating peripheral nerves. Elders with decreased tolerance to cold may be unable to tolerate even brief applications of therapeutic cold modalities.[3,5,7,9,12,26,32]

Cold modalities may be used to decrease edema, pain, and spasticity during range of motion prior to application of the orthosis. Cryotherapy does not increase soft-tissue extensibility and may reduce circulation, oxygen, and nutrition to healing tissues. Refer to Table 3-3 for a comparison of the therapeutic effects of cryotherapy and thermotherapy.

Review Questions

1. What are six handling characteristics of thermoplastics?
2. What are six performance characteristics of thermoplastics?
3. At what temperature range are LTT materials softened?
4. What steps are involved in making a pattern for an orthosis?
5. What equipment can be used to soften thermoplastic materials?
6. How can a therapist prevent a tacky thermoplastic from sticking to the hair on a person's arms?
7. What are the purposes of using a heat gun?
8. Why should a therapist use a bonding agent?
9. Why should the edges of an orthosis be rolled or flared?
10. What is the AOTA position on the use of PAMs by occupational therapy practitioners?
11. What is the depth of penetration to skin and subcutaneous tissue obtained with superficial agents?
12. How can PAMs be used in preparation for orthotic intervention?

References

1. Agnew PJ, Maas F: Compliance in wearing wrist working splints in rheumatoid arthritis, *Occup Ther J Res* 15(3):165–180, 1995.
2. American Occupational Therapy Association: Position paper: physical agent modalities, *Am J Occup Ther* 57:650, 2003.
3. Belanger AY: *Evidenced-based guide to therapeutic physical agents*, Philadelphia, 2002, Lippincott Williams & Wilkins.
4. Berger S: Personal communication, 1995.
5. Bracciano A: *Physical agent modalities: theory and application for the occupational therapist*, Thorofare, NJ, 2002, Slack.
6. Callinan N, Mathiowetz V: Soft versus hard resting hand splints in rheumatoid arthritis: pain relief, preference and compliance, *Am J Occup Ther* 50(5):347–353, 1996.
7. Cameron M: *Physical agents in rehabilitation: from research to practice*, ed 4, St Louis, 2013, Elsevier.
8. Fleming ND, Mills C: Helping students understand how they learn, *The Teaching Professor* volume:3–4, 1993.
9. Hayes KW: *Manual for physical agents*, ed 5, Upper Saddle River, NJ, 2000, Prentice-Hall.
10. Jack M: Latex allergies: a new infection control issue, *Can J Infect Control* 9(3):67–70, 1994.
11. Jansen CW, Olson SL, Hasson SM: The effect of use of a wrist orthosis during functional activities on surface electromyography of the wrist extensors in normal subjects,, *J Hand Ther* 10(4): 283–289, 1997.
12. Kahn J: *Principles and practices of electrotherapy*, ed 4, Philadelphia, 2000, Churchill Livingstone.
13. Lee DB: Objective and subjective observations of low-temperature thermoplastic materials, *J Hand Ther* 8(2):138–143, 1995.

14. McKee P, Morgan L: Orthotic materials. In McKee P, Morgan L, editors: *Orthotics in rehabilitation*, Philadelphia, 1998, FA Davis.

15. Melvin JL: *Rheumatic disease in the adult and child: occupational therapy and rehabilitation*. Philadelphia, 1989, FA Davis.

16. Nordenskiöld U: Elastic wrist orthoses: reduction of pain and increase in grip force for women with rheumatoid arthritis, *Arthritis Care Res* 3(3):158–162, 1990.

17. North Coast Medical: *Hand therapy catalog*, San Jose, CA, 1999, NCM.

18. North Coast Medical: *Hand therapy catalog*, San Jose, CA, 2006, NCM.

18. *Orfit splinting materials*, Gilroy, CA, 2012-2013, North Coast Medical (Volume 1).

19. Personius CD: Patients, health care workers, and latex allergy, *Med Lab Obs* 27(3):30–32, 1995.

20. Preston Sammons Rolyan: *Hand rehab products for hand rehabilitation*, Bolingbrook, IL, 2006, Patterson Medical Products.

21. Racelis MC, Lombardo K, Verdin J: Impact of telephone reinforcement of risk reduction education on patient compliance, *J Vasc Nurs* 16(1):16–20, 1998.

22. Schneiders AG, Zusman M, Singer KP: Exercise therapy compliance in acute low back pain patients, *Manual therapy* 3(3):147–152, 1998.

23. Schultz-Johnson K: Splinting: a problem-solving approach. In Stanley BG, Tribuzi SM, editors: *Concepts in hand rehabilitation*, Philadelphia, 1992, FA Davis.

24. Schultz-Johnson K: Personal communication, 1999.

25. Schultz-Johnson K: Personal communication, 2006.

26. Shankar K, Randall KD: *Therapeutic physical modalities*, Philadelphia, 2002, Hanley & Belfus.

27. Shurr DG, Michael JW: *Prosthetics and orthotics*, Upper Saddle River, NJ, 2002, Prentice Hall.

28. Stern EB, Callinan N, Hank M, et al.: Neoprene splinting: dermatological issues, *Am J Occup Ther* 52(7):573–578, 1998.

29. Stern EB, Sines B, Teague TR: Commercial wrist extensor orthoses: hand function, comfort and interference across five styles, *J Hand Ther* 7:237–244, 1994.

30. Stern EB, Ytterberg S, Krug HE, et al.: Finger dexterity and hand function: effect of three commercial wrist extensor orthoses on patients with rheumatoid arthritis, *Arthritis Care Res* 9(3):197–205, 1996.

31. Stern EB, Ytterberg SR, Krug HE, et al.: Commercial wrist extensor orthoses: a descriptive study of use and preference in patients with rheumatoid arthritis, *Arthritis Care Res* 10(1):27–35, 1997.

32. Sussman C, Bates-Jensen BM: *Wound care: a collaborative practice manual for physical therapists and nurses*, Philadelphia, 1998, Lippincott Williams & Wilkins.

33. Wilton JC: *Hand splinting principles of design and fabrication*, Philadelphia, 1997, Saunders.

APPENDIX 3-1 LABORATORY EXERCISE

Laboratory Exercise 3-1 Low-Temperature Thermoplastics

Cut small squares of different thermoplastic materials. Soften them in water, and experiment with the plastics so that you can answer the following questions for each type of thermoplastic material.

Name of the thermoplastic material: _____

1. Does it contour and drape to the hand?	Yes ○	No ○
2. Does it appear to be strong when cool?	Yes ○	No ○
3. Can its edges be rolled easily?	Yes ○	No ○
4. Does it discolor when heated?	Yes ○	No ○
5. Does it take fingerprints easily?	Yes ○	No ○
6. Does it bond to itself?	Yes ○	No ○
7. Can it revert to original shape after being reheated several times?	Yes ○	No ○

APPENDIX 3-2   FORM

FORM 3-1* Hints for drawing and fitting a splint pattern

- Explain the pattern-making process to the person.
- Ask or assist the person to remove any jewelry from the area that will be in the orthosis.
- Wash the area that will be fitted with an orthosis if it is dirty.
- If applying an orthosis over bandages or foam, cover the extremity with stockinette or a moist paper towel to prevent the plastic from sticking to the bandages.
- Position the affected extremity on a paper towel in a flat, natural resting position. The wrist should be in a neutral position with a slight ulnar deviation. The fingers should be extended and slightly abducted.
- To trace the outline of the person's extremity, keep the pencil at a 90-degree angle to the paper.
- Mark the landmarks needed to draw the pattern before the person removes the extremity from the paper.
- For a more accurate pattern, the paper towel can be wet and placed on the area for evaluation of the pattern, or aluminum foil can be used.
- Folding the paper towel to mark adjustments in the pattern can help with evaluation of the pattern.
- When evaluating the pattern fit of a forearm-based orthosis on the person, look for the following:
  - Half the circumference of body parts for the width of troughs
  - Two-thirds the length of the forearm
  - The length and width of metacarpal or palmar bars
  - The correct use of hand creases for landmarks
  - The amount of support to the wrist, fingers, and thenar and hypothenar eminencies
- When tracing the pattern onto the thermoplastic material, do not use an ink pen because the ink may smear when the material is placed in the hot water to soften. Rather, use a pencil, grease pencil, or awl to mark the pattern outline on the material.

APPENDIX A

Sources of Vendors

AliMed
1-800-225-2610
http://www.alimed.com/online-catalog.aspx
Email: psteam@alimed.com

Benik Corporation
1-800-442-8910
http://benik.com/
Email: info@benik.com

Biodex Medical Systems
1-800-224-6339
http://biodex.com/physical-medicine
Email: info@biodex.com

BSN Medical
1-800-552-1157
http://www.bsnmedical.com
Email: BSNcorporate@bsnmedical.com

Chattanooga Group
1-866-512-2764
http://www.chattmed.com

Chesapeake Medical Products
1-888-560-2674
http://www.chesapeakemedical.com

Core Products International, Inc.
(877) 249-1251
http://www.coreproducts.com/

DeRoyal
1-800-251-9864
http://www.deroyal.com/
Email: customerservice@deroyal.com

Dynasplint
1-800-638-6771
http://www.dynasplint.ca/en/
Email: info@dynasplint.com

Empi
1-800-328-2536
http://www.djoglobal.com
Email: support@empi.com

Joint Active Systems
1-800-879-0117
http://www.jointactivesystems.com/For-Professionals/
Email: info@jointactivesystems.com

Joint Jack Company
(860) 906 1113
http://jointjackcompany.com/
Email: jointjack2@aol.com

North Coast Medical, Inc.
1-800-821-9319
http://www.ncmedical.com/
Email: custserv@ncmedical.com

Restorative Care of America, Inc. (RCAI)
1-800-627-1595
http://www.rcai.com/

Patterson Medical
1-800-343-9742
http://www.pattersonmedical.com/

Smith & Nephew, Inc.
1-800-558-8633
http://smith-nephew.com/us/professional/

Tetra Medical Supply Corporation
1-800-621-4041
http://www.tetramed.com/
Email: tetra@tetramed.com

3-Point Products
1-410-604-6393
http://www.3pointproducts.com/
Email: service@3pointproducts.com

U.E. Tech
1-800-736-1894
http://www.uetech.com/
Email: karen@uetech.com

CHAPTER 4

Anatomic and Biomechanical Principles Related to Orthotic Provision

Brenda M. Coppard, PhD, OTR/L, FAOTA

Key Terms

Aponeurosis
degrees of freedom
dorsal
grasp
mechanical advantage
plasticity
prehension
pressure
radial
stress
three-point pressure
torque
ulnar
viscoelasticity
volar
zones of the hand

Chapter Objectives

1. Define the anatomical terminology used in orthotic prescriptions.
2. Relate anatomy of the upper extremity to orthotic design.
3. Identify arches of the hand.
4. Identify creases of the hand.
5. Articulate the importance of the hand's arches and creases to orthotic intervention.
6. Recall actions and nerve innervations of upper extremity musculature.
7. Differentiate among prehensile and grasp patterns of the hand.
8. Apply basic biomechanical principles to orthotic design.
9. Describe the correct width and length for a forearm orthosis.
10. Describe uses of padding in an orthosis.
11. Explain the reason that orthotic edges should be rolled or flared.
12. Relate contour to orthotic fabrication.
13. Describe the change in skin and soft tissue mechanics with scar tissue, material application, edema, contractures, wounds, and infection.

Troy is a new practitioner in a rural hospital. He commonly receives referrals to see clients who are initially patients at larger health facilities post surgery and who then opt for therapy at the local, smaller and rural hospital. Troy has a strong knowledge base of anatomic and biomechanical principles. He often reflects back on his hours when he studied diligently, and he is happy that he did so for this client population!

Basic Anatomical Review for Orthotic Intervention

Orthotic intervention requires sound knowledge of anatomic terminology and structures, biomechanics, and the way in which pathologic conditions impact function. Knowledge of anatomic structures is necessary in the choice and fabrication of an orthosis. Anatomic knowledge also influences the therapeutic intervention and home program. The following is a brief overview of anatomic terminology, proximal-to-distal structures, and landmarks of the upper extremity pertinent to the orthotic process. The overview is neither comprehensive nor all-inclusive. For more depth and breadth in anatomic review, access an anatomy text, anatomic atlas, anatomy website, or computer programs that show anatomic structures.

Terminology

Knowing anatomic location terminology is extremely important when a therapist receives a prescription for an orthosis or is reading professional literature about orthotic interventions. In rehabilitation settings, the word *arm* usually refers to the segment of the upper extremity from the shoulder to the elbow (humerus). The term *antecubital fossa* refers to the depression at the bend of the elbow. *Forearm* is used to describe the portion of the upper extremity from the elbow to the wrist, which includes the radius and ulna. *Carpal* or *carpus* refers to the wrist or the carpal bones. A variety of terms are used to refer to the thumb and fingers. Such terms include *thumb, index, middle* or *long, ring,* and *little fingers.* A numbering system is used to refer to the digits (Figure 4-1). The thumb is digit I, the index finger is digit II, the middle (or long) finger is digit III, the ring finger is digit IV, and the little finger is digit V.

The terms *palmar* and **volar** are used interchangeably and refer to the front or anterior aspect of the hand and forearm in relationship to the anatomic position. The term **dorsal** refers to the back or posterior aspect of the hand and forearm in relationship to the anatomic position. The term **radial** indicates the thumb side, and the term **ulnar** refers to the side of the fifth digit (little finger). Therefore, when a therapist receives an order for a dorsal wrist orthosis, the physician has ordered an orthosis that is to be applied on the back of the hand and wrist. Another example of location terminology in an orthotic prescription is a radial gutter thumb immobilization (spica) orthosis. This type of orthosis is applied to the thumb side of the hand and forearm.

Literature addressing hand injuries and rehabilitation protocols often refers to zones of the hand. Figure 4-2 diagrams the **zones of the hand.**[18] Table 4-1 presents the zones' borders. Therapists should be familiar with these zones for understanding literature, conversing with other health providers, and documenting pertinent information.

Shoulder Joint

The shoulder complex comprises seven joints, including the glenohumeral, suprahumeral, acromioclavicular, scapulocostal, sternoclavicular, costosternal, and costovertebral

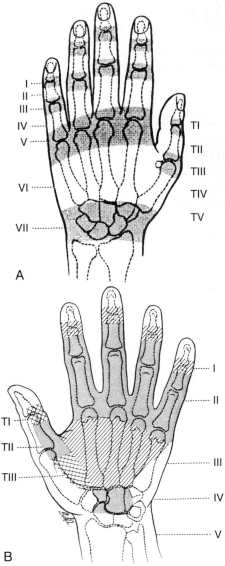

A

B

Figure 4-2 Zones of the hand for **(A)** extensor and **(B)** flexor tendons. (From Kleinert HE, Schepel S, Gill T: Flexor tendon injuries, *Surg Clin North Am* 61(2):267, 1981.)

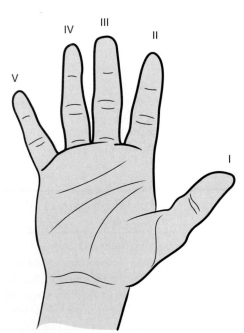

Figure 4-1 Numbering system used for the digits of the hand.

joints.[10] The suprahumeral and scapulocostal joints are pseudojoints, but they contribute to the shoulder's function. Mobility of the shoulder is a compilation of all seven joints. Because the shoulder is extremely mobile, stability is sacrificed. This is evident when one considers that the head of the humerus articulates with approximately a third of the glenoid fossa. The shoulder complex allows motion in three planes, including flexion, extension, abduction, adduction, and internal and external rotation.

The scapula is intimately involved with movement at the shoulder. *Scapulohumeral rhythm* is a term used to describe the coordinated series of synchronous motions, such as shoulder abduction and elevation.

A complex of ligaments and tendons provides stability to the shoulder. Shoulder ligaments are named according to the bones they connect. The ligaments of the shoulder complex include the coracohumeral ligament and the superior, middle, and inferior glenohumeral ligaments.[17] The rotator cuff muscles contribute to the dynamic stability of the shoulder by compressing the humeral head into the glenoid fossa.[28] The rotator cuff muscles include the supraspinatus, infraspinatus, teres minor, and subscapularis. Table 4-2 lists the muscles involved with scapular and shoulder movements.

Elbow Joint

The elbow joint complex consists of the humeroradial, humeroulnar, and proximal radioulnar joints. The humeroradial joint is an articulation between the humerus and the radius. The humeroradial joint has two degrees of freedom

that allow for elbow flexion and extension and forearm supination and pronation. The humerus articulates with the ulna at the humeroulnar joint. Flexion and extension movements take place at the humeroulnar joint. Elbow flexion and extension are limited by the articular surfaces of the trochlea of the ulna and the capitulum of the humerus.

The medial and lateral collateral ligaments strengthen the elbow capsule. The radial collateral, lateral ulnar, accessory lateral collateral, and annular ligaments constitute the ligamentous structure of the elbow.

Muscles acting on the elbow can be categorized as functional groups: flexors, extensors, flexor-pronators, and extensor-supinators. Table 4-3 lists the muscles in these groups and their innervation.

Wrist Joint

The wrist joint is frequently incorporated into an orthotic design. A therapist must be knowledgeable of the wrist joint structure to appropriately choose and fabricate an orthosis that meets therapeutic goals and objectives. The osseous structure of the wrist and hand consists of the ulna, radius, and eight carpal bones. Several joints are associated with the wrist complex, including the radiocarpal, midcarpal, and distal radioulnar joints.

The carpal bones are arranged in two rows (Figure 4-3). The proximal row of carpal bones includes the scaphoid (navicular), lunate, and triquetrum. The pisiform bone is considered a sesamoid bone.[28] The distal row of carpal bones comprises the trapezium, trapezoid, capitate, and

Table 4-1	Tendon Injury Zones of the Hand	
	FLEXOR TENDON ZONE BORDERS	**EXTENSOR TENDON ZONE BORDERS**
Zone I	Extends flexor digitorum profundus (FDP) distal to flexor digitorum superficialis (FDS) on middle phalanx	Over the distal interphalangeal (DIP) joints
Zone II (no man's land)	Extends from proximal end of the digital fibrous sheath to the distal end of the A1 pulley	Over the middle phalanx
Zone III	Extends from proximal end of the finger pulley system to the distal end of the transverse carpal ligament	Over the apex of the proximal interphalangeal (PIP) joint
Zone IV	Entails the carpal tunnel, extending from the distal to the proximal borders of the transverse carpal ligament	Over the proximal phalanx
Zone V	Extends from the proximal border of the transverse carpal ligament to the musculotendinous junctions of the flexor tendons	Over the apex of the metacarpophalangeal (MCP) joint
Zone VI	—	Over the dorsum of the hand
Zone VII	—	Under the extensor tendon retinaculum
Zone VIII	—	The distal forearm
Thumb zone TI	Distal to the interphalangeal (IP) joint	Over the IP joint
Thumb zone TII	Annular ligament to IP joint	Over the proximal phalanx
Thumb zone TIII	The thenar eminence	Over the MCP joint
Thumb zone TIV	—	Over the first metacarpal
Thumb zone TV	—	Under the extensor tendon retinaculum
Thumb zone TVI	—	The distal forearm

Table 4-2   Muscles Contributing to Scapular and Shoulder Motions

MOVEMENT	MUSCLES	INNERVATION
Scapular elevation	Upper trapezius	Accessory, CN 1
	Levator scapulae	third and fourth cervical; dorsal scapular
Scapular depression	Lower trapezius	Accessory CN 1
Scapular lateral rotation	Serratus anterior	Long thoracic
Scapular medial rotation	Rhomboids	Dorsal scapular
Scapular abduction	Serratus anterior	Long thoracic
Scapular adduction	Middle and lower trapezius	Accessory CN 1
	Rhomboids	Dorsal scapular
Shoulder flexion	Anterior deltoid	Axillary
	Coracobrachialis	Musculocutaneous
Shoulder extension	Teres major	Lower subscapular
	Latissimus dorsi	Thoracodorsal
Shoulder abduction	Middle deltoid	Axillary
	Supraspinatus	Suprascapular
Shoulder adduction	Pectoralis major	Medial and lateral
	Latissimus dorsi	Pectoral
	Teres major	Thoracodorsal
	Coracobrachialis	Lower subscapular
		Musculocutaneous
Shoulder external rotation	Infraspinatus	Suprascapular
	Teres minor	Axillary

Table 4-3   Elbow and Forearm Musculature Actions and Nerve Supply

MUSCLE GROUP	INNERVATION
Flexors	
Biceps	Musculocutaneous
Brachialis	Musculocutaneous, radial
Brachioradialis	Radial
Extensors	
Triceps	Radial
Anconeus	Radial
Supinators	
Supinator	Posterior
Interosseous branch of supinator	Radial
Pronators	
Pronator teres	Median
Pronator quadratus	Anterior
Interosseous branch of pronator quadratus	Median

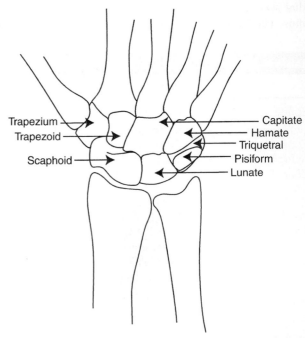

Figure 4-3 Carpal bones. Proximal row: Scaphoid, lunate, pisiform, and triquetrum. Distal row: Trapezium, trapezoid, capitate, and hamate. (From Pedretti LW, editor: *Occupational therapy: practice skills for physical dysfunction*, ed 4, St Louis, 1996, Mosby, p 320.)

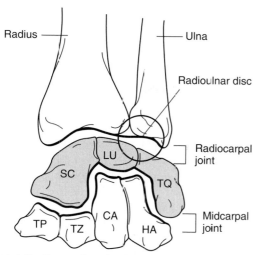

Figure 4-4 Radiocarpal and midcarpal joints. (From Norkin C, Levangie P: *Joint structure and function: a comprehensive analysis,* Philadelphia, 1983, FA Davis, p 217.)

hamate. The distal row of carpal bones articulates with the metacarpals.

The radius articulates with the lunate and scaphoid in the proximal row of carpal bones. This articulation is the radiocarpal joint, which is mobile. The radiocarpal joint (Figure 4-4) is formed by the articulation of the distal head of the radius and the scaphoid and lunate bones. The ulnar styloid is attached to the triquetrum by a complex of ligaments and fibrocartilage. The ligaments bridge the ulna and radius and separate the distal radioulnar joint and the ulna from the radiocarpal joint. Motions of the radiocarpal joint include flexion, extension, and radial and ulnar deviation. The majority of wrist extension occurs at the midcarpal joint with less movement occurring at the radiocarpal joint.[17]

The midcarpal joint (see Figure 4-4) is the articulation between the distal and proximal carpal rows. The joint exists, although there are no interosseous ligaments between the proximal and distal rows of carpals.[8] The joint capsules remain separate. However, the radiocarpal joint capsule attaches to the edge of the articular disk, which is distal to the ulna.[23] The wrist motions of flexion, extension, and radial and ulnar deviation also take place at this joint. The majority of wrist flexion occurs at the radiocarpal joint. The midcarpal joint contributes less movement for wrist flexion.[17]

The distal radioulnar joint is an articulation between the head of the ulna and the distal radius. Forearm supination and pronation occur at the distal radioulnar joint.

Wrist stability is provided by the close-packed positions of the carpal bones and the interosseous ligaments.[28] The intrinsic intercarpal ligaments connect carpal bone to carpal bone. The extrinsic ligaments of the carpal bones connect with the radius, ulna, and metacarpals. The ligaments on the volar aspect of the wrist are thick and strong, providing stability. The dorsal ligaments are thin and less developed.[28] In addition, the intercarpal ligaments of the distal row form a stable fixed transverse arch.[12] Ligaments of the wrist cover

the volar, dorsal, radial, and ulnar areas. The ligaments in the wrist serve to stabilize joints, guide motion, limit motion, and transmit forces to the hand and forearm. These ligaments also assist in prevention of dislocations. The wrist contributes to the hand's mobility and stability. Having two **degrees of freedom** (movements occur in two planes), the wrist is capable of flexing, extending, and deviating radially and ulnarly.

Finger and Thumb Joints

Cutaneous and Connective Coverings of the Hand

The skin is the protective covering of the body. There are unique characteristics of volar and dorsal skin, which are functionally relevant. The skin on the palmar surface of the hand is thick, immobile, and hairless. It contains sensory receptors and sweat glands. The palmar skin attaches to the underlying palmar **aponeurosis**, which facilitates grasp.[7] Palmar skin differs from the skin on the dorsal surface of the hand. The dorsal skin is thin, supple, and quite mobile. Thus, it is often the site for edema accumulation. The skin on the dorsum of the hand accommodates to the extremes of the fingers' flexion and extension movements. The hair follicles on the dorsum of the hand assist in protecting as well as activating touch receptors when the hair is moved slightly.[7]

Palmar Fascia

The superficial layer of palmar fascia in the hand is thin. Its composition is highly fibrous and is tightly bound to the deep fascia. The deep fascia thickens at the wrist and forms the palmar carpal ligament and the flexor retinaculum. The fascia thins over the thenar and hypothenar eminences but thickens over the midpalmar area and on the volar surfaces of the fingers. The fascia forms the palmar aponeurosis and the fibrous digital sheaths.[8]

The superficial palmar aponeurosis consists of longitudinal fibers that are continuous with the flexor retinaculum and palmaris longus tendon. The flexor tendons course under the flexor retinaculum. With absence of the flexor retinaculum, as in carpal tunnel release, bowstringing of the tendons may occur at the wrist level (Figure 4-5). The distal borders of the superficial palmar aponeurosis fuse with the fibrous digital sheaths. The deep layer of the aponeurosis consists of transverse fibers, which are continuous with the thenar and hypothenar fascias. Distally, the deep layer forms the superficial transverse metacarpal ligament.[8] The extensor retinaculum is a fibrous band that bridges over the extensor tendons. The deep and superficial layers of the aponeurosis form this retinaculum.

Functionally, the fascial structure of the hand protects, cushions, restrains, conforms, and maintains the hand's arches.[7] Therapists may fabricate orthoses for persons with Dupuytren disease, in which the palmar fascia thickens and shortens.

Joint Structure

Orthoses often immobilize or mobilize joints of the fingers and thumb. Therefore, therapists must have knowledge of these joints. The hand skeleton comprises five polyarticulated rays (Figure 4-6). The radial ray or first ray (thumb) is the shortest and includes three bones: a metacarpal and two phalanges. Joints of the thumb include the carpometacarpal (CMC) joint, the metacarpophalangeal (MCP) joint, and the interphalangeal (IP) joint (see Figure 4-6). Functionally, the thumb is the most mobile of the digits. The thumb significantly enhances functional ability by its ability to oppose the pads of the fingers, which is needed for prehension and

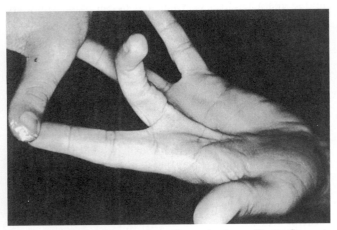

Figure 4-5 Bowstringing of the flexor tendons. (From Stewart-Pettengill KM, van Strien G: Postoperative management of flexor tendon injuries. In Mackin EJ, Callahan AD, Skirven TM, et al., editors: *Rehabilitation of the hand: surgery and therapy,* ed 5, St Louis, 2002, Mosby, p. 434.)

grasp. The thumb has three degrees of freedom, allowing for flexion, extension, abduction, adduction, and opposition. The second through fifth rays comprise four bones: a metacarpal and three phalanges. Joints of the fingers include the MCP joint, proximal interphalangeal (PIP) joint, and the distal interphalangeal (DIP) joint. The digits are unequal in length. However, their respective lengths contribute to the hand's functional capabilities.

The thumb's metacarpotrapezial or CMC joint is saddle shaped and has two degrees of freedom, allowing for flexion, extension, abduction, and adduction movements. The CMC joints of the fingers have one degree of freedom to allow for small amounts of flexion and extension.

The fingers' and thumb's MCP joints have two degrees of freedom: flexion, extension, abduction, and adduction. The convex metacarpal heads articulate with shallow concave bases of the proximal phalanges. Fibrocartilaginous volar plates extend the articular surfaces on the base of the phalanges. As the finger's MCP joint is flexed, the volar plate slides proximally under the metacarpal. This mechanism allows for significant range of motion. The volar plate movement is controlled by accessory collateral ligaments and the metacarpal pulley for the long flexor tendons to blend with these structures.

During extension, the MCP joint is able to move medially and laterally. During MCP extension, collateral ligaments are slack. When digits II through V are extended at the MCP joints, finger abduction movement is free. Conversely, when the MCP joints of digits II through V are flexed abduction is extremely limited. The medial and lateral collateral ligaments of the metacarpal heads become taut and limit the distance by which the heads can be separated for abduction to occur. Mechanically, this provides stability during grasp.

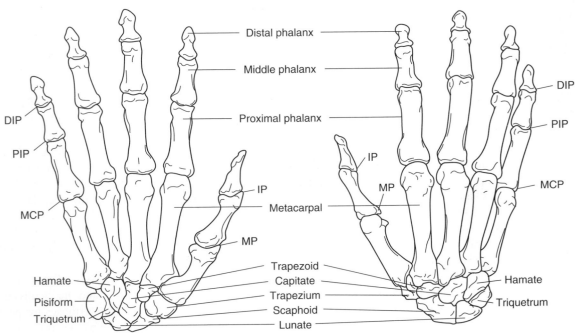

Figure 4-6 Joints of the fingers and thumb.

Digits II through V have two IP joints: a PIP joint and a DIP joint. The thumb has only one IP joint. The IP joints have one degree of freedom, contributing to flexion and extension motions. IP joints have a volar plate mechanism similar to the MCP joints, with the addition of check reign ligaments. The check reign ligaments limit hyperextension.

Table 4-4 provides a review of muscle actions and nerve supply of the wrist and hand.[13] Muscles originating in the forearm are referred to as extrinsic muscles. Intrinsic muscles originate within the hand. Each group contributes to upper extremity function.

Extrinsic Muscles of the Hand

Extrinsic muscles acting on the wrist and hand can be further categorized as extensor and flexor groups. Extrinsic muscles of the wrist and hand are listed in Box 4-1. Extrinsic flexor muscles are most prominent on the medial side of the upper forearm. The function of extrinsic flexor muscles includes flexion of joints between the muscles' respective origin and insertion. Extrinsic muscles of the hand and forearm accomplish flexion and extension of the wrist and the phalanges (fingers). For example, the flexor digitorum superficialis (FDS) flexes the PIP joints of digits II through V, whereas the flexor digitorum profundus (FDP) primarily flexes the DIP joints of digits II through V.

Because these extrinsic muscle tendons pass on the palmar side of the MCP joints, they tend to produce flexion of these joints. During grasp, flexion of the MCPs is necessary to obtain the proper shape of the hand. However, flexion of the wrist is undesirable because it decreases the grip force. The synergic contraction of the wrist extensors during finger flexion prevents wrist flexion during grasp. The force of the extensor contraction is proportionate to the strength of the grip. The stronger the grip, the stronger the wrist extensors contract.[25] Digit extension and flexion are a combined effort from extrinsic and intrinsic muscles.

At the level of the wrist, the extensor tendons organize into six compartments.[16] The first compartment consists of tendons from the abductor pollicis longus (APL) and extensor pollicis brevis (EPB). When the radial side of the wrist is palpated, it is possible to feel the taut tendons of the APL and EPB.

The second compartment contains tendons of the extensor carpi radialis longus (ECRL) and brevis (ECRB). A therapist can palpate the tendons on the dorsoradial aspect of the wrist by applying resistance to an extended wrist.

The third compartment houses the tendon of the extensor pollicis longus (EPL). This tendon passes around the Lister tubercle of the radius and inserts on the dorsal base of the distal phalanx of the thumb.

The fourth compartment includes the four extensor digitorum communis (EDC) tendons and the extensor indicis

Table 4-4 Wrist and Hand Musculature Actions and Nerve Supply

MUSCLE	ACTIONS	NERVE
Flexor carpi radialis	Wrist flexion, wrist radial deviation	Median
Palmaris longus	Wrist flexion, tenses palmar fascia	Median
Flexor carpi ulnaris	Wrist flexion, wrist ulnar deviation	Ulnar
Extensor carpi radialis longus (ECRL)	Wrist radial deviation, wrist extension	Radial
Extensor carpi radialis brevis (ECRB)	Wrist extension, wrist radial deviation	Radial
Extensor carpi ulnaris (ECU)	Wrist extension, wrist ulnar deviation	Radial
Flexor digitorum superficialis (FDS)	Finger proximal interphalangeal (PIP) flexion	Median
Flexor digitorum profundus (FDP)	Finger distal interphalangeal (DIP) flexion	Median, ulnar
Extensor digitorum communis (EDC)	Finger metacarpophalangeal (MCP) extension	Radial
Extensor indicis proprius (EIP)	Index finger MCP extension	Radial
Extensor digiti minimi (EDM)	Little finger MCP extension	Radial
Interosseous	Finger MCP abduction	Ulnar
Dorsal palmar	Finger MCP adduction	Ulnar
Lumbricals	Finger MCP flexion and interphalangeal (IP) extension	Median, ulnar
Abductor digiti minimi	Little finger MCP abduction	Ulnar
Opponens digiti minimi	Little finger opposition	Ulnar
Flexor digiti minimi	Little finger MCP flexion	Ulnar
Flexor pollicus longus	Thumb IP flexion	Median
Flexor pollicus brevis	Thumb MCP flexion	Median, ulnar
Extensor pollicis longus (EPL)	Thumb IP extension	Radial
Extensor pollicis brevis (EPB)	Thumb MCP extension	Radial
Abductor pollicis longus (APL)	Thumb radial abduction	Radial
Abductor pollicis brevis	Thumb palmar abduction	Median
Adductor pollicis	Thumb adduction	Ulnar
Opponens pollicis	Thumb opposition	Median

Box 4-1   Extrinsic Muscles of the Wrist and Hand

- Extensor digitorum
- Extensor pollicis longus (EPL)
- Flexor digitorum profundus (FDP)
- Flexor pollicis longus
- Extensor digiti minimi (EDM)
- Extensor carpi radialis longus (ECRL)
- Extensor carpi ulnaris (ECU)
- Palmaris longus
- Flexor digitorum superficialis (FDS)
- Extensor pollicis brevis (EPB)
- Extensor indicis proprius (EIP)
- Abductor pollicis longus (APL)
- Extensor carpi radialis brevis (ECRB)
- Flexor carpi radialis
- Flexor carpi ulnaris

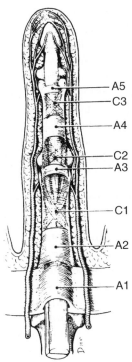

Figure 4-7 Annular (A) and cruciate (C) pulley system of the hand. The digital flexor sheath is formed by five annular (A) pulleys and three cruciate (C) bands. The second and fourth annular pulleys are the most important for function. (From Tubiana R, Thomine JM, Mackin E: *Examination of the hand and wrist,* St Louis, 1996, Mosby, p 81.)

proprius (EIP) tendon, which are the MCP joint extensors of the fingers.

The fifth compartment includes the extensor digiti minimi (EDM), which extends the little finger's MCP joint. The EDM acts alone to extend the little finger.

The sixth compartment consists of the extensor carpi ulnaris (ECU), which inserts at the dorsal base of the fifth metacarpal. A taut tendon can be palpated over the ulnar side of the wrist just distal to the ulnar head.

Unlike the other fingers, the index and little fingers have dual extensor systems comprising the EIP and the EDM in conjunction with the EDC. The EIP and EDM tendons lie on the ulnar side of the EDC tendons. Each finger has a FDS and FDP tendon. Five annular (or A) pulleys and four cruciate (or C) pulleys prevent the flexor tendons from bowstringing (Figure 4-7).

In relationship to orthotic fabrication, when pathology affects extrinsic musculature, the orthotic design often incorporates the wrist and hand. This wrist-hand orthotic design is necessary because the extrinsic muscles cross the wrist and hand joints.

Intrinsic Muscles of the Hand and Wrist

The intrinsic muscles of the thumb and fingers are listed in Box 4-2. The intrinsic muscles are the muscles of the thenar and hypothenar eminences, the lumbricals, and the interossei. Intrinsic muscles can be grouped according to those of the thenar eminence, the hypothenar eminence, and the central muscles between the thenar and hypothenar eminences. The function of these intrinsic hand muscles produces flexion of the proximal phalanx and extension of the middle and distal phalanges, which contribute to the precise finger movements required for coordination.

The thenar eminence comprises the opponens pollicis, flexor pollicis brevis, adductor pollicis, and abductor pollicis brevis. The thenar eminence contributes to thumb opposition, which functionally allows for grasp and prehensile

Box 4-2   Intrinsic Muscles of the Hand

Central Compartment Muscles	Thenar Compartment Muscles	Hypothenar Compartment Muscles
Lumbricals	Opponens pollicis	Opponens digiti minimi
Palmar interossei	Abductor pollicis brevis	Abductor digiti minimi
Dorsal interossei	Adductor pollicis	Flexor digiti minimi brevis
	Flexor pollicis brevis	Palmaris brevis

patterns. The thumb seldom acts alone except when pressing objects and playing instruments.[25] However, without a thumb the hand is virtually nonfunctional.

The hypothenar eminence includes the abductor digiti minimi, the flexor digiti minimi, the palmaris brevis, and the opponens digiti minimi. Similar to the thenar muscles, the hypothenar muscles also assist in rotating the fifth digit during grasp.[3]

The muscles of the central compartment include lumbricals and palmar and dorsal interossei. The interossei muscles are complex with variations in their origins and insertions.[3] There are four dorsal interossei and three palmar interossei muscles. The four lumbricals are weaker than the interossei.

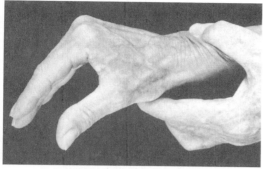

Figure 4-8 Intrinsic plus position of the hand. Metacarpophalangeal (MCP) flexion with proximal interphalangeal (PIP) extension. (From Tubiana R, Thomine JM, Mackin E: *Examination of the peripheral nerve function in the upper extremity,* St Louis, 1996, Mosby, p 308.)

The lumbricals originate on the radial aspect of the FDP tendons and insert on the extensor expansion of the finger. They are the only muscles in the human body with a moving origin and insertion. The primary function of the lumbricals is to flex the MCP joints.[28]

Normally, the interossei extend the PIP and DIP joints when the MCP joint is in extension. The dorsal interossei produce finger abduction, and the palmar interossei produce finger adduction. Functionally, the first dorsal interossei is a strong abductor of the index finger, which assists in properly positioning the hand for pinching. Research shows the interossei are active during grasp and power grip in addition to pinch.[19] With function of the interossei and lumbricals, a person is able to place the hand in an intrinsic plus position. An intrinsic plus position is established when the MCP joints are flexed and the PIP joints are fully extended (Figure 4-8). Some injuries may result in an intrinsic minus hand caused by paralysis or contractures (Figure 4-9). With an intrinsic minus hand, the person loses the cupping shape of the hand.[3] In addition, the intrinsic musculature may waste or atrophy. In relationship to orthotic provision, if intrinsic muscles are solely affected, the orthotic design often involves only immobilizing or mobilizing the finger joints as opposed to incorporating the wrist. To facilitate function and prevent deformity, joint positioning in orthoses frequently warrants an intrinsic plus posture rather than an intrinsic minus position.

Arches of the Hand

To have a strong functional grasp, the hand uses the following three arches: (1) the longitudinal arch, (2) the distal transverse arch, and (3) the proximal transverse arch (Figure 4-10). Because of their functional significance, these arches require care during the orthotic fabrication process for their preservation. Therapists should never position the hand in a flat posture in an orthosis because doing so compromises function and creates deformity. Especially in cases of muscle atrophy (as with a tendon or nerve injury), the orthosis should maintain the integrity and mobility of the arches.

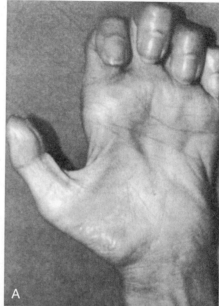

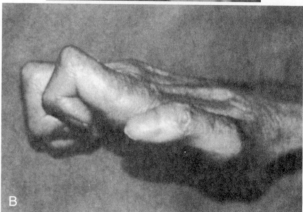

Figure 4-9 A, Intrinsic minus position of the hand. **B,** Notice loss of normal arches of the hand and wasting of all intrinsic musculature resulting from a long-standing low median and ulnar nerve palsy. (From Aulicino PL: Clinical examination of the hand. In Mackin EJ, Callahan AD, Skirven TM, et al., editors: *Rehabilitation of the hand: surgery and therapy,* ed 5, St Louis, 2002, Mosby, p 130.)

The proximal transverse arch is fixed and consists of the distal row of carpal bones. The proximal transverse arch is a rigid arch acting as a stable pivot point for the wrist and long-finger flexor muscles.[12] The transverse carpal ligament and the bones of the proximal transverse arch form the carpal tunnel. The finger flexor tendons pass beneath the transverse carpal ligament. The transverse carpal ligament provides mechanical advantage to the finger flexor tendons by serving as a pulley.[2]

The distal transverse arch, which deepens with flexion of the fingers, is mobile and passes through the metacarpal heads.[2] An orthosis must allow for the functional movement of the distal arch to maintain or increase normal hand function.[12]

The longitudinal arch allows the DIP, PIP, and MCP joints to flex.[16] This arch follows the longitudinal axes of each

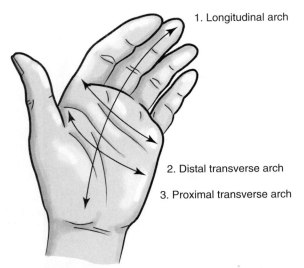

Figure 4-10 Arches of the hand. *1,* Longitudinal arch; *2,* distal transverse arch; *3,* proximal transverse arch.

finger. Because of the mobility of their base, the first, fourth, and fifth metacarpals move in relationship to the shape and size of an object placed in the palm. **Grasp** is the result of holding an object against the rigid portion of the hand provided by the second and third digits. The flattening and cupping motions of the palm allow the hand to pick up and handle objects of various sizes.

Anatomic Landmarks of the Hand

Creases of the Hand

The creases of the hand are critical landmarks for orthotic pattern making and molding. Therefore, knowledge of the creases and their functional implications is important. Three flexion creases are located on the palmar surface of digits II through V, and additional creases are located on the palmar surface of the hand and wrist (Figure 4-11).

The three primary palmar creases are the distal, proximal, and thenar creases. As shown in Figure 4-11, the distal palmar crease extends transversely from the fifth MCP joint to a point midway between the third and second MCP joints.[9] This crease is the landmark for the distal edge of the palmar portion of an orthosis intended to immobilize the wrist while allowing motion of the MCPs. By positioning the orthosis proximal to the distal palmar crease, the therapist makes full MCP joint flexion possible. Proximal to the distal palmar crease is the proximal palmar crease, which is used as a guide during orthotic fabrication. An orthosis must be proximal to the proximal palmar crease at the index finger or the MCP joint will not be free to move into flexion.

The thenar crease begins at the proximal palmar crease near the radial side of the second digit and curves around the base of the thenar eminence (see Figure 4-11).[9] To allow for thumb motion, this crease should define the limit of the orthosis' edge. If the orthosis extends beyond the thenar

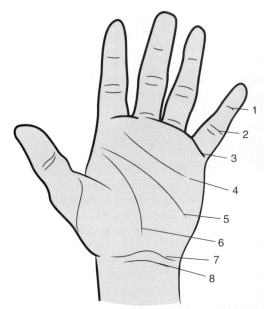

Figure 4-11 Creases of the hand *1,* Distal digital (distal interphalangeal [DIP]) crease; *2,* middle digital (proximal interphalangeal [PIP]) crease; *3,* proximal digital (metacarpophalangeal [MCP]) crease; *4,* distal palmar crease; *5,* proximal palmar crease; *6,* thenar crease; *7,* distal wrist crease; *8,* proximal wrist crease.

crease toward the thumb, thumb opposition and palmar abduction of the CMC joint are inhibited.

The two palmar (or volar) wrist creases are the distal and proximal wrist creases. The distal wrist crease extends from the pisiform bone to the tubercle of the trapezium (see Figure 4-11) and forms a line that separates the proximal and distal rows of the carpal bones. The proximal wrist crease corresponds to the radiocarpal joint and delineates the proximal border of the carpal bones, which articulates with the distal radius.[9] The distal and proximal wrist creases assist in locating the axis of the wrist motion.[13] Wrist creases serve as a guide when fabricating hand based orthoses that allow for wrist motion. Such wrist creases should not be covered by the orthosis in order to allow for full wrist flexion and extension.

The three digital palmar flexion creases are on the palmar aspect of digits II through V (see Figure 4-11). The distal digital crease (or DIP crease) marks the DIP joint axis, and the middle digital crease (or PIP crease) marks the PIP joint axis. The proximal digital crease (or MCP crease) is distal to the MCP joint axis at the base of the proximal phalanx. The creation of the proximal and distal palmar creases results from the thick palmar skin folding due to the force allowing full MCP flexion.[2] The flexion axis of the IP joint of the thumb corresponds to the IP crease of the thumb. Similarly, the MCP crease describes the axis of thumb MCP joint flexion.

The creases are close to but not always directly over bony joints.[12] When providing an orthosis to immobilize a particular joint, the therapist must be sure to include the corresponding joint flexion crease within the orthosis so as to provide adequate support for immobilization. Conversely, when attempting to mobilize a specific joint, the therapist must not incorporate the corresponding flexion crease in the orthosis to allow for full range of motion.[16] When one is working with persons who have moderate to severe edema, the creases may dissipate. Creases may also dissipate with disuse associated with paralysis or disuse resulting from pain, stiffness, or psychological problems.

Grasp and Prehensile Patterns

The normal hand can perform many prehensile patterns in which the thumb is a crucial factor. Therapists must be knowledgeable about prehensile and grasp patterns, especially when providing orthoses to assist the performance of these patterns.

Even though hand movements are extremely complex, they can be categorized into several basic prehensile and grasp patterns, including fingertip prehension, palmar prehension, lateral prehension, cylindrical grasp, spherical grasp, hook grasp,[25] and intrinsic plus grasp.[5] Figure 4-12 depicts these types of prehensile and grip patterns. Therapists should keep in mind that finer prehensile movements require less strength than grasp movements. Pedretti[22] remarked, "The grasp and prehension patterns that may be provided by hand orthoses are determined by the muscles that are functioning, potential and present deformities, and how the hand is to be used."

Fingertip **prehension** is the contact of the pad of the index or middle finger with the pad of the thumb.[25] This movement, which clients use to pick up small objects such as beads and pins, is the weakest of the pinch patterns and

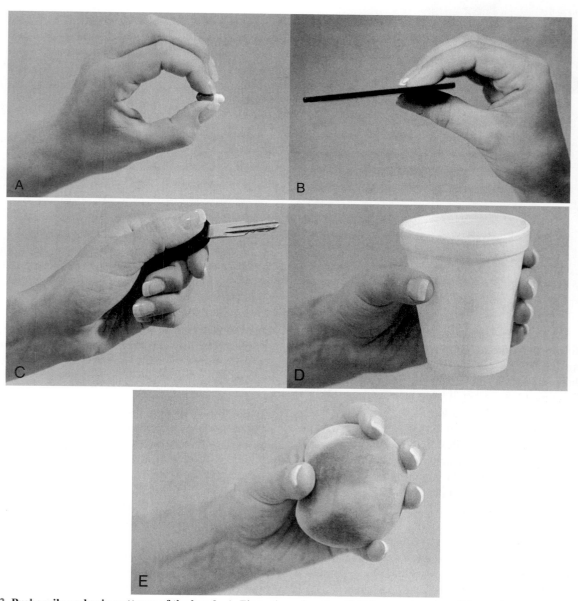

Figure 4-12 Prehensile and grip patterns of the hand. A, Fingertip prehension. **B,** Palmar prehension. **C,** Lateral prehension. **D,** Cylindrical grasp. **E,** Spherical grasp.

Continued

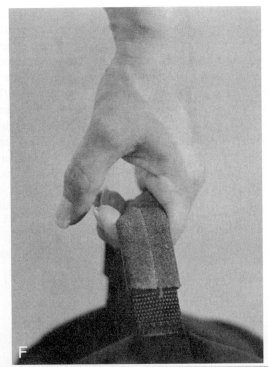

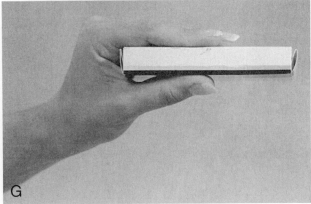

Figure 4-12, cont'd F, Hook grasp. **G,** Intrinsic plus grasp.

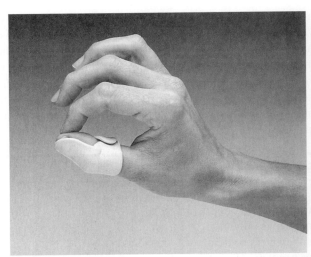

Figure 4-13 Static orthosis to block the thumb interphalangeal (IP) joint in slight flexion to facilitate tip pinch. (From Pedretti LW, editor: *Occupational therapy: practice skills for physical dysfunction,* ed 4, St Louis, 1996 Mosby, p 327.)

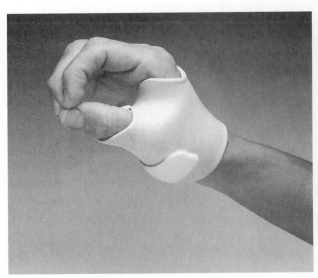

Figure 4-14 Thumb spica orthosis to facilitate palmar prehension by positioning the thumb in opposition to the index and long fingers. (From Pedretti LW, editor: *Occupational therapy: practice skills for physical dysfunction,* ed 4, St Louis, 1996, Mosby, p 327.)

requires fine motor coordination. An orthosis to facilitate the fingertip prehension for a person with arthritis may include a static orthosis to block (stabilize) the thumb IP joint in slight flexion (Figure 4-13).[5]

Palmar prehension, also known as the *tripod* or *three jaw chuck pinch,*[5,13] is the contact of the thumb pad with the pads of the middle and index fingers. People use palmar prehension for holding pencils and picking up small spherical objects. Orthoses to facilitate palmar prehension include thumb spica orthoses that position the thumb in palmar abduction, which may be hand or forearm based (Figure 4-14).

Lateral prehension, the strongest of the pinch patterns, is the contact between the thumb pad and the lateral aspect of the index finger.[25] Clients typically use this pattern for holding keys. Orthoses that position the hand for lateral prehension include thumb spica orthoses that place the thumb in slight radial abduction (Figure 4-15).

Cylindrical grasp is used for holding cylindrical-shaped objects, such as soda cans, pan handles, and cylindrical tools.[25] The object rests against the palm of the hand, and the adducted fingers flex around the object to maintain a grasp. Orthotic provision to encourage such motions as thumb opposition or finger and thumb joint flexion may contribute to a person's ability to regain cylindrical grasp (Figure 4-16).

The spherical grasp is used to hold round objects, such as tennis balls and baseballs.[25] The object rests against the palm of the hand, and the abducted five digits flex around the object. Orthoses that enhance spherical grasp may include orthoses addressing such motions as finger and thumb abduction (Figure 4-17).

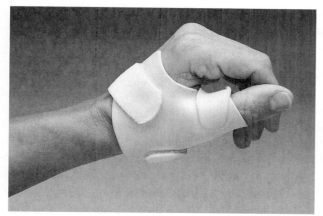

Figure 4-15 Thumb spica orthosis to facilitate lateral prehension by positioning the thumb in lateral opposition to the index finger. (From Pedretti LW, editor: *Occupational therapy: practice skills for physical dysfunction,* ed 4, St Louis, 1996, Mosby, p 327.)

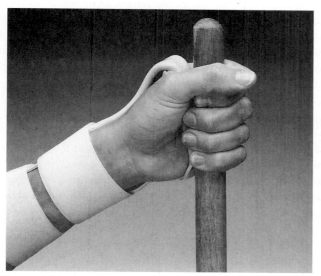

Figure 4-16 This dorsal wrist orthosis stabilizes the wrist to increase grip force and minimizes coverage of the palm. (From Pedretti LW, editor: *Occupational therapy: practice skills for physical dysfunction,* ed 4, St Louis, 1996, Mosby, p 328.)

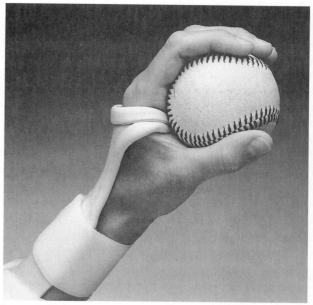

Figure 4-17 This dorsal wrist orthosis stabilizes the wrist and allows metacarpophalangeal (MCP) mobility required for a spherical grasp. (From Pedretti LW, editor: *Occupational therapy: practice skills for physical dysfunction,* ed 4, St Louis, 1996, Mosby, p 328.)

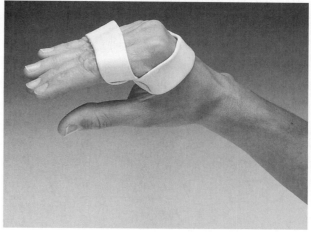

Figure 4-18 Figure-eight orthosis to facilitate an intrinsic plus grasp. (From Pedretti LW, editor: *Occupational therapy: practice skills for physical dysfunction,* ed 4, St Louis, 1996, Mosby, p 328.)

The hook grasp, which is accomplished with the fingers only, involves the carrying of such items as briefcases and suitcases by the handles.[25] The PIPs and DIPs flex around the object, and the thumb often remains passive in this type of grasp. With ulnar and median nerve damage, this position may be avoided rather than encouraged. However, for PIP and DIP joints lacking flexion a therapist may fabricate dynamic flexion orthoses to gain range of motion in these joints.

The intrinsic plus grip is characterized by MCP flexion and PIP and DIP extension. The thumb is positioned in palmar abduction for opposition with the third and fourth fingers.[5] This grasp is helpful in holding flat objects, such as books, trays, or sandwiches. The intrinsic plus grip is not present with ulnar and median nerve injuries. A therapist may facilitate the grasp by using a figure-eight orthosis, shown in Figure 4-18.

Biomechanical Principles for Orthotic Intervention

Orthotic fabrication involves application of external forces on the hand, and thus understanding basic biomechanical principles is important for the therapist when constructing and fitting orthoses. Correct biomechanics of orthotic design results in an optimal fit and reduces risks of skin irritation and pressure areas, which ultimately may lead to client comfort, compliance, and function. In addition, knowledgeable manipulation of biomechanics increases the orthoses' efficiency and improves orthoses' durability while decreasing cost and frustration.[15]

Three-Point Pressure

Most orthoses use a three-point pressure system to affect a joint motion. A **three-point pressure** system consists of three individual linear forces in which the middle force is directed in an opposite direction from the other two forces, as depicted in Figure 4-19. Three-point pressure systems in orthoses are used for different purposes.[2,15] For example, an orthosis affecting extension or flexion of a joint exerts forces in one plane or unidirectionally, as shown in Figure 4-20. Three-point systems can be applied to multiple directions. In other words, an orthosis may immobilize one joint while mobilizing an adjacent joint. An example of a multidirectional three-point pressure system is a circumferential wrist orthosis, shown in Figure 4-21.

Mechanical Advantage

Orthoses incorporate lever systems, which incorporate forces, resistance, axes of motion, and moment arms. Orthoses that serve as levers use a proximal input force (F_i), two moment arms, and an axis or fulcrum to move a distal output force.[15] Similar to a teeter-totter, the force side of an orthosis' lever equals the resistance side of the lever. The sum of the proximal (F_i) and the distal (F_o) forces equals the magnitude (F_m) of the middle opposing force. The system's balance is defined as:

$$F_i \times d_i = F_o \times d_o$$

In this equation, F_i is the input force and d_i is the input distance (or the proximal force moment arm). F_o is the resistance (or output) force, and d_o is the output distance (or the resistance moment arm). **Mechanical advantage** is defined as:

$$\frac{d_i}{d_o}$$

Mechanical advantage principles can be applied and adjusted when the therapist is designing an orthosis. For example, when designing a volar-based wrist immobilization orthosis, increasing the length of the forearm trough decreases force on the proximal anterior forearm (Figure 4-22). Mechanical advantage results in a more comfortable orthosis for the client. Application of this concept involves consideration of the anatomic segment length in designing the orthosis. The length of an orthosis' forearm trough should be approximately two-thirds the length of the forearm. Persons wearing volar-based orthoses should be able to flex their elbows fully without interference.[4] The width of a thumb or forearm trough should be half the circumference of the thumb or forearm. The muscle bulk of an extremity gradually increases more proximal to the body, and the orthosis' trough should widen proportionately in the proximal area. When making an orthotic pattern, the therapist attempts to maintain one-half the circumference of the thumb or forearm for a correct fit.

Torque

Torque is a biomechanical principle defined as the "extent to which a force tends to cause rotation of an object (body part) about an axis."[21] Other terms used synonymously include *moment arm* or *moment of force*. Torque is the product of the applied force (F) multiplied by the perpendicular distance

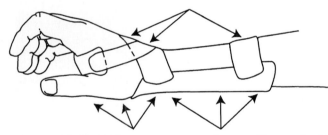

Figure 4-19 Three-point pressure system is created by a orthosis' surface and properly placed straps to secure the orthosis and ensure proper force for immobilization. (From Pedretti LW, editor: *Occupational therapy: practice skills for physical dysfunction,* ed 4, St Louis, 1996, Mosby, p 336.)

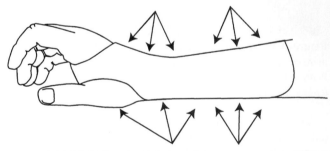

Figure 4-21 Multidirectional three-point pressure systems. (From Pedretti LW, editor: *Occupational therapy: practice skills for physical dysfunction,* ed 4, St Louis, 1996, Mosby, p 336.)

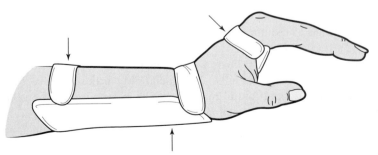

Figure 4-20 Unidirectional three-point pressure system. (From Fess EE, Philips CA: *Hand splinting: principles and methods,* ed 2, St Louis, 1987, Mosby, p 4.)

from the axis of rotation to the line of application of force (d). The equation for torque is:

$$Torque = F \times d$$

It is important to consider torque for dynamic or mobilization orthoses (see Chapter 12).

Pressure and Stress

There are four ways in which skin and soft tissue can be damaged by force or **pressure**:

- Degree
- Duration
- Repetition
- Direction

Degree and Duration of Stress

Generally, low **stress** can be tolerated for longer periods of time, whereas high stress over long periods of time causes damage.[6] It must be noted that *low stress* and *high stress* are generic and imprecise terms. Generally the tissue that least tolerates pressure is the skin. Skin becomes ischemic as load increases. Low stress can be damaging if it is continuous and can eventually cause capillary damage and lead to ischemia. The effects of continuous low force from constricting circumferential bandages and orthoses and their straps can be damaging at times. However, if a system can be devised to distribute pressure over a larger area of skin, a higher load can be exerted on a ligament, adhesion, tendon, or muscle. Such an orthotic design may include a longer trough or a circumferential component.

Repetitive Stress

If a stress is repetitively applied in moderate amounts, it can lead to inflammation and skin breakdown.[6] An example of a repetitive stress may be seen in a person wearing a dynamic flexion orthosis that has rubber band traction. If the person continually flexes the finger against the tension, the tissue may become inflamed after some time. If inflammation or redness occurs, the tension is adjusted by relaxing the traction. Persons with traumatic hand injuries or pathology may not be able to tolerate the repetitive

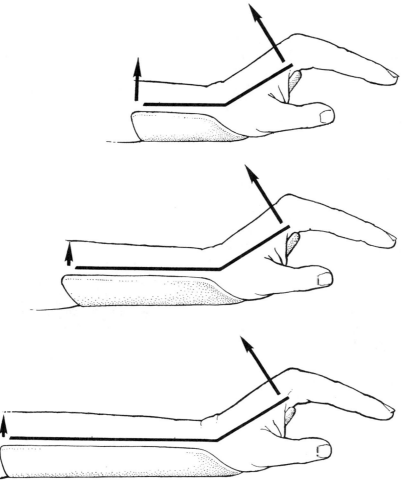

Figure 4-22 A longer forearm trough decreases the resultant pressure caused by the proximally transferred weight of the hand to the anterior forearm. (From Fess EE, Gettle KS, Philips CA, et al: Mechanical principles. In Fess EE, Philips CA, editors: *Hand splinting: principles and methods,* ed 3, St Louis: Mosby, p 167.)

CHAPTER 5

Clinical Examination and Implications for Orthotic Intervention

Brenda M. Coppard, PhD, OTR/L, FAOTA

Key Terms

Assessment of Motor and Process Skills (AMPS)
Canadian Occupational Performance Measure (COPM)
Protocols
Reliability
Responsiveness
Validity
verbal analog scale (VeAS)
visual analog scale (ViAS)

Chapter Objectives

1. List components of a thorough clinical examination as related to orthotic intervention.
2. Describe components of a history, an observation, and palpation.
3. Describe the resting hand posture.
4. Relate how skin, vein, bone, joint, muscle, tendon, and nerve assessments are relevant to orthotic intervention.
5. Identify specific assessments that can be used in a clinical examination prior to orthotic intervention.
6. Explain the three phases of wound healing.
7. Recognize the signs of abnormal illness behavior.
8. Explain how a therapist assesses a person's knowledge of orthotic precautions and wear and care instructions.

Katrina is a therapist who recently switched practice from pediatrics to an outpatient rehabilitation clinic. During her first week, she receives a referral for Agatha, an 82-year-old female with a flare up of rheumatoid arthritis. Prior to scheduling an appointment with Agatha, Katrina conceptualizes her screening and assessment plan.

Clinical Examination

A thoughtfully selected battery of clinical assessments is crucial to therapists' and physicians' intervention plans. A thorough, organized, and clearly-documented examination is the basis for the development of an intervention plan. In today's health care system, therapists complete examinations that are time and cost efficient. This chapter addresses components of the assessment process in relationship to orthotic provision.

Time-efficient, informal assessments may indicate the level of hand and upper extremity function initially. The results may prompt a therapist to select more sophisticated testing procedures, as indicated by the person's condition.[24] Generally, initial and discharge evaluations are most comprehensive in scope, whereas regular reassessments are usually more focused.

Reassessments typically occur at consistent intervals of time. For example, if Joe is evaluated at his Monday appointment, the therapist may reevaluate Joe every Monday or every other Monday thereafter. On some occasions, a case manager may request the therapist to reevaluate a client. However, the time span between assessments is based on the person's condition and progress. For example, a person with a peripheral nerve injury may be reevaluated once every 3 weeks because of the slow nature of nerve healing. Another person being rehabilitated after a burn injury may be reevaluated every week because his condition changes more quickly, thereby affecting his functional ability.

The assessment process for the upper extremity incorporates data from an interview, observation, palpation, and a selection of tests that are objective, valid, and reliable. Form 5-1 is a check-off sheet therapists can use when evaluating a person with upper extremity dysfunction. Ancillary tools (such as radiographs, computerized tomography [CT] scans, magnetic resonance imaging [MRI] scans, electrodiagnostics, and laboratory tests) assist in confirming the diagnosis and provide the therapist with a broader context of the person's condition(s).[48]

History

Beginning with a medical history, the therapist gathers data from various sources. Depending on the setting, the therapist may have access to the person's medical chart, surgical or radiologic reports, and the physician's referral or prescription. The person's age, gender, and diagnosis are typically easy to obtain from these sources. Client age is important because some congenital anomalies and diagnoses are unique to certain age groups. Age may also affect prognosis or length of recovery. Some problems are unique to gender.

From available sources, the therapist seeks out the person's past medical history, the dates of occurrences, current medical status and treatment. The history includes invasive and noninvasive treatments. Conditions such as diabetes, epilepsy, kidney or liver dysfunction, arthritis, and gout should be reported, because they can directly or indirectly influence rehabilitation (including orthotic intervention). The therapist determines whether the current upper extremity problem is the result of neurologic or orthopedic dysfunction, or a combination of both. For example, Ken fell and sustained a traumatic brain injury and experienced upper extremity fractures. Some conditions are solely orthopedic in nature resulting from trauma affecting soft tissue (i.e., tendon laceration, burn). The nature of dysfunction helps the therapist determine the orthotic approach.

With postoperative persons, therapists must know the anatomic structures involved and the surgical procedures performed. Be aware that some physicians may prefer to follow conventional rehabilitative programs for certain diagnostic populations. Other physicians may prefer to follow rehabilitative programs that they developed for specific postoperative diagnostic populations. Whether standardized or nonstandardized, these programs are known as **protocols.** Protocols delineate which types of orthoses, exercises, and therapeutic interventions are appropriate in rehabilitation programs. Protocols indicate the timing of interventions.

Interview

The therapist collects the person's history at the time of the initial evaluation. The goal of the interview is for the therapist to determine the impact of the condition on the person's functioning, family, economic status, and social/emotional well-being. Most important, therapists ask what a person's goals are.[48] At the beginning of the interview, complete introductions and explain what occupational therapy is and what the purpose of evaluation and intervention are. In addition, the therapist creates a teaching/learning environment directed at the client's learning style. For example, a therapist tells a person that she should feel comfortable about asking any questions concerning therapy, evaluation, or intervention.

Therapists may obtain co-histories from family, parents, friends, and caretakers of children and persons who are unable to communicate or who have cognitive impairments and are unreliable or questionable self-reporters. The therapist obtains the following information by asking the person a variety of questions:

- Age
- Date of injury
- Hand dominance
- Avocation interests
- Subjective complaints
- Support systems
- Vocation
- Method of injury
- Functional abilities
- Family composition
- Social history
- Interventions to date

Therapists ask about general health and about prior orthopedic, neurologic, psychologic, or cardiopulmonary conditions.[19] Habits and conditions such as smoking,[40,49] stress,[17] obesity,[68] and depression[58] may influence rehabilitation.[45] The therapist asks the client about any previous upper extremity conditions and dates of onset in order to assess the current condition. The therapist inquires about prior interventions and their results. The therapist determines clients' insight into their condition by asking them to describe what they understand about their condition or diagnosis.

After background information is gleaned, the client should be asked open-ended questions about the present signs and symptoms. Probing questions about the current condition suggests to the therapist the client's level of irritability.[48] If a client reports minimal pain at rest, transient pain upon movement and symptoms that are not easily provoked, the person is said to have low irritability. If pain is present upon resting, pain increases with movement, and decreased mobility is noted, the person has a highly irritable condition. Determining the irritability level determines how aggressively the surgeon and therapist may perform evaluations and interventions.

Observation

Observations are noted immediately when the person walks into a clinic or during the first meeting between the therapist and client. For example, the therapist observes how the person carries the upper extremity, looking for reduced reciprocal arm swing, guarding postures, and involuntary movements, such as tremors or tics.[52] Facial tics may be a sign of a neurologic or psychological problem. Further information is gleaned from observing facial movements, speech patterns, and affect. For example, if there is a facial droop, the therapist may suspect that the client has Bell palsy or has had a stroke. The therapist always observes the person's ability to answer questions and follow instructions.

A general inspection of the person's upper quarter (including the neck, shoulder, elbow, forearm, wrist, and hand) and joint attitude is noted. The therapist notes the posture of the affected extremity and looks for any postural asymmetry and guarded or protective positioning. A normal hand at rest assumes a posture of 10 to 20 degrees of wrist extension, 10 degrees of ulnar deviation, slight flexion and abduction of the thumb, and approximately 15 to 20 degrees of flexion of the metacarpophalangeal (MCP) joints. The fingers in a resting posture exhibit a greater composite flexion to the radial side of the hand (scaphoid bone) (Figure 5-1).[2] The thumbnail usually lies perpendicular to the index finger. Observations of hand postures influences planning for orthotic provision because a person's hand often deviates from the normal resting posture in the presence of injury or disease.

A variety of presentations observed by the therapist contributes to the overall clinical picture of the person. The following are noteworthy observational points[19,48]:

- Position of hand in relationship to the body: protective or guarding posture
- Diminished or absent reciprocal arm swing
- Quality of movement
- Hand arches and creases
- Muscle atrophy
- Contractures
- Nails: ridged or smooth
- Edema, hematoma (blood clot), ecchymosis (bruise)
- Finger pads: thin or smooth (loss of rugal folds, fingerprint lines)

- Lesions: scars, abrasions, burns, wounds
- Abnormal web spaces
- Heberden or Bouchard nodes
- Neurologic deficit postures: claw hand, wrist drop, simian hand
- Color: pale, red, blue
- Grafts or sutures
- External devices: percutaneous pins, external fixator, orthoses, slings, braces
- Deformities: boutonniere, mallet finger, intrinsic minus hand, swan neck
- Pilomotor signs: appearance of "goose pimples" or hair standing on end
- Joint deviation or abnormal rotation

Palpation

After a general inspection of the client, the therapist palpates the affected areas when appropriate. A therapist palpates any area in which the person describes symptoms, including any area that is swollen or abnormal.[52] Muscle bulk is palpated on each extremity to compare proximal and distal muscles, and to compare right and left. Muscle tone is best assessed through passive range of motion (PROM). When assessing tone, the therapist coaches the client to relax the muscles so that the most accurate results are obtained. The client's skin is examined. In the presence of ulcers, gangrene, inflammation, or neural or vascular impairment, skin temperature may change and can be felt during palpation.[45] In the presence of

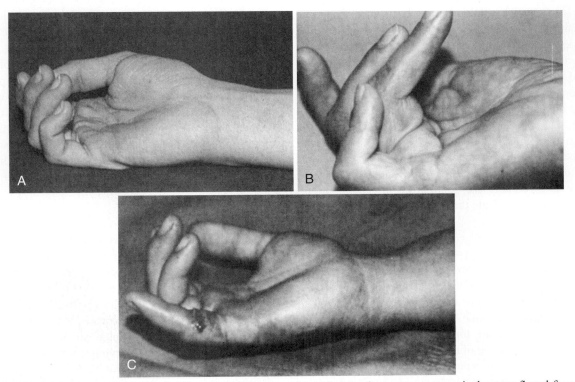

Figure 5-1 Resting posture of the hand. A, Normal resting posture. Note that the fingers are progressively more flexed from the radial aspect to the ulnar aspect of the hand. **B,** This normal hand posture is lost because of contractures of the digits as a result of Dupuytren disease. **C,** Loss of the normal hand posture is due to a laceration of the flexor tendons of the fifth digit. (From Hunter JM, Mackin EJ, Callahan AD, editors: *Rehabilitation of the hand: surgery and therapy,* ed 4, St Louis, 1996, Mosby, p 55.)

infection, draining wounds, or sutured sites, therapists wear sterile gloves and follow universal precautions.

Assessments

Assessment selection is a critical step in formulating appropriate interventions. There are more than 100 assessments in the musculoskeletal literature.[57] Several factors are considered when selecting an assessment, including content, methodology, and clinical utility.[57] In order to critically choose assessment tools used for practice, one must understand the tool's psychometric development.

Content of an assessment is what the tool attempts to measure. Content is separated into three categories: type, scale, and interpretation. The type of content can be focused on data gathered by the clinician or data reported by the client. The scale of the content refers to the measurements or questions that constitute the tool and how they are measured. Content interpretation addresses how scores or measures pertain to "excellent" or "poor" outcomes.[57]

Methodology of the tool relates to validity, reliability, and responsiveness. **Validity** is the extent to which the assessment measures what it intends to measure. Table 5-1 lists and defines the various types of validity. **Reliability** is the consistency of the assessment. Table 5-2 lists and defines the types of reliability. **Responsiveness** refers to the assessment's sensitivity to measure differences in status.[57]

Clinical utility refers to the degree the tool is easy to administer and the degree of ease the client experiences in completing the assessment. Utility is a subjective component addressing the degree to which the tool is acceptable to the client and the degree to which the tool is feasible to the therapist. Factors that impact clinical utility include training for competent administration, cost and administration, documentation and interpretation time.[57]

Assessment tools are categorized in several ways. There are standardized and nonstandardized assessment tools. Some assessments are norm based, whereas others are criterion based. Bear-Lehman and Abreu[3] suggest that evaluation is a quantitative and qualitative process. Thus, therapists who select assessments that produce precise, objective, and quantitative measurement decrease subjective judgments and increase their ability to obtain reproducible findings. However, therapists are cautioned to reject the tendency to neglect important information about their clients that may not be quantifiable.[3] Qualitative information—such as attitude, pain response, coping mechanisms, and locus of control (center of responsibility for one's behavior)—influence the evaluation process. "The selection of the hand assessment tools to be used, the art of human interaction between the therapist and the client, the art of evaluating the client's hand as a part, but also as an integrated whole, are part of the subjective processes involved in hand assessment."[3] Even objective evaluation tools require the comprehension and motivation of the client.

Unfortunately, there is no universally accepted upper extremity assessment tool. Depending on the setting, a battery of assessments may be developed by facility or department practitioners. In other settings, therapists use their clinical reasoning to determine what battery of assessments will be used with each person. A theoretical perspective and a diagnostic population can influence the evaluation selection.[3] For example, one facility's assessment reflects a biomechanical perspective, whereas another facility's assessment reflects a neurodevelopmental perspective.

The sections that follow explore common assessments performed as part of an upper extremity battery of evaluations. There is a gamut of assessments for particular conditions not presented in this text.[35]

Pain

Several options for evaluating pain exist, including interview questions, rating scales, body diagrams, and questionnaires.

Table 5-1	Definitions of Types of Validity
TYPE OF VALIDITY	**DEFINITION**
Construct validity	The degree to which a theoretical construct is measured by the tool
Content validity	The degree to which the items in a tool reflect the content domain being measured
Face validity	Determination if a tool appears to be measuring what it is intended to measure
Criterion validity	The degree to which a tool correlates with a "gold standard" or criterion test (It can be assessed as concurrent or predictive validity.)
Concurrent validity	The degree to which the scores from a tool correlate with a criterion test when both tools are administered relatively at the same time

Table 5-2	Definitions of Types of Reliability
TYPE OF RELIABILITY	**DEFINITION**
Inter-rater reliability	The degree to which two raters can obtain the same ratings for a given variable
Test/retest reliability	The degree to which a test is stable based on repeated administrations of the test to the same individuals over a specified time interval
Internal consistency	The degree to which each item of a test measures the same trait
Intra-rater reliability	The degree to which one rater can reproduce the same score in administering the tool on multiple occasions to the same individual

Box 5-1 lists questions related to pain that can be asked of the client.[22] Therapists often use a combination of pain measures to obtain an accurate representation of the client's pain.[31]

The **verbal analog scale (VeAS)** is used to determine the person's perception of pain intensity. The client rates pain on a scale from 0 to 10 (0 refers to no pain, and 10 refers to the worst pain ever experienced). Reliability scores for retesting under the VeAS are moderate to high, ranging from 0.67 to 0.96.[26,29] When correlated with the **visual analog scale (ViAS)**, the VeAS had a reliability score of 0.79 to 0.95.[26,29]

Box 5-1   Assessment Questions Relating to Pain*

Location and Nature of Pain
- Where do you feel uncomfortable (pain)?
- Does your discomfort (pain) feel deep or superficial?
- Is your problem (pain) constant or intermittent? If constant, does it vary in intensity?
- How long does your discomfort (pain) last?
- What is the frequency of your discomfort (pain)?
- How long have you had this problem (pain)?
- Are you experiencing discomfort (pain) right now?

Pain Manifestations
- How would you describe your discomfort (pain): throbbing, aching/sharp, dull, electrical, and so on?
- Does the discomfort (pain) move or spread to other areas?
- Does movement aggravate the discomfort (pain)?
- Do certain positions aggravate the discomfort (pain)? If yes, can you show me the movement or postures that cause the discomfort (pain)?
- Do you have stiffness with your discomfort (pain)?
- Do you have discomfort (pain) at rest?
- Do you have discomfort (pain) during the morning or night?
- Does the discomfort (pain) wake you from sleep?
- Do you have discomfort (pain) during particular activities?
- Do you experience discomfort (pain) after performing particular activities?
- What makes your discomfort (pain) worse?
- What helps relieve your discomfort (pain)?
- What have you tried to reduce your discomfort (pain)?
- What worked to reduce your discomfort (pain)?

*Therapists working with persons experiencing chronic pain may find that focusing on pain and repeating the word pain over and over is not beneficial. Therapists may select questions according to their judgment and substitute alternative words for pain when necessary.

Finch and colleagues[26] reported that a three-point change in score is necessary to establish a true pain intensity change. Thus, the VeAS may be limited to detect small changes, and clients with cognitive deficits may have trouble following instructions to complete the VeAS.[26,27]

A ViAS is also used to rate pain intensity. A client refers to a 10-cm horizontal line, with the left side of the line representing "no pain" and the right side representing "pain as bad as it could be." The client indicates pain level by marking a slash on the line, which represents the pain experienced. The distance from no pain to the slash is measured and recorded in centimeters (Figure 5-2). The ViAS "may have a high failure rate because patients may have difficulty interpreting the instructions."[67] Some errors occur due to changes in length of the line resulting from photocopying.[31] The VeAS and ViAS are unidimensional assessments of pain (i.e., intensity).[31] Although test-retest is not applicable to self-reported measures, researchers demonstrated a high range of test-retest reliability (ICC = 0.71 to 0.99).[19,26,29] When compared to the VeAS, concurrent validity measures ranged from 0.71 to 0.78.[19]

A body diagram consists of outlines of a body with front and back views (Figure 5-3). The person is asked to shade or color in the location of pain that corresponds to the body part experiencing pain. Colored pencils corresponding to a legend can be used to represent different intensities or types of pain, such as numbness, pins and needles, burning, aching, throbbing, and superficial.

Self-report questionnaires are commonly used. Such questionnaires such as the Short Form-36 (SF-36), Disabilities of the Arm, Shoulder, and Hand (DASH), and disease or condition-specific questionnaires exist.[22]

Therapists may use a more formal pain assessment, such as the McGill Pain Questionnaire (MPQ)[23] or the Schultz Pain Assessment.[67] Although formal assessments usually take more time to administer than screening tools, they comprehensively assess many aspects of pain.[46]

Melzack[38] developed the MPQ, which is widely used in clinical practice and for research purposes. The MPQ consists of a pain rating index, total number of word descriptors, and a present pain index. In its original version, the MPQ required 10 to 15 minutes to administer. The MPQ is a valid and reliable assessment tool. High internal consistency within the MPQ exists with correlations of 0.89 to 0.90.[38] Test-retest reliability scores for the MPQ are reported as 70.3%.[38]

For assessment of pediatric pain, self-reporting measures are considered the gold standard.[43] A therapist determines the child's concepts of quantification, classification,

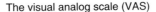
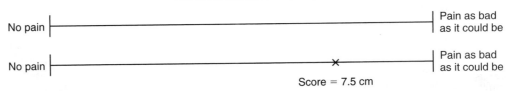

Figure 5-2 The visual analog scale (ViAS) and an example of a completed ViAS with a score of 7.5.

and matching prior to administering simple pain intensity scales.[13] Nonverbal scales using facial expressions and the ViAS are commonly used. Children's ability to report pain is affected by their stage in child development. Table 5-3 outlines ages and recommendations associated with the various types of reporting in children.

Skin

A thorough examination of the surface condition and contour of the extremity may define possible pathologic conditions, which may influence orthotic design. During the examination the therapist observes and documents the skin's color, temperature, and texture. The therapist observes the skin for muscle atrophy, scarring, edema, hair patterns, sweat patterns, and abnormal masses. Clients with fragile skin (especially persons who are older, who have been taking steroids for a long time, or who have diabetes) require careful monitoring. For these persons, the therapist carefully considers the orthotic material to prevent harm to the already fragile skin (see Chapter 15).

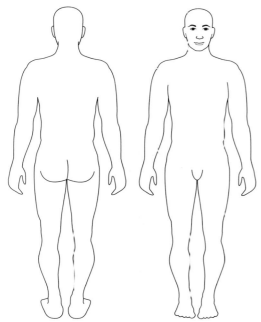

Figure 5-3 Example of a body diagram.

Table 5-3	Children's Report of Pain
AGE	**REPORT**
2 years	Presence and location of pain
3 to 4 years	Presence, location, and intensity of pain
	3-years-old: Use a three-level pain intensity scale
	4-years-old: Use a four- to five-item scale
5 years	Begin to use pain rating scales
8 years	Rate quality of pain

Data from O'Rourke D: The measurement of pain in infants, children, and adolescents: from policy to practice, *Physical Therapy* 84:560-570, 2004.

With regard to skin, many clients are aware if they have skin allergies. Some are allergic to bandages, adhesive, and latex (all of which can be used in the orthotic process). To avoid skin reactions, the therapist asks each client to disclose any types of allergy before choosing orthotic materials. When persons are unsure of skin allergies, the therapist should be aware that thermoplastic material, padding, and strapping supplies may create an allergic reaction. Therapists educate persons to monitor for any rashes or other skin reactions that develop from wearing an orthosis. The client experiencing a reaction should generally discontinue wearing the orthosis and report immediately to the therapist.

Veins and Lymphatics

Normally the veins on the dorsum of the hand are easy to see and palpate. They are cordlike structures. Any tenderness, pain, redness, or firmness along the course of veins is noted.[45] Venous thrombosis, subcutaneous fibrosis, or lymphatic obstruction causes edema.[42]

Wounds

The therapist measures wounds or incisions (usually in centimeters) and assesses discharge from wounds for color, amount, and odor. If there is concern about the discharge being a sign of infection, a wound culture is obtained by the medical staff to identify the source of infection, and appropriate medication is prescribed. Wounds are classified by color: black, yellow, or red.[14] A black wound consists of dark, thick eschar, which impedes epithelialization. A yellow wound ranges in color from ivory to green-yellow (e.g., colonization with pseudomonas). Typically, yellow wounds are covered with purulent discharge. A red wound indicates the presence of granulation tissue and is normal. Red wounds should be protected from mechanical forces, such as tapes, dressings, whirlpool agitation, and so on.[62]

Many wounds consist of a variety of colors.[14] Treatment focuses on treating the most serious color initially. For example, in the presence of eschar (common after thermal and crush injuries) a wound takes on a white or yellow-white color. Part of the intervention regimen for eschar is mechanical, chemical, or surgical debridement, which usually must be done before orthotic prescription. Debridement may result in a yellow wound. The yellow wound is managed by cleansing and dressing techniques to assist in the removal of debris. Once the desired red wound bed is achieved, it is protected by dressings.[64]

Because open wounds threaten exposure to the person's body fluids, the therapist follows universal precautions. The following precautions were derived from the Centers for Disease Control (CDC)[50]:

- Wear gloves for all procedures that may involve contact with body fluids.
- Change gloves after contact with each person.
- Wear masks for procedures that may produce aerosols or splashing.

perform.

Proximal musculature affects distal musculature tension in persons experiencing spasticity. For example, wrist position influences the amount of tension placed on finger musculature. When the therapist attempts to increase wrist extension in the presence of spasticity, the wrist, hand, and fingers must be incorporated into the orthotic design. If the orthotic design addresses only wrist extension, the result may be increased finger flexion. Conversely, if the orthotic

(Figure 5-5). This mapping pists, clients, case managers, and employers.[59] The Semmes-Weinstein Monofilament Test is the most reliable sensation test available and is often used as the comparison for concurrent validity studies.[15]

Therapists searching for objective sensory assessment data should be aware that "tests that were considered objective in the past can be demonstrated to be subjective in application dependent on the technique of the examiner."[5,6] For

- Wear protective eyewear or face shields for procedures generating droplets or splashing.
- Wear gowns or aprons for procedures that may produce splashing or contamination of clothing.
- Wash hands immediately after removal of gloves and after contact with each person.
- Replace torn gloves immediately.
- Replace gloves after punctures, and discard the instru-

10 the new collagen fibers begin to align parallel to the longitudinal collagen bundles of the tendon ends.[34]

The final stage is the maturation (remodeling) phase. This phase is seen typically after day 21 and can last up to 1 or 2 years after the injury.[53,54,56,62] During the maturation stage, the tensile strength continually increases. Initially, the scar may appear red, raised, and thick, but with maturation a normal scar softens and becomes more pliable. The maturation phase for healing tendons is lengthier than time needed

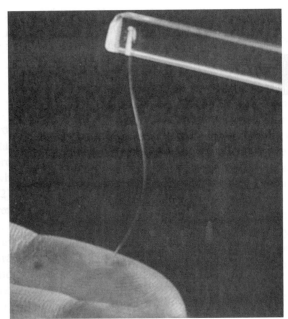

Figure 5-5 The monofilament collapses when a force dependent on filament diameter and length is reached, controlling the magnitude of the applied touch pressure. (From Hunter JM, Mackin EJ, Callahan AD, editors: *Rehabilitation of the hand: surgery and therapy,* ed 4, St Louis, 1996, Mosby, p 76.)

example, when administering the Semmes-Weinstein Monofilament Test, if the stimulus is applied too quickly, "the force can result in an overshoot beyond the desired stimulus"[6] and affect the test results. In addition, even when the Semmes-Weinstein Monofilament Test is administered with excellent technique, the cooperation and comprehension of the client are required.

When peripheral nerve injuries have occurred or are suspected, a Tinel test can be conducted. A Tinel test can be performed in two ways. The first method involves gently tapping over the suspected entrapment site to help determine whether entrapment is present. The second method consists of tapping the nerve distal to proximal. The location where the paresthesias are felt is considered the level to which a nerve has regenerated after Wallerian degeneration has occurred. A person has a positive Tinel sign if tingling or shooting sensations in one of two areas occurs: (1) at the site of tapping or (2) in a direction distally from the tapped area.[45] If the person experiences paresthesia or hyperparesthesia in a direction proximal to the tapped area, the Tinel test is negative.

A Phalen sign is present if a person feels similar symptoms to a positive Tinel test while resting elbows on the table and flexing the wrists for 15 to 60 seconds.[51] Phalen sign may indicate a median nerve problem. Tinel and Phalen signs can be positive in normal subjects.[52]

Cervical nerve problems are ruled out before a diagnosis of peripheral nerve injury is made.[37] For example, a person may have signs similar to carpal tunnel syndrome in conjunction with complaints of neck pain. In the absence of a

cervical nerve screen, the person may be misdiagnosed with carpal tunnel syndrome when the cause of the problems is actually cervical nerve involvement. In the absence of electrical studies, some physicians make the diagnosis of nerve compression!

During the fitting process, hand orthoses may cause pressure and friction on vulnerable areas with impaired sensibility. If a person has decreased sensibility, the therapist uses an orthotic design with long, well-molded components. The reason for using such an orthosis is to distribute the forces of the orthosis over as much surface area as possible, thereby decreasing the potential for pressure areas.

When an orthosis is placed across the wrist, the superficial branch of the radial nerve is at risk of compression. If the radial edge of the forearm orthosis stops beyond the midlateral forearm near the dorsum of the thumb, the superficial branch of the radial nerve can be compressed.[11] During the evaluation of orthotic fit, therapists should be aware of the signs of compression of the superficial branch of the radial nerve. Orthoses that cause compression require adjustments to decrease the pressure near the dorsum of the thumb.

Vascular Status

To understand the vascular status of a diseased or injured hand, the therapist monitors the skin's color and temperature and checks for edema. The therapist clearly defines areas of questionable tissue viability and adapts orthoses to prevent obstruction of arterial and venous circulation. To assess radial and ulnar artery patency, the therapist uses an Allen test.[48]

A therapist can take circumferential measurements proximal and distal to the location of orthotic application. Then, after applying the orthosis to the extremity, the therapist measures the same areas and compares them with the previous measurements. An increase in measurements taken while the orthosis is on indicates that the orthosis is exerting too much force on the underlying tissues. This situation poses a risk for circulation. When fluctuating edema is present, the therapist should make the orthotic design larger. A well-fitting circumferential orthosis, sometimes in conjunction with a pressure garment, can control or eliminate fluctuating edema. In addition, fluctuating edema may signal poor compliance with elevation. A sling and education about its use may assist in edema control.

The therapist can also use the Fingernail Blanch Test to assess circulation.[2] Long-lasting blanched areas of the fingertips indicate restricted circulation.

When a therapist applies an orthosis to the upper extremity, the skin should maintain its natural color. Red or purple areas indicate obstructed venous circulation. Dusky or white areas indicate obstructed arterial circulation. Orthoses causing circulation problems must be modified or discontinued.

Range of Motion and Strength

The therapist records active and passive motions when no contraindications are present (Figure 5-6) and takes

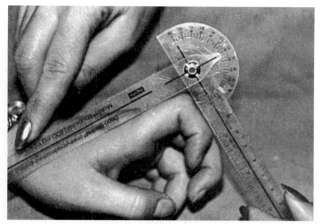

Figure 5-6 Goniometric measurements of active and passive motion are taken regularly when no contraindications are present (From Hunter JM, Mackin EJ, Callahan AD, editors: *Rehabilitation of the hand: surgery and therapy,* ed 4, St Louis, 1996, Mosby, p 34.)

measurements on both extremities for a baseline data comparison. The therapist also records total active motion (TAM) and total passive motion (TPM).[48] Grasp and pinch strengths are completed and documented only when no contraindications are present (Figure 5-7 and Figure 5-8). Manual muscle testing (MMT) assesses muscle strength but should be done only when there are no contraindications. For example, if a person with rheumatoid arthritis in an exacerbated state is being evaluated, MMT should be avoided to prevent further exacerbation of pain and swelling.

Coordination and Dexterity

Hand coordination and dexterity are needed for many functional performance tasks, and it is important to evaluate them. Many standardized tests for coordination and dexterity exist, including the Nine Hole Peg Test (Figure 5-9), Minnesota Rate of Manipulation Test (MRMT), Crawford Small Parts Dexterity Test, Purdue Peg Board Test, Rosenbusch Test of Dexterity, and Valpar Component Work Samples (VCWS)

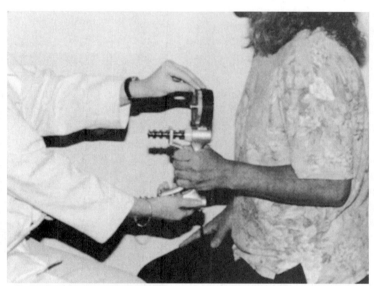

Figure 5-7 Therapists use the Jamar dynamometer to obtain reliable and accurate grip strength measurements. (From Tubiana R, Thomine JM, Mackin E: *Examination of the hand and wrist,* St Louis, 1996, Mosby, p 344.)

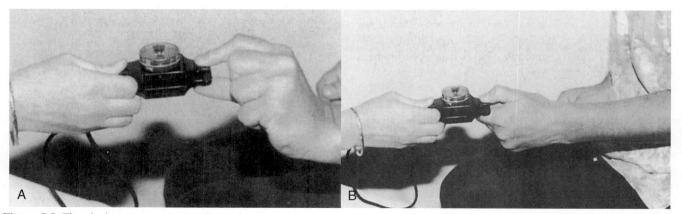

Figure 5-8 The pinch meter measures pulp pinch **(A)** and lateral pinch **(B).** (From Tubiana R, Thomine JM, Mackin E: *Examination of the hand and wrist,* St Louis, 1996, Mosby, p 344.)

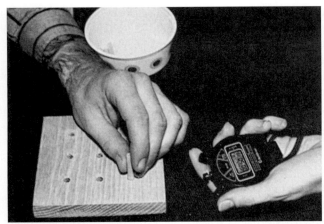

Figure 5-9 The Nine Hole Peg Test is a quick test for coordination. (From Hunter JM, Mackin EJ, Callahan AD, editors: *Rehabilitation of the hand: surgery and therapy,* ed 4, St Louis, 1996, Mosby, p 1158.)

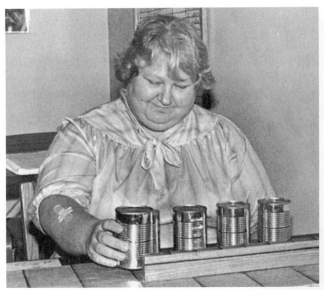

Figure 5-10 The Jebsen-Taylor Hand Test assesses the ability to perform prehension tasks. (From Hunter JM, Mackin EJ, Callahan AD, editors: *Rehabilitation of the hand: surgery and therapy,* ed 4, St Louis, 1996, Mosby, p 98.)

tests. Most dexterity tests are based on time measurements, and normative data are available for all of these tests. In particular, the VCWS use methods time measurement (MTM). MTM is a method of analyzing work tasks to determine how long a trained worker will require to complete a certain task at a rate that can be sustained for an 8-hour workday.

The Sequential Occupational Dexterity Assessment (SODA) was developed in the Netherlands.[60] The SODA is a test to measure hand dexterity and the client's perception of difficulty and pain while performing four unilateral and eight bilateral activity of daily living (ADL) tasks.[36] In a study conducted by Massey-Westropp and colleagues[36] on 62 clients with rheumatoid arthritis, they concluded that: "The SODA is also valid and reliable for assessing disability in a clinical situation that cannot be generalized to the home."[36] More research is needed to test such findings.

Function

Function is assessed by observation, interview, task performance, and standardized testing. Close observation during the interview and orthotic fabrication gives the therapist information regarding the person's views of the injury and disability. The therapist also observes the person for protected or guarded positioning, abnormal hand movements, muscle substitutions, and pain involvement during functional tasks. During evaluation, the person's willingness for the therapist to touch and move the affected extremity is noted.

During the initial interview, the therapist questions the person about the status of ADLs, instrumental activities of daily living (IADLs), and avocational and vocational activities. The therapist notes problem areas. Having clients perform tasks as part of an evaluation may result in more information, particularly when self-reporting is questioned by the therapist.

The therapist may use standardized hand function assessments. The Jebsen-Taylor Hand Function Test is helpful

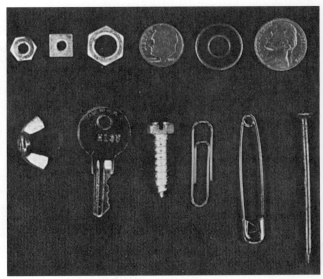

Figure 5-11 Items used in the Dellon modification of the Moberg Pick-up Test. (From Hunter JM, Mackin EJ, Callahan AD, editors: *Rehabilitation of the hand: surgery and therapy,* ed 3, St Louis, 1990, Mosby, p 608.)

because it gives objective measurements of standardized tasks with norms the therapist uses for comparison (Figure 5-10).[30] The Dellon modification of the Moberg Pick-up Test evaluates hand function when the person grasps common objects (Figure 5-11).[39] Similar objects in the test require the person to have sensory discrimination and prehensile abilities.[10]

Other functional outcome assessments that may be used include the **Canadian Occupational Performance Measure (COPM)**; the **Assessment of Motor and Process Skills (AMPS)**; the DASH, the SF-36, Handwriting Assessment Battery (HAB), and Manual Ability Measure (MAM).

The COPM is a client-centered outcome measure used to assess self-care, productivity, and leisure.[33] Clients rate their performance and satisfaction with performance on a 1 to 10 point scale. The result is a weighted individualized client goal plan.[32] It is a top-down assessment, which is done before administration of tests to evaluate performance components. Test-retest reliability was reported as ICC = 0.63 for performance and ICC = 0.84 for satisfaction—as cited in Case-Smith, "Validity was estimated by correlating COPM change scores with changes in overall function as rated by caregivers (r = 0.55, r = 0.56), therapist (r = 0.30, r = 0.33), and clients (r = 0.26, r = 0.53)."[12,47]

The DASH is a standardized questionnaire rating disability and symptoms related to upper extremity conditions. The DASH includes 30 pre-determined questions that explore function within performance areas. The client rates current ability to complete particular skills, such as opening a jar or turning a key, on a scale of 1 (no difficulty) to 5 (unable). Beaton and colleagues[4] studied reliability and validity of the DASH. Excellent test-retest reliability was reported (ICC = 0.96) in a study of 86 clients. Concurrent validity was established with correlations with other pain and function measures (r > 0.69).

The SF-36 measures eight aspects of health that contribute to quality of life.[66] The SF-36 "yields an eight scale profile of functional health and well being scores, as well as psychometrically based physical and mental health summary measures and a preference based health utility index."[65] Reliability scores range from r = 0.43 to r = 0.96.[8] Evidence of content, concurrent, criterion, construct, and predictive evidence of validity have been established.[65] The tool has been translated for use in more than 60 countries and languages.

The HAB consists of three sections with items from eight subtests.[21] Each subtest results in a profile of performance related to pen control and manipulation, writing speed, and legibility. Administration of the HAB requires approximately 20 minutes and another 15 minutes to score. Although the HAB demonstrates excellent inter-rater reliability, further testing is needed.

The MAM is available in two versions: MAM-16 (16 items) and MAM-36 (36 items).[44] The MAM is occupation-based in that the assessment items are everyday tasks, such as eating a sandwich, cutting meat, and wringing a towel. Clients use a four-point ordinal rating scale that asks how easy or hard it is to perform such tasks (1 = cannot do, 2 = very hard, 3 = a little hard, 4 = easy). Administration takes approximately 15 minutes. The MAM-36 is appropriate to use with clients who have neurologic and musculoskeletal disorders.[13]

Both the COPM and AMPS may take more time to administer than other tools. In addition, therapists using these tests should be trained in their administration, scoring, and interpretation.

Work

Evaluations of paid and unpaid work entail assessment of the work to be done and how the work is performed.[41] It is estimated that 36% of all functional capacity evaluations (FCEs) are conducted because of upper extremity and hand injuries.[41]

Some facilities use a specific type of FCE system, such as the Blankenship System or the Key Method. Standardized testing includes the Work Evaluations Systems Technologies II (WEST II), the EPIC Lift Capacity (ELC), the Bennett Hand Tool Dexterity Test, the Purdue Pegboard, the MRMT, and the VCWS. Commercially-available computerized tests can be administered in work evaluations. Isometric, isoinertial, and isokinetic tests can be performed on equipment tools manufactured by Cybex, Biodex, and Baltimore Therapeutic Equipment (BTE). FCEs frequently assess abnormal illness behavior and often include observation, psychometric testing, and physical or functional testing. New and experienced therapists should have specialized training in administering and interpreting FCEs because of the standardized nature of the examination and the legal implications of these assessments.[41]

Other Considerations

The person's motivation, ability to understand and carry out instructions, and compliance may affect the type of orthosis the therapist chooses. The therapist considers a person's vocational and avocational interests when designing an orthosis. Some persons wear more than one orthosis throughout the day to allow for completion of various activities. In addition, some persons wear one orthotic design during the day and a different design at night.

Related to motivation may be the presence or absence of a third-party payment source. Whenever possible, the therapist discusses payment issues with the client before completing the initial visit. If a third party is paying for the client's services, the therapist first determines whether that source intends to pay for any or all of the orthotic fabrication services. At times, some clients are very motivated to adhere to the rehabilitation program if they have to self-pay for the services. In other cases, where third-party reimbursement is quite good and the client is temporarily on a medical leave from work, the client may be less motivated and perhaps show signs of abnormal illness behavior. Terms such as *malingering, secondary gain, hypochondriases, hysterical neurosis, conversion, somatization disorder, functional overlay,* and *nonorganic pain* have been used to describe abnormal illness behaviors.[41] Gatchel and colleagues[28] reported the following red flags, which can assist the therapist in identifying such abnormal behaviors[7]:

- Client agitates other clients with disruptive behaviors.
- Client has no future work plan or changes to previous work plan.
- Client is applying for or receiving Social Security or long-term disability.
- Client opposes psychological services and refuses to answer questions or fill out forms.
- Client has obvious psychosis.
- Client has significant cognitive or neuropsychological deficits.
- Client expresses excessive anger at persons involved in case.
- Client is a substance abuser.

- Client's family is resistant to his or her recovery or return to work.
- Client has young children at home or has a short-term work history for primarily financial reasons.
- Client perpetually complains about the facility, staff, and program rather than being willing to deal with related physical and psychological issues.
- Client is chronically late to therapy and is noncompliant with excuses that do not check out.
- Client focuses on pain complaints in counseling sessions rather than dealing with psychological issues.

Orthotic Precautions

During the orthotic assessment, the therapist is aware of orthotic precautions. An ill-fitting orthosis can harm a person. Several precautions are outlined in Form 5-2, which a therapist can use as a check-off sheet. The therapist must not only educate a client about appropriate precautions but evaluate the client's understanding of them. The client's understanding can be assessed by having him or her repeat important precautions to follow or by role-playing (e.g., "If this happens, what will you do?"). In follow-up visits, the client can be questioned again to determine whether precautions are understood. Form 5-3 lists orthotic fabrication hints to follow. Adherence to the hints assists in avoiding situations that result in clients experiencing problems with their orthoses.

Pressure Areas

After fabricating an orthosis, the therapist does not allow the person to leave until the orthosis has been evaluated for problem areas. A general guideline is to have the person wear the orthosis at least 20 to 30 minutes after fabrication. Red areas should not be present 20 minutes after removal of the orthosis. Orthoses often require some adjustment. After receiving assurance that no pressure areas are present, the therapist instructs the person to remove the orthosis and to call if any problems arise. Persons with fragile skin are at high risk of developing pressure areas. The therapist provides the person with thorough written and verbal instructions on the wear and care of the orthosis. The instructions should include a phone number for emergencies. During follow-up visits, the therapist inquires about the orthotic fit to determine whether adjustments are necessary in the design or wearing schedule.

Edema

The therapist completes an evaluation for excessive tightness of the orthosis or straps. Often edema is caused by inappropriate strapping, especially at the wrist or over the MCP joints. Strapping systems are evaluated and modified if they are contributing to increased edema. If the orthosis is too narrow, it may also inadvertently contribute to increased edema. Persons can usually wear orthoses over pressure garments if necessary. However, therapists must monitor circulation closely.

The therapist assesses edema by taking circumferential or volumetric measurements (Figure 5-12).[61] When taking volumetric measurements, the therapist administers the test according to the testing protocol and then compares the involved extremity measurement with that of the uninvolved extremity. If edema fluctuates throughout the day, it is best to fabricate the orthosis when edema is present so as to ensure

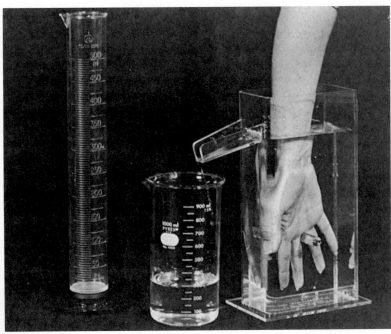

Figure 5-12 The volumeter measures composite hand mass via water displacement. (From Hunter JM, Mackin EJ, Callahan AD, editors: *Rehabilitation of the hand: surgery and therapy,* ed 3, St Louis, 1990, Mosby, p 63.)

that the orthosis accommodates the edema fluctuation. When edema is minimal but fluctuates during the day, the orthotic design must be wider to accommodate the edema.[11]

Orthotic Regimen

Upon provision of an orthosis, the therapist determines a wearing schedule for the client. Most diagnoses allow persons to remove the orthoses for some type of exercise and hygiene. The therapist provides a written orthotic schedule and reviews the schedule with the person, nurse, and caregiver responsible for putting on and taking off the orthosis. If the person is confused, the therapist is responsible for instructing the appropriate caregiver regarding proper orthotic wear and care. The therapist must evaluate the client's or caregiver's understanding of the wearing schedule.

Clients wearing mobilizing (dynamic) orthoses follow several general precautions. A therapist must be cautious when instructing a client to wear a mobilizing (dynamic) orthosis during sleep. Because of moving parts on mobilization orthoses, the person could accidentally scratch, poke, or cut himself or herself. Therefore, therapists must design orthoses with no sharp edges and must consider the possibility of using elastic traction (see Chapter 12).

Typically, persons should wear mobilizing (dynamic) orthoses for a few minutes out of each hour and gradually work up to longer time periods. As with all orthoses, a therapist never fabricates a mobilizing (dynamic) orthosis without checking its effect on the person. The therapist considers the diagnosis and appropriately schedules orthotic wearing. Often, but not always, an orthotic regimen allows for times of rest, exercise, hygiene, and skin relief. The therapist considers the client's daily activity schedule when designing the orthotic regimen. However, intervention goals must sometimes supersede the desire for the client to perform activities. In addition, the therapist uses clinical judgment to determine and adjust the orthotic wearing schedule and reevaluates the orthosis consistently to alter the intervention plan as necessary.

Adherence

On the basis of the initial interview and statements from conversations, the therapist determines whether compliance with the wearing schedule and rehabilitation program is a problem. (Chapter 6 contains strategies to help persons with adherence and acceptance.) If the hand (or wrist, elbow, shoulder, etc.) demonstrates that the orthosis is not achieving its goal, the therapist must check that the orthosis is well designed and fits properly and then determine whether the orthosis is being worn. If the therapist is certain about the design and fit, adherence is probably poor. Clients returning for follow-up visits must bring their orthoses. The therapist can generally determine whether a client is wearing the orthosis by looking for signs of normal wear and tear. Signs include dirty areas or scratches in the plastic, soiled straps, and nappy straps (caused by pulling the strap off the Velcro hook).

Orthotic Care

Therapists are responsible for educating persons about orthotic care. An evaluation of a person's understanding of orthotic care is completed before the client leaves the clinic or is discharged. Assessment is accomplished by asking the client to repeat instructions or demonstrate orthotic care. To keep the orthosis clean, washing the hand with warm water and a mild soap and cleansing the orthosis with rubbing alcohol are effective. The person or caregiver thoroughly dries the hand and orthosis before reapplication. Chlorine occasionally removes ink marks on the orthosis. Rubbing alcohol, chlorine bleach, and hydrogen peroxide are good disinfectants to use on the orthosis for infection control.

Persons should be aware that heat may melt their orthoses and should be careful not to leave their orthoses in hot cars, on sunny windowsills, or on radiators. Therapists discourage persons from making self-adjustments, including the heating of orthoses in microwave ovens (which may cause orthoses to soften, fold in on themselves, and adhere). If the person successfully softens the plastic, a burn could result from the application of hot plastic to the skin. However, clients are encouraged to make suggestions to improve an orthosis. Therapists, especially novice therapists, tend to ignore the client's ideas. Not only does this send a negative message to the client but clients often have wonderful ideas that are too beneficial to discount.

SELF-QUIZ 5-1*

For the following questions, circle either true (T) or false (F).

1. T F All physicians follow the same protocol for postoperative conditions.
2. T F Motivation may affect the person's adherence for wearing an orthosis, and thus determining the person's motivational level is an important task for the therapist.
3. T F The resting hand posture is 10 to 20 degrees of wrist extension, 10 degrees of ulnar deviation, 15 to 20 degrees of metacarpophalangeal (MCP) flexion, and partial flexion and abduction of the thumb.
4. T F Proximal musculature never affects distal musculature.
5. T F Therapists should encourage persons to carry their affected extremities in guarded or protective positions to ensure that no further harm is done to the injury.
6. T F A general guideline for evaluating orthotic fit is to have the person wear the orthosis for 20 minutes and then remove the orthosis. If no reddened areas are present after 20 minutes of orthosis removal, no adjustments are necessary.
7. T F All orthoses require 24 hours of wearing to be most effective.
8. T F Every person should receive an orthotic wearing schedule in written and verbal forms.
9. T F For infection control purposes, persons and therapists should use extremely hot water to clean orthoses.
10. T F Strength of a healing tendon is stronger when the tendon is immobilized rather than mobilized.
11. T F A red wound is a healthy wound.
12. T F A score of 10 on a verbal analog scale (VeAS) indicates that pain does not need to be addressed in the intervention plan.
13. T F Strapping, padding, and thermoplastic materials may cause a skin allergic reaction in some persons.
14. T F Assessments of function include the Nine Hole Peg Test and the Semmes-Weinstein Monofilament Test.

*See Appendix A for the answer key.

Summary

Evaluation before orthotic provision is an integral part of the orthotic provision process. The evaluation process includes report reading, observation, interview, palpation, and formal and informal assessments. Evaluation before, during, and after orthotic provision results in the therapist's ability to understand how the orthosis affects function and how function affects the orthosis. A thorough evaluation process ultimately results in client satisfaction.

Review Questions

1. What are components of a thorough hand examination before orthotic fabrication?
2. What is the posture of a resting hand?
3. What information should a therapist obtain about the person's history?
4. What sources can therapists use to obtain information about persons and their conditions?
5. What should a therapist be noting when palpating a client?
6. What observations should be made when a client first enters a clinic?
7. What types of formal upper extremity assessments for function are available?
8. What procedure can a therapist use when assessing whether a newly fabricated orthosis fits well on a person?
9. What precautions should a therapist keep in mind when designing and fabricating an orthosis?
10. How can a therapist evaluate a client's understanding of an orthotic wearing schedule?
11. What safeguard can a therapist employ to avoid skin reactions from orthotic materials?

References

1. American Society for Surgery of the Hand: *The hand*, New York, 1983, Churchill Livingstone.
2. Aulicino PL, DuPuy TE: Clinical examination of the hand. In Hunter JM, Schneider LH, Mackin EJ, et al.: *Rehabilitation of the hand: surgery and therapy*, ed 3, St Louis, 1990, Mosby.
3. Bear-Lehman J, Abreu BC: Evaluating the hand: issues in reliability and validity, *Phys Ther* 69(12):1025–1031, 1989.
4. Beaton DE, Katz JN, Fossel AH, et al.: Measuring the whole or the parts? Validity, reliability, and responsiveness of the Disabilities of the Arm, Shoulder and Hand outcome measure in different regions of the upper extremity, *J Hand Ther* 14(2):128–146, 2001.
5. Bell-Krotoski JA: Sensibility testing: current concepts. In Hunter JM, Mackin EJ, Callahan AD, editors: *Rehabilitation of the hand*, ed 4, St Louis, 1995, Mosby.
6. Bell-Krotoski JA, Buford WL: The force/time relationship of clinically used sensory testing instruments, *J Hand Ther* 10(4):297–309, 1997.
7. Blankenship KL: *The Blankenship system: functional capacity evaluation, the procedure manual*, Macon, GA, 1989, Blankenship Corporation, Panaprint.
8. Brazier JE, Harper R, Jones N, et al.: Validating the SF-36 Health Survey Questionnaire: new outcome measure for primary care, *Br Med J* 305:160–164, 1992.

9. Cailliet R: *Hand pain and impairment*, ed 4, Philadelphia, 1994, FA Davis.

10. Callahan AD: Sensibility testing: clinical methods. In Hunter JM, Schneider LH, Macklin EJ, et al.: *Rehabilitation of the hand: surgery and therapy*, ed 3, St Louis, 1990, Mosby.

11. Cannon NM, Foltz RW, Koepfer JM, et al.: *Manual of hand splinting*, New York, 1985, Churchill Livingstone.

12. Case-Smith J: Outcomes in hand rehabilitation using occupational therapy services, *AJOT* 57:499–506, 2003

13. Chen C, Bode K: Psychometric validation of Manual Ability Measure (MAM-36) in patients with neurologic and musculoskeletal disorders, *Arch Phys Med Rehabil* 91(3):414–420, 2010.

14. Cuzzell JZ: The new RYB color code: next time you assess an open wound, remember to protect red, cleanse yellow and debride black, *Am J Nurs* 88(10):1342–1346, 1988.

15. Dannenbaum RM, Michaelsen SM, Desrosiers J, et al.: Development and validation of two new sensory tests of the hand for patients with stroke, *Clin Rehabil* 16(6):630–639, 2002.

16. de Klerk AJ, Jouck LM: Primary tendon healing: an experimental study, *S Afr Med J* 62(9):276–281, 1982.

17. Ebrecht M, Hextall J, Kirtley LG, et al. editors: Perceived stress and cortisol levels predict speed of wound healing in healthy male adults, *Psychoneuroendocrinology* 29(6):798–809, 2004.

18. Ellem D: Assessment of the wrist, hand and finger complex, *J Man Manip Ther* 3(1):9–14, 1995.

19. Enebo BA: Outcome measures for low back pain: pain inventories and functional disability questionnaires, *J Chiropractic Technique* 10:68–74, 1998.

20. Evans RB, McAuliffe JA: Wound classification and management. In Mackin EJ, Callahan AD, Skirven TM, et al. editors: *Rehabilitation of the hand and upper extremity*, ed 5, St Louis. 2002, Mosby, pp 311–330.

21. Faddy K, McCluskey A, Lannin NA: Interrater reliability of a new handwriting assessment battery for adults, *Am J Occup Ther* 62(5):595–599, 2008.

22. Fedorczyk JM: Pain management: principles of therapist's intervention. In Skirven TM, Osterman AL, Fedorczyk JM, et al editors: *Rehabilitation of the hand: surgery and therapy*, ed 6, St Louis, 2011, Mosby.

23. Fedorczyk JM, Michlovitz SL: Pain control: putting modalities in perspectives. In Hunter JM, Mackin EJ, Callahan AD, (Eds) *Rehabilitation of the hand: surgery and therapy*, St Louis, 1999, Mosby.

24. Fess EE: Documentation: Essential elements of an upper extremity assessment battery. In Hunter JM, Mackin EJ, Callahan AD, editors: *Rehabilitation of the hand*, ed 4, St Louis, 1995, Mosby.

25. Fess EE, Gettle KS, Philips CA, et al.: *Hand and upper extremity splinting: principles and methods*, ed 3, St Louis, 2005, Elsevier Mosby.

26. Finch E, Brooks D, Stratford PW, et al.: *Physical rehabilitation outcome measures: a guide to enhanced clinical decision making*, ed 2, Baltimore, 2002, Lippincott, Williams & Wilkins.

27. Flaherty SA: Pain measurement tools for clinical practice and research, *AANA Journal* 64:133–140, 1996.

28. Gatchel R, Mayer T, Capra P, et al.: Million Behavioral Health Inventory: its utility in predicting physical function in patients with low back pain, *Arch Phys Med Rehabil* 67(12):879–882, 1996.

29. Good M, Stiller C, Zauszniewski JA, et al.: Sensation and distress of pain scales: reliability, validity, and sensitivity, *J Nurs Meas* 9(3):219–238, 2001.

30. Jebsen RH, Taylor N, Trieschmann RB, et al.: An objective and standardized test of hand function, *Arch Phys Med Rehabil* 50(6):311–319, 1969.

31. Kahl C, Cleland JA: Visual analogue scale, numeric pain rating scale and the McGill Pain Questionnaire: an overview of psychometric properties, *Phys Ther Reviews* 10:123–128, 2005.

32. Law M, Baptiste S, Carswell A, et al.: *Canadian occupational performance measures*, ed 3, Ottawa, Ontario, 1998, CAOT.

33. Law M, Baptiste S, McColl M, et al.: The Canadian Occupational Performance Measure: an outcome measure for occupational therapy, *Can J Occup Ther* 57(2):82–87, 1990.

34. Lindsay WK: Cellular biology of flexor tendon healing. In Hunter JM, Schneider LH, Mackin EJ, editors: *Tendon surgery in the hand*, St Louis, 1987, Mosby.

35. Macdermid JC: Outcome measurement in upper extremity practice. In Skirven TM, Osterman AL, Fedorczyk JM, et al.: *Rehabilitation of the hand: surgery and therapy*, ed 6, St Louis, 2011, Mosby.

36. Massy-Westropp N, Krishnan J, Ahern M: Comparing the AUSCAN osteoarthritis hand index, Michigan hand outcomes questionnaire, and sequential occupational dexterity assessment for patients with rheumatoid arthritis, *J Rheumatol* 31(10):1996–2001, 2004.

37. McClure P: Upper quarter screen. In Skirven TM, Osterman AL, Fedorczyk JM, et al. editors: *Rehabilitation of the hand: surgery and therapy*, ed 6, St Louis, 2011, Mosby.

38. Melzack R: The McGill pain questionnaire: major properties and scoring methods, *Pain* 1:277–299, 1975.

39. Moberg E: Objective methods for determining the functional value of sensibility in the hand, *J Bone Joint Surg Br* 40:454–476, 1958.

40. Mosely LH, Finseth F: Cigarette smoking: impairment of digital blood flow and wound healing in the hand, *Hand* 9:97–101, 1977.

41. Mueller BA, Adams ED, Isaac CA: Work activities. In Van Deusen J, Brunt D, editors: *Assessment in occupational therapy and physical therapy*, Philadelphia, 1997, WB Saunders.

42. Neviaser RJ: Closed tendon sheath irrigation for pyogenic flexor tenosynovitis, *J Hand Surg* 3:462–466, 1978.

43. O'Rourke D: The measurement of pain in infants, children, and adolescents: from policy to practice, *Phys Ther* 84:560–570, 2004.

44. Rallon CR, Chen CC: Relationship between performance based and self-reported assessment of hand function, *Am J Occup Ther* 62(5):574–579, 2008.

45. Ramadan AM Hand analysis. In Van Deusen J, Brunt D, editors: *Assessment in occupational therapy and physical therapy*, Philadelphia, 1997, WB Saunders.

46. Ross RG, LaStayo PC: Clinical assessment of pain. In Van Deusen J, Brunt D, editors: *Assessment in occupational therapy and physical therapy*, Philadelphia, 1997, WB Saunders.

47. Sanford J, Law M, Swanson L, et al: Assessing clinically important change on an outcome of rehabilitation in older adults. Paper presented at the Conference of the American Society of Aging. San Francisco, 1994.

48. Seftchick JL, Detullio LM, Fedorczyk JM, et al.: Clinical examination of the hand. In Skirven TM, Osterman AL, Fedorczyk JM, et al. editors: *Rehabilitation of the hand: surgery and therapy*, ed 6, St Louis, 2011, Mosby.

49. Siana JE, Rex S, Gottrup F: The effect of cigarette smoking on wound healing, *Scand J Plast Reconstr Surg Hand Surg* 23(3):207–209, 1989.

50. Singer DI, Moore JH, Byron PM: Management of skin grafts and flaps. In Hunter JM, Mackin EJ, Callahan AD, editors: *Rehabilitation of the hand: surgery and therapy*, ed 4, St Louis, 1995, Mosby.

51. Skirven TM, Osterman AL: Clinical examination of the wrist. In Skirven TM, Osterman AL, Fedorczyk JM, et al. editors: *Rehabilitation of the hand: surgery and therapy*, ed 6, St Louis, 2011, Mosby.

52. Smith GN, Bruner AT: The neurologic examination of the upper extremity, *Physical Medicine and Rehabilitation: State of the Art Reviews* 12(2):225–241, 1998.

53. Smith KL: Wound care for the hand patient. In Hunter JM, Schneider LH, Macklin EJ, et al. editors: *Rehabilitation of the hand: surgery and therapy*, ed 3, St Louis, 1990, Mosby.

54. Smith KL: Wound care for the hand patient. In Hunter JM, Mackin EJ, Callahan AD, editors: *Rehabilitation of the hand: surgery and therapy*, ed 4, St Louis, 1995, Mosby.

55. Smith KL: Wound healing. In Stanley BG, Tribuzi SM, editors: *Concepts in hand rehabilitation*, Philadelphia, 1992, FA Davis.

56. Staley MJ, Richard RL, Falkel JE: Burns. In O'Sullivan SB, Schmidtz TJ, editors: *Physical rehabilitation: assessment and treatment*, ed 3, Philadelphia, 1988, FA Davis.

57. Suk M, Hanson B, Norvell D, et al.: *Musculo-skeletal outcome measures and instruments*, Switzerland, 2005, AO Publishing.

58. Tarrier N, Gregg L, Edwards J, et al.: The influence of pre-existing psychiatric illness on recovery in burn injury patients: the impact of psychosis and depression, *Burns* 31:45–49, 2005.

59. Tomancik L: *Directions for using Semmes-Weinstein monofilaments*, San Jose, CA, 1987, North Coast Medical.

60. Van Lankveld W, van't Pad Bosch P, Bakker J, et al.: Sequential occupational dexterity assessment (SODA): a new test to measure hand disability, *J Hand Ther* 9(1):27–32, 1996.

61. Villeco JP: Edema: therapist's management. In Skirven TM, Osterman AL, Fedorczyk JM, et al. editors: *Rehabilitation of the hand: surgery and therapy*, ed 6, St Louis, 2011, Mosby.

62. Von Der Heyde RL: Evans RB: Wound classification and management. In Skirven TM, Osterman AL, Fedorczyk JM, et al.: *Rehabilitation of the hand: surgery and therapy*, ed 6, St Louis, 2011, Mosby.

63. Wadsworth CT: Wrist and hand examination and interpretation, *J Orthop Sports Phys Ther* 5(3):108–120, 1983.

64. Walsh M, Muntzer E: Wound management. In Stanley BG, Tribuzzi SM, editors: *Concepts in hand rehabilitation*, Philadelphia, 1992, FA Davis.

65. Ware JE: SF-36 health survey update. In Maruish ME, editor: ed 3, The use of psychological testing for treatment planning and outcomes assessment, volume 3, Mahwah, NJ, 2004, Lawrence Erlbaum Associates, pp 693–718.

66. Ware JE, Snow KK, Kosinski M, et al.: *SF-36 health survey: manual and interpretation guide*, Lincoln, RI, 2000, QualityMetric, Inc.

67. Weiss S, Falkenstein N: *Hand rehabilitation: a quick reference guide and review*, ed 2, St Louis, 2005, Mosby.

68. Wilson JA, Clark JJ: Obesity: impediment to postsurgical wound healing, *Adv Skin Wound Care* 17:426–435, 2004.

APPENDIX 5-1 FORMS

FORM 5-1 Hand Evaluation Check-off Sheet

Person's History: Interviews, Chart Review, and Reports:

○ Age
○ Vocation
○ Date of injury and surgery
○ Method of injury
○ Hand dominance
○ Treatment rendered to date (surgery, therapy, and so on)
○ Medication
○ Previous injury
○ General health
○ Avocational interests
○ Family composition
○ Subjective complaints
○ Support systems
○ Activity of daily living (ADL) responsibilities before and after injury
○ Impact of injury on family, economic status, and social well-being
○ Reimbursement
○ Motivation

Observation:

○ Walking, posture
○ Facial movements
○ Speech patterns
○ Affect
○ Hand posture
○ Cognition

Palpation:

○ Muscle tone
○ Muscle symmetry
○ Scar density/excursion
○ Tendon nodules
○ Masses (ganglia, fistulas)

Assessments for:

○ Pain
○ Skin and allergies
○ Wound healing/wound status
○ Bone
○ Joint and ligament
○ Muscle and tendon
○ Nerve/sensation
○ Vascular status
○ Skin turgor and trophic status
○ Range of motion
○ Strength
○ Coordination and dexterity
○ Function
○ Reimbursement source
○ Vocation

Follow-Up Considerations:

○ Orthosis fit
○ Compliance

FORM 5-2 Orthotic Precaution Check-off Sheet

○ Account for bony prominences such as the following:
  - Metacarpophalangeal (MCP), proximal interphalangeal (PIP), and distal interphalangeal (DIP) joints
  - Pisiform bone
  - Radial and ulnar styloids
  - Lateral and medial epicondyles of the elbow
○ Identify fragile skin, and select the orthotic material carefully. Monitor the temperature of the thermoplastic material closely before applying the material to the fragile skin.
○ Identify skin areas having impaired sensation. The orthotic design should not impinge on these sites.
○ If fluctuating edema is a problem, consider pressure garment wear in conjunction with an orthosis.
○ Do not compress the superficial branch of the radial nerve. If the radial edge of a forearm orthosis impinges beyond the middle of the forearm near the dorsal side of the thumb, the branch of the radial nerve may be compressed.

FORM 5-3 Hints for Orthotic Provision

○ Give the person oral and written instructions regarding the following:
- Wearing schedule
- Care of the orthosis
- Purpose of the orthosis
- Responsibility in therapy program
- Phone number of contact person if problems arise
- Actions to take if skin reactions such as the following occur: rashes, numbness, reddened areas, pain increase because of orthotic application

○ Evaluate the orthosis after the person wears it at least 20 to 30 minutes and make necessary adjustments.

○ Position all joints incorporated into the orthosis at the correct therapeutic angle(s).

○ Design the orthosis to account for bony prominences such as the following:
- Metacarpophalangeal (MCP), proximal interphalangeal (PIP), and distal interphalangeal (DIP) joints
- Pisiform
- Radial and ulnar styloids
- Lateral and medial epicondyles of the elbow

○ If fluctuating edema is a problem, make certain the orthotic design can accommodate the problem by using a wider design. Consider a pressure garment to wear under the orthosis.

○ Make certain the orthotic design does not mobilize or immobilize unnecessary joint(s).

○ Make certain the orthosis does not impede or restrict motions of joints adjacent to the orthosis.

○ Make certain the orthosis supports the arches of the hand.

○ Take into consideration the creases of the hand for allowing immobilization or mobilization, depending on the purpose of the orthosis.

○ Make certain the orthosis does not restrict circulation.

○ Make certain application and removal of the orthosis are easy.

○ Secure the orthosis to the person's extremity using a well-designed strapping mechanism.

○ Make certain the appropriate edges of the orthosis are flared or rolled.

CHAPTER 6

Clinical Reasoning for Orthotic Fabrication

Helene Lohman, OTD, OTR/L, FAOTA
Linda S. Scheirton, PhD

Key Terms
adherence
client safety
clinical reasoning
documentation
Health Insurance Portability and Accountability Act (HIPPA)
intervention process
orthotic intervention error

Chapter Objectives
1. Describe clinical reasoning approaches and their application to orthotic intervention.
2. Identify essential components of an orthotic referral.
3. Discuss reasons for the importance of communication with the physician about an orthotic referral.
4. Discuss diagnostic implications for orthotic provision.
5. List helpful hints regarding the hand evaluation for orthotic provision.
6. Explain factors the therapist considers when selecting an orthotic intervention approach and design.
7. Describe what therapists problem solve during orthotic fabrication.
8. Describe areas that require monitoring after orthotic fabrication is completed.
9. Describe the reflection process of the therapist before, during, and after orthotic fabrication.
10. Discuss important considerations concerning an orthotic-wearing schedule.
11. Identify conditions that determine orthotic discontinuation.
12. Identify patient safety issues related to orthotic intervention errors.
13. Discuss factors that affect orthotic cost and payment.
14. Discuss how the Health Insurance Portability and Accountability Act (HIPAA) regulations influence orthotic provision in a clinic.
15. Discuss documentation of orthotic intervention.

Susan works in a therapy department at a critical access hospital located in a rural area where she follows a variety of patients. On Friday Susan came to work expecting it to be like any other day. She was surprised when she had a walk-in patient with a post-flexor tendon repair and an order to fabricate a dorsal-block orthosis. Susan had no experience in treating a client with a post-flexor tendon repair. Although she had made a couple of orthoses before, she had never fabricated a dorsal-block orthosis. Susan did not have much time to think about the orthosis because she had a tight schedule that day. Susan thought, "I have made other orthoses, and although I don't know how to do this one, I can figure it out because I am familiar with basic orthotic skills." Susan consulted books and quickly called a therapist who informally mentored her. Susan then successfully fabricated the dorsal-block orthosis.

In clinical practice there is no simple design or type of orthosis that applies to all diagnoses. Orthotic design and wearing protocols vary because each injury is unique. **Clinical reasoning** about which orthosis to fabricate involves considering the physician's referral, the surgical and rehabilitation protocol, the therapist's conceptual model, the assessment of the client's needs based on objective and subjective data gathered during the evaluation process, and knowledge about the payment source.

Instructors often teach students only one way to do something when in reality there may be multiple ways to achieve a goal. For example, this book emphasizes the typical methods that generalist clinicians use to fabricate common orthoses. Learning a foundation for orthotic fabrication is important. In clinical practice, however, the therapist should use a problem-solving approach and apply clinical reasoning to address the needs of each client who requires an orthosis. Clinical reasoning may include integration of knowledge of biomechanics, anatomy, kinesiology, psychology, conceptual models, and pathology. Clinical reasoning also involves orthotic intervention protocols and techniques, clinical experience, and awareness of the client's motivation, adherence, and lifestyle (occupational) needs.

This chapter first overviews clinical reasoning models and then addresses approaches to clinical reasoning from the moment the therapist obtains an orthotic referral until the client's discharge. This chapter also presents prime questions to facilitate the clinical reasoning process that therapists undertake during intervention planning throughout the course of therapy.

Clinical Reasoning Models

Clinical reasoning helps therapists approach the complexities of clinical practice. Clinical reasoning involves professional thinking during evaluation and intervention.[44] Professional thinking is the ability to distinctly and critically analyze the reasons for whatever actions therapists make and to reflect on the decisions afterward.[46] Skilled therapists reflect throughout the entire orthotic **intervention process** (reflection in action), not solely after the orthosis is completed (reflection on action).[51] Clinical reasoning also entails understanding the meaning a disability, such as a hand injury, has from the client's perspective.[39]

With clinical reasoning, therapists consider available evidence in the literature to critically reflect on whether orthoses can help their clients. Based on a review of various studies,[8] therapists consider client characteristics and outcomes with orthotic intervention. Therapists analyze how the clients that they are following relate to those discussed in the studies.

Various approaches to clinical reasoning are depicted in the literature. Facione discussed an "argument and heuristic analysis model of decision making" for critical thinking.[21] System 1 involves automatic quick reactive thinking, and System 2 involves logical reflective thinking. Both types of critical thinking can be utilized with orthotic fabrication. Therapists apply System 1 to think quickly as the working time with thermoplastic materials is very short. Yet to appropriately fabricate orthoses, therapists must use System 2 to logically and reflectively consider factors such as which orthosis to provide, length of provision, wearing schedule, and principles of fabrication.

One clinical reasoning model in occupational therapy literature includes interactive, narrative, pragmatic, conditional, and procedural reasoning. Although each of these approaches is distinctive, experienced therapists often shift from one type of thinking to another to critically analyze complex clinical problems,[24] such as orthotic intervention.

Interactive reasoning involves getting to know the client as a human being so as to understand the impact that the hand condition has on the client's life.[24] Understanding the impact can help identify the proper orthosis to fabricate. For example, for a client who is very sensitive about appearance after a hand injury, the therapist may select a skin-tone thermoplastic material that blends with the skin and attracts less attention than a white thermoplastic material.

With narrative reasoning, the therapist reflects on the client's occupational story (or life history), taking into consideration activities, habits, and roles.[44] For assessment and intervention, the therapist first takes a top-down approach[59] by considering the roles that the client had prior to the hand condition and the meaning of occupations in the client's life. The therapist also considers the client's future and the impact that the therapist and the client can have on it.[24] For example, through discussion or a formal assessment interview, a therapist learns that continuation of work activities is important to a client with carpal tunnel syndrome. Therefore, the therapist fabricates a wrist immobilization orthosis to position the wrist in neutral and has the client practice typing while wearing the orthosis.

With pragmatic reasoning, the therapist considers practical factors, such as payment, public policy regulations, documentation, availability of equipment, and the expected discharge environment. Pragmatic reasoning includes considerations of the therapist's values, knowledge, and skills.[44,50] For example, a therapist may need to review the literature and research evidence if the therapist is unknowledgeable about a particular diagnosis that requires an orthosis. If a therapist does not have the expertise to fabricate an orthosis for a client with a complicated injury, the therapist might consider referring the client to another therapist who has the expertise.

In addition, a therapist may need to make ethical decisions, such as whether to fabricate an orthosis for a terminally ill 98-year-old client. This ethical decision involves the therapist's values about age and terminal conditions. In today's ever-changing health care environment, there is a trend toward cost containment. Budgetary shortages may require therapists to ration clinical services. Prospective payment systems for reimbursing the costs of rehabilitation, such as in skilled nursing facilities (SNFs), are a reality. Therapists fabricate orthoses quickly and efficiently to save costs. The information provided throughout this book may assist with pragmatic reasoning.

With conditional reasoning, the therapist reflects on the client's "whole condition" by considering the client's life before the injury, the disease or trauma, current status, and possible future life status.[40] Reflection is multidimensional and includes the condition that requires orthotic intervention, the meaning of having the condition or dysfunction, and the social and physical environments in which the client lives.[23] The therapist then envisions how the client's condition might change as a result of orthotic provision and therapy. Finally, the therapist realizes that success or failure of the intervention ultimately depends on the client's adherence to the orthotic requirements.[24,44] Evaluation and intervention with this clinical reasoning model begin with a top-down approach, considering the meaning of having an injury in the context of a client's life.

Box 6-1	Examples of Incomplete and Complete Orthotic Referrals

Incomplete Referral	Complete Referral
From the Office of Dr. S. Name: Mrs. P. MR. Number: 415672 Age: 51 Diagnosis: de Quervain tenosynovitis Date: August 12th Fabricate a left hand orthosis Dr. S.	From the Office of Dr. S. Date: August 12th Name: Mrs. P. MR. Number: 415672 Age: 51 Diagnosis: de Quervain tenosynovitis Fabricate a volar-based thumb immobilization orthosis L UE with the wrist in 15 degrees dorsiflexion, the thumb CMC joint in 40 degrees palmar abduction and the MCP joint in 10 degrees flexion. Dr. S.

CMC, Carpometacarpal; *L*, left; *MCP*, metacarpophalangeal; *UE*, upper extremity.

for requesting this information (Box 6-1). The therapist prepares a list of questions before calling; and if the physician is not available, the therapist conveys the list to the physician's administrative assistant, nurse, or physician assistant and agrees on a specific time to call again. Sometimes the contact client at the physician office can read the chart notes or fax an operative report to the therapist. With electronic medical records, access to radiographic reports, operative reports, and any other relevant reports may be accessible for review. The therapist must never rely solely on the client's perception of the diagnosis and orthotic requirements.

In some cases, the physician expects the therapist to have the clinical reasoning skills to select the appropriate orthosis for the specific clinical diagnosis. Sometimes a therapist receives a physician's order for an inappropriate orthosis, a nontherapeutic wearing schedule, or a less than optimal material. The therapist is responsible to always scrutinize each physician referral. If the referral is inappropriate, the therapist should apply clinical reasoning skills to determine the appropriate orthotic intervention approach. The therapist makes successful independent decisions with a knowledge base about the fundamentals of orthotic intervention and with the ability to locate additional information. Then the therapist calls the physician's office and diplomatically explains the problem with the referral and suggests a better orthotic intervention approach and rationale.

Diagnostic Implications for Orthotic Provision

The therapist identifies the client's diagnosis after reviewing the orthotic order. Often, the therapist can begin the clinical reasoning process by using a categorical orthotic intervention approach according to the diagnosis. The first category involves chronic conditions, such as hemiplegia. In such a situation, an orthosis may prevent skin maceration or contracture. The second category involves a traumatic or acute condition that may encompass surgical or nonsurgical intervention. For example, the client may have tendinosis and require a nonsurgical orthotic intervention for the affected extremity.

Regardless of whether the condition is acute or chronic, it is important that the therapist have an adequate knowledge of diagnostic protocols. By knowing protocols, therapists are aware of precautions for orthotic intervention. For example, for a client with carpal tunnel syndrome, the therapist knows to place the wrist in a neutral position. If the therapist placed the wrist in a functional position of 30 degrees extension, it could cause more pain by putting too much pressure on the median nerve. Therapists should keep abreast of current intervention trends through review of evidence in literature, continuing education, and communication with physicians. In all cases, the orthotic provision approach is individually tailored to each client, beginning with categorization by diagnosis and then adapting the approach according to the client's performance, cognition, and occupational needs.

Factors Influencing the Orthotic Approach

The following sections offer specific hints that elaborate on areas of the orthotic evaluation the therapist can use with clinical reasoning. (See Chapter 5 for essential components to include in a thorough hand evaluation.)

Age

The client's age is important for many reasons. Barring other problems, most children, adolescents, and adults can wear orthoses according to the respective protocol. An infant or toddler, however, can usually get out of any orthosis at any time or place. Extraordinary and creative methods are often necessary to keep orthoses on these youngsters.[4] Older clients, especially those with diminished functional and cognitive capacities, may require careful monitoring by the caregiver to ensure a proper fit and adherence with the wearing schedule. For more information about working with older adults refer to Chapter 15 and for pediatrics refer to Chapter 16.

Occupation

From the interview with the client, family, and caregiver (and from the medical record review), the therapist surmises the impact that an orthosis may have on occupational function, economic status, and social well-being. The therapist carefully considers the meaning that the upper extremity condition has for the client, how the client has dealt with medical conditions in the past, how the client's condition may change as a result of the orthotic provision, and the client's social environment. Thus, when choosing the orthotic design and material, the therapist considers the client's lifestyle needs.

The following are some specific questions to reflect on when determining lifestyle needs:

- What valued occupations, such as work or sports, will the client engage in while wearing the orthosis?
- Do special considerations exist because of rules and regulations for work or sports?
- In what type of environment will the client wear the orthosis? For example, will the orthosis be used in extreme temperatures? Will the orthosis get wet?
- Will the orthosis impede a hand function necessary to the client's job or home activities?
- What is the client's normal schedule, and how will wearing an orthosis impact that schedule?

If a physician refers a client for a wrist immobilization orthosis because of wrist strain, the therapist might contemplate the following question: Is the client a construction worker who does heavy manual work or a computer operator who does light, repetitious work? A construction worker may require an orthosis of stronger material with extremely secure strapping. The computer operator may benefit from lighter, thinner thermoplastic material with wide soft straps. In some situations, the client may best benefit from a prefabricated orthosis.

The therapist determines the client's activity status, including when the client is wearing an orthosis that does not allow for function or movement (such as a positioning orthosis). If the client must return to work immediately, albeit in a limited capacity, the orthosis must always be secure. Proper instructions regarding appropriate care of the limb and the orthosis are necessary. This care may involve elevation of the affected extremity, wound management, and periodic range of motion (ROM) exercises while the client is working.

When the client plans to continue in a sports program (professional, school, or community-based), the therapist checks the rules and regulations governing that particular sport. Rules and regulations usually prevent athletes from wearing hard thermoplastic material during participation in the sport, unless the orthotic design includes exterior and interior padding. Therapists need to communicate with the coach or referee to determine appropriateness of an orthosis[67] and perhaps consider alternative interventions, such as applying Kinesio tape to the area.

Expected Environment

The therapist must consider the client's discharge environment. Some clients return to their own homes and have families and friends who can lend assistance if necessary. For those clients returning to inpatient units or nursing homes, therapists consider instructing the staff in the care and use of the orthoses. If clients return to psychiatric units or prison wards, consider whether supervision is necessary so that orthoses are not used as weapons to harm themselves or others.

Activities of Daily Living Responsibilities

The therapist considers the following question: Is the client able to successfully complete all activities of daily living (ADLs) and instrumental activities of daily living (IADLs) if an orthosis needs to be worn? For example, the therapist may consider how a client can successfully prepare a meal wearing an orthosis that immobilizes one extremity. In that case, the therapist may address one-handed meal-preparation techniques.

Client Adherence and Motivation

Orthotic provision requires adherence on many levels including attending therapy sessions, following wearing schedules and home programs, and adhering to safety expectations.[45] The terminologies of adherence and compliance are often discussed interchangeably, but there are differences with the definitions. Compliance can be perceived as follow through with intervention instructions. **Adherence** can be perceived as more client-centered as the client collaborates with the intervention. Adherence is currently the more utilized term.[36] The World Health Organization (WHO) defines adherence as "numerous health-related behaviours"[66] and discusses five dimensions of adherence related to factors and interventions which include: "(1) social economic, (2) health system and health care team, (3) therapy, (4) condition, and (5) patient."[66] Other considerations affecting adherence with intervention regimens include external factors, such as socioeconomic status and family support. Internal factors such as the client's perception of the severity of the condition are also considered. Knowledge, beliefs, and attitudes about the condition can influence adherence.[9,26]

There is a limited amount of research investigating how adherence relates to clients with hand injuries[25,34] or with orthotic provision. A recent systematic review[45] considered adherence with orthotic wear in adults. Six studies met the selection criteria for a total of 490 subjects. The author concluded that there was "no consistent correlation [with adherence to orthotic wear] to age or gender" or to "socioeconomic and condition related factors."[45] However, the author found some evidence supporting the importance of intervention factors (such as the comfort of the orthosis) and impact of the orthosis on lifestyle and occupations.

Another factor addressed in research is the psychosocial construct of locus of control, which proposes a relationship between a client's perception of control over intervention outcomes and the likelihood that the client will adhere to intervention. This perception of control can be internally or externally based.[9] For example, an internally-motivated client would follow an orthotic schedule based on self-motivation. An externally-motivated client may need encouragement from the therapist or caregiver to follow an orthotic-wearing schedule. Often not discussed with adherence are organizational variables and clinic environment issues, such as transportation problems, interference with daily schedule, wait time, inconsistent therapists, and clinic location.[34]

The therapist can positively influence the client's adherence and motivation to wear an orthosis. Establishing goals together may encourage the client to follow through with the intervention. Perhaps completing an occupation-focused assessment, such as the Canadian Occupational Performance Measure (COPM), can encourage the client to wear the orthosis.[35] If the goals determined by the COPM are improvement of hand function, the therapist discusses how the orthosis will meet these goals. Furthermore, it is important for the therapist to examine intervention goals in relation to the client's goals, because there might be disparity between them.[34] Sometimes the client will have input about the orthotic design, which should be considered seriously by the therapist. Therapists should convey to clients that success with rehabilitation and orthoses involves shared responsibility. To attain the therapeutic goal, the therapist must always reiterate the client's responsibilities in the intervention plan.

In addition, the therapist should perceive the client as a whole individual with a lifestyle beyond the clinic, not just as a client with an injury. Paramount to adherence is education about the medical necessity of wearing the orthoses. The therapist should consider the client's perspectives on the impact of the orthoses on lifestyle. Education should be repetitive throughout the time the client wears the orthosis.[26,54] When the therapist and the physician communicate clearly about the type of orthosis necessary, the client receives consistent information regarding the rationale for wearing the orthosis. Showing the way the orthosis works and explaining the goal of the orthosis enhances client adherence.

Adherence involves both therapist and client (Box 6-2).[34] Rather than labelling the client as noncompliant or uncooperative, therapists must make a serious attempt to help the client better cope with the injury. The therapist should be an empathetic listener as the client learns to adjust to the diagnosis and to the orthosis. The therapist can ask questions of the patient to assist the therapist in eliciting pertinent information from clients about orthotic adherence, fit, and follow-up (Box 6-3).

Others can also have an impact on client adherence. Sometimes a peer wearing an orthosis can be a positive role model to help a client who is not adhering to the plan. A supportive spouse or caregiver encourages adherence, and physician support influences adherence. Sometimes a client may need more structured psychosocial support from mental health personnel.

Selection of an appropriate design may alleviate a client's difficulty in adjusting to an injury and wearing an orthosis.

Box 6-2   Examples of Factors That May Influence Adherence with Orthotic Wear

Organizational/Clinic Environment
- Time involved with orthotic wear
- Interference with life tasks
- Inconsistent therapists
- Transportation issues
- Long wait time for therapy
- Inconvenient clinic location
- Noisy clinic with little privacy

Client
- Belief in the efficacy of wearing an orthosis
- Belief in one's ability to follow through with the orthosis-wearing schedule
- Poor social support

Intervention
- Orthosis is uncomfortable
- Orthosis is cumbersome
- Orthosis is poorly made

Therapeutic Relationship and Communication
- Inconsistent communication between therapists and physicians concerning the orthosis
- Poor understanding, difficulty reading, or being forgetful about instructions on orthotic wear and care

Adapted from Kirwan T, Tooth L, Harkin C: Compliance with hand therapy programs: therapists' and patients' perceptions, *J Hand Ther* 15(1):31-40, 2002.

Box 6-3   Questions for Follow-up Telephone Calls or Email Communication Regarding Clients with Orthoses

The following open- and closed-ended questions may assist the therapist in eliciting pertinent information from clients about orthotic adherence, fit, and follow-up. Closed-ended questions usually elicit a brief response, often a yes or no.
- Have you been wearing your orthosis according to the schedule I gave you? If no, why aren't you wearing your orthosis?
- Have you noticed any reddened or painful areas after removing your orthosis? If so, where?
- Is the orthosis easy to put on and take off?
- Are there any tasks you want to do but cannot do when wearing your orthosis?
- Do you have any concerns about your orthotic-wearing schedule or care?
- Are there any broken or faulty components on your orthosis?
- Do you have any questions for me?
- Do you know how to reach me?
- Have you noticed any increased swelling or pain since you've been wearing the orthosis?
  Open-ended questions elicit a qualitative response that may give the therapist more information.
- Will you tell me about a typical day and when you put your orthosis on and take it off?
- What concerns, if any, might you have about your orthotic wear and care schedule?
- What precautions have you been taking in regard to monitoring your orthotic wear?
- How is the orthosis affecting your activities at home and at work?
- Are there any areas to improve with our clinic management, which would help with your follow-through with orthotic wear?
- Can you tell me how you would contact me if you need to do so?
- Do you have any questions for me?

Therapists should ask themselves many questions as they consider the best design. (See the questions listed in the section on procedural reasoning in Table 6-1.)

In addition to orthotic design, material selection (e.g., soft versus hard) may influence satisfaction with an orthosis.[12] People with rheumatoid arthritis who wear a soft prefabricated orthosis consider comfort and ease of use when involved in activities, which are important factors for orthotic satisfaction.[55] (See the discussion of advantages and disadvantages of prefabricated soft orthoses in Chapter 3.)

Making the orthosis aesthetically pleasing helps with adherence. A client is less likely to wear an orthosis that is messy or sloppy. This is especially true of children and adolescents for whom personal appearance is often an important issue. Therapists need to think of an orthosis as a representation of their work, because other people will see it in public and may inquire about it.

Thermoplastic and strapping materials are now available in a variety of colors. Clients, both children and adults, who are coping successfully with the injury may want to have fun with the orthosis and select one or more colors. However, a client who is having a difficult time adjusting to the injury may not want to wear an orthosis in public at all, let alone an orthosis with a color that draws more attention.

Finally, fabrication of a correct-fitting orthosis on the first attempt eases a client's anxiety. The therapist is responsible for listening to the client's complaints and adjusting the orthosis. A therapist's attitude about orthotic adjustments makes a difference. If the therapist seems relaxed, the client may consider adjustment time a normal part of the orthotic fabrication process. Encouraging effective communication with the client facilitates understanding and satisfaction about orthotic provision.

Cognitive Status

When a client is unable to attend to the therapy program and follow the orthotic intervention regimen because of cognitive status, the therapist must educate the family, caregiver, or staff members. Education includes medical reasons for the orthotic provision, wearing schedule, home program, precautions, and cleaning. Education leads to better cooperation. Sometimes the therapist selects designs and techniques to maximize the client's independence. For example, instructions are written directly on the orthosis. Symbols, such as suns and moons to represent the time of day, can be used in written instructions of wearing schedules.[52] Simple communication strategies (such as showing the client a sheet with a smiley face, neutral face, or frowning face) can be used to determine how the client feels about orthotic comfort.

Orthotic Intervention Approach and Design Considerations

The five approaches to orthotic design are dorsal, palmar, radial, ulnar, and circumferential. The therapist must determine the type of orthosis to fabricate, such as a mobilization orthosis or immobilization orthosis. Understanding the purpose of the orthosis clarifies these decisions. For example, when working with a client who has a radial nerve injury, the therapist may choose to fabricate a dorsal torque transmission orthosis (wrist flexion: index-small finger metacarpophalangeal [MCP] extension/index-small finger MCP flexion, wrist extension torque transmission orthosis)[3] to substitute for the loss of motor function in the wrist and MCP extensors. On the basis of clinical reasoning, the therapist may also choose to fabricate a palmar-based wrist extension immobilization orthosis once the client regains function of the MCP extensors. The wrist orthosis allows the client to engage in functional activities.

In addition to the information that the therapist obtains from a thorough evaluation, other factors dictate orthosis choice. To determine the most efficient and effective orthosis choice, the therapist must consider the physician's orders, the diagnosis, the therapist's judgment, the payment source, and the client's function.

Physician's Orders

Physicians often predetermine the orthotic-application approach on the basis of their training, surgical technique, and evidence in the literature. As discussed, sometimes the therapist may apply clinical reasoning to determine a different orthotic design or material than what was ordered. In that case, the therapist calls the physician.

Diagnosis

Frequently, the diagnosis mandates the approach to orthotic design. The diagnosis determines the number of joints that the therapist must involve. The least number of joints possible should be restricted while allowing the orthosis to accomplish its purpose. Diagnosis also determines positioning and whether the orthosis should be of the mobilization or immobilization type. For example, using one early mobilization protocol for a flexor tendon repair, the therapist places the orthosis on the dorsum of the forearm and hand to protect the tendon and to allow for rubber band traction. The wrist and MCP joints should be in a flexed position. (Alternatively, some physicians now prefer a neutral wrist position to block extension.) These orthoses protect the repair and allow early tendon glide. In this example, the repaired structures and the need to begin tendon gliding guide the approach. (See Chapter 12 for more information on mobilization orthotic fabrication with tendon repairs.)

Therapist's Judgment

The therapist determines the orthotic design and type on the basis of knowledge and experience. For example, after a carpal tunnel release, the therapist can place a wrist immobilization orthosis dorsally or volarly directly over the surgical

Table 6-2   Common Positioning Choices in Orthotic Design

ORTHOSIS	VOLAR	DORSAL	RADIAL	ULNAR
Hand immobilization hand orthosis	X	X	—	—
Wrist immobilization orthosis	X	X	—	X
Thumb orthosis	X	X	X	—
Ulnar nerve orthosis (anticlaw)	—	X	—	X
Radial nerve orthosis	—	X	—	—
Median nerve orthosis (thumb CMC palmar abduction mobilization orthosis)	X	X	X	—
Elbow positioning orthosis	X	X	—	—
Mobilization hand extension orthosis	—	X	—	—
Mobilization hand flexion orthosis	X	—	—	—

CMC, Carpometacarpal.

site. As an advocate of early scar management, the therapist chooses a palmar orthosis and adds silicone elastomer or Otoform to the orthosis.

Client's Function

The client's primary task responsibilities may influence the type of orthosis. A construction worker's wrist has different demands placed on it than the wrist of a computer operator with the same diagnosis. Not only does the therapist choose different materials for each client, but the design approach may be different. A thumb-hole volar wrist immobilization orthosis decreases the risk of the orthosis migrating up the arm during the construction worker's activities, because it tightly conforms to the hand. The computer operator may prefer a dorsal wrist immobilization orthosis to allow adequate sensory feedback and unimpeded flexibility of the digits during keyboard use. (See Chapter 7 for patterns of wrist orthoses.)

Table 6-2 outlines a variety of positioning choices for orthotic design. However, therapists should not view these suggestions as strict rules. For example, a skin condition (such as eczema) may necessitate that a mobilization extension orthosis be volarly-based rather than dorsally-based.

Clinical Reasoning Considerations for Designing and Planning the Orthosis

The orthotic designing and planning process involves many clinical decisions about materials and techniques the therapist can use. (Refer to chapters throughout this book for more specific information about materials and techniques.) Initial considerations are often related to infection control procedures.

Infection-Control Procedures

The therapist considers whether dressing changes are necessary. If so, the therapist follows universal precautions and maintains a sterile environment. The therapist should be aware that skin maceration under an orthosis can occur more easily in the presence of a draining wound. With skin maceration, the therapist first carefully applies a dressing to absorb the fluid. Orthotic fabrication should take place over the dressing, and the therapist should instruct the client in how to apply new dressings at appropriate intervals.[53] Before the application of the thermoplastic material, the therapist can place a stockinette over the client's bandages to prevent the thermoplastic material from sticking to the bandages.

If the client has a draining or infected wound, the therapist does not use regular strapping material to hold the orthosis in place to absorb bacteria. Instead, the therapist uses gauze bandages that are replaced at each dressing change. If a client is unwilling or unable to change a dressing, the therapist can instruct a family member or friend to do so. If assistance is not possible, the client may need to visit the therapist more frequently.

Time Allotment for Orthotic Fabrication and Client and Nursing or Caregiver Education

The therapist considers the time required for orthotic fabrication and education. Fabrication time varies according to the complexity of the orthosis and the client's ability to comply with the fabrication process. For example, squirmy babies and people with spasticity are more difficult to fabricate an orthosis for and require more time. In these cases, it may be beneficial to have an additional staff member or a caregiver help position the client.

Orthotic fabrication time is also dependent on the therapist's experience. If possible, a beginning therapist should schedule a large block of time for orthotic fabrication. As therapists gain clinical experience, they require less time to fabricate orthoses. With any orthotic application, the therapist should allow enough time for educating the client, family, and caregiver about the wear schedule, precautions, and their responsibility in the rehabilitation process. As discussed, education helps with adherence.

Batteson[7] found that in an institutional setting, a nurse training program (developed by the occupational therapist) that addressed orthotic fabrication was very helpful in increasing adherence with an orthotic-wearing schedule. This program included orthotic rationale, common orthotic care questions, and familiarization with thermoplastic materials. A nurse liaison was identified to deal specifically with the client's orthosis concerns. In addition, an orthotic resource file developed by the therapist was made available to the nurses. A similar system could be created on the computer.

Post-Fabrication Monitoring

The therapist uses clinical reasoning skills to thoroughly evaluate and monitor the fabricated orthosis. In particular, the therapist must be aware of pressure areas and edema.

Monitoring Pressure

Regardless of its purpose or design, the orthosis requires monitoring to determine effects on the skin. A client wearing an orthosis is superimposing a hard lever system on an existing lever system that is covered by skin, a living tissue that requires an adequate blood supply. The therapist must therefore follow mechanical principles during orthotic fabrication to avoid excessive pressure on the skin. With fabrication, therapists weigh the pros and cons of the amount of orthotic coverage. With minimal coverage from an orthosis, there is increased mobility. Increased coverage by an orthosis allows for more protection and better pressure distribution. To reduce pressure, the therapist designs an orthosis that covers a larger surface area.[22] Warning signs of an ill-fitting orthosis are red marks, indentations, and ulcerations on the skin.

A well-fitting orthosis, after its removal, may leave a red area on the client's skin. This normal response to the pressure of the orthosis disappears within seconds. When an orthosis exerts too much pressure on one area (usually occurs over a bony prominence) the redness may last longer. For clients of color, in whom redness is not easily visible, the therapist may lightly touch the skin to determine the presence of hot spots or warmer skin. Another way to check skin temperature is with a thermometer. With any orthosis, the therapist checks the skin after 20 to 30 minutes of wearing time before the client leaves the clinic. If red areas are present after 20 to 30 minutes of wearing the orthosis, adjustments need to be made.

A client with intact sensibility who has an ill-fitting orthosis usually requests an adjustment or simply discards the orthosis because it is not comfortable. For a condition in which sensation is absent, vigorous orthotic monitoring is critical.[10,22] The therapist teaches the client and the family to remove the orthosis every 1 to 2 hours to check the skin so as to avoid skin breakdown.

Monitoring for Skin Maceration

Wet, white, macerated skin can occur when the skin under an orthosis holds too much moisture. Skin maceration occurs for many reasons, such as a child drooling on an orthosis. When this happens to a client with intact skin who has simply

forgotten to remove the orthosis, the therapist can easily correct the problem by washing and drying the area. Educating the client about proper care of the hand and providing a polypropylene stockinette to absorb moisture should resolve this situation.

Monitoring Edema

A therapist frequently needs to fabricate an orthosis for an edematous extremity. Edema is often present after surgery, in the presence of infection, with severe trauma (e.g., from a burn), or with vascular or lymphatic compromise. A well-designed, well-fitting orthosis can reduce edema and prevent the sequelae of tissue damage and joint contracture. A poorly-designed or ill-fitting orthosis can contribute to the damaging results of persistent edema. Generally, the design and fit principles already discussed in this text apply.

The therapist considers the method used to hold the orthosis in place. Soft, wide straps accommodate increases in edema and are better able to distribute pressure than rigid, non-yielding Velcro straps.[13] When too tight, strapping can contribute to pitting edema as a result of hampered lymphatic flow.[15] For severe edema, the therapist may gently apply a wide elastic wrap to keep the orthosis in place. The continuous contact of the wrap helps reduce edema.[15] Therapists should be cautioned that straps applied at intervals may further restrict circulation and cause "windowpane" edema distally and between the straps. When using Ace wraps or compressive gauze, the therapist must apply them in a spiral pattern and use gradient distal-to-proximal pressure. The therapist must properly monitor the orthosis and wrap to ensure that the wrap does not roll or bunch.[36] Pressure created by rolling or bunching could cause constriction and further edema and stiffness.

If the lymphatic system is not damaged, edema reduction usually begins relatively quickly with appropriate wound healing (i.e., no infection), proper elevation, and gentle active exercises as permitted. As edema resolves, the therapist remolds the orthosis to fit the new configuration of the extremity. The therapist asks the client with severe edema to return to the clinic daily for monitoring and intervention. When the edema appears to be within the normal postoperative range, the therapist asks the client to return to the clinic in 3 to 5 days for an orthotic check. Helping the client understand the frequency and purpose of the orthotic adjustments is also important. Again, education is an important part of the edema-reduction regimen.[38]

Monitoring Physical and Functional Status

When a client's physical or functional status changes, an orthotic adjustment is often necessary. If a client is receiving intervention for a specific injury and it is effective, the orthosis requires adjustments in conjunction with improvement. For example, if a client has a median nerve injury in which the thumb has an adduction contracture, the therapist fabricates a thumb carpometacarpal (CMC) palmar abduction mobilization orthosis[3] to gradually widen the tight web space. As intervention progresses and thumb motions increase, the therapist adjusts the orthosis to accommodate the gains in motion.[48]

Evaluation and Adjustment of Orthoses

After fabricating the orthosis, the therapist carefully evaluates the design to determine fit and necessary adjustments. The therapist looks carefully at the orthosis when the client is and is not wearing it and considers whether the orthosis serves its purpose. The orthosis should be functional for the client and should accomplish the goals for which it was intended. It should also have a design that uses correct biomechanical principles and should be cosmetically appealing. (Refer to specific chapters in this book for hints and orthosis-evaluation forms.)

Therapists learn from self-reflection before, during, and after each orthosis is made. Reflection helps fine-tune critical thinking skills. The following are reflective questions that the therapist can consider after orthotic fabrication:
* Did the orthosis accomplish the purpose for which it was intended?
* Is it correctly fitted according to biomechanical principles?
* Did I select the best materials for the orthosis?
* Did I take into consideration fluctuating edema?
* Is it cosmetically appealing?
* Is it comfortable for the client and free of pressure areas?
* Have I addressed how orthotic intervention impacts the client's valued occupations?
* Have I addressed functional considerations?
* What would I do differently if I were to refabricate this orthosis?
* Did I properly educate the client/caregiver about the orthosis?

If major adjustments are required, the therapist should avoid using a heat gun except to smooth the orthotic edges. If the therapist has selected the appropriate simple orthotic design and has used a thermoplastic product that is easily reheatable and remoldable, the water-immersion method is the best way to adjust the orthosis. Years of experience demonstrate that reheating the entire orthosis in water and reshaping it is more efficient than spot heating. The activity of the therapist reheating and adjusting one spot often affects the adjacent area, thereby producing another area requiring adjustment. This cycle may not end until the orthosis is useless. When possible, the therapist should use an orthosis product that is reheatable in water and easily reshapable to obtain a proper fit for the client.

Orthotic-Wearing Schedule Factors

Development of an orthotic-wearing schedule for a client is sometimes extremely frustrating for a novice therapist, because there are no magic numbers or formulas for each type of orthosis or diagnostic population. The therapist tailors and customizes the wearing schedule to the individual and exercises clinical judgment. Only general guidelines for orthotic-wearing schedules exist.

In the case of joint limitation, the therapist increases the wearing frequency and time as much as the client can tolerate. Alternatively, the therapist adjusts the intervention plan to try a different orthosis. If motion is increasing steadily, the therapist may decrease the orthotic-wearing time, allowing the client to engage in function by using the limited joint or joints. If the orthosis improves function or the extremity requires protection, the client wears the orthosis when necessary. The following are questions to consider when determining a wearing schedule:
* What is the purpose of the orthosis?
* Does the therapist anticipate that the client will be compliant with an orthotic-wearing schedule?
* Does the client have any medical contraindications or precautions for removing the orthosis?
* Which variables may affect the client's tolerance of the orthosis?
* Does the client need assistance to apply or remove the orthosis?
* Is the orthosis for day or night use, or both?
* Does the client need to apply or remove the orthosis for functional activities?
* How often does the client need to perform exercise and hygiene tasks?

Answers to these questions should guide the development of a wearing schedule. The therapist should keep in mind that the wearing schedule may require adjustment as the client's condition progresses. In any situation, the therapist should discuss the wearing schedule with the client and caregiver (Box 6-4).

Discontinuation of an Orthosis

No distinct rules exist concerning discontinuation of an orthosis. Frequently the physician makes the decision to discontinue an orthosis. Other times the physician defers to the clinical judgment of the therapist to determine when an orthosis is no longer beneficial. Specific protocols, such as for a flexor tendon repair, indicate when an orthosis is discontinued. In such cases, the therapist should contact the physician for a discharge order. Sometimes physicians order an orthosis to be discontinued "cold turkey." If the therapist clinically reasons that the client would benefit from being weaned off the orthosis, the physician should be contacted. The therapist should communicate the rationale for the weaning and ask for approval. The following are questions to consider when making the clinical decision to discontinue an orthosis:
* Have the client and the caregivers been compliant with the orthotic-wearing schedule? If not, why?
* What are the original objectives for orthotic provision, and has the client accomplished them?

Box 6-4   Sample Wearing Schedule

Person's name:

Name of orthosis:

The purpose of this orthosis is to maintain the hand in a functional position.

Prescribed wearing schedule:

8 AM to 12 PM On*

12 PM to 2 PM Off Provide PROM

2 PM to 6 PM On*

6 PM to 8 PM Off Provide PROM

8 PM to 12 AM On*

12 AM to 2 AM Off Provide PROM

2 AM to 6 AM On*

6 AM to 8 AM Off Provide PROM

Wear the orthosis on the right upper extremity. Please contact J. Smith at [phone number] in the Occupational Therapy Department if any of the following occur:

- Pink or reddened areas
- Complaints of increased pain because of the orthosis
- Increased swelling with orthotic wear
- Skin rash
- Complaints of decreased sensation because of the orthosis

---

*Skin check to be performed.

PROM, Passive range of motion.

- Will the same objectives be compromised or accomplished without an orthosis?

Adherence of the person and the caregiver is essential for success with an orthotic-wearing regimen. If the client is not wearing the orthosis, the therapist first uses clinical reasoning to identify the reasons for nonadherence. For example, the nonadherence of an older client in an institutional setting could be the result of one or more of the following factors:

- Poor communication among the staff about the wearing schedule
- Poor staff follow-through with the wearing schedule
- The older adult's lack of understanding about the orthosis' purpose
- Discomfort of the orthosis
- The older adult's fear of hidden costs associated with the orthosis
- The older adult's dislike of the orthosis' cosmetic appearance

Reasons for nonadherence could be beyond this list, and it would be up to the therapist to ascertain the problem. After identifying the reason or reasons for nonadherence, the therapist can work on possible solutions.

An important factor in determining when to discontinue the orthosis is a careful review of the orthosis' objectives. For example, a therapist fabricates a mobilization orthosis for a client who has a proximal interphalangeal (PIP) soft-tissue flexion contracture of the middle finger. The objective is mobilization of the PIP joint to help correct the flexion deformity. Gradually, the orthosis facilitates lengthening of the restricting structures and extension is restored. By monitoring ROM and evaluating the orthosis' line of pull, the therapist determines that the orthosis has maximally helped the client and that the original intervention objectives were accomplished. At this time, the therapist calls the physician for an order to discontinue the orthosis.

Therapists must consider whether accomplishment of the objectives is possible without the orthosis. Timely discontinuation of any orthosis is important. Therapists should keep in mind that inappropriately-provided or poorly-fabricated orthoses can restrict movement, make postural compromises by causing atrophy in one muscle group and overuse in another, and injure other parts of the anatomy. In addition, preventing the client's dependence on an orthosis is important. When the client has the functional capabilities, therapists should adjust the orthotic-wearing schedule to gradually wean the client away from the orthosis.[47]

Cost and Payment Issues

Two issues exist regarding the cost of orthoses. First, how does the therapist arrive at the price of an orthosis? Second, how does the therapist receive payment for an orthosis? To calculate the price of an orthosis, the therapist totals the direct and indirect costs (Box 6-5). Direct costs include items such as the thermoplastic material, strapping material, stockinette, rivets, shipping costs, tax, and so on. A hospital or clinic purchases supplies at wholesale cost. However, a percentage markup may appear on the cost. (This assists with replenishing the inventory.) Indirect costs include non-disposable supplies (such as scissors and fry pans), the time required for the average therapist to make the orthosis, and overhead costs (such as rent and electricity).

As a result of tighter control of health-care dollars many therapists are finding that payment for orthoses is becoming increasingly difficult. It is important that when necessary the therapist take an active role in the outcome of a payment policy of an insurance plan regarding the orthoses. This may help obtain payment for the orthosis. For example, the therapist communicates with the case manager the purpose of the orthosis.

The therapist must remember, however, that the plan belongs to the client, not to the therapist. If a particular insurance plan reimburses costs partially or not at all, the therapist should inform the client of the responsibility for paying the balance of the cost. Some facilities make accommodations for people who are uninsured or underinsured and need orthotic provision, or there might be a pro bono clinic available in the area. In addition, the therapist should provide specific documentation to insurance companies about the affected extremity and the type of orthosis and purpose of the orthosis.[20]

It is important that therapists know how to effectively navigate the system to receive payment for orthotic fabrication. If an orthosis is ordered, it needs to be made. The therapist and the client should work out financial aspects with the facility and communicate with the appropriate clients, such

---

Box 6-5   Hints for Determining Direct and Indirect Costs

Direct Costs	Indirect Costs

• Thermoplastic Material
  • Know cost of sheet
  • Estimate how much of the sheet you used
  • Determine cost (¼ sheet used)
• Strapping
  • Know cost per inch
  • Charge for number of inches used
• Padding
  • Know cost per square inch
  • Charge for number of square inches used
• Chemicals (cold spray, glue, solvent, and so on)
  • Usually a small set amount is charged whenever chemicals are used
• Other materials (finger loops, outrigger kit, D-rings, and so on)
  • Charge the purchase amount
• Time
  • Know cost per unit of time
  • Charge for number of units used to make the orthosis
	• Lighting, space, fry pan, hydrocollator, scissors, heat gun, shipping, handling, and storage charges for materials
	• Indirect costs are usually figured in a percentage markup of the direct costs of an orthosis (for example, a 10% markup cost)

as billing personnel. Payment is always determined by the payer source. Generally, when billing, insurance companies expect a line item bill detailing all charges applied including therapy codes, such as Current Procedural Terminology (CPT) codes[14] and supply charges. CPT codes are numeric codes covering tasks and services for payment.

In an inpatient setting, costs for orthoses are often bundled and payment is determined by pre-set contracted amounts. Medicare patients are paid according to diagnostic-related group (DRG) categories. Regardless, therapists still figure the direct and indirect costs for the materials and fabrication process. After the insurance company is billed, the company pays based on a DRG or a cost outlier, which is payment for services that are costlier than others in the DRG. A cost outlier method may be applied in instances where the DRG payment is significantly below the expenses spent on intervention with the particular client. Some facilities negotiate reduced rates for clients who self-pay for services.[41]

For outpatient services, coding systems are also used for payment of orthoses. With Medicare Part B (outpatient therapy) therapists access Level I and Level II codes of the Healthcare Common Procedure Coding System (HCPCS) codes[14] and the terminology "orthotics" is used with billing—not "splinting." For Level I codes, therapists utilize the Medicare Physician Fee Schedule (MPFS) to determine the proper CPT codes. Different pricing exists for the MPFS between states. With orthotics, the most frequently-used code is 97760 covering "orthotics management and training" and another commonly-utilized CPT code is 97762 covering "adjustments/modifications of an orthosis or prosthetic."[2] Level II HCPCS codes address products and supplies including orthotics.[14] Coverage for orthotic materials is located in section "A" and for orthotic procedural codes in section "L." L-codes "give a brief description of the device and state whether the device needs to be molded to a patient, custom fabricated, custom fitted, or have no fitting specifications."[11] For example L3808 denotes a "Wrist hand finger orthosis, rigid without joints, may include soft interface material; straps, custom fabricated, includes fitting and adjustment."[27] L-codes are commonly used with billing from other insurers besides Medicare, and in that case other payers may have different L-code lists. Additionally, payers often have their own negotiated rates of payment.[16] There are specific guidelines for filing a claim depending upon the setting where the services are provided, such as for hospital outpatient, SNF Part B, in private practice, or in a physician's office practice.

For some clients with upper extremity problems that occurred on the job, rehabilitation is reimbursed from the worker's compensation system. Therapists must keep in mind that in every state worker's compensation laws are interpreted differently. Therefore, it is important to be familiar with the state guidelines. Most state worker's compensation plans cover medical costs related to the injury, such as medical care (including receiving an orthosis), vocational rehabilitation, and temporary disability. (The amount varies from state to state.)[5] Many states have adopted a managed care system. With case managers, the therapist should provide consistent and clear communication about the client's progress.

Some insurance companies simply refuse to pay for orthoses, and others ask for so much documentation that more time is required to prepare the bill than to make the orthosis. For example, some insurance companies ask therapists for original invoices for the purchase of thermoplastic and strapping materials. Developing outcome studies or finding evidence in the literature may help obtain payment from insurers. Giving these outcomes to insurers will increase their understanding of the importance of orthotic intervention in its relation to function. The American Society of Hand Therapists[3] published *Splint Classification Systems*, a book about naming and designing orthoses. This book helps terminology become more uniform.[3]

Policy Regulations: The Health Insurance Portability and Accountability Act

This broad health legislation enacted in 1996 covers many areas with Title II, or Administrative Simplification, influencing therapy practice. Title II includes three main parts: Transaction Rule, Privacy Rule, and Security Rule. The first

Box 6-6 Client Protections

The following are key client protections with a brief description:

- Access to medical records: See or obtain copies of medical records, and ask for corrections of errors.
- Notice of privacy practice: Covered providers must provide information on how personal medical information will be used and patient rights under HIPPA regulations.
- Limits on use of personal medical information: Sets guidelines on minimal standards of health care information sharing.
- Prohibition on marketing: Sets guidelines on disclosing of client information for marketing purposes.
- Stronger state laws: State laws that are stronger than HIPAA are followed.
- Confidential communications: Clients can request that confidentiality be kept (e.g., asking the therapist to call his or her work instead of home).
- Complaints: Clients have a right to file a formal complaint.

part, Transaction Rule, affects billing procedures. It mandates uniform national requirements for formats and codes for electronic transmission.[65]

Privacy Rule is another major component of Administrative Simplification and directly influences clinical practice. Privacy rules involve protection of client-identifying or confidential information and client rights about their health information. These rules regulate how protected health information (PHI) or any client-identifying information is presented in written, verbal, or electronic format.[60] Therapists should obtain the client's consent prior to using PHI for intervention, payment, or health care operations. However, if a client objects or fails to provide consent, therapists are permitted to use PHI for intervention, payment, or health care operations without the client's consent. In most other circumstances, with very few exceptions, therapists may not disclose PHI without the client's written authorization to do so.[61]

Numerous privacy rights with respect to the client's health information are written into the regulations. For example, clients have a right to request to see their medical record. See Box 6-6 for a listing of client protections. Therapy clinics should have policies in place to protect the privacy of client information. Requiring working charts to be kept in a locked cabinet with the documents shredded after intervention completion is an example of an internal policy protecting privacy.[17] Other guidelines for protecting client privacy apply to usage of electronic health records (EHRs). Some areas of client information are excluded from the law, such as allowing clients to sign in for intervention, calling out a client's name to go into the orthotic fabrication room, or sharing information with another health professional about the orthosis.[17,57] However, reasonable efforts to avoid these types of disclosures should be taken. For instance, instead of calling out, "Mr. Edward Jones, the therapist will see you now to customize your resting hand orthosis," a better approach would be, "Edward, the therapist will see you now."

Incidental disclosures (information that is heard with reasonable efforts to not be overheard) or sharing information that is limited are not considered in violation of the **Health Insurance Portability and Accountability Act (HIPAA)** law.[57] An example of an incidental disclosure is an occupational therapist discussing information about an orthosis bill with the secretary in the waiting room. These disclosures are not considered liable under the law as long as there are no other reasonable options (i.e., no other area for individual privacy to discuss the bill).[56] Because therapy often takes place in an open area with several people involved in conversations, some of which potentially involve sharing of PHI, it needs to be clear in the consent form about the clinic setup.[43] Therapists working in clinics with an open area can employ simple strategies to allow more privacy, such as partitioning off a private area or using a private room available for intervention, communicating with lower voices, and being careful with leaving sensitive messages on answering machines.[68] As York states, "creating a culture of privacy and maintaining good rapport with patients will go a long way to preventing HIPAA complaints as well as other types of legal problems."[68]

The third main part of Administrative Simplification, the Security Rule, involves the policies and procedures that a facility has in place to protect the PHI through "administrative, technical and physical safeguards."[65] The Security Rule mainly focuses on "electronic protected health information,"[65] such as who has access to computer data in a clinic. The simplification provisions include national identifiers for health care providers and practitioners.[62] Finally, therapists must keep abreast of their state privacy laws. If they are stricter, they take priority over the HIPAA regulations.[68]

Documentation

Orthotic application must be well documented. **Documentation** assists in third-party payment and communication with other health care providers, helps ascertain the medical-legal necessity, and demonstrates the efficacy of the intervention. This section overviews general documentation principles to be used with orthotics whether documentation is in written or in electronic format.

Orthotic documentation should be specific and should include several elements, such as the onset of the medical condition that warrants an orthosis; the medical necessity for the orthosis; the level of function before the orthosis; the client's rehabilitation potential with the orthosis; and type, purpose, and anatomical location of the orthosis. Therapists should also document that they have communicated with the client an oral and written wearing schedule and have had discussions about precautions. Any input that the client provides to the intervention plan, such as mutual goal setting, should be documented.

Orthotic documentation, including goal setting, should be related to function. It is not sufficient to document that a client's ROM has improved to a certain level as a result of wearing an orthosis. The therapist should specifically document how the improved ROM has helped the client perform specific functional activities. For example, the therapist may document that because of improved wrist motion from wearing an orthosis, the client is able to use the computer at work.

As with any documentation, the therapist should consider legal implications. Documentation should be thorough, complete, and objective. The therapist should always remember, "If it wasn't documented it didn't happen." For example, the therapist should document the specific measurements by which the hand is positioned and an orthosis fabricated for a client who has de Quervain tenosynovitis. Also for example, if the client has a reddened area as a result of wearing an orthosis, the specific location and size of the reddened area as well as any orthotic adjustments made should be documented. Any communication or advice about the orthosis from the physician should be documented with the time and date of the call.[19]

Documentation for follow-up visits should include the date and time that the client is supposed to return and a notation that the date and time has been discussed with the client. This helps protect the therapist if there are claims of negligence with follow-up care.[19] Documentation for follow-up visits should also include any changes in the orthotic design and wearing schedule. In addition, the therapist should note whether problems with adherence are apparent. Documenting evidence of adherence includes documenting instructions provided and objective client's or caregiver's behavior that contradicts instructions. For example, the therapist might document that the client stated that he or she did not follow the orthotic-wearing schedule. Another example is documenting objective observations of dates and times that the orthotic-wearing schedule is not being followed for a client in a SNF. In this case the therapist may further educate the caregivers and note when and what type of education was completed. If the caregivers still do not properly follow the schedule, the therapist should come up with another plan and involve the caregivers in the decision-making process to ensure adherence.

Another objective observation for a client followed in any setting is notation of signs of wear, such as scratching, light soil, or strap wear. With documentation, it is inappropriate to criticize other health care professionals, such as documenting that contractures developed as a result of the nursing staff who did not apply an orthosis.[19]

The therapist should perform orthotic reassessments regularly until completion of the client's weaning from the orthosis or discharge from services. Documentation after the reassessments should be timely and based on guidelines from the insurer.[19] Finally, the therapist should keep in mind that different facilities use different methods to document, and the therapist should be familiar with the routine method of the facility. (See Examples 6-1 and 6-2 for illustrations of a narrative and a SOAP note for an orthosis, respectively.)

Orthotic Intervention Error and Client Safety Issues

Orthotic intervention errors occur in occupational therapy.[49] Examples of these errors include fabricating the wrong type of orthosis for the condition or failure to follow through with the orthotic-wearing schedule. Either of these errors could cause client harm, such as severe pain or breakdown of the skin. Although many errors are the direct result of individual failure, most errors are caused by system problems. System errors may occur due to diagnostic error, equipment/product failure, or miscommunication of medical orders, to name a few.

Orthotic intervention errors can easily result from incorrect or inadequate communication. A physician, for example, may order a right hand orthosis when it is meant for the left hand. If the therapist fails to question the physician order, an orthosis may be fabricated for the wrong site. Wrong patient, wrong site, or wrong procedure is one of the leading sentinel events reported to the Joint Commission on Accreditation of Healthcare Organizations (JCAHO).[31] According to data collected by the JCAHO, team miscommunication is at the root of a great proportion of all errors made in health care.[32] Occupational therapists often lack assertiveness when communicating with physicians, and this failure to adequately communicate can result in patient harm.[37]

Understanding the nature of hierarchic organizational structures and the need for coordination of care through "interdisciplinary care management" and "coordinated communication" are vital to **client safety.**[29] Occupational therapists need to participate in team training.[33] Team training allows therapists to have the knowledge, skill and attitude competencies,[42] as well as assertiveness and adaptability capability to enhance team effectiveness and the culture of safety.[18]

To create this culture of safety, occupational therapists must also debunk or dispel the myth of performance perfection. To err is human! After all, health care delivery is a very complex system. In complex systems, errors are inevitable regardless of how well-trained, well-intentioned, or ultracareful the individual therapist may be. In the case of the therapist acting on the physician's wrong order, it would be unjust to simply require the last treating practitioner to be fully accountable for the error. In this situation, blaming and sanctioning would only encourage the therapist and/or physician to hide the error rather than disclose and report it.

Today's undisclosed near miss or minor error can become tomorrow's egregiously harmful error. Only by acknowledging error can health practitioners individually and collectively learn from that error and make individual and system practice changes to prevent errors in the future. Furthermore, truthful disclosure of error to clients by the therapist or a disclosure team is not only an ethical obligation but organizations (such as The Joint Commission, the University of Michigan Health System, and the Veterans Health Administration) and a number of states (such as Nevada, Florida, California, and Pennsylvania) now mandate disclosure.[30,63]

Part of the disclosure process should be expressions of sympathy and a formal and authentic apology. There is an advocacy organization, The Sorry Works! Coalition[58] that provides disclosure and apology educational programs to practitioners to assist them in communicating with clients that have been harmed by an error.[58,64] In the past, health care practitioners were actually cautioned by their malpractice insurance carriers not to apologize, because an apology might increase the chances of being sued.[6] Currently, at least 36 states have enacted statutes that prevent some or all information given in an apology from being used if a client sues

a practitioner.[28] Clients want to receive apologies and to be told the truth when an error occurs that causes them harm. A number of health care organizations that have instituted disclosure programs now have evidence that disclosing errors can lower liability lawsuit expenses.

Ultimately, creating an environment where practitioners are encouraged and supported for promoting safety, reporting errors, and truthfully disclosing them to clients is everyone's goal. This practice safety goal should always be a guidepost for clinical reasoning when orthotic fabrication failures occur.

SELF-QUIZ 6-1*

Circle either true (T) or false (F) with regard to the following questions.

1. T F An infant can follow an orthotic-wearing program without extraordinary methods.
2. T F Determining a client's lifestyle needs for orthotic design and material is important.
3. T F Paramount to a client's cooperation is education about the medical necessity for wearing an orthosis.
4. T F If a client has a wound that requires dressing changes, the therapist should fabricate the orthosis over the dressing and instruct the client to apply new dressings at appropriate intervals.
5. T F The only sign of an ill-fitting orthosis is red marks.
6. T F A well-fitting orthosis, upon removal, may leave a red area on the client's skin.
7. T F In the presence of severe edema, the therapist should use circumferential straps.
8. T F The therapist should use a heat gun for all necessary adjustments.
9. T F If motion is decreased because of joint limitation, the therapist should decrease the frequency or time the client wears the orthosis.
10. T F When deciding to discontinue an orthosis, the therapist must consider the original objectives of the orthotic fabrication.
11. T F To calculate the cost of an orthosis, the therapist should consider the direct and indirect costs.
12. T F Payment is always determined by the payer source.
13. T F If a client develops a reddened area because of wearing an orthosis, the therapist should just document that fact and note specifics about location or size of the affected area.
14. T F Calling out a client's name in a waiting room to go back into the orthotic fabrication area is considered in violation of HIPAA.

*See Appendix A for the answer key

Review Questions

1. How would a therapist apply the various clinical reasoning models to orthotic provision?
2. What does an orthosis referral include?
3. How can the therapist facilitate communication with the physician's office about the orthosis referral?
4. Why is knowing the client's age important to the therapist when fabricating an orthosis?
5. Which lifestyle needs of the client must the therapist consider with orthotic provision?
6. How can the therapist enhance the adherence of a client wearing an orthosis?
7. What are the infection-control procedures that a therapist should follow with orthotic provision?
8. What should therapists monitor when providing an orthosis for a client during the following conditions: pressure, edema, and physical status of a client?
9. What are the four directions of orthotic design?
10. What are some helpful hints for making adjustments after orthotic fabrication?
11. What are the factors that the therapist should consider when establishing a client on an orthotic-wearing schedule?
12. What are the factors that a therapist should consider for orthosis discontinuation?
13. What are the cost and payment issues the therapist must keep in mind?
14. How might HIPAA influence communication with clients about orthoses in a clinical setting?
15. What documentation issues should the therapist be aware of with orthotic intervention?

References

1. Abraham, M: *CPT 2013 Current procedural terminology standard edition*, Chicago, 2012, American Medical Association.
2. American Occupational Therapy Association (AOTA): *Coding and Billing FAQs*. Retrieved from http://www.aota.org/en/Advocacy-Policy/Federal-Reg-Affairs/Coding/FAQ.aspx, 2007.
3. American Society of Hand Therapists: *Splint classification systems*, Garner, NJ, 1992, The American Society of Hand Therapists.
4. Armstong J: Splinting the pediatric patient. In Fess EE, Gettle KS, Philips CA, et al, editors: *Hand and upper extremity splinting: principles and methods*, ed 3, St Louis, 2005, Elsevier Mosby, pp 480–516.
5. Bailey DM: Legislative and reimbursement influences on occupational therapy: changing opportunities. In Neistadt ME, Crepeau EB, editors: *Willard & Spackman's occupational therapy*, ed 9, Philadelphia, 1998, Lippincott, pp 763–772.
6. Banja J: Does medical error disclosure violate the medical malpractice insurance cooperation clause? In Henriksen K, Battles JB, Marks ES, et al, editors: *Advances in Patient safety: from research to implementation (Volume 3: Implementation Issues)*, Rockville, MD, 2005, Agency for Healthcare Research and Quality (US).
7. Batteson R: A strategy to improve nurse/occupational therapist communication for managing clients with splints, *Br J Occup Ther* 60:451–454, 1997.
8. Benner P, Hughes RG, Sulphen M: Chapter 6: clinical reasoning, decision making, and action: thinking critically and clinically. In Hughes RG, editor: *Patient safety and quality: an evidence-based handbook for nurses*, Rockville, MD, 2008, Agency for Healthcare Research and Quality.
9. Bower KA: Compliance as a patient education issue. In Woldum KM, Ryan-Morrell V, Towson MC, et al, editors: *Patient education: foundations of practice*, Rockville, MD, 1985, Aspen Publications, pp 45–111.
10. Brand PW, Hollister A: *Clinical mechanics of the hand*, ed 2, St Louis, 1993, Mosby.
11. Brown JG: Medicare orthotics, Department of Health and Human Services, Office of Inspector General. http://oig.hhs.gov/oei/reports/oei-02-95-00380.pdf. Accessed February 14, 2014.
12. Callinan NJ, Mathiowetz V: Soft versus hard resting hand splints in rheumatoid arthritis: pain relief, preference, and compliance, *Am J Occup Ther* 50(5):347–353, 1996.
13. Cannon NM, Foltz RW, Koepfer JM, et al.: *Manual of hand splinting*, New York, 1985, Churchill Livingstone.
14. Centers for Medicare & Medicaid Services: HCPCS—general information, *CMS.gov* (website). https://www.cms.gov/MedHCPCSGenInfo/. Accessed February 14, 2014.
15. Colditz JC: Therapist's management of the still hand. In Mackin EJ, Callahan AD, Skirven TM, et al, editors: *Rehabilitation of the hand and upper extremity*, ed 5, St Louis, 2002, Mosby, pp 1021–1049.
16. Cooper: Personal communication, 2012.
17. Costa DM, Whitehouse D: HIPAA and fieldwork, *OT Practice* 8(17):23–24, 2003.
18. Dingley C, Daugherty K, Derieg MK, et al: Improving patient safety through provider communication strategy enhancements. In Henriksen K, Battles JB, Keyes MA, et al., editors, Advances in Patient Safety: New Directions and Alternative Approaches (Vol. 3). Rockville (MD): Agency for Healthcare Research and Quality (US); Available from: http://www.ncbi.nlm.nih.gov/books/NBK43663/
19. Ekelman-Ranke BR: Documentation in the age of litigation, *OT Practice* 3(3):20–24, 1998.
20. Evans RB: Personal communication, February 7, 1995.
21. Facione NC, Facione PA: Critical thinking and clinical judgement. In Facione NC, Facione PA, editors: *Critical thinking and clinical reasoning in the health sciences: an international multidisciplinary teaching anthology*, Milbrae, CA, 2008, The California Academic Press.
22. Fess EE, Gettle KS, Philips CA, et al.: *Hand and upper extremity splinting: principles and methods*, ed 3, St Louis, 2005, Elsevier Mosby.
23. Fleming MH: Conditional reasoning: creating meaningful experiences. In Mattingly C, Fleming MH, editors: *Clinical reasoning: forms of inquiry in a therapeutic practice*, Philadelphia, 1994, FA Davis, pp 197–235.
24. Fleming MH: The therapists with the three-track mind, *Am J Occup Ther* 45:1007–1014, 1991.
25. Groth GN, Wilder DM, Young VL: The impact of compliance of rehabilitation of patients with mallet finger injuries, *J Hand Ther* 7(1):21–24, 1994.
26. Groth GN, Wulf MB: Compliance with hand rehabilitation: health beliefs and strategies, *J Hand Ther* 8(1):18–22, 1995.
27. Buck, C: *2014 HCPCS level II*, ed 1, St. Louis, 2013, Saunders.
28. Ho B, Liu E: Does sorry work? The impact of apology laws on medical malpractice, *J Risk Uncertain* 43:141–167, 2011.
29. Joint Commission on Accreditation of Health Care Organizations: *Patient safety: essentials for healthcare*, ed 3, Oakbrook, IL, 2005, Joint Commission Resources.
30. Joint Commission on Accreditation of Healthcare Organizations: *Patient safety essentials for health care*, ed 5, Oakbrook, IL, 2009, Joint Commission Resources.
31. Joint Commission on Accreditation of Healthcare Organizations: Summary Data of Sentinel Events Reviewed by the Joint Commission, 2004–2011, http://www.jointcommission.org/assets/1/18/2011_Stats_Summary.pdf
32. Joint Commission on Accreditation of Healthcare Organizations: Sentinel Event Data—Root Causes by Event Type, *The Joint Commission* (website). http://www.jointcommission.org/Sentinel_Event_Statistics/. Accessed February 14, 2014.
33. King HB, Battles J, Baker DP, et al.: TeamSTEPPS™: team strategies and tools to enhance performance and patient safety. In Henriksen K, Battles JB, Keyes MA, et al, editors: Advances in patient safety: new directions and alternative approaches, (Vol. 3: Performance and Tools). Rockville, MD, 2008, Agency for Healthcare Research and Quality (US).
34. Kirwan T, Tooth L, Harkin C: Compliance with hand therapy programs: therapists' and patients' perceptions, *J Hand Ther* 15(1):31–40, 2002.
35. Law M, Baptiste S, Carswell A, et al.: *Canadian occupational performance measure*, ed 3, Ottawa, ON, 1998, CAOT Publications.
36. Loue S, Sajatovic M: Adherence. *Encyclopedia of aging and public health*, ed 1, New York, Springer.
37. Cochran TM, Mu K, Lohman H, et al.: Physical therapists' perspectives on practice errors in geriatric, neurologic, or orthopedic settings, *Physiother Theory Pract* 25(1):1–13, 2009.
38. Mackin EJ, Callahan AD, Skirven TM, et al, editors: *Rehabilitation of the hand and upper extremity*, ed 5, St Louis, 2002, Mosby.
39. Mattingly C: The narrative nature of clinical reasoning, *Am J Occup Ther* 45:998–1005, 1991.
40. Mattingly C, Fleming MH: *Clinical reasoning: forms of inquiry in a therapeutic practice*, Philadelphia, 1994, FA Davis.
41. McCreery R: *Personal communication*, March 2012.

42. Mu K, Lohman H, Scheirton L, et al.: Improving client safety: strategies to prevent and reduce practice errors in occupational therapy, *Am J Occup Ther* 65(6):69–76, 2011.

43. Murer CG: Trends and issues: protecting patient privacy, *Rehab Management* 15(3):46–47, 2002.

44. Neistadt ME: Teaching clinical reasoning as a thinking frame, *Am J Occup Ther* 52:211–229, 1998.

45. O'Brien L: Adherence to therapeutic splint wear in adults with acute upper limb injuries: a systematic review, *Hand Ther* 15:3–10, 2010.

46. Parham D: Towards professionalism: the reflective therapist, *Am J Occup Ther* 41:555–560, 1987.

47. Pascarelli E, Quilter D: *Repetitive strain injury*, New York, 1994, John Wiley & Sons.

48. Reynolds CC: Preoperative and postoperative management of tendon transfers after radial nerve injury. In Hunter JM, Mackin EJ, Callahan AD, editors: *Rehabilitation of the hand*, ed 4, St Louis, 1995, Mosby, pp 753–763.

49. Scheirton LS, Mu K, Lohman H: Occupational therapists' responses to practice errors in physical rehabilitation settings, *Am J Occup Ther* 57(3):307–314, 2003.

50. Schell BA, Cervero RM: Clinical reasoning in occupational therapy: an integrated review, *Am J Occup Ther* 47:605–610, 1993.

51. Schon DA: *Educating the reflective practitioner*, San Francisco, 1987, Jossey-Bass.

52. Schultz-Johnson K: *Personal communication*, March 1999.

53. Skotak CH, Stockdell SM: Wound management in hand therapy. In Cromwell FS, Bear-Lehman J, editors: *Hand rehabilitation in occupational therapy*, Binghamton, NY, 1988, Haworth Press, pp 17–35.

54. Southam MA, Dunbar JM: Integration of adherence problems. In Meichenbaum D, Turk DC, editors: *Facilitating treatment adherence*, New York, 1987, Plenum Publishing.

55. Stern EB, Ytterberg SR, Krug HE, et al.: Commercial wrist extensor orthoses: a descriptive study of use and preference in patients with rheumatoid arthritis, *Arthritis Care Res* 10(1):27–35, 1997.

56. Sullivan JM: *Personal communication,* October 12, 2004.

57. Sullivan JM: *The OT's guide to HIPAA: the impact of privacy laws on the practice of occupational therapy*, Minneapolis, MN, 2004, The American Occupational Therapy Association.

58. Wojcieszak D: *Sorry works! Making disclosure a reality for healthcare organizations* (website): http://sorryworks.net/. Accessed February 14, 2014.

59. Trombly C: Anticipating the future: assessment of occupational function, *Am J Occup Ther* 47:253–257, 1993.

60. U.S. Department of Health & Human Services: Fact sheet: Protecting the privacy of patients' health information. http://dlthede.net/informatics/chap20ehrissues/privacyfactsapril03.pdf.

61. U.S. Department of Health & Human Services: What is the difference between "consent" and "authorization" under the HIPAA Privacy Rule? http://www.hhs.gov/ocr/privacy/hipaa/faq/authorizations/264.html.

62. U.S. Department of Health & Human Services: Health information privacy: HIPAA administrative simplification statute and rules, *HHS.gov* (website). http://www.hhs.gov/ocr/privacy/hipaa/administrative/index.html. Accessed February 14, 2014.

63. Veterans Health Administration 2008 [Need full ref]

64. Wojcieszak D, Saxton JW, Finkelstein MM: *Sorry works! Disclosure, apology, and relationships prevent medical malpractice claims*, Bloomington, IN, 2007, AuthorHouse.

65. Wilson HP: HIPAA: the big picture for home care and hospice, *Home Health Care Mang Pract* 16(2):127–137, 2004.

66. World Health Organization: Adherence to long-term therapies: evidence for action (website): http://www.who.int/entity/chp/knowledge/publications/adherence_full_report.pdf?ua=1

67. Wright HH, Rettig A: Management of common sports injuries. In Mackin EJ, Callahan AD, Skirven TM, et al.: *Rehabilitation of the hand and upper extremity*, ed 5, St Louis, 2005, Mosby, pp 2076–2109.

68. York AM: HIPAA smarts: top 10 privacy musts, *Rehab Management* 16(2):44–45, 2003.

Note: This chapter includes content from previous contributions from Sally E. Poole, MA, OTR, CHT and Joan L. Sullivan, MA, OTR, CHT.

APPENDIX 6-1   CASE STUDIES

CASE STUDY 6-1

Read the following scenario, and answer the questions based on information in this chapter.

Steven, a 46-year-old construction worker who has problems with alcohol consumption, awakened from a drinking binge after he fell asleep with his arm over the top of a chair to find that his right hand and wrist were limp. He showed his wife how he could no longer extend his wrist to do activities and stated, "Maybe I had a stroke." Hoping that his function would improve, he waited a few days and then decided to see his primary physician. Steven asserted to his physician that he thought he had a stroke and was concerned about his ability to do work. The physician examined Steven's arm and stated, "I can't say for certain whether it was a small stroke or a nerve injury. In the past with issues like this, I have referred patients to an occupational therapist at an outpatient therapy clinic." Occupational therapy was ordered for intervention and orthotic fabrication. The order was vague as to what type of orthosis.

You are a new therapist at the outpatient clinic. Initial evaluation reveals decreased sensation in the pathway of the radial nerve, absent wrist extension, metacarpophalangeal (MCP) finger extension, and thumb abduction and extension. Please refer to Chapter 13 for information on nerve injuries.

1. What injury do you assume Steven has sustained, and how did he sustain it?
2. How do you clarify the physician's order if you are unsure about it?
3. As a new therapist unsure about which one, where would you find the information about an appropriate orthosis for this patient?
4. After completion of the orthosis, you send Steven home with a home exercise program and instructions about orthotic wear. What type of education and orthotic-wearing schedule will you provide? Why?
5. Upon return to the clinic, Steven states that he does not like wearing the orthosis because, as he states, "It does not fit with my macho image, and it seems like it is taking forever to do any good." He reports minimal wear of the orthosis. How will you handle his nonadherence?

*See Appendix A for the answer key.

CASE STUDY 6-2

Read the following scenario, and answer the questions based on information in this chapter.

Marie, a 57-year-old woman, is employed as a department store clerk. She works part-time, except for during the winter holiday season. She has been in good health with the exception of having diabetes, which is well regulated. Her job demands involve unloading boxes, stocking new merchandise, and operating a cash register. During the winter holiday season, Marie worked 40-hour weeks. In addition, she was busy at home decorating and baking. One week prior to Christmas she noted pain radiating up her dominant right forearm and around the radial styloid.

Marie complained to her employer of pain when moving the thumb and when turning her forearm up. Marie was seen by the company physician, who diagnosed her condition as de Quervain tenosynovitis. She was provided with a prefabricated thumb immobilization orthosis, which she did not wear due to it being uncomfortable and causing some chafing on the volar surface of the thumb IP joint. Two weeks later, when symptoms did not improve, the company physician ordered occupational therapy. The order read: "Fabricate an R thumb orthosis and provide a home exercise program." The following initial therapy note purposely displays flawed documentation.

10-13

Client was followed on 10-13 for fabrication of an orthosis and to provide a home exercise program. Client was wearing a prefabricated orthosis. Reddened areas were noted on the thumb. Client was instructed in a home exercise program, orthotic precautions, and a wearing schedule. It doesn't appear that the client will be compliant with wearing the orthosis.

Results of the evaluation are as follows:

ROM	All ROM was WNL except for the following:
	• Thumb:
	  • DIP flexion, 0-50; MP flexion, 0-30; palmar abduction, 0-30
	  • Radial abduction, 0-30; Opposition: to ring finger
	• Wrist:
	  • Flexion, 0-50; extension, 0-40; ulnar deviation, 0-15; radial deviation, 0-15
	  • FA: supination, 0-45

Strength:	• Grasp strength: R UE, 35#s; L UE, 52#s • Pinch strength: Lateral, tip, and key pinch R UE, 5#s; L UE, 10#s
Edema evaluation:	• Edema noted around area of radial styloid. Circumferential measurement at that area: R UE, 10 cm; L UE, 9 cm.
Volometer reading:	• R UE, 420; L UE, 380
Circulation:	• WNL for Allen testing. Temperature: WNL
Sensory evaluation:	• WNL to Semmes-Weinstein Monofilament Test

DIP, Distal interphalangeal; *FA,* forearm; *IP,* interphalangeal; *L,* left; *MP,* metacarpal; *R,* right; *ROM,* range of motion; *UE,* upper extremity; *WNL,* within normal limits.

Goals

• Long-term goal: Patient will follow provided orthotic-wearing schedule by discharge from therapy.
• Short-term goal: Patient will show decreased symptoms from de Quervain tenosynovitis.

To encourage clinical reasoning skills, answer the following questions about the case. See Chapter 8 for specifics about orthoses for de Quervain tenosynovitis.

1. List a minimum of five areas of the documentation that could be improved by being more specific or more complete.
2. On the basis of the interactive clinical reasoning approach, what are two questions that will facilitate an understanding of the impact that having de Quervain tenosynovitis and wearing an orthosis has on Marie's work and home life?
3. What are some concerns about adherence you may have based on Marie's history with her prefabricated orthosis? How will you approach any adherence concerns?
4. Considering that the referral came from work, what type of insurance might Marie have?

---

*See Appendix A for the answer key.

APPENDIX 6-2   EXAMPLES

EXAMPLE 6-1

The following is an initial progress note (IPN) following orthotic fabrication. Although this note is an exemplar for written documentation, the same information should be included in electronic format.

February 24, 20__, 4:00 PM

   This 42-year-old female was seen by an occupational therapist for fabrication of a right wrist immobilization orthosis on the dominant R UE. Client has a history of carpal tunnel syndrome since August 20, 20__. Client reports being independent in ADLs, work, and leisure tasks before condition developed. Client displays problems related to carpal tunnel syndrome including decreased R grip strength, R hand swelling at end of day, pain, tingling, decreased sensation in the area of the median nerve, and a positive Phalen sign. (Refer to the summary report of the Semmes-Weinstein Monofilament Test.) Client displays problems with cooking meals and typing on computer at work. Client currently requires help from her daughter for such tasks as opening cans and jars and cutting food with a knife. Client is employed as a secretary, and job demands primarily involve computer work. At work, client tolerates 20 minutes of typing on computer before pain and tingling develop in the R hand. Client stated, "It is difficult for me to type on the computer and cook a meal." B UE AROM was WNL except for the following R UE motions:

- Thumb: Opposition to ring finger—unable to oppose little finger
- R finger TAMs (Normal = 250 to 265 degrees):
  - Index = 230 degrees
  - Middle = 230 degrees
  - Ring = 240 degrees
  - Little = 270 degrees
- R wrist:
  - Flexion = 0 to 50 degrees (Normal = 0 to 80 degrees)
  - Wrist extension (WNL)
  - Radial deviation = 0 to 15 degrees (Normal = 0 to 20 degrees)
  - Ulnar deviation (WNL)

Grip strength was tested with Jamar dynamometer. R grip strength = 30 pounds (10th percentile for age and gender) and L grip strength = 64 pounds (Normal = 75th percentile for age and gender). MMT results are as follows:

- R abductor pollicis = 3 (fair)/5, L = 5 (normal)/5
- R opponens pollicis = 3 (fair)/5, L = 5 (normal)/5

   A R volar-based, neutral wrist immobilization orthosis was fabricated. Client presented with no pressure marks or rash after orthotic application. Client was evaluated for functional hand motions while wearing the orthosis. The orthosis did not restrict finger and thumb motions. Client received verbal and written instructions about orthotic-wearing schedule and a form to document wearing adherence. Client was able to independently don and doff her orthosis. Client received verbal and written instructions for a home exercise program, orthosis precautions, and ergonomic adaptations for home and work environments. Client's understanding of all instructions appeared to be good. Client will be followed two more times per physician order to monitor orthosis and program and ergonomic adaptations.

OT Goals

LTGs: Client will report a decrease in R hand pain and tingling so as to complete home and work activities independently by [date].

   STGs:

- Client will independently complete computer tasks at work while wearing R wrist orthosis for 3 hours daily and taking hourly exercise breaks by [date].
- Client will independently cook a meal while wearing R wrist orthosis and report reduced pain by [date].
- Client will properly position B UEs during computer work activities and utilize ergonomic office equipment by [date].
- Client will comply with orthotic-wearing schedule 90% of the time as evidenced by the orthotic-wearing schedule adherence sheet by [date].

ADL, Activity of daily living; *AROM,* active range of motion; *B,* bilateral *L,* left; *LTG,* long-term goal; *MMT,* manual muscle testing; *OT,* occupational therapy; *R,* right; *STG,* short-term goal; *TAM,* total active motion; *UE,* upper extremity; *WNL,* within normal limits.

EXAMPLE 6-2

The following is an OT SOAP note. Although this note is an exemplar for written documentation, the same information can be included in electronic format.

February 24, 20__, 4:00 PM

S (subjective): "My right hand tingles and hurts all the time." Client also reports difficulty cooking meals and typing on the computer while at work.

O (objective): Client presents with an Hx of carpal tunnel symptoms in dominant, R, hand since August 20, 20__. Client reports being independent in ADLs, work, and leisure tasks before condition developed. Client displays a positive R Phalen sign with decreased sensation in the R median nerve distribution area. (Refer to Semmes-Weinstein Monofilament Test summary sheet.) B UE AROM was WNL, except for the following motions:

R thumb opposition to ring finger—unable to oppose little finger
R finger TAMs (Normal = 250 to 265 degrees):

- Index = 230 degrees
- Middle = 230 degrees
- Ring = 240 degrees
- Little = 270 degrees
- R wrist: Flexion = 0 to 50 degrees (Normal = 0 to 80 degrees)
- Wrist extension (WNL)
- Radial deviation = 0 to 15 degrees (Normal = 0 to 20 degrees)
- Ulnar deviation (WNL)

Grip strength was tested with Jamar dynamometer. R grip strength = 30 pounds (10th percentile for age and gender). L grip strength = 64 pounds (75th percentile for age and gender). MMT results as follows:

- Abductor pollicis: R = 3 (fair)/5, L = 5 (normal)/5
- Opponens pollicis: R = 3 (fair)/5, L = 5 (normal)/5

Client displays problems related to carpal tunnel syndrome including decreased R grip strength, R hand swelling at end of day, and problems with cooking meals and typing on computer at work. Client currently requires help from her daughter for such tasks as opening cans and jars and cutting food with a knife. At work, client tolerates 20 minutes of typing on computer before pain and tingling develop in the R hand.

A R volar-based, neutral wrist immobilization orthosis was fabricated. Client presented with no pressure marks or rash after orthotic application. Client was evaluated for functional hand motions while wearing the orthosis. The orthosis does not restrict finger and thumb motions. Client received verbal and written instructions about orthotic-wearing schedule and a form to document wearing adherence. Client was able to independently don and doff orthosis. Client received verbal and written instructions for a home exercise program, orthosis precautions, and ergonomic adaptations for home and work environments. Client's understanding of all instructions appeared to be good.

A (assessment): Client seems to have a good rehabilitation potential as she reports motivation to comply with OT intervention. Client is able to complete functional activities while wearing the R wrist immobilization orthosis. Symptoms may decrease with orthosis wear and with implementation of the home exercise program and ergonomic home and work adaptations.

P (plan): Client will be followed two more times per physician order to monitor orthosis and program and ergonomic adaptations.

OT Goals

LTGs: Client will report a decrease in R hand pain and tingling so as to complete home and work activities independently by [date].

STGs:
- Client will independently complete computer tasks at work while wearing R wrist orthosis for 3 hours daily and taking hourly exercise breaks by [date].
- Client will independently cook a meal while wearing R wrist orthosis and report reduced pain by [date].
- Client will properly position B UEs during computer work activities and utilize ergonomic office equipment by [date].
- Client will comply with orthotic-wearing schedule 90% of the time as evidenced by the orthotic-wearing schedule adherence sheet by [date].

(John Smith, OTR)

ADL, Activity of daily living; *AROM*, active range of motion; *B*, bilateral; *Hx*, history; *L*, left; *LTG*, long-term goal; *OT*, occupational therapy; *OTR*, *registered occupational therapist*; *R*, right; *STG*, short-term goal; *TAM*, total active motion; *UE*, upper extremity; *WNL*, within normal limits.

Orthosis for Conditions and Populations

CHAPTER 7

Orthoses for the Wrist

Helene Lohman, OTD, OTR/L, FAOTA,
with contributions from Robert Gilmore, OTS

Key Terms
carpal tunnel syndrome (CTS)
circumferential
complex regional pain syndrome (CRPS) type I
dorsal
forearm trough
hypothenar bar
metacarpal bar
radial nerve injuries
rheumatoid arthritis (RA)
tendinopathy
ulnar
volar

Chapter Objectives
1. Discuss diagnostic indications for wrist immobilization orthoses.
2. Identify reasons to provide serial orthotic intervention with wrist immobilization orthoses.
3. Identify major features of wrist immobilization orthoses.
4. Describe the fabrication process for a volar or dorsal wrist orthosis.
5. Relate hints for a proper fit to a wrist immobilization orthosis.
6. Review precautions for wrist immobilization orthotic intervention.
7. Use clinical reasoning to evaluate a problematic wrist immobilization orthosis.
8. Use clinical reasoning to evaluate a fabricated wrist immobilization orthosis.
9. Apply knowledge about the application of wrist immobilization orthoses to case studies.
10. Explain the importance of evidence-based practice with wrist orthotic provision.
11. Describe the appropriate use of prefabricated wrist orthoses.

You are dining with your good friend, Maria. She tells you she has been experiencing night pain in her right wrist, thumb, index, and middle fingers. You ask her to describe the pain, and she says it feels like pins and needles and sometimes her fingers become numb. Immediately you ask her what she's been doing lately. She recently got a part-time job as a grocery checker. Her job involves much pinching, flexion, and ulnar deviation of her wrist during scanning of items. You suspect she might have carpal tunnel syndrome (CTS) and advise her to see her physician. A week later you see Maria again. She informs you that she was diagnosed with CTS and asks you what types of therapy could help alleviate the symptoms. You tell her that based on evidence, an effective intervention in early stages of CTS is to wear an orthosis that positions her wrist in neutral.

Maintaining the wrist in proper alignment is essential because the wrist is important to the health and balance of the entire hand. During functional activities, the wrist is positioned in extension for grasp and prehension. Therefore, the wrist extension immobilization type 0 orthosis[3] or the wrist cock-up orthosis is the most common orthosis fabricated in clinical practice. Wrist immobilization orthoses usually maintain the wrist in either a neutral or a mildly extended position, depending on the protocol for a particular diagnostic condition and the person's intervention goals. A wrist immobilization orthosis positions the wrist while allowing full metacarpophalangeal (MCP) flexion and thumb mobility. Thus, the person can continue to perform functional activities with the added support and proper positioning of the wrist that the orthosis provides. Positioning the wrist in 0 to 30 degrees of wrist extension in a orthosis promotes functional hand patterns for completing functional activities.[43,54]

Therapists fabricate wrist immobilization orthoses to provide volar; dorsal; ulnar; circumferential forearm, wrist, and hand; and occasionally for radial support (Figure 7-1 to Figure 7-4). Therapists also use wrist immobilization orthoses as bases for mobilization and static progressive orthotic intervention (see Chapter 12). Although some wrist immobilization orthoses are commercially available, they cannot provide the exact fit of custom-made orthoses. However, commercially-available orthoses made from soft material may be more comfortable in certain situations, especially in a work or sports setting. Commercially-available orthoses are not as restrictive and allow more functional hand

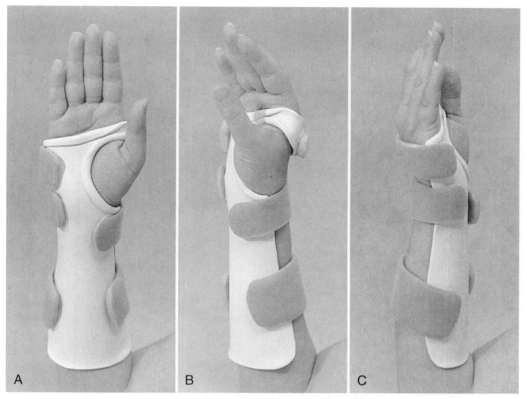

Figure 7-1 A volar wrist immobilization orthosis.

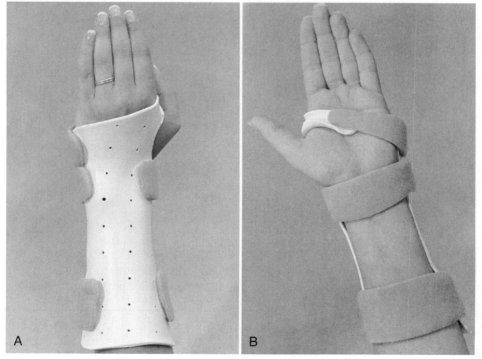

Figure 7-2 A dorsal wrist immobilization orthosis.

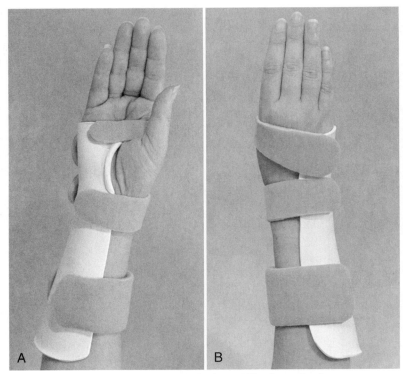

Figure 7-3 An ulnar wrist immobilization orthosis.

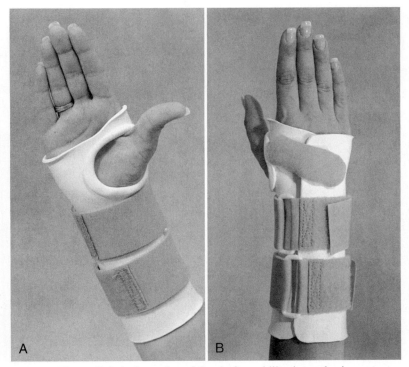

Figure 7-4 A circumferential wrist immobilization orthosis.

use.[68] Some people with rheumatoid arthritis (RA) may also prefer the comfort of a soft wrist orthosis due to its ability to reduce pain and provide stability during functional activities.[7,47,67]

This chapter primarily gives an overview for wrist immobilization orthoses according to type, features, and diagnoses. The chapter addresses technical tips, troubleshooting tips, the use of prefabricated orthoses, the impact on occupations, and the application of a wrist mobilization and serial static approach.

Volar, Dorsal, Ulnar, and Circumferential Wrist Immobilization Orthoses

In clinical practice, the therapist must decide whether to fabricate a volar, dorsal, ulnar, or circumferential wrist immobilization orthosis. Each has advantages and disadvantages.[17]

Volar

The **volar** wrist immobilization orthosis (see Figure 7-1) depends on a dorsal wrist strap to hold the wrist in extension in the orthosis. An appropriate design furnishes adequate support for the weight of the wrist and hand. In cases in which the weight of the hand (flaccidity) must be held by the orthosis or in which the person is pulling against it (spasticity), the strap may not be adequate to hold the wrist in the orthosis. However, a well-designed volar wrist orthosis with a properly placed wide wrist strap will support a flaccid wrist.[62] The volar design is best suited for circumstances that require rest or immobilization of the wrist when the person still has muscle control of the wrist.[17]

In one study, the volar wrist orthosis allowed the hand the best dexterity of custom-made wrist orthoses. A volar wrist orthosis' greatest disadvantage is interference with tactile sensibility on the palmar surface of the hand and the loss of the hand's ability to conform around objects.[62] In the presence of edema, one must use this design carefully because the dorsal strap can impede lymphatic and venous flow.[17] To address the presence of edema, a strap adaptation is made by fabricating a continuous strap. The therapist applies self-adhesive Velcro hooks along the radial and ulnar borders of the orthosis, which are attached by a flexible fabric to create a soft dorsal shell.

Dorsal

Some therapists fabricate **dorsal** orthoses with a large palmar bar that supports the entire hand. This large palmar bar tends to distribute pressure well and is necessary for comfort and function. However, a large palmar bar does not free up the palmar surface as much for sensory input as a dorsal orthosis fabricated with a thinner palmar bar (see Figure 7-2). Dorsal wrist orthoses designed with a standard strap configuration can be better tolerated by persons who have edematous hands because of the pressure distribution. Either the volar or the dorsal design may be used as a base for mobilization (dynamic) orthotic intervention. However, these designs can sometimes lead to orthotic migration and suboptimal orthotic performance.

Ulnar

The **ulnar** wrist orthosis is easy to don and doff and can be applied if the person warrants more protection on the ulnar side of the hand, such as with sports injuries (see Figure 7-3). This ulnar orthotic design is sometimes used for a person who has **carpal tunnel syndrome (CTS)** or ulnar wrist pain.[40] It can also be used as a base for mobilization orthoses.

Circumferential

A **circumferential** orthosis is helpful to prevent migration, especially when used as a base for mobilization orthoses.

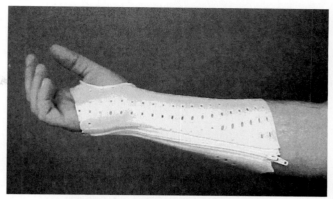

Figure 7-5 A "zipper" orthosis option for making a circumferential orthosis (Sammons Preston & Rolyan). (From Bednar JM, Von Lersner-Benson C: Wrist reconstruction: salvage procedures. In Mackin EJ, Callahan AD, Shirven TM, et al., editors: *Rehabilitation of the hand and upper extremity,* ed 5, St Louis, 2002, Mosby, p. 1200.)

Circumferential wrist orthoses also provide good forearm support, control edema, provide good pressure distribution, and eliminate edge pressure.[63] Some people may feel more confined in a circumferential orthosis. When fabricating a circumferential orthosis, the therapist is conscious of a possible pressure area over the distal ulna and checks that the fingers and thumb have full motion (see Figure 7-4).[38] One among many circumferential orthosis options is a "zipper" orthosis made from perforated thermoplastic material (Figure 7-5).

Features of the Wrist Immobilization Orthosis

Understanding the features of a wrist immobilization orthosis helps therapists design orthotic interventions appropriately. Whether fabricating a volar, dorsal, ulnar, or circumferential wrist orthosis, the therapist must be aware of certain features of the various components of the wrist immobilization orthosis—such as a forearm trough, metacarpal bar, and hypothenar bar (Figure 7-6 and Figure 7-7).[23] With a volar or dorsal immobilization orthosis, the **forearm trough** should be two-thirds the length of the forearm and one-half the circumference of the forearm to allow for appropriate pressure distribution. It is sometimes necessary to notch or flare the area near the distal ulna on the forearm trough to avoid a pressure point.

The **hypothenar bar** helps to place the hand in a neutral resting position by preventing extreme ulnar deviation. The hypothenar bar should not inhibit MCP flexion of the ring and little fingers. The metacarpal bar supports the transverse metacarpal arch. When supporting the palmar surface of the hand, the metacarpal bar is sometimes called a *palmar bar.* With a volar wrist immobilization orthosis, the therapist positions this bar proximal to the distal palmar crease and distal and ulnar to the thenar crease to ensure full MCP flexion. On the ulnar side of the hand, it is especially important that the metacarpal bar be positioned proximal to the distal palmar crease to allow full little finger metacarpal flexion.

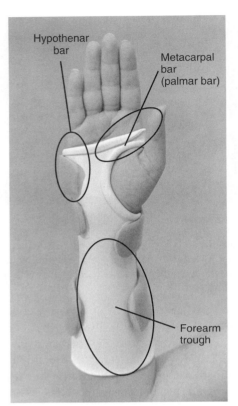

Figure 7-6 A volar wrist immobilization orthosis with identified components.

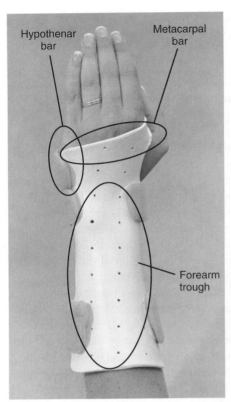

Figure 7-7 A dorsal wrist immobilization orthosis with identified components.

On the radial side, it is important for the position of the metacarpal bar to be below the distal palmar crease and distal to the thenar crease to allow adequate index and middle MCP flexion and thumb motions. On a dorsal wrist immobilization orthosis, the therapist positions this bar slightly proximal to the MCP heads on the dorsal surface of the hand when it winds around to the palmar surface. The same principles apply when positioning the metacarpal bar on the volar surface of the hand (proximal to the distal palmar crease, and distal and ulnar to the thenar crease).

The therapist should also carefully consider the application of straps to the wrist orthosis. Straps are applied at the level of the metacarpal bar, exactly at the wrist level, and at the proximal end of the orthosis. The straps attach to the orthosis with pieces of self-adhesive Velcro hook. The therapist should note that the larger the piece of self-adhesive hook Velcro, the larger the interface between it and the thermoplastic material. This larger interface helps ensure that it remains in place and does not peel off. With the identification of the potential for pressure or shear problems, the therapist applies padding to the orthosis (see Figures 7-1, 7-6).

Diagnostic Indications

The clinical indications for the wrist immobilization orthosis vary according to the diagnosis. The therapist can apply the wrist immobilization orthosis for any upper extremity condition that requires the wrist to be in a static position. Application of this orthosis addresses a variety of goals, depending on the client's intervention needs. These goals include decreasing wrist pain or inflammation, providing support, enhancing digital function, preventing wrist deformity, minimizing pressure on the median nerve, and minimizing tension on involved structures.

In some cases, a wrist mobilization orthosis serial static approach is used to increase passive range of motion (PROM). Specific diagnostic conditions that may require a wrist immobilization orthosis can include, but are not limited to, tendinopathy, distal radius or ulna fracture, wrist sprain, radial nerve palsy, carpal ganglion, stable wrist fracture, wrist arthroplasty, and nerve compression at the wrist (CTS and Guyon canal syndrome). Wrist orthoses for complex regional pain syndrome (CRPS) type I (reflex sympathetic dystrophy) may be applied if the person is posturing in flexion, but application of orthoses for this condition is controversial because immobilization may increase the pain cycle.[20]

The specific wrist positioning depends on the diagnostic protocol, physician referral, and person's intervention goals. When the goal is functional hand use during orthotic wear, the therapist avoids extreme wrist flexion or extension because either position disrupts the normal functional position of the hand. Extreme positions can contribute to the development of CTS.[23,24] An exception to this rule is when the orthotic goal is to increase PROM. In that case, an extreme position may be indicated. However, extreme positions may preclude function. The therapist must judge whether the trade-off is worth the loss of function.[63]

The therapist performs a thorough hand evaluation before fitting a person with a wrist immobilization orthosis and provides the person with a wearing schedule, instructions about orthotic maintenance and precautions, and an exercise program based on particular needs. Physicians and experienced therapists may have detailed guidelines for positioning and wearing schedules. Every hand is slightly different and thus orthotic positioning and wearing protocols vary. Table 7-1 lists suggested wearing schedules and positioning protocols

of common hand conditions that may require wrist immobilization orthoses.

Wrist Orthotic Intervention for Carpal Tunnel Syndrome

In recent guidelines for the treatment of CTS from the American Academy of Orthopaedic Surgeons (AAOS), wrist orthotic intervention continues to be recommended specifically for conservative management of mild to moderate CTS.[1] Additionally, recent quality measures for CTS

Table 7-1 Conditions That May Require a Wrist Immobilization Orthosis

HAND CONDITION	SUGGESTED WEARING SCHEDULE	TYPE OF ORTHOSIS AND WRIST POSITION
Nerve Compression		
Carpal tunnel syndrome (CTS) (median nerve compression)	There is no consistent protocol for orthotic provision with CTS. Some therapists determine the wear schedule based on what activities are irritating for the person. For example, if activities during the day are irritating the person, the orthosis should be worn during the day. Some therapists start with wear during sleep and increase the time if the orthosis does not decrease symptoms. Often during an acute flare-up the person wears the wrist immobilization orthosis continuously for 4 to 6 weeks with removal for hygiene and range of motion (ROM) exercises. The orthotic wearing schedule gradually decreases. An orthosis may be suggested in lieu of steroid injection. However, if the person undergoes steroid injection, the orthosis may be worn only at night.	Volar, dorsal, or ulnar gutter orthosis with the wrist in a neutral position.
Carpal tunnel release surgery	There is no consistent protocol for orthotic provision with carpal tunnel release surgery. Some physicians have the orthosis fabricated preoperatively, and some are fabricated immediately postoperatively. Some physicians do not prescribe orthoses at all. Others may recommend a wrist immobilization orthosis 1 week after surgery with the therapist providing instructions for an orthotic wearing schedule (which includes orthotic application during sleep, during strenuous activities, and for support throughout the healing phase). Orthosis is weaned when appropriate to prevent adhesion formation.	A volar orthosis with the wrist in neutral or slightly extended position.
Radial nerve palsy	Some physicians may suggest a wrist immobilization orthosis that maintains the wrist in a functional position and substitutes for the loss of the radial nerve by placing the wrist in extension. This static orthosis may be worn at night. Many other orthotic options for radial nerve palsy besides a static wrist orthosis are discussed in Chapter 13.	Volar or dorsal, 15 to 30 degrees of wrist extension. For night splinting a resting hand orthosis is appropriate for positioning the MCPs in extension and thumb MP and IP in extension to use in conjunction with a day wrist orthosis (see Chapter 9).
Tendinitis/Tenosynovitis		
Any inflammation or degradation of the tendon and tendon sheath within the wrist	The person wears a wrist immobilization orthosis to avoid painful activity with removal for hygiene and ROM exercises followed by gradual wearing of the orthosis.	Volar or dorsal, 20 to 30 degrees of wrist extension.
Wrist synovitis	The person wears a wrist immobilization orthosis continuously during acute flare-ups with removal for hygiene and ROM exercises.	Volar, 0 to 15 degrees of extension.

Table 7-1   Conditions That May Require a Wrist Immobilization Orthosis—cont'd

HAND CONDITION	SUGGESTED WEARING SCHEDULE	TYPE OF ORTHOSIS AND WRIST POSITION
Rheumatoid Arthritis Periods of swelling, wrist subluxation, and joint inflammation	The person continuously wears a wrist immobilization orthosis with established periods for ROM exercises and hygiene during the orthotic wearing schedule. If MCP joints are developing an ulnar drift and IP joints are not involved, the therapist may fabricate a wrist orthosis that includes the MCP joints.	Volar in extension up to 30 degrees based on person's comfort level. During the early stage of the development of metacarpal ulnar drift, position close to neutral.
Wrist fractures	After the removal of the cast and healing of the fracture, the therapist fabricates a wrist immobilization orthosis. Usually the therapist discontinues the orthosis use as soon as possible to encourage functional movement. Sometimes the therapist may need to fabricate serial orthoses if the wrist does not have enough functional extension.	Dorsal, volar, or circumferential (if more support is needed) maximum passive extension the person can tolerate up to 30 degrees.
Wrist Sprain Any grade I or grade II tear of the ligament	The person wears a wrist immobilization orthosis continuously for 3 to 6 weeks. The physician may allow removal during bathing, depending on severity.	Choose approach as needed for function. Location of ligament may help dictate position. The orthosis should remove stress (tension from ligament).
Other Complex regional pain syndrome (CRPS) type I	The person wears a wrist immobilization orthosis during functional activities only if these activities are painful without the orthosis.	Volar, in extension as person tolerates. A circumferential wrist orthosis might also be used as it helps avoid pressure on the edges, and problems with edema.

recommend orthotic intervention for conservative management.[48] Orthotic intervention of the wrist as close as possible to zero degrees (neutral) avoids added pressure on the median nerve[10,24,35,36,48] and may help with blood circulation.[50] See Table 7-2 for expert opinion guidelines for CTS.

One must be careful when applying prefabricated wrist immobilization orthoses for CTS because some orthoses place the wrist in a functional position of 20 to 30 degrees of extension.[48,52,77] Therefore, if it is possible to adjust the wrist angle of the orthosis, it should be modified to a neutral position. Some of the prefabricated orthoses have a compartment in which a metal or thermoplastic insert is placed, and the insert allows adjustments for wrist position. However, prefabricated orthoses that have their angles adjusted may become unstable, less rigid, and less comfortable than a custom-molded orthosis.[74] Based on some research, custom-made orthoses that hold the wrist and MCPs in neutral are more effective in treating the symptoms of CTS and improving function in individuals than prefabricated wrist

cock-up orthoses. Both orthoses were effective in decreasing symptoms among the subjects, but individuals wearing the custom wrist orthosis demonstrated greater pinch and grip strength than those wearing the prefabricated wrist cock-up orthoses.[8]

Another consideration with the wrist immobilization orthosis provision is the amount of finger flexion allowed. Recent research evidence suggests that finger flexion affects carpal tunnel pressure, especially if fingers fully flex to form a fist.[4,8] The rationale is because the lumbrical muscles may sometimes enter the carpal tunnel with finger flexion.[16,64] When orthoses are provided to clients with CTS, they should be instructed to not flex their fingers "beyond 75% of a full fist."[4] Therefore, therapists should check finger position with orthotic provision. Osterman and colleagues[52] advised therapists to fabricate a volar wrist orthosis with a metacarpal block to decrease finger flexion if CTS symptoms are not improving (Figure 7-8).

When fabricating an orthosis for a person who has CTS, the therapist considers home and occupational demands

Table 7-2 Suggested Guidelines for Carpal Tunnel Syndrome Treatments*

AUTHOR'S CITATION	SUMMARY OF RECOMMENDATIONS

Keith MW, Masear V, Chung KC, et al: American Academy of Orthopaedic Surgeons clinical practice guideline on the treatment of carpal tunnel syndrome, *J Bone Joint Surg Am* 92(1):218-219, 2010. *Recommendations accepted by the American Academy of Orthopaedic Surgeons (AAOS)	• Both surgical and nonsurgical (oral and local steroids, orthotic intervention, and ultrasound) treatments can be effective for carpal tunnel syndrome (CTS).
	 • There is minimal evidence suggesting a specific treatment when CTS coexists with other conditions, such as diabetes, radiculopathy, hypothyroidism, rheumatoid arthritis (RA), pregnancy, and polyneuropathy.
	 • The wrist should not be immobilized postoperatively after a routine carpal tunnel release.
	 • No recommendation available for the use or nonuse of the following:
	   • Electric stimulation
	   • Iontophoresis
	   • Massage therapy
	   • Exercise
	   • Phonophoresis
	   • Systemic steroid injection
	   • Weight reduction

Nuckols T, Harber P, Sancin K, et al: Quality measures for the diagnosis and non-operative management of carpal tunnel syndrome in occupational settings, *J Occup Rehabil* 21(1):100-119, 2011.	• Forty measures/concerns related to the evaluation and treatment of CTS were reviewed and evaluated by a panel of experts.
	 • Non-operative recommendations:
	   • Orthoses should be utilized with the wrist in a neutral position. Orthoses should be worn for at least 6 weeks following diagnosis of CTS.
	   • Pharmacology agents including nonsteroidal anti-inflammatory drugs (NSAIDs), muscle relaxants, opioids, and diuretics should not be used by individuals with CTS.
	   • Steroid injections should only be utilized when the risks have been discussed with patient. Steroid injections should be limited to four occurrences.
	 • "Exposures to vibration, force, and repetition should be minimized (p. 105)."
	 • Returning to work following CTS treatment should be accompanied by a follow-up evaluation from a physician.

*This table does not necessarily reflect evidence-based practice but should be referred to as "expert opinion."

carefully, keeping in mind that the wrist contributes to the overall function of the hand.[61] If an orthosis is worn at work, durability of the orthosis and the ability to wash it may be salient. Some people may benefit from the fabrication of two orthoses (one for work and one for home), especially if their job demands are in an unclean environment. Many computer operators tolerate orthoses that support the wrist position in the plane of flexion and extension but allow 10 to 20 degrees of radial and ulnar deviation for effective typing on the computer. Fabricating a slightly wider **metacarpal bar** on a custom-made wrist orthosis allows for a small area of mobility on the radial and ulnar sides of the hand.[60] However, with this orthotic adaptation the client is instructed to be cautious when using a wrist orthosis with repetitive activity because it may cause proximal muscle pain or inflammation due to the altered biomechanics of the upper extremity. If increased pain or inflammation occurs, the therapist instructs the client to decrease orthotic use at the computer and have the client try "pretending that the orthosis is on."[20] Finally, the client simulates work and home tasks while wearing the wrist immobilization orthosis, and the therapist checks for functional fit.[60]

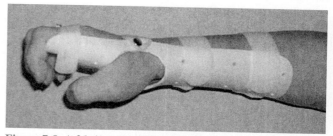

Figure 7-8 A fabricated wrist immobilization (lumbrical positioning) orthosis with the wrist and metacarpophalangeals (MCPs) in a neutral position (From Brininger TL, Rogers JC, Holm MB, et al: Efficacy of fabricated customized splint and tendon and nerve gliding exercises for the treatment of carpal tunnel syndrome: a randomized controlled trial. *Arch Phys Med Rehabil* 88(11):1429-1436, 2007.)

Therapists take into account orthotic-wearing schedules. Options prescribed include nighttime wear only, wear during activities that irritate the condition, a combination of the latter two schedules, or constant wear. Based on a review of recent evidence, Ono, Chapham, and Chung[50] recommended minimally a nighttime wearing schedule and that clinical judgment be used to determine if daytime wear is appropriate. Furthermore, a recent review of randomized control studies regarding the effectiveness of orthotic intervention for individuals with CTS identified that there was a significant benefit of nighttime wear compared to no therapy at all.[30] Individuals who sleep with the wrist flexed or extended may benefit from nighttime wearing.[60] In another study, subjects were found to benefit most from full-time wear of the orthosis, but adherence to the wearing schedule was an issue.[74] Length of time for orthotic wear may be prescribed by the person's physician. It is generally suggested that the orthosis be worn for six to eight weeks with effectiveness of wear shown for up to one year.[41]

An exercise program issued with an orthosis may be an effective conservative treatment.[58] In one study (n = 197), a conservative treatment program for CTS that combined nerve and tendon gliding exercises with wrist immobilization orthotic intervention was found to be more effective in helping people avoid surgery than orthotic wear alone. It is hypothesized that these exercises help improve the excursion of the median nerve and flexor tendons because the exercises may contribute to the remodeling of the adhered tenosynovium.[58] Akalin and colleagues[2] (n = 28) also studied tendon and nerve gliding exercises with orthotic intervention compared to orthotic intervention alone. Ninety-three percent of the orthotic intervention and exercise group participants reported good to excellent results compared to 72% of the orthosis-only group participants. However, the researchers did not consider the results statistically significant. More recently, researchers (n = 53) considered orthotic intervention and paraffin therapy along with either nerve or tendon gliding.[29] The group who wore orthoses, had paraffin therapy, and completed tendon gliding exercises exhibited significant improvements with their scores for functional status over the group who wore orthoses, had paraffin therapy, and completed nerve gliding exercises.[29] Another study found that for mild to moderate CTS, a wrist orthosis combined with lumbrical muscle stretches was more effective in the long term than orthotic intervention alone or stretches alone. Further research suggested that exercise programs in addition to orthotic intervention are effective in CTS symptom management but are not effective replacements of orthoses.[8] These studies accentuate the value of early conservative intervention.

Other effective intervention measures for CTS are the modification of activities (so that the person does not make excessive wrist and forearm motions, especially wrist flexion). It is also important to avoid sustained pinch or grip activities and to use good posture whenever possible with all activities of daily living (ADLs). Because CTS is generically a disease of decreased blood supply to the soft tissues, an environment that is cold will additionally deprive nerves of blood. Thus, staying warm is an important part of CTS care, and orthoses provide local warmth.[62] When conservative measures are ineffective, additional medical management includes corticosteroid injection or the possibility of surgery.

There are several goals of wrist orthotic intervention after carpal tunnel release surgery. Goals include:

- Minimizing pressure on the median nerve
- Preventing bowstringing of the flexor tendons[19]
- Providing support during stressful activities
- Maintaining gains from exercise[45,63]
- Resting the extremity during the immediate healing phase

Some therapists do not provide a wrist immobilization orthosis postoperatively to clients because of concerns about the impact of immobilization on joint stiffness and muscle shortening.[28] Findings from one study[19] (n = 50) suggest that orthotic intervention post-surgery resulted in joint stiffness as well as delays with returning to work, recovering grip and pinch strength, and resuming ADLs. These researchers concluded that if an orthotic intervention is used, it should be applied for 1 week only postoperatively to prevent tendon bowstringing and nerve entrapment.

Orthotic intervention postoperatively may be recommended to prevent extreme nighttime wrist postures (flexion and extension) or to manage inflammation.[28] Therapists instruct the person to gradually wean away from wearing the orthosis (when the orthosis is no longer meeting the person's therapeutic goals) in order to prevent stiffness and allow the person to return to work and ADLs more quickly. Weaning is often done over the course of 1 week, gradually decreasing the hours of orthotic wear.[62]

A series of studies were conducted to examine orthotic intervention for CTS compared to other interventions, such as surgery or steroid injections (see Table 7-3, which outlines the research evidence). The majority of studies comparing orthotic intervention to surgery favored surgery as the most effective treatment for CTS.[25,73] Orthotic intervention did show some promising results, but was not as strong in efficacy as surgery. For example, with the Gerristen and colleagues[25] study, (n = 178) after 18 months 75% of the subjects improved with orthotic wear as compared to 90% of the surgery group. The researchers recommended that orthotic intervention is beneficial while waiting for surgery, or if a client does not desire surgery. When considering the results of this study, therapists should recognize that 75% improvement with orthotic intervention is a high success rate and is less risky than having surgery. Some people do not want therapy, orthotic intervention, and activity modification and, therefore, may best benefit from a surgical approach.[62] However, a consideration about surgery for CTS is the severity of nerve damage. If the CTS results in moderate to severe nerve damage, there is the risk of possibly losing thenar muscle function, which is functionally devastating.[20]

Therapists and physicians must be aware of current evidence that can influence intervention approaches. Therapists need to critically question how the research was performed and be aware of limitations. As McClure[42] stated, "these details are important in deciding whether my patient is similar enough to those in the study to use these results with her."

Table 7-3 Evidence-Based Practice about Wrist Orthotic Intervention

AUTHOR'S CITATION	DESIGN	NUMBER OF PARTICIPANTS	DESCRIPTION	RESULTS	LIMITATIONS
Baker NA, Moehlingm KK, Rubinstein EN, et al: The comparative effectiveness of combined lumbrical muscle splints and stretches on symptoms and function in carpal tunnel syndrome, Arch Phys Med Rehabil 93(1):1-10, 2012.	Randomized clinical trial	124 volunteer subjects with mild to moderate CTS	Subjects participated in a 4-week program of night orthotic intervention with either a prefabricated wrist cock-up or custom fabricated lumbrical orthosis in neutral along with daily lumbrical stretches (either general or intensive). Subjects were randomly divided into four groups: 1. Lumbrical orthotic/lumbrical stretch group (intensive lumbrical intervention) 2. Lumbrical orthotic/general stretch group 3. General orthotic lumbrical stretch group 4. General orthotic/general stretch group	Subjects were evaluated with the Carpal Tunnel Symptom Severity and Function Questionnaire (CTQ) and the Disabilities of the Arm, Shoulder, and Hand (DASH) questionnaire. Researchers concluded that orthotic intervention along with the lumbrical stretches was more effective than orthotic intervention alone or stretches alone. The authors also concluded that it may take several months to resolve CTS symptoms and that function may show continual improvement after symptoms have halted. Subjects were followed up at 4, 12, and 24 weeks. At 24 weeks, the group with the general orthosis along with lumbrical stretches demonstrated continual functional improvement. Surgery following these conservative interventions was only 25.5%.	Inclusion criteria did not specifically involve subjects with lumbrical tightness, nor did inclusion criteria require electrodiagnostic nerve conduction studies to confirm CTS. Subjects self-reported adherence to the study regimen. Subjects followed a prescribed regimen for only a 1 week time-frame, which might have biased later results. There was no control group.
Huisstede BM, Hoogvliet P, Randsdorp MS, et al: Carpal tunnel syndrome. Part I: effectiveness of nonsurgical treatments—a systematic review, Arch Phys Med Rehabil 91(7):981-1004, 2010.	Literature review of randomized control trials	Participants differed depending upon the study referenced. Data sources include the Cochrane Library, PubMed, EMBASE, CINAHL, and PEDro. 20 randomized controlled trials were collected.	Criteria for inclusion were: a. Participants with CTS b. CTS not caused by acute trauma or systematic disease c. An intervention for CTS with results on pain and function reported following the intervention Evidence was reviewed from the 20 randomized control trials (RCTs) by two independent reviewers. Topics of the RCTs included nonsurgical treatments, such as orthotic intervention, oral medications, ultrasound, yoga, laser therapy, chiropractic treatment, ergonomic keyboards, corticosteroid injection, tendon and nerve gliding exercises, different modalities, and other non-traditional therapeutic procedures.	Evidence obtained from the RCT reviews include but were not limited to the following: • Limited evidence for the effectiveness of full-time orthotic wear compared to an orthosis worn at nighttime only for patients with CTS. • No significant differences were noted in the outcomes with the addition of nerve and tendon gliding exercises to an orthotic regimen in the treatment of CTS. • The effectiveness of other therapies including magnetic therapy, cupping therapy, heat wrap therapy, and massage therapy demonstrated varied results in the treatment of CTS. • Specific study reviews are available within the main text of the article.	One limitation was the diminished quality of the RCTs in terms of research outcomes, study integrity, and reliability. Different methods for reviewing different sources were used because of the difference in credibility and validity of the sources.

Table 7-3 Evidence-Based Practice about Wrist Orthotic Intervention—cont'd

AUTHOR'S CITATION	DESIGN	NUMBER OF PARTICIPANTS	DESCRIPTION	RESULTS	LIMITATIONS
Ono S, Clapham PJ, Chung KC: Optimal management of carpal tunnel syndrome, *Int J Gen Med* 3: 255-261, 2010.	Systematic review of evidence-based articles	25 studies met inclusion criteria including 13 randomized control trials and 12 systematic reviews	Two independent reviewers selected articles for review based on specific inclusion criteria: a. Type of article b. Publication in English c. Published from 2007-2010 d. Sample consisting of individuals with CTS e. The evaluation of efficacy of one or more treatment options All relevant studies that met the inclusion criteria were included in the final review.	Early surgical release is beneficial for individuals with CTS "with or without median nerve denervation (255)." Orthotic intervention and steroid injections have an early but temporary benefit in the treatment of CTS. Further research is needed to determine the efficacy of ultrasound in the treatment of individuals with CTS. Future research is also needed to explore the cost/benefit analysis of treatments, including surgery, given the trend of rising health care costs.	One limitation is that efficacy of treatments factored in the cost of the procedure/ treatment, and was not based solely on functional outcomes following the treatment.
Brininger TL, Rogers JC, Holm MB, et al: Efficacy of fabricated customized splint and tendon and nerve gliding exercises for the treatment of carpal tunnel syndrome: a randomized controlled trial, *Arch Phys Med Rehabil* 88(11):1429-1436, 2007.	Randomized factorial design 2X2X3	61 participants with mild to moderate CTS symptoms	The goal of this study was to compare the effects of a custom-made neutral wrist and metacarpophalangeal (MCP) orthosis and a prefabricated wrist cock-up orthosis in the treatment of CTS. The researchers examined the effect of tendon and nerve gliding exercises in addition to the two different orthosis groups. Along with a baseline, results were assessed at 4 and 8 weeks. Specific measurements included the Moberg Pick-up Test, grip strength, tip, palmar, and lateral pinch strengths.	The neutral wrist and MCP orthosis produced a greater reduction in symptoms than the prefabricated wrist cock-up orthosis. Both orthotic groups, regardless of exercises performed, demonstrated a decrease in the severity of symptoms. The tendon and nerve gliding exercises did not appear to have a significant impact on improvement of symptoms for either group.	About 40% of the subjects in the study had previously been treated with orthoses and anti-inflammatory medications for symptoms. Steroid injections and anti-inflammatory medications were not withheld during the study.

Citation	Design	Sample	Methods	Results	Limitations
Finsen V, Zeitlmann H: Carpal tunnel syndrome during pregnancy, Scand J Plast Reconstr Surg Hand Surg 40(1):41-45, 2006.	Single group pre/post test	30 pregnant women identified to have CTS symptoms by a positive Tinnel sign and Phalen test	Participants were asked to record the intensity of their symptoms on a 1-10 pain scale throughout their pregnancy and after. Participants were provided with a wrist orthosis and a diary to record subjective information.	Most CTS symptoms appeared during the 31st week of pregnancy. Five participants requested a release operation during the third trimester. The average pain score remained fairly consistent throughout the final trimester (between 5 and 6). The average pain score declined quickly after delivery. Seven days after delivery the average pain score was 2.4. The pain score correlated positively with the increase and decrease in weight of the pregnant participants.	Incidence of carpal tunnel syndrome in pregnant individuals varies. Participants in the study were often difficult to contact by telephone. Subjective comments and symptoms recorded in subject's diaries were vague.
Werner RA, Franzblau A, Gell N: Randomized controlled trial of nocturnal splinting for active workers with symptoms of carpal tunnel syndrome, Arch Phys Med Rehabil 86(1):1-7, 2005.	Randomized controlled trial	112 participants	Study performed in a Midwest auto plant. Workers with CTS symptoms were included in the study. The treatment group was instructed to wear a customized wrist orthosis in a neutral posture at night for 6 weeks. Both groups viewed a video on workplace ergonomics and repetitive strain injuries. Outcome measures were assessed at 3, 6, and 12 months.	The 6-week trial of wrist orthotic intervention reduced discomfort scores, showed a trend in improvement of the Levine symptom severity scores among the participants in the treatment group and effects lasted throughout the 12-month period.	This study included several limitations that could have affected the interpretation of the results. CTS was not diagnosed in participants before inclusion in the study. The sample size was small. The lack of complete data at the 3 and 6 month appointments limited the interpretation of the outcomes. The loss of study subjects by the 3-month mark when optimal effects would have been expected may have confounded the analysis. Missing data in the regression model may have biased the analysis.

Continued

Table 7-3 Evidence-Based Practice about Wrist Orthotic Intervention—cont'd

AUTHOR'S CITATION	DESIGN	NUMBER OF PARTICIPANTS	DESCRIPTION	RESULTS	LIMITATIONS
Graham RG, Hudson DA, Solomons M, et al: A prospective study to assess the outcome of steroid injections and wrist splinting for the treatment of carpal tunnel syndrome, Plast Reconstr Surg 113(2): 550-556, 2004.	Prospective outcome study	75 patients with 99 affected hands were involved in the study.	The protocol used in this study combined steroid injection with orthotic intervention for CTS. Each patient involved in the study received up to three betamethasone injections depending on the severity of their symptoms and wore a neutral wrist orthosis continuously for 9 weeks. Following the intervention, patients still experiencing symptoms received an open carpal tunnel release. Those who were asymptomatic received follow-up visits for 1 year. Patients who experienced a relapse after conservative treatment were scheduled for surgery.	In the conservative treatment group, only seven patients with ten affected hands remained asymptomatic 1 year after the start of the study. Of the original treatment group, 10.1% of the patients' symptoms were alleviated on a long-term basis using steroid injection and orthotic intervention alone. Of those patients that improved using conservative methods, most had shorter symptom duration (2.9 months versus 8.5 months) and less sensory involvement than those who did not improve with conservative methods. The researchers suggest that patients presenting with CTS receive one steroid injection and wear a neutral wrist orthosis for 3 weeks to determine whether or not a conservative approach might work for them or if they are good candidates for surgery	One limitation of the study was the fluctuation of the participants from beginning to end. Also, only patients experiencing symptoms for longer than 6 weeks were entered in the study. If patients with shorter symptom duration were included in the study, orthotic intervention may have shown greater efficacy.
Gerritsen AA, Korthals-de Bos IB, Laboyrie P, et al: Splinting for carpal tunnel syndrome: prognostic indicators of success, J Neurol Neurosurg Psychiatry 74:1342-1344, 2003.	Randomized controlled trial	89 patients were randomized to the treatment group.	Participants in the randomized treatment group were instructed to wear a neutral wrist orthosis at night for 6 weeks. Eighty-three participants attended follow-up sessions at 12 months after the initial intervention. Those patients (n = 33) who sought other types of treatment were not considered in the study's results.	Predicted probabilities of success of orthotic intervention at 12 months follow up: | DURATION OF COMPLAINTS	SEVERITY OF PARAESTHESIA AT NIGHT	PREDICTED PROBABILITY OF SUCCESS AT 12 MONTHS	ACTUAL SUCCESS AT 12 MONTHS
---	---	---	---
> 1 year	> 6	5%	13% (2/16)
> 1 year	≤ 6	19%	12% (2/17)
≤ 1 year	> 6	28%	23% (6/26)
≤ 1 year	≤ 6	62%	67% (16/24)		The small number of participants involved in this study may have decreased detection of associations between the outcome and certain potential prognostic indicators. Authors cited this study as exploratory in nature.

Reference	Study Type	Sample	Methods	Results	Limitations
Celiker R, Arslan S, Inanici F: Corticosteroid injection vs. nonsteroidal anti-inflammatory drug and splinting in carpal tunnel syndrome, Phys Med Rehabil 81 (3):182-186, 2002.	Prospective unblended randomized clinical trial	37 hands of 23 patients; none had thenaratrophy.	Subjects were randomly assigned to either group A or group B. Group A was treated with a custom-made neutral wrist orthosis for night use only and acemetacine (120 mg/day). Intervention with group B included (40 mg methyl-prednisolone acetate) injected into the area of the carpal tunnel. Pre- and post-treatment measures included: VAS Symptom Severity Scale, median nerve conduction studies, and Phalen and Tinel tests.	Before treatment, Phalen test was positive in 13 (81.3%) hands in group A and 14 (66.6%) hands in group B. Following treatment, Phalen test was negative for all hands in group A and positive in three (14.3%) hands in group B. These findings were not statistically significant between groups. Scores from the VAS were not statistically significant between groups. Evaluation with the Symptom Severity Scale showed statistically significant improvement for both groups. Nerve conduction studies were statistically significant in improvement for both groups. In patients with symptom duration less than 9 months, orthotic intervention and steroid injection resulted in significant improvement in median nerve motor and sensory distal latencies. However, changes in conduction studies were not significant in clients with symptoms lasting more than 9 months.	Because of the short duration (8 weeks) of the study, long-term effects of the two treatment groups cannot be predicted. Results are derived from almost exclusively males and may not generalize beyond that population. This study also may not apply to those with severe CTS because patients with thenar atrophy were excluded from the study.
Walker WC, Metzler M, Cifu DX, et al: Neutral wrist splinting in carpal tunnel syndrome: a comparison of night-only versus full-time wear instructions, Arch Phys Med Rehabil 81(4):424-429, 2000.	Randomized clinical trial	21 patients participated; 17 completed the study.	Subjects were randomly assigned to one of two groups; night-only wear or full-time wear. Participants were instructed to wear a custom-made thermoplastic neutral-positioned wrist orthosis. A self-administered symptom questionnaire assessed symptom severity and functional deficits in CTS.	Six weeks of neutral wrist orthotic intervention in this study was associated with improved symptoms and functional and median nerve impairments. Despite a small sample size, there was a greater physiologic outcome in full-time orthotic wearers. More frequent wear lessened median nerve impairment.	This study was performed using a participant sample from the Veterans Administration consisting of predominantly male subjects (16 to 1). CTS appears more frequently in females. Possibly decreasing the ability to generalize findings from the study. This study also lacked a nonintervention control group due to ethical considerations. This study could have benefitted from a longer study period and larger sample size.

CTS, Carpal tunnel syndrome.

Awareness of current research also points to the fact that many of these studies emphasize the importance of orthotic intervention with early intervention for mild to moderate CTS[50] because orthoses are less beneficial with ongoing parasthesias.[11]

Wrist Orthotic Intervention for Radial Nerve Injuries

Radial nerve injuries most commonly occur from fractures of the humeral shaft, fractures and dislocation of the elbow, or compressions of nerve.[65] Other reasons for radial nerve injuries include lacerations, gunshot wounds, explosions, and amputations. The classic picture of a radial nerve injury is a wrist drop position whereby the wrist and MCP joints are unable to actively extend. If the wrist is involved, sometimes a physician may order a wrist orthosis to place the wrist in a more functional position. The exact wrist positioning is highly subjective, and it is up to the therapist and the client to decide on the amount of extension that maximizes function.

Commonly, 30-45 degrees of extension is considered a position of function for this condition because it facilitates optimum grip and pinch.[13] If a night static wrist orthosis is fabricated it should include the MCPs in extension as well as the thumb MP and IP in extension. Although a wrist orthosis is one option for this condition, there are many other options that therapists should critically consider. These include the location of the orthosis (volar versus dorsal), type of orthosis (e.g., wrist immobilization, tenodesis, or mobilization), and whether to fabricate one or two orthoses. More details about these other types of orthotic intervention options for a radial nerve injury are discussed in Chapter 13.

Wrist Orthotic Intervention for Tendinopathy and Tenosynovitis

Tendinopathy (deterioration of the tendon along with tiny micro tears surrounding the tendon) and tenosynovitis (inflammation of the tendon and its surrounding synovial sheath)[49] are painful conditions that benefit from conservative management, including wrist orthotic intervention. These conditions commonly occur because of cumulative and repetitive motions in work, home, and leisure activities. Having tendinopathy and tenosynovitis can result in an overuse cycle. The overuse cycle begins with friction, microscopic tears, pain, and limitations in motion, followed by resting the involved area, avoidance of use, and development of weakness. When activities resume, the cycle repeats itself.[32] The term tendinopathy is used to refer to many tendon problems and can involve the muscles on the volar (flexor muscles) and dorsal (extensor muscles) surfaces of the forearm. A common site for tendinopathy is the lateral and medial elbow and rotator cuff tendons of the upper extremity.[33]

Tendinopathy often leads to substitution patterns and muscle imbalance.[32] Resting the hand in an orthosis helps to take tension off the muscle-tendon unit. Orthotic intervention for tendinopathy or tenosynovitis minimizes tendon excursion and thus decreases friction at the insertion of the muscles. Orthotic intervention can serve as a reminder to decrease engagement in painful activities. It is beneficial to ask clients to pay attention to those activities that are limited by an orthosis because they are often aggravating factors for tendinopathy. Clients should become more cognizant of aggravating activities and modify them so as not to enhance the condition.[62] Clients should also be cautioned not to tense their muscles and thus fight against the orthosis when wearing it or it may aggravate the tendinopathy. Rather, the muscles should be relaxed. Orthoses provided for tendinopathy or tenosynovitis during acute flare-ups are worn as needed to avoid pain. Orthotic intervention to avoid pain is beneficial, but continuous orthotic usage prevents the nourishment of collagen that is associated with pain-free arcs of motion. Therefore orthotic provision for these conditions should allow for removal for hygiene and pain-free range of motion (ROM) exercises followed by gradual weaning.[20]

Generally, when fabricating orthoses for flexor carpi radialis (FCR) or flexor carpi ulnaris (FCU) tendinopathy, it is recommended that the person's wrist be positioned at neutral or 10 degrees of flexion[20] to rest the tendons.[31] Therapists can fabricate a volar wrist orthosis for FCR and an ulnar gutter wrist orthosis for FCU. Wrist extensor tendinopathy can be fabricated in 20 to 30 degrees of wrist extension, because this normal resting position provides a balance between the flexors and extensors.

Wrist Orthotic Intervention for Rheumatoid Arthritis

For some conditions—such as **rheumatoid arthritis (RA)**—therapists fabricate wrist immobilization orthoses in functional positions of 0 to 30 degrees of wrist extension, thus promoting synergistic wrist-extension and finger-flexion patterns. This position allows the greatest level of function with grip for ADLs.[43,54]

Wearing a wrist orthosis may be used to control pain during activities,[34] and doing so is especially helpful in protecting the wrist during demanding tasks.[67] For people with radiocarpal or mid carpal arthritis, a wrist orthosis fabricated out of thin 1/16-inch thermoplastic material is recommended.[34] For a total wrist arthrodesis, a volar wrist orthosis is provided when the cast is removed (usually at about week 6 to 8 postoperative). This volar wrist orthosis is worn full-time for 8 to 12 weeks.[5]

Wrist orthotic intervention for someone with RA can be quite challenging because of the tendency for the carpal structures of the rheumatoid arthritic wrist to sublux volarly and ulnarly.[22] In addition, there can be related digital involvement to consider, such as MCP volar subluxation and/or ulnar drift. In the early stages of this ulnar drift, the wrist joint should be positioned as close to neutral with respect to radial and ulnar deviation as can be comfortably tolerated. However, some experts recommend positioning the wrist in slight ulnar deviation to promote more neutral MCP positioning.[20] With consistent access to the person, the therapist can progress the wrist into neutral on successive visits. This position helps eliminate the development of a zigzag deformity. The zigzag deformity develops when the carpal bones deviate ulnarly and the metacarpals deviate radially, which exacerbates the ulnar deviation of the MCP joints.[22]

If the MCP joints but not the interphalangeal (IP) joints are involved, the therapist may consider fabricating a wrist orthosis in a neutral position that extends beyond the distal palmar crease and ends proximal to the proximal interphalangeal (PIP) crease. This orthosis supports the MCP joints (Figure 7-9).[55] Another recommendation for someone with

a zigzag deformity is to fabricate an orthosis on the entire hand (see Chapter 9).

When fabricating a wrist orthosis for a person with RA, the therapist uses a thermoplastic material with a high degree of conformability and drapability to help prevent pressure areas. However, when additional assistance is not available, the long working time that highly rubber-based thermoplastic materials provide helps the therapist create a more cosmetic and well-fitting orthosis.[62] The therapist carefully monitors for the development of pressure areas over many of the small bones of the hand and wrist, as shown in Figure 7-10.[22] Another consideration for orthosis fabrication for an individual who has RA is to use an orthotic sock or stockinette underneath the orthosis. If the individual has been on a steroid regimen for a long period of time, the skin is likely to be thinner and more fragile, which increases the potential for superficial burns during the orthotic intervention process.[13] Finally, some people with RA may prefer a prefabricated orthosis that is easy to apply and is perceived to be more comfortable than a fabricated orthosis because it is made out of softer material and has more flexibility. Further discussion later in this chapter addresses the functional implications of commercial or prefabricated wrist orthoses with RA.

Wrist Orthotic Intervention for Fractures

Orthoses for Colles fractures are individualized, based on the person's skeletal and soft tissue status. The initial goal of rehabilitation after a fracture of the distal radius is to regain functional wrist extension.[39] To achieve this goal, fabricate the orthosis to position the wrist in slight extension. Wrist orthotic intervention post-fracture provides protection, pain relief, and rest to the extremity.[46] Custom fabricated orthoses are best because prefabricated

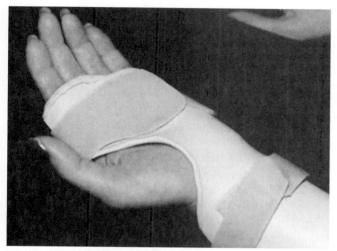

Figure 7-9 An orthosis for a zigzag deformity. (From Philips CA: *Therapist's management of patients with rheumatoid arthritis.* In Hunter JM, Mackin EJ, Callahan AD, editors: *Rehabilitation of the hand,* ed 4, St Louis, 1995, Mosby, pp. 1345-1350.)

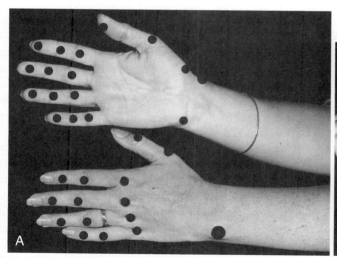
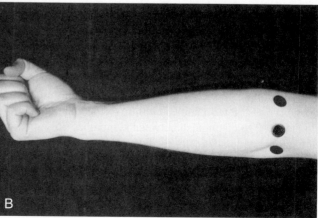

Figure 7-10 Potential areas of fingers, hand, wrist, and forearm include: dorsal metacarpophalangeal (MCP) joints, thumb web space, ulnar styloid, radial styloid, thumb carpometacarpal (CMC) joint, center of palm (especially with flexion wrist contractures), proximal edge of orthosis. (From Fess EE, Gettle KS, Phillips CA, et al: *Hand and upper extremity rehabilitation: Principles and methods,* ed 3, St Louis, 2005, Mosby.)

orthoses may not fit comfortably and may block ROM of the fingers and thumb.[38] Sometimes a serial static orthotic intervention approach may be necessary to regain PROM. (Refer to the discussion later in this chapter for more details about serial static orthotic intervention and also see Chapter 12.)

The therapist fabricates a well-designed custom dorsal or volar orthosis. Moscony[46] recommends a volar wrist orthosis after the removal of a cast for approximately 1 to 2 weeks, whereas Laseter[38] recommends fabricating a dorsal wrist orthosis because it helps control edema and allows for functional motions of the finger joints. If the person needs more support, a circumferential wrist orthosis may be considered.[38] Using a circumferential orthosis is highly supportive and very comfortable. The circumferential orthosis tends to limit forearm rotation more than a volar or dorsal wrist orthosis does.[63] The client is weaned away from any orthosis as soon as possible.[38,39] To encourage regaining function, Weinstock[76] recommends that the orthosis be part of intervention until 30 to 45 degrees of active extension is obtained. If PROM of the wrist/forearm remains limited after approximately 6 to 8 weeks, it may be appropriate to discuss the possibility of mobilization orthotic provision with the physician (see Chapter 12).

Wrist Orthotic Intervention for Sprains

A grade I sprain results in a substance tear with minimal fiber disruption and no obvious tear of the fibers. A mild grade II sprain results in tearing of the ligament fibers. Persons with grade I and II sprains may benefit from wearing a wrist immobilization orthosis. With grade I sprains, the person will likely wear the orthosis for 3 weeks. For grade II sprains, 6 weeks of wear may be indicated. This wrist orthosis helps rest the hand during the acute healing phase and removes stress from the healing ligament.

Wrist Orthotic Intervention for Complex Regional Pain Syndrome Type I (Reflex Sympathetic Dystrophy)

Complex regional pain syndrome describes a complex grouping of symptoms impacting an extremity and characterized by extreme pain, diffuse edema, stiffness, trophic skin changes, and discoloration.[37,72] **Complex regional pain syndrome (CRPS) type I** is a term coined by the World Health Organization (WHO) to distinguish between sympathetically mediated and non-sympathetically mediated pain. CRPS type I is a sympathetically mediated pain.[44,56] CRPS type I refers to pain from a minor injury that lasts longer and hurts more than is anticipated. Type II refers to pain related to a nerve injury. Symptoms are similar for both types of pain.[56]

Orthotic intervention may be a part of the rehabilitation program. However, the current approach is that orthoses are only suggested if it is painful for the person to perform functional movements.[20] The therapist applies clinical reasoning

skills to determine which orthosis meets the various therapeutic goals. (See the discussion on the use of resting hand orthoses with this condition in Chapter 9.) Purposes for providing wrist immobilization orthoses in addition to pain relief are for muscle spasm relief and for regaining a functional resting wrist position.[37,59,75] Recovering a functional resting hand position is important for normal hand motions and for the prevention of deforming forces as a result of muscle imbalance. To increase wrist extension to a more functional position, the therapist may need to provide serial wrist orthoses.

Wrist Joint Contracture: Serial Orthotic Intervention with a Wrist Orthosis

When a wrist is not properly moving (such as after removal of a cast for a Colles fracture), the therapist may consider serial wrist orthotic intervention.[57] With serial orthotic intervention, the therapist intermittently remolds the orthosis to facilitate increases in wrist extension (Figure 7-11). The orthosis is first applied with the wrist positioned at the maximal amount of extension that the current soft-tissue length allows and the person can tolerate. The person is instructed to wear the orthosis for long periods of time, with periodic removal for exercise and hygiene, until the wrist is able to move beyond that amount of extension.

The orthosis is readjusted to position the soft tissues at their maximum length.[17] Positioning living tissue at maximum length causes the tissue to remodel to a longer length.[61] This process is repeated until optimal wrist extension is regained. Thus, serial orthotic intervention is beneficial for PROM limitations because it provides long periods of low load stress at or near the end of the soft-tissue length.[61] Serial wrist orthotic intervention is only one approach that can improve wrist PROM. Other approaches include fabricating a static progressive orthosis and an elastic tension orthosis (see Chapter 12).

Fabrication of a Wrist Immobilization Orthosis

The initial step in the fabrication of a wrist immobilization orthosis (after evaluation of the person's hand) is the drawing of a pattern. Pattern making is important in customizing an orthosis because every person's hand is different in shape and size. Pattern making also saves time and minimizes waste of materials.

A common mistake of a novice therapist during fabrication of a wrist immobilization pattern is drawing the forearm trough narrower than the natural curve of the forearm muscle-bulk contour. This mistake can occur with anyone but especially with a person who has a large forearm. If the forearm trough is not one-half the circumference of the forearm, the orthosis will not provide adequate support. In addition, the therapist must follow the natural angle of the MCP heads with the pattern.

A volar wrist immobilization pattern presents another orthotic intervention option (Figure 7-12, *A*). It is sometimes

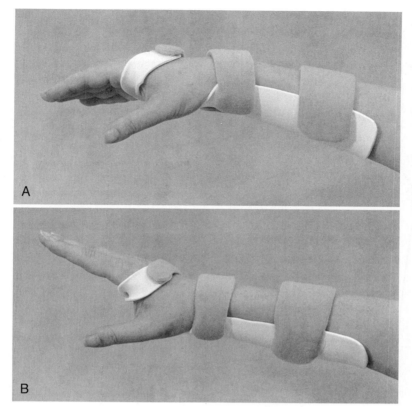

Figure 7-11 A and **B,** Serial wrist orthotic intervention.

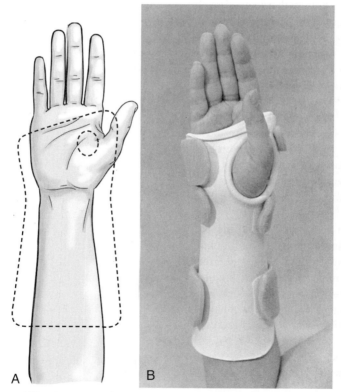

Figure 7-12 A, A volar wrist immobilization pattern for a thumb-hole orthosis. **B,** A volar wrist immobilization thumb-hole orthosis.

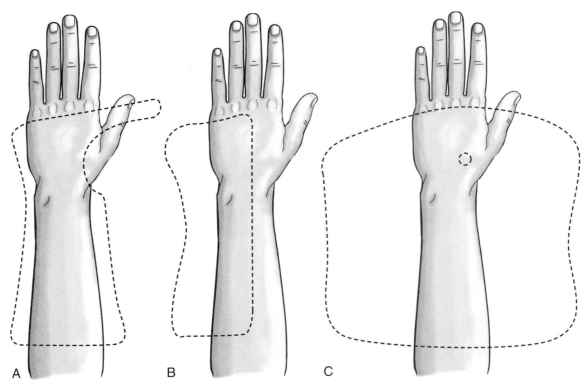

Figure 7-13 A, A dorsal wrist immobilization pattern. **B,** An ulnar wrist immobilization pattern. **C,** A circumferential wrist immobilization pattern.

called a *thumb-hole wrist orthosis.*[66] The therapist constructs the orthosis by punching a hole with a leather punch in the heated thermoplastic material and pushing the thumb through the hole. The therapist rolls the material away from the thumb and thenar eminence far enough that it does not interfere with functional thumb movement and yet allows adequate wrist support (see Figure 7-12, *B*). In one research study, this thumb-hole wrist orthosis was found to be the most restrictive of wrist motion and slowest with dexterity performance compared with volar and dorsal wrist orthoses with metacarpal bars.[66] Figure 7-13, *A,* shows a pattern for a dorsal wrist immobilization orthosis. Figure 7-13, *B,* is a pattern for an ulnar wrist immobilization orthosis. Figure 7-13, *C,* depicts a pattern for a circumferential wrist immobilization orthosis.

Novice therapists may learn to fabricate orthosis patterns by following detailed written instructions and looking at pictures of patterns. As therapists gain experience, they can easily draw patterns without copying from pictures. (See Figures 7-1, 7-2, 7-3, and 7-4 for pictures of completed orthosis products.) The following instruction is for construction of a volar wrist immobilization orthosis (see Figure 7-6 and Figure 7-14) and is similar to instruction for a dorsal wrist immobilization orthosis (see Figure 7-7 and Figure 7-13, *A*). Table 7-4 overviews safety considerations for any wrist orthotic provision.

1. Position the person's hand palm down on a piece of paper. The wrist should be as neutral as possible with respect to radial and ulnar deviation. The fingers should be in a natural resting position (not flat) and slightly

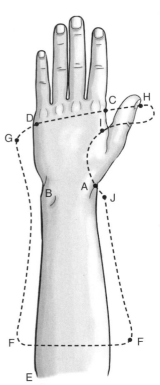

Figure 7-14 A detailed pattern for a volar wrist immobilization orthosis.

abducted. Draw an outline of the hand and forearm to the elbow.

2. While the person's hand is still on the paper, mark an A at the radial styloid and a B at the ulnar styloid.

Table 7-4   Patient Safety Considerations for Wrist Orthotic Intervention

ORTHOTIC FABRICATION	ORTHOTIC WEARING
• Avoid pressure points around the radial and ulnar styloids, the first web space, and the dorsal portion of the metacarpals. • Be aware of the temperature of the thermoplastic material when molding on the patient's wrist. Use a cool damp paper towel or stockinette as protection during the fabrication process. • Never apply the heat gun to the orthosis while the patient is wearing the orthosis. • Monitor wrist position while the thermoplastic material is cooling because sometimes patients reposition during the process. • For individuals with thin skin, consider lining the orthosis with padding or an orthotic liner to reduce pressure or skin irritation, or have the person wear a stockinette.	• Patient should be instructed to monitor skin for redness and report immediately to the therapist any irritation(s). • Educate the patient on the importance of following the orthotic wearing schedule. • Provide patient with information regarding safe storage and cleaning of the orthosis. • Instruct the patients to never make their own adjustments to the orthosis and to inform the therapist of any discomfort.

Mark the second and fifth metacarpal heads C and D, respectively. Mark the olecranon process of the elbow E. Remove the hand from the pattern. Mark two-thirds the length of the forearm on each side with an X. Place another X on each side of the pattern about 1 to 1½ inches outside and parallel to the two previous X markings for the approximate width of the orthosis, and label each F. These markings are to accommodate for the side of the forearm trough.

3. Draw an angled line connecting the marks of the second and fifth metacarpal heads (C to D). Extend this line approximately 1 to 1½ inches from the ulnar side of the hand, and mark it G. On the radial side of the hand, extend the line straight out approximately 2 inches, and mark it H.

4. On the ulnar side of the orthosis, extend the metacarpal line from G down the hand and forearm of the orthotic pattern, making sure the pattern follows the person's forearm muscle bulk. End this line at F.

5. Measure and place an I approximately ¾ inch below the mark for the head of the index finger (C). Extend a line parallel from I to the line between C and H. Curve this line to meet H. This area represents the extension of the metacarpal bar and usually measures approximately ¾ inch down from C to the outline on the other side of the metacarpal bar. Draw a curved line that simulates the thenar crease from I to A. Extend the line past A about 1 inch, and mark it J.

6. Draw a line from J down the radial side of the forearm, making sure the line follows the increasing size of the forearm. Curve out like drawing a "bell" to ensure that the orthosis design is adequate to fit the forearm. To ensure that the orthosis is two-thirds the length of the forearm, end the line at F.

7. For the bottom of the orthosis, draw a straight line connecting both F marks.

8. Make sure the pattern lines are rounded at H, G, J, and the two Fs to prevent any pressure or discomfort.

9. Cut out the pattern.

10. Position the person's upper extremity with the elbow resting on a pad (folded towel or foam wedge) on the table and the forearm in a neutral position—rather than in supination or pronation, which results in a poorly-fitted orthosis. Make sure that the fingers are relaxed and the thumb is lightly touching the index finger. Place the wrist immobilization pattern on the person as shown in Figure 7-15, A. Check that the wrist has adequate support, with the pattern ending just proximal to the MCP joint. On the dorsal surface of the hand, check whether the hypothenar bar on the ulnar side of the hand ends just proximal to the fifth metacarpal head. The metacarpal bar on the radial side of the hand should point to the triquetrum or distal ulna bone after it wraps through the first web space. On the volar surface of the hand, check below the thumb carpometacarpal (CMC) joint to determine whether the pattern provides enough support at the wrist joint. Make sure the forearm trough is two-thirds the length and one-half the width of the forearm. Make necessary adjustments (i.e., additions or deletions) on the pattern.

11. Trace the pattern onto the sheet of thermoplastic material.

12. Heat the thermoplastic material.

13. Cut the pattern out of the thermoplastic material.

14. Measure the person's wrist using a goniometer to determine whether the wrist has been placed in the correct position. The therapist should instruct and practice with the person maintaining the correct position (see Figure 7-15, B).

15. Reheat the thermoplastic material.

16. Mold the form onto the person's hand. To fit the orthosis on the person, place the person's elbow in a resting position on a pad on the table with the forearm in a neutral position. Make sure the fingers are relaxed and the thumb is lightly touching the index finger (see Figure 7-15, C). The advantage of this approach is that the therapist can better monitor the wrist position visually during orthosis formation.

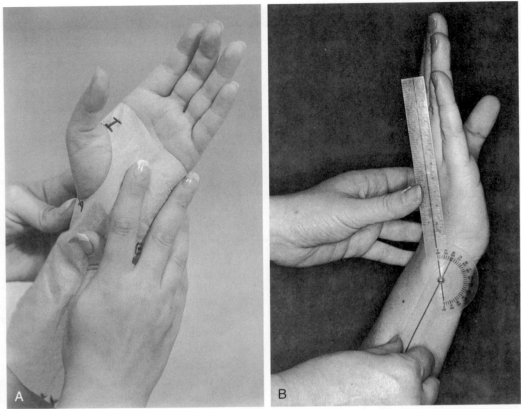

Figure 7-15 A, Placing of the wrist immobilization pattern on the person. **B,** Before forming the orthosis, the therapist should measure the person's wrist with a goniometer to obtain the correct amount of extension.

17. Make sure that the wrist remains correctly positioned as the thermoplastic material hardens. During the formation phase, roll the metacarpal bar just proximal to the distal palmar crease, and roll the thermoplastic material toward the thenar crease. Flare the distal end of the orthosis on a flat surface to prevent skin breakdown (see Figure 7-15, *D*).
18. Make necessary adjustments on the orthosis (see Figure 7-15, *E* and *F*).
19. Cut the Velcro into approximately ½-inch oval shaped pieces for the metacarpal bar area and 1½-inch oval pieces for the forearm trough. Heat the adhesive with a heat gun to encourage adherence before putting them on the orthosis. Using a solvent on the thermoplastic material, scratch the thermoplastic material to remove some of the non-stick coating to help with adherence of the Velcro pieces (see Figure 7-15, *G*). For an adult, add two 2-inch straps on the forearm trough and one narrower strap on the dorsal surface of the hand, thus connecting the metacarpal bar on the radial side to the hypothenar bar on the ulnar side of the hand. A child's orthosis requires straps that are narrower than an adult's. The strap placed at the wrist is located exactly at the wrist joint and not proximal to it to ensure a good fit (see Figure 7-15, *H*).

Technical Tips for a Proper Fit

- Choose a thermoplastic material that has a high degree of conformability to allow a close fit and to prevent migration. Some therapists may prefer a rubber-based moderate drape thermoplastic material.
- Use caution when cutting a pattern out of thermoplastic material that stretches easily. Leave stretchable thermoplastic material flat on the table when cutting to prevent the material from stretching and the orthosis from losing the original shape of the pattern.
- When positioning the client, one option is to position the person's elbow joint on a towel with the elbow flexed 90 degrees and the forearm in neutral. Another option is to position the person's forearm resting on a rolled towel on a table in a supinated position, allowing the wrist to fall into extension. The first position allows for more careful observation of wrist position, but the orthotic material may stretch. The second option provides a more comfortable relaxed position for the person.
- Mold the orthosis sequentially. For a volar wrist immobilization orthosis, form the hypothenar bar (Figure 7-16, *A*), wrap the metacarpal bar around the palm to the dorsal side of the hand (see Figure 7-16, *B*), roll down the metacarpal bar (see Figure 7-16, *C*), and then form the thenar area (see Figure 7-16, *D*). See the

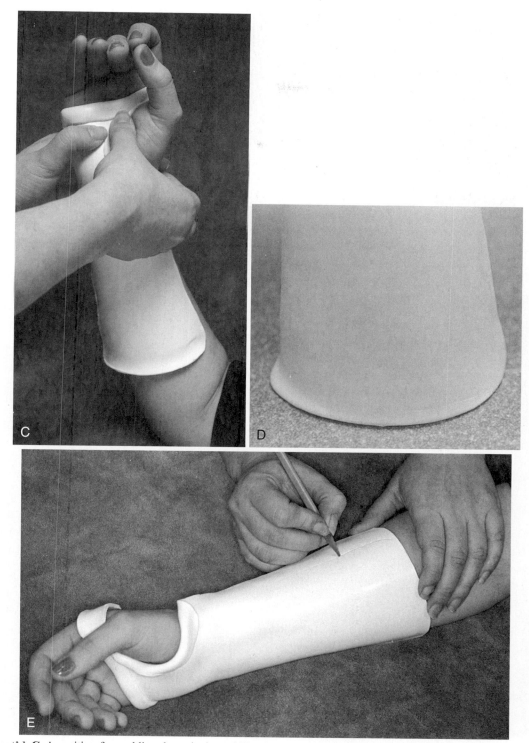

Figure 7-15, cont'd C, A position for molding the wrist immobilization orthosis. **D,** Flaring the distal end of the orthosis on a flat surface. **E,** Marking of the orthosis to make an adjustment.

specific comments in this section for hints about each of these areas.

- As the orthosis is being formed, be sure to follow the natural curves of the longitudinal, distal, and proximal arches. Having the person lightly touch the thumb to the index finger during molding helps conform the orthosis to the arches

of the hand (see Figure 7-15, C). Mold the thermoplastic material to conform naturally to the center of the palm. Be careful not to flatten the transverse arch, which could cause metacarpal contractures. However, overemphasizing the transverse carpal arch can create a focal pressure point in the central palm that will be intolerable for the person.

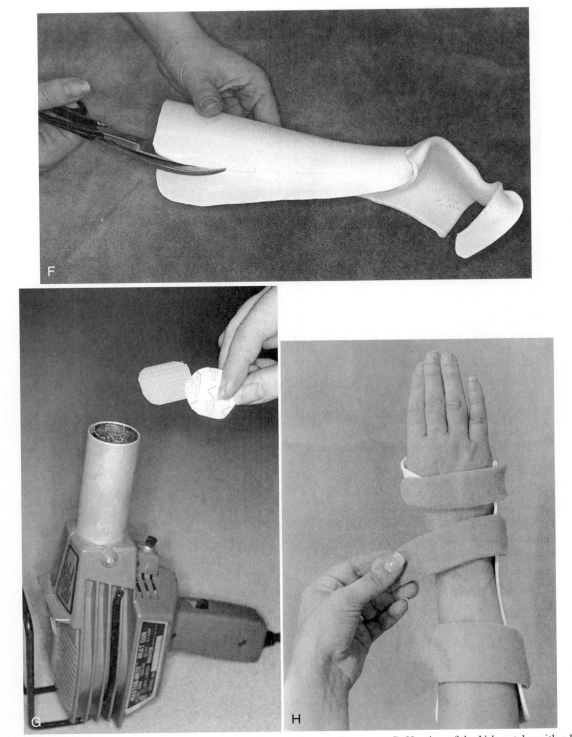

Figure 7-15, cont'd F, Cutting off excess thermoplastic material to make an adjustment. **G,** Heating of the Velcro tabs with a heat gun to help them adhere to the orthosis. **H,** The therapist should place two straps on the forearm trough with one at the wrist level and one strap on the dorsal surface of the hand that connects the metacarpal bar to the hypothenar bar.

- For a volar wrist immobilization orthosis, position the metacarpal bar on the volar surface just proximal to the distal palmar crease. This position allows adequate wrist support and full MCP flexion. In addition, make sure the metacarpal bar follows the natural angle of the distal transverse arch (see Figure 7-16, *B*). On the dorsal

surface, position the metacarpal bar just proximal to the natural angle of the MCP heads. A correctly conformed dorsal metacarpal bar helps to hold the wrist in the correct position. If the metacarpal bar does not conform and there is a gap, the wrist will be mobile. For comfort, some clients may prefer that the metacarpal bar is

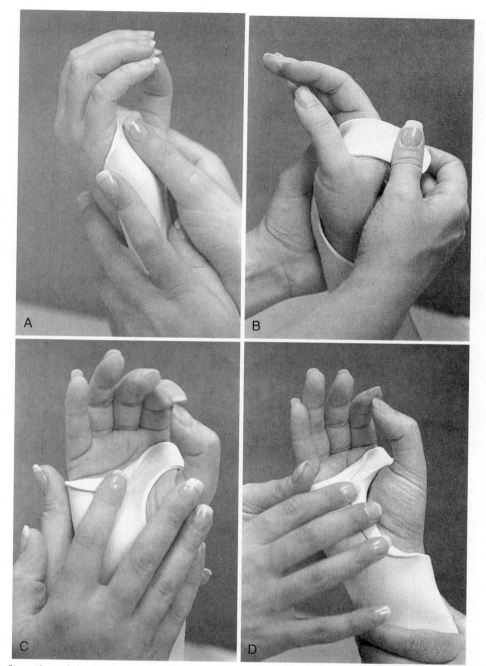

Figure 7-16 A, The formation of the hypothenar bar. **B,** Wrapping the metacarpal bar around the palm. **C,** Rolling the metacarpal bar. **D,** Forming the thenar area.

shorter and the strap longer on the dorsal surface due to the bony prominence of the metacarpals on the dorsum of the hand.

- Always determine whether the person has full finger flexion when wearing the orthosis by having him or her flex the MCP joints. If any areas of the metacarpal bar are too high, the therapist makes adjustments.
- Make sure the hand and wrist are positioned correctly by taking into consideration the position of a normal resting hand. On volar and dorsal wrist immobilization orthoses, the metacarpal bar (which wraps around the radial side of the hand) and the hypothenar bar (on the ulnar side)

help position and hold the wrist (Figure 7-17). If adequate support is lacking on either side, the wrist may be in an incorrect position.

- A frequent fabrication mistake is to allow the wrist to deviate radially or ulnarly. This mistake can occur because of a lack of careful monitoring of the person's wrist position as the thermoplastic material is cooling. The therapist should closely monitor the wrist position in any orthosis that positions the wrist in neutral, because it is easy for the wrist to move in slight flexion. A quick spot check before the thermoplastic material is completely cool can address this problem.

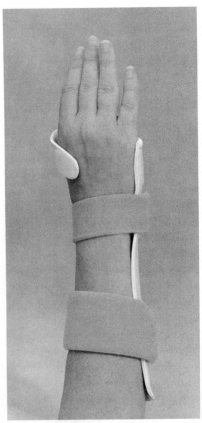

Figure 7-17 The metacarpal bar and hypothenar bar help position and hold the wrist.

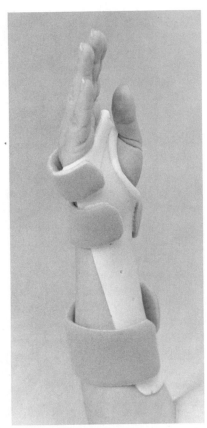

Figure 7-18 This forearm trough was twisted.

- If a mistake occurs with an orthotic material that easily stretches, be extremely careful with adjustments to avoid further compromising of wrist position. For thermoplastic material with memory, remold the entire orthosis rather than spot heating the wrist area because doing the latter tends to cause the material to buckle. Sometimes adjustments can be done by heating the entire orthosis made from material without memory.
- After the formation of the palmar and wrist part of the orthosis is complete, the therapist can begin to work on other areas of the orthosis, such as the forearm trough. A problem that can easily be corrected just before the thermoplastic material is cooled is twisting of the forearm trough. If this problem is not corrected, the orthosis will end up with one edge of the forearm trough higher than the other (Figure 7-18).
- After the thermoplastic material has cooled, determine whether the person can fully oppose the thumb to all fingers. The thenar eminence should not be restricted or flattened. Wrist support should be adequate to maintain the angle of the wrist. To check whether the thenar eminence area is rolled enough, have the person move the thumb in opposition to the little finger, and sustain the hold while evaluating the roll. Also observe that the thenar crease is visible, to allow for full thumb mobility. Adjustments should be made to allow complete thumb excursion. Otherwise, a potential for a pressure sore to develop exists, especially in the area of the thumb web space (Figure 7-19).

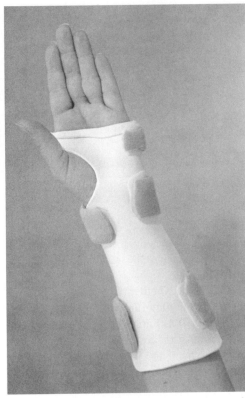

Figure 7-19 This thenar web space was not rolled enough to allow full thumb excursion.

- Occasionally after the thermoplastic material is cooled, the therapist will note areas that are too tight in the forearm trough, which can potentially result in pressure sores. To easily correct this problem, the therapist pulls apart the sides of the forearm trough.

Trouble Shooting Wrist Immobilization Orthoses

A careful practitioner must continuously think of precautions, such as checking for pressure areas. Precautions for making a wrist immobilization orthosis include the following:

- Be aware of and make adjustments for potential pressure points on the radial styloid, on the ulnar styloid, at the first web space, and over the dorsal aspects of the metacarpals. The thumb web space is a prime area for skin irritation because it is so tender. Some people cannot tolerate plastic in the first web space. The thermoplastic material must be cut back and replaced with soft strapping. Others can tolerate the plastic if it is rolled and extremely thin.[63] Instruct the person to monitor the skin for reddened areas and to communicate immediately about any irritation that occurs.
- Control edema before orthotic provision. For persons with sustained edema, avoid using constricting wrist orthoses. Instead, fabricate a wider forearm trough with wide strapping material.[14] Dorsal orthoses are better for edematous hands.[17,38] Carefully monitor persons who have the potential for edematous hands and make necessary orthotic adjustments. As discussed earlier, a "continuous strap" made out of flexible fabric is a good strapping option to help manage edema.
- For persons with little subcutaneous tissue and thin skin, carefully monitor the skin for pressure areas. Lining the orthosis with padding may help, but several adjustments may be necessary for a proper fit. Fabricating the orthosis over a thick orthotic liner, QuickCast liner, or a piece of stockinette can prevent skin irritation during orthotic fabrication.
- Make sure the orthosis provides adequate support for functional activities.

Prefabricated Orthoses

Prefabricated or commercially-available wrist orthoses are commonly used in the treatment of CTS and RA.[22,67,78] A variety of prefabricated wrist orthoses are available, as shown in Figure 7-20.

As discussed, conservative management of CTS includes positioning the wrist as close to neutral as possible to maximize the space in the carpal tunnel. The supportive metal or thermoplastic stay in most prefabricated wrist orthoses positions the wrist in extension. Therefore, an adjustment must be made to position the wrist in the desired neutral position. However, care must be taken when adjustments are made to ensure that the orthosis adequately fits and supports the hand.

Several options for prefabricated wrist orthoses are marketed for CTS. Options for the work environment include padding to reduce trauma from vibration, leather for added durability, and metal internal pieces that act to position the wrist. Prefabricated wrist immobilization orthoses are also effective for symptoms of CTS during pregnancy (Figure 7-20).[2]

Fabricating an orthosis for a person who has RA is most effective in the early stages and incorporates positioning, immobilization, and the assumed comfort of neutral warmth from a soft orthosis. The effects of RA can result in decreased joint stability, leading to decreased grip strength and the more obvious finger deformities.[22] When persons with RA wear elastic wrist orthoses, they help decrease pain during ADLs.[67] Prefabricated wrist orthoses marketed for persons with RA are designed for easy application and to decrease ulnar deviation. Some orthoses include correction or protection for finger joints as well as for the wrist joint.

Therapists need to determine whether or not to fabricate a custom wrist orthosis or to use a commercial prefabricated wrist orthosis. There are many factors to consider with this decision, such as the impact of the prefabricated or custom orthosis on hand function, pain reduction, and degrees of immobilization that the orthosis provides.[8,53,70,71] Research helps therapists select the best orthosis for their clients. Collier and Thomas[18] studied the degree of immobilization of a custom volar wrist orthosis as compared to three commercial prefabricated wrist orthoses. They found that the custom wrist orthosis allowed "significantly less palmar flexion and significantly more dorsiflexion" than the commercial orthoses. Thus, custom thermoplastic orthoses may block wrist motion better than prefabricated orthoses, which are more flexible.

Other studies considered the effect of commercial prefabricated orthoses on grip and dexterity,[12,67,70,71] work performance,[53] and proximal musculature.[9] Continued research needs to be done to analyze the efficacy of commercial orthoses, especially as newer ones are developed. Furthermore, as Stern and colleagues[69] found, no single type of wrist orthosis will be appropriate for all clients and that satisfaction with a prefabricated orthosis is often associated with therapeutic benefits, comfort, and utility. Therefore, it benefits therapists to stock a variety of prefabricated orthosis options in the clinic[67] or therapists can provide information to clients so that they can procure the right orthosis for themselves. Box 7-1 provides some questions for therapists to contemplate when considering a prefabricated wrist orthosis or custom-made wrist orthosis. This information can also be used to educate clients to procure the right prefabricated orthosis for themselves.

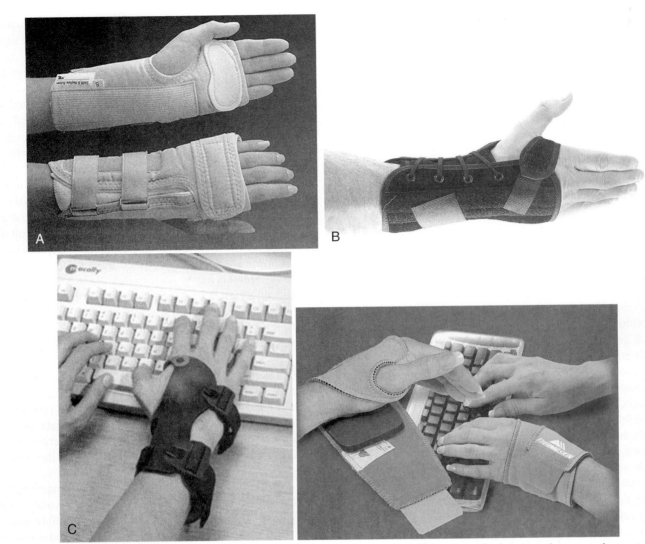

Figure 7-20 A, This wrist orthosis has D-ring straps (Rolyan D-Ring Wrist Brace). **B,** This wrist orthosis has a unique strapping system with laces (Sammons Preston Rolyan Laced Wrist Support). **C,** This light weight orthosis can be used for carpal tunnel and other repetitive injuries (Exolite Wrist Brace). **D,** This orthosis is made of a Neoprene blend, which allows circulation to the skin (Termoskin Wrist Brace). **E,** This orthosis is a prefabricated orthosis commonly used to relieve carpal tunnel syndrome and other conditions affecting the wrist. (**D,** Courtesy of Sammons Preston Rolyan, Bolingbrook, IL.)

Box 7-1   Questions to Determine Use of Custom-Made versus Prefabricated Wrist Orthosis

- Is time a factor? (Consider providing prefabricated orthoses; although with experience a custom orthosis can be made in a short time period.)
- Is cost a factor? (Consider costs with custom orthoses versus prefabricated orthoses.)
- Is fit a factor? (Consider whether the prefabricated orthosis is restricting too much motion, such as thumb opposition, or chafes the hand.[67] Or consider whether it is really doing what it is supposed to do, such as keeping the hand in neutral with carpal tunnel syndrome (CTS).[74])
- Is only wrist support required? (Consider either a custom or a prefabricated orthosis.)
- Is restriction of motion a factor? (Consider a custom orthosis.)
- Does the person need the orthosis only for pain relief, such as with arthritis? (Consider a prefabricated orthosis or a custom-made orthosis with padding.)

- Is the person involved in sports? (Consider a soft prefabricated orthosis to avert injury to other people.[6])
- Is wrist and hand edema a factor? (Consider fabricating a custom dorsal wrist orthosis, taking edema into consideration.)
- Is the weight of the orthosis a factor? (Consider custom fabricating an orthosis out of lighter thermoplastic material [$\frac{1}{16}$ inch] or a lightweight prefabricated orthosis.)
- What are the occupational demands of the person? (Consider a custom-fabricated orthosis if heavy labor is part of the person's life or a prefabricated orthosis if demands are minimal.[34] Consider the material out of which the prefabricated orthosis is fabricated. A prefabricated orthosis out of leather may provide adequate durability, support, protection, and comfort for job demands.)
- Has any research evidence on the orthoses being considered been accessed?

Impact on Occupations

For people with the diagnoses discussed in this chapter, supporting the wrist while allowing finger and thumb motions enables them to continue their life occupations. For example, a person with CTS wears a wrist orthosis to avoid extreme wrist positions when working and doing other occupations.

A person with arthritis obtains support and pain relief from wearing a wrist orthosis while doing functional activities. A person undergoing serial orthotic intervention after a Colles fracture to decrease stiffness will eventually be able to better perform meaningful occupations. Wrist orthoses can help many people maintain or eventually improve their functional abilities.

SELF-QUIZ 7-1*

In regard to the following questions, circle either true (T) or false (F).

1. T F Wrist immobilization orthoses can be volar, dorsal, ulnar, or circumferential.
2. T F A wrist immobilization orthosis usually decreases wrist pain or inflammation, provides support, enhances digital function, and prevents wrist deformity.
3. T F All prefabricated orthoses are made to correctly fit someone who has carpal tunnel syndrome (CTS).
4. T F Some research suggests the value of early conservative intervention with orthotic intervention.
5. T F After removal of a cast for a Colles fracture, if motion is limited in the wrist, the therapist may consider serial orthotic intervention.
6. T F The therapist must follow standard intervention protocols exactly for any diagnosis that requires a wrist immobilization orthotic application.
7. T F With a wrist immobilization orthosis, the therapist usually positions the wrist in extreme extension, which promotes functional movement.
8. T F The hypothenar bar on a wrist immobilization orthosis helps to position the hand in a neutral resting position by preventing extreme ulnar deviation.
9. T F The therapist should position the volar wrist immobilization orthosis distal to the distal palmar crease.
10. T F If a mistake is made during fabrication of a volar wrist immobilization orthosis, in getting the correct wrist extension the therapist should spot heat the wrist area to make an adjustment.
11. T F People with CTS should be encouraged to perform strong finger flexion while wearing their orthoses to allow for finger mobility.

*See Appendix A for the answer key.

Summary

As this chapter content reflects, appropriate wrist alignment is very important to maintaining a functional hand. A well-fitted orthosis can be a key element to assist with recovery from many conditions. Therefore, therapists should be aware of diagnostic indications, types, parts, and appropriate fabrication for wrist orthotic intervention. As always in clinical practice, the therapist needs to apply clinical reasoning, because each case is different. Finally, therapists should consider the person's occupations when providing a wrist orthosis.

Review Questions

1. What are three main indications for use of a wrist immobilization orthosis?
2. When fabricating a wrist orthosis for a person with RA, what are some of the common deformities that can influence orthotic intervention?
3. When might a therapist consider serial orthotic intervention with a wrist immobilization orthosis?
4. What are the goals of wrist orthotic intervention with a Colles fracture?
5. What is the advantage of a volar wrist immobilization orthosis?
6. What is a disadvantage of a dorsal wrist immobilization orthosis?
7. What purpose does the hypothenar bar serve on a wrist immobilization orthosis?
8. What are two positions that the therapist can use for molding a static wrist orthosis, and what are the advantages of each?
9. Which precautions are unique to static wrist immobilization orthoses?
10. What are four questions that therapists could consider when deciding on a prefabricated wrist orthosis versus a custom fabricated wrist orthosis?
11. What are some findings from the evidence that support wrist orthotic intervention for CTS?

References

1. American Academy of Orthopaedic Surgeons: *Clinical practice guideline on the treatment of carpal tunnel syndrome*, Rosemont, IL, 2008, American Academy of Orthopaedic Surgeons (AAOS).

2. Alakin E, El O, Peker O, et al.: Treatment of carpal tunnel syndrome with nerve and tendon gliding exercises, *American J Phys Med Rehabil* 81(2):108–113, 2002.

3. Bailey J, Cannon N, Colditz J, et al.: *Splint classification system*, Chicago, 1992, Am Soc Hand Therap.

4. Apfel E, Johnson M, Abrams R: Comparison of range-of-motion constraints provided by prefabricated splints used in the treatment of carpal tunnel syndrome: a pilot study, *J Hand Ther* 15(3):226–233, 2002.

4a. Baker NA, Moehlingm KK, Rubinstein EN, Wollstein R, Gustafsonk N,P, Baratz M: The comparative effectiveness of combined lumbrical muscle splints and stretches on symptoms and function in carpal tunnel syndrome, *Archives of Physical Medicine and Rehabilitation* 93(1):1–10, 2012.

5. Bednar JM, Von Lersner-Benson C: Wrist reconstruction: salvage procedures. In Mackin EJ, Callahan AD, Skirven TM, et al.: *Rehabilitation of the hand and upper extremity*, ed 5, St Louis, 2002, Mosby, pp 1195–1202.

6. Bell-Krotoski JA, Breger-Stanton DE: Biomechanics and evaluation of the hand. In Mackin EJ, Callahan AD, Skirven TM, et al, editor: *Rehabilitation of the hand and upper extremity*, ed 5, St Louis, 2002, Mosby, pp 240–262.

7. Biese J: Therapist's evaluation and conservative management of rheumatoid arthritis in the hand and wrist. In Mackin EJ, Callahan AD, Skirven TM, et al.: *Rehabilitation of the hand and upper extremity*, ed 5, St Louis, 2002, Mosby, pp 1569–1582.

8. Brininger TL, Rogers JC, Holm MB, et al.: Efficacy of fabricated customized splint and tendon and nerve gliding exercises for the treatment of carpal tunnel syndrome: a randomized controlled trial, *Arch Phys Med Rehabil* 88(11):1429–1436, 2007.

9. Bulthaup S, Cipriani DJ, Thomas JJ: An electromyography study of wrist extension orthoses and upper-extremity function, *Am J Occup Ther* 53(5):434–444, 1999.

10. Burke D, Burke MM, Steward GW, et al.: Splinting for carpal tunnel syndrome: in search of the optimal angle, *Arch Phys Med Rehabil* 75(11):1241–1244, 1994.

11. Burke FD, Ellis J, McKenna H, et al.: Primary care management of carpal tunnel syndrome, *Postgrad Med J* 79(934):433–437, 2003.

12. Burtner PA, Anderson JB, Marcum ML, et al.: A comparison of static and dynamic wrist splints using electromyography in individuals with rheumatoid arthritis, *J Hand Ther* 16(4):320–325, 2003.

13. Cannon, et al.: *Diagnosis and treatment manual for physicians and therapists*, ed 4, Indianapolis, 2013, The Hand Rehabilitation Center of Indiana.

14. Cannon NM: *Manual of hand splinting*, New York, 1985, Churchill Livingstone.

15. Celiker R, Arslan S, Inanici F: Corticosteroid injection vs. nonsteriodal antiinflammatory drug and splinting in carpal tunnel syndrome, *Am J Phys Med Rehabil* 81(3):182–186, 2002.

16. Cobb TK, An KN, Cooney WP: Effect of lumbrical muscle incursion within the carpal tunnel on carpal tunnel pressure: a cadaveric study, *J Hand Surg Am* 20(2):186–192, 1995.

17. Colditz JC: Therapist's management of the stiff hand. In Mackin EJ, Callahan AD, Skirven TM, et al.: *Rehabilitation of the hand and upper extremity*, ed 5, St Louis, 2002, Mosby, pp 1021–1049.

18. Collier SE, Thomas JJ: Range of motion at the wrist: a comparison study of four wrist extension orthoses and the free hand, *Am J Occup Ther* 56(2):180–184, 2002.

19. Cook AC, Szabo RM, Birkholz SW, et al.: Early mobilization following carpal tunnel release: a prospective randomized study, *J Hand Surg Br* 20(2):228–230, 1995.

20. Cooper C: Personal communication, January 2012.

21. Courts RB: Splinting for symptoms of carpal tunnel syndrome during pregnancy, *J Hand Therapy* 8:31–34, 1995.

22. Dell PC, Dell RB: Management of rheumatoid arthritis of the wrist, *J Hand Ther* 9(2):157–164, 1996.

23. Fess EE, Gettle KS, Philips CA, et al.: *Hand splinting principles and methods*, ed 3, St Louis, 2005, Elsevier Mosby.

23a. Finsen V, Zeitlmann H: Carpal tunnel syndrome during pregnancy, *Scandinavian Journal of Plastic and Reconstructive Surgery and Hand Surgery* 40:41–45, 2006.

24. Gelberman RH, Hergenroeder PT, Hargens AR, et al.: The carpal tunnel syndrome: a study of carpal canal pressures, *J Bone Joint Surg Am* 63(3):380–383, 1981.

25. Gerritsen AA, de Vet HC, Scholten RJ, et al.: Splinting vs surgery in the treatment of carpal tunnel syndrome: a randomized controlled trial, *JAMA* 288(10):1245–1251, 2002.

26. Gerritsen AA, Korthals-de Bos IB, Laboyrie PM, et al.: Splinting for carpal tunnel syndrome: prognostic indicators of success, *J Neurol Neurosurg Psychiatry* 74(9):1342–1344, 2003.

27. Graham RG, Hudson DA, Solomons M, et al.: A prospective study to assess the outcome of steroid injections and wrist splinting for the treatment of carpal tunnel syndrome, *Plast Reconstr Surg* 113(2):550–556, 2004.

28. Hayes EP, Carney K, Mariatis Wolf J, et al.: Carpal tunnel syndrome. In Mackin EJ, Callahan AD, Skirven TM, et al.: *Rehabilitation of the hand and upper extremity*, ed 5, St Louis, 2002, Mosby, pp 643–659.

29. Horng YS, Hsieh SF, Tu YK, et al.: The comparative effectiveness of tendon and nerve gliding exercises in patients with carpal tunnel syndrome, *Am J Phys Med Rehabil* 90(6):435–442, 2011.

30. Huisstede BM, Hoofvliet P, Randsdorp MS, et al.: Carpal tunnel syndrome. Part I: effectiveness of nonsurgical treatments—a systematic review, *Arch Phys Med Rehabil* 91(7):981–1004, 2010.

31. Idler RS: Helping the patient who has wrist or hand tenosynovitis. Part 2: managing trigger finger, de Quervain's disease, *J Musculoskelet Med* 14(2):62–65, 1997. 68, 74–75.

32. Kasch MC: Therapist's evaluation and treatment of upper extremity cumulative-trauma disorders. In Mackin EJ, Callahan AD, Skirven TM, et al, editors. *Rehabilitation of the hand and upper extremity*, ed 5, St Louis, 2002, Mosby, pp 1005–1018.

32a. Keith MW, et al.: Clinical practice guideline on the treatment of carpal tunnel syndrome, *The Journal of Bone and Joint Surgery, Incorporated* 92:218–219, 2010.

33. Khan KM, Cook JL, Taunton JE, et al.: Overuse tendinosis, not tendonitis part 1: a new paradigm for a difficult clinical problem, *Phys Sportsmed* 28(5):38–48, 2000.

34. Kozin SH, Michlovitz SL: Traumatic arthritis and osteoarthritis of the wrist, *J Hand Ther* 13(2):124–135, 2000.

35. Kulick RG: Carpal tunnel syndrome, *Orthop Clin North Am* 27(2):345–354, 1996.

36. Kuo MH, Leong CP, Cheng YF, et al.: Static wrist position associated with least median nerve compression: sonographic evaluation, *Am J Phys Med Rehabil* 80(4):256–260, 2001.

37. Lankford LL: Reflex sympathetic dystrophy. In Hunter JM, Mackin EJ, Callahan AD, editors: *Rehabilitation of the hand: surgery and therapy*, ed 4, St Louis, 1995, Mosby, pp 779–815.

38. Laseter GF: Therapist's management of distal radius fractures. In Mackin EJ, Callahan AD, Skirven TM, et al.: *Rehabilitation of the hand and upper extremity*, ed 5, St Louis, 2002, Mosby, pp 1136–1155.

39. Laseter GF, Carter PR: Management of distal radius fractures, *J Hand Ther* 9(2):114–128, 1996.

40. LaStayo P: Ulnar wrist pain and impairment: a therapist's algorithmic approach to the triangular fibrocartilage complex. In Mackin EJ, Callahan AD, Skirven TM, et al, editors. *Rehabilitation of the hand and upper extremity*, ed 5, St Louis, 2002, Mosby, pp 1156–1170.

41. LaBlanc KE, Cestia W: Carpal tunnel syndrome, *Am Fam Physician* 83(8):952–958, 2011.

42. McClure P: Evidence-based practice: an example related to the use of splinting in a patient with carpal tunnel syndrome, *J Hand Ther* 16(3):256–263, 2003.

43. Melvin JL: *Rheumatic disease in the adult and child: occupational therapy and rehabilitation*, ed 3, Philadelphia, 1989, FA Davis.

44. Mersky H, Bogduk N: *Classification of chronic pain: descriptions of chronic pain syndromes and definitions of pain terms*, ed 2, Seattle, 1994, IASP Press.

45. Messer RS, Bankers RM: Evaluating and treating common upper extremity nerve compression and tendonitis syndromes... without becoming cumulatively traumatized, *Nurse Pract Forum* 6(3):152–166, 1995.

46. Moscony AMB: Common wrist and hand fractures. In Cooper C, editor: *Fundamentals of hand therapy: clinical reasoning and treatment guidelines for common diagnoses of the upper extremity*, St Louis, 2007, Elsevier.

47. Nordenskiold U: Elastic wrist orthoses: reduction of pain and increase in grip force for women with rheumatoid arthritis, *Arthritis Care Res* 3(3):158–162, 1990.

48. Nuckols T, Harber P, Sandin K, et al.: Quality measures for the diagnosis and non-operative management of carpal tunnel syndrome in occupational settings, *J Occup Rehabil* 21(1):100–119, 2011.

49. Tendinopathy, *Online medical information* (website). http://online-medical-information.com/tendinopathy/tendinopathy.html. Accessed February 16, 2014.

50. Ono S, Chapham PJ, Chung KC: Optimal management of carpal tunnel syndrome, *Int J Gen Med* 3:235–261, 2010.

51. O'Connor D, Mullett H, Doyle M, et al.: Minimally displaced Colles' fractures: a prospective randomized trial of treatment with a wrist splint or a plaster cast, *J Hand Surgery Br* 28(1):50–53, 2003.

52. Osterman AL, Whitman M, Porta LD: Nonoperative carpal tunnel syndrome treatment, *Hand Clin* 18(2):279–289, 2002.

53. Pagnotta A, Baron M, Korner-Bitensky N: The effect of a static wrist orthosis on hand function in individuals with rheumatoid arthritis, *J Rheumatol* 25(5):879–885, 1998.

54. Palmer AK, Werner FW, Murphy D, et al.: Functional wrist motion: a biomechanical study, *J Hand Surg Am* 10(1):39–46, 1985.

55. Philips CA: Therapist's management of patients with rheumatoid arthritis. In Hunter JM, Mackin EJ, Callahan AD, editors: *Rehabilitation of the hand: surgery and therapy*, ed 4, St Louis, 1995, Mosby, pp 1345–1350.

56. Phillips EM: Stages of CRPS/RSD (website) Retrieved from http://www.rsdinfo.com/stages_of_crps_rsd.htm. Accessed on June 5, 2014.

57. Reiss B: Therapist's management of distal radial fractures. In Hunter JM, Mackin EJ, Callahan AD, editors: *Rehabilitation of the hand: surgery and therapy*, ed 4, St Louis, 1995, Mosby, pp 337–351.

58. Rozmaryn LM, Dovelle S, Rothman ER, et al.: Nerve and tendon gliding exercises and the conservative management of carpal tunnel syndrome, *J Hand Ther* 11(3):171–179, 1998.

59. Saidoff DC, McDonough AL: *Critical pathways in therapeutic intervention: upper extremity*, St Louis, 1997, Mosby.

60. Sailer SM: The role of splinting and rehabilitation in the treatment of carpal and cubital tunnel syndromes, *Hand Clin* 12(2):223–241, 1996.

61. Schultz-Johnson K: Splinting the wrist: mobilization and protection, *J Hand Ther* 9(2):165–176, 1996.

62. Schultz-Johnson K: Personal communication, April 2006.

63. Schultz-Johnson K: Personal communication, April 1999.

64. Siegel DB, Kuzma G, Eakins D: Anatomic investigation the role of the lumbrical muscles in carpal tunnel syndrome, *J Hand Surg Am* 20(5):860–863, 1995.

65. Skirven T: Nerve injuries. In Stanley BG, Tribuzi SM, editors: *Concepts in hand rehabilitation*, Philadelphia, 1992, FA Davis, pp 323–352.

66. Stein CM, Svoren B, Davis P, et al.: A prospective analysis of patients with rheumatic diseases attending referral hospitals in Harare, Zimbabwe, *J Rheumatol* 18(12):1841–1844, 1991.

67. Stern EB: Grip strength and finger dexterity across five styles of commercial wrist orthoses, *Am J Occup Ther* 50(1):32–38, 1996.

68. Stern EB, Sines B, Teague TR: Commercial wrist extensor orthoses: hand function, comfort, and interference across five styles, *J Hand Ther* 7(4):237–244, 1994.

69. Stern EB, Ytterberg SR, Krug HE, et al.: Commercial wrist extensor orthoses: a descriptive study of use and preference in patients with rheumatoid arthritis, *Arthritis Care Res* 10(1):27–35, 1997.

70. Stern EB, Ytterberg SR, Krug HE, et al.: Finger dexterity and hand function: effect of three commercial wrist extensor orthoses on patients with rheumatoid arthritis, *Arthritis Care Res* 9(3):197–205, 1996.

71. Stern EB, Ytterberg SR, Krug HE, et al.: Immediate and short-term effects of three commercial wrist extensor orthoses on grip strength and function in patients with rheumatoid arthritis, *Arthritis Care Res* 9(1):42–50, 1996.

72. Taylor-Mullins PA: Reflex sympathetic dystrophy. In Stanley BG, Tribuzi SM, editors: *Concepts in hand rehabilitation*, Philadelphia, 1992, FA Davis, pp 446–471.

73. Verdugo FJ, Salinas RS, Castillo J, et al.: Surgical versus non-surgical treatment for carpal tunnel syndrome (Cochrane Review). In *The cochrane library*, Issue Chichester, UK, 2004, John Wiley & Sons.

74. Walker WC, Metzler M, Cifu DX, et al.: Neutral wrist splinting in carpal tunnel syndrome: a comparison of night-only versus full-time wear instructions, *Arch Phys Med Rehabil* 81(4):424–429, 2000.

75. Walsh MT, Muntzer E: Therapist's management of complex regional pain syndrome (reflex sympathetic dystrophy). In Mackin EJ, Callahan AD, Skirven TM, et al, editors: *Rehabilitation of the hand and upper extremity*, ed 5, St Louis, 2002, Mosby, pp 1707–1724.

76. Weinstock TB: Management of fractures of the distal radius: therapists commentary, *J Hand Ther* 12(2):99–102, 1999.

77. Weiss ND, Gordon L, Bloom T, et al.: Position of the wrist associated with the lowest carpal-tunnel pressure: implications for splint design, *J Bone Joint Surg Am* 77(11):1695–1699, 1995.

78. Williams K: Carpal tunnel syndrome captivates American industry, *Advance for Directors of Rehabilitation* 12:13–18, 1992.

APPENDIX 7-1   CASE STUDIES

CASE STUDY 7-1*

Read the following scenario, and use your clinical reasoning skills to answer the questions based on information in this chapter.

Beth is a homemaker who began experiencing carpal tunnel syndrome (CTS) symptoms of numbness, grasp weakness, and parastheias over the distribution of the median nerve. Beth went to her family physician, whose nurse provided her with a quick remedy. Not being familiar with the correct wrist positioning for CTS, the nurse placed a strip of thermoplastic material stretching down the dorsal aspect of Beth's forearm, wrist, and hand and wrapped it in gauze. After a while Beth began to complain about the thermoplastic strip feeling awkward during activities, such as using a knife to cut meat, because it was not supporting the wrist. Eventually Beth began to wake up in the middle of the night, noticing that her hand was again numb. Beth returned to her family physician. This time he referred her to a neurologist, who diagnosed her with CTS. The neurologist provided a cortisone shot and referred her to occupational therapy. The occupational therapist requested an order for a custom orthosis. At that point, Beth had doubts about wearing the orthosis. She asked for valid reasons for the custom orthosis versus a prefabricated orthosis. She stated in frustration, "Why don't I just go ahead and have surgery!"

1. Provide two reasons that the thermoplastic strip was not the best choice. _____
    _____
    _____

2. Describe the correct position for the custom orthosis that the therapist should fabricate for Beth. _____
    _____
    _____

3. What would be the suggested wearing schedule? _____
    _____
    _____

4. What precautions are important with orthotic wear? _____
    _____
    _____
    _____

5. How should the therapist address Beth's concerns about getting a custom orthosis and surgery? Include in the answer how you might present the research evidence to Beth. _____
    _____
    _____
    _____

6. Explain two advantages of using a custom-made orthosis compared to a prefabricated orthosis for CTS. _____
    _____
    _____
    _____

*See Appendix A for the answer key.

CASE STUDY 7-2*

Read the following scenario, and use your clinical reasoning skills to answer the questions based on information from this chapter.

Megan is a 52-year-old woman who was walking outside at dusk with a friend. She came up to an intersection without seeing the curb, and she fell with her right hand stretched out in front of her. She went to the emergency room, and a closed reduction approach with casting was utilized for her non-displaced Colles fracture. After her cast was removed, the physician ordered therapy for edema and pain control, range of motion (ROM), and fabrication of a wrist orthosis for the right upper extremity.

1. Megan comes to therapy with her right wrist in 15 degrees flexion. Her wrist can be passively extended to neutral. Describe the orthotic position for her right hand and the rationale for the position. _____ _____ _____

2. As Megan's ROM improves, how should the therapist revise the position of the orthosis? _____ _____ _____

3. At what point should the therapist discontinue wrist orthotic intervention? _____ _____ _____

*See Appendix A for the answer key.

APPENDIX 7-2 LABORATORY EXERCISES

Laboratory Exercise 7-1

1. Practice making a wrist immobilization orthotic pattern on another person. Use the detailed instructions provided to draw the pattern.
2. Using the outline for the left and right hand, draw a wrist immobilization pattern without the detailed instructions.

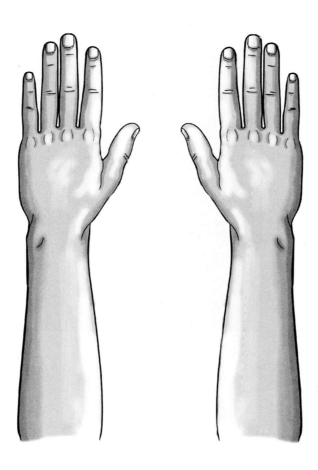

Laboratory Exercise 7-2

Orthosis A

1. What problems can you identify regarding this orthosis?
2. What problems may arise from continual orthotic wear?

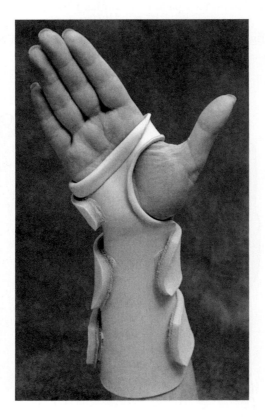

Orthosis B

You are supervising a student in clinical practice. You ask the student to practice making a wrist immobilization orthosis before actually fabricating an orthosis on a person. Orthosis B is a picture of the student's orthosis.

1. What problems should you address with the student regarding the orthosis?

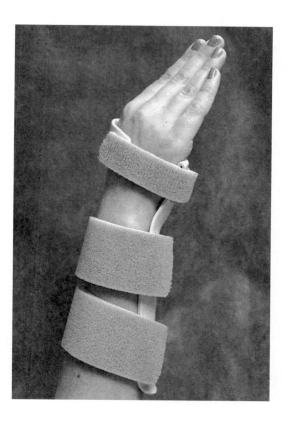

Orthosis C

Orthosis C was made for a 54-year-old man working as a bus driver. The person works full-time and has wrist extensor tendinopathy.

1. What problems can you identify regarding this orthosis?
2. What problems may arise from continual orthotic wear?

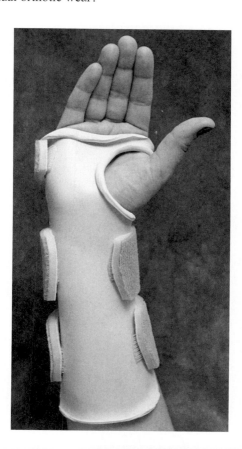

Laboratory Exercise 7-3

Practice fabricating a wrist immobilization orthosis on a partner. Before starting, determine the correct position for your partner's hand. Measure the angle of wrist extension with a goniometer to ensure a correct position. After fitting your orthosis and making all adjustments, use Form 7-1 as a self-evaluation of the wrist immobilization orthosis, and use Grading Sheet 7-1 as a classroom grading sheet.

Laboratory Exercise 7-4

The following picture is a volar-based wrist immobilization orthosis. Identify the parts of the orthosis that the arrows are pointing to.

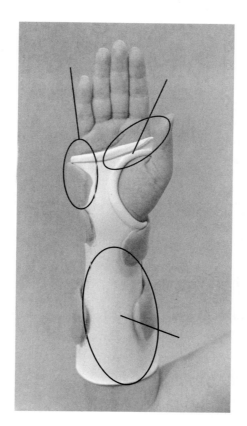

APPENDIX 7-3   FORMS AND GRADING SHEETS

FORM 7-1 Wrist immobilization orthosis

Name: _____

Date: _____

Type of cone wrist and hand orthosis:

Volar platform ○   Dorsal platform ○

Wrist position: _____

After the person wears the orthosis for 30 minutes, answer the following questions. (Mark NA for non-applicable situations.)

Evaluation Areas				Comments
Design				
1. The wrist position is at the correct angle.	Yes ○	No ○	NA ○	
2. The wrist has adequate support.	Yes ○	No ○	NA ○	
3. The sides of the thenar and hypothenar eminences have support in the correct position.	Yes ○	No ○	NA ○	
4. The thenar and hypothenar eminences are not restricted or flattened.	Yes ○	No ○	NA ○	
5. The orthosis is two-thirds the length of the forearm.	Yes ○	No ○	NA ○	
6. The orthosis is one-half the width of the forearm.	Yes ○	No ○	NA ○	
Function	Yes ○	No ○	NA ○	
1. The orthosis allows full thumb motions.	Yes ○	No ○	NA ○	
2. The orthosis allows full metacarpophalangeal (MCP) joint flexion of the fingers.	Yes ○	No ○	NA ○	
3. The orthosis provides wrist support that allows functional activities.	Yes ○	No ○	NA ○	
Straps	Yes ○	No ○	NA ○	
1. The straps are secure and rounded.	Yes ○	No ○	NA ○	
Comfort	Yes ○	No ○	NA ○	
1. The orthosis edges are smooth with rounded corners.	Yes ○	No ○	NA ○	
2. The proximal end is flared.	Yes ○	No ○	NA ○	
3. The orthosis does not cause impingements or pressure sores.	Yes ○	No ○	NA ○	
4. The orthosis does not irritate bony prominences.	Yes ○	No ○	NA ○	
Cosmetic Appearance	Yes ○	No ○	NA ○	
1. The orthosis is free of fingerprints, dirt, and pencil and pen marks.	Yes ○	No ○	NA ○	
2. The thermoplastic material is not buckled.	Yes ○	No ○	NA ○	
Therapeutic Regimen	Yes ○	No ○	NA ○	
1. The person has been instructed in a wearing schedule.	Yes ○	No ○	NA ○	
2. The person has been provided orthotic precautions.	Yes ○	No ○	NA ○	
3. The person demonstrates understanding of the education.	Yes ○	No ○	NA ○	
4. Client/caregiver knows how to clean the orthosis.	Yes ○	No ○	NA ○	
5. The person is able to recognize signs of pressure and impingement.	Yes ○	No ○	NA ○	

Discuss possible orthotic adjustments or changes that you should make based on the self-evaluation. (What would you do differently next time?)

_____
_____
_____
_____

Discuss possible areas to improve with clinical safety when fabricating the orthosis.

_____
_____
_____
_____

GRADING SHEET 7-1*

Wrist Immobilization Orthosis

Name: _____

Date: _____

Type of wrist immobilization orthosis:

Volar ○   Dorsal ○

Wrist position: _____

Grade:

1 = Beyond improvement, not acceptable
2 = Requires maximal improvement
3 = Requires moderate improvement
4 = Requires minimal improvement
5 = Requires no improvement

Evaluation Areas						**Comments**
Design						
1. The wrist position is at the correct angle.	1	2	3	4	5	
2. The wrist has adequate support.	1	2	3	4	5	
3. The sides of the thenar and hypothenar eminences have support in the correct position.	1	2	3	4	5	
4. The orthosis is one-half the width of the forearm.	1	2	3	4	5	
5. The thenar and hypothenar eminences are not restricted or flattened.	1	2	3	4	5	
6. The orthosis is two-thirds the length of the forearm.	1	2	3	4	5	
Function						
1. The orthosis allows full thumb motion.	1	2	3	4	5	
2. The orthosis allows full metacarpophalangeal (MCP) joint flexion of the fingers.	1	2	3	4	5	
3. The orthosis provides wrist support that allows functional activities.	1	2	3	4	5	
Straps						
1. The straps are secure and rounded.	1	2	3	4	5	
Comfort						
1. The orthosis edges are smooth with rounded corners.	1	2	3	4	5	
2. The proximal end is flared.	1	2	3	4	5	
3. The orthosis does not cause impingements or pressure sores.	1	2	3	4	5	
4. The orthosis does not irritate bony prominences.	1	2	3	4	5	
Cosmetic Appearance						
1. The orthosis is free of fingerprints, dirt, and pencil and pen marks.	1	2	3	4	5	
2. The thermoplastic material is not buckled.	1	2	3	4	5	

*See Appendix C for a perforated copy of this grading sheet.

CHAPTER 8

Thumb Immobilization Orthoses

Helene Lohman, OTD, OTR/L, FAOTA

Key Terms

de Quervain tenosynovitis
hypertonicity
osteoarthritis
rheumatoid arthritis (RA)
scaphoid fracture
ulnar collateral ligament (UCL) injury (skier's thumb or gamekeeper's thumb)

Chapter Objectives

1. Discuss important functional and anatomic considerations for orthotic intervention of the thumb.
2. Explain appropriate thumb and wrist positions in a thumb immobilization orthosis.
3. Identify the three components of a thumb immobilization orthosis.
4. Describe the reasons for supporting the joints of the thumb.
5. Discuss the diagnostic indications for a thumb immobilization orthosis.
6. Discuss the process of pattern making and orthotic fabrication for a thumb immobilization orthosis.
7. Describe elements of a proper fit of a thumb immobilization orthosis.
8. Explain general and specific patient safety precautions for a thumb immobilization orthosis.
9. Use clinical reasoning to evaluate fit problems of a thumb immobilization orthosis.
10. Use clinical reasoning to evaluate a fabricated thumb immobilization orthosis.
11. Apply knowledge about thumb immobilization orthotic intervention to a case study.
12. Recognize the importance of evidence-based practice with thumb immobilization orthotic provision.
13. Describe the appropriate use of prefabricated thumb orthoses.

On a winter vacation, Jill fell while snow skiing down a steep slope. She attempted to brace herself with an outstretched hand and thumb abducted. Jill's thumb bent backward upon hitting the ground. After being helped down the slope, Jill was seen by a local orthopaedic physician who diagnosed her with skier's thumb. The physician referred Jill to a local occupational therapy clinic where she was fitted her with a hand-based thumb orthosis. The physician suggested that she follow up with additional physician monitoring and therapy once she returned to her home state.

A commonly prescribed orthosis is the thumb palmar abduction immobilization orthosis.[2] Other names for this orthosis are the *thumb spica orthosis,* the *short or long opponens orthosis,*[51] the *CMC-MCP immobilization orthosis,*[61] or the *thumb gauntlet orthosis.* The purpose of this orthosis is to immobilize, protect, rest, and position one or all of the thumb carpometacarpal (CMC), metacarpophalangeal (MCP), and interphalangeal (IP) joints while allowing the other digits to be free. Thumb immobilization orthoses can be divided into two broad categories: (1) forearm based and (2) hand based. Forearm-based thumb orthoses stabilize the wrist and the thumb. Stabilizing the wrist is beneficial for a painful wrist and the orthosis provides support. The hand-based thumb spica orthoses provide stabilization for the thumb while allowing for wrist mobility.

Forearm-based or hand-based thumb immobilization orthoses are often used to help manage different conditions that affect the thumb's CMC, MCP, or IP joints. These conditions include but are not limited to: de Quervain tenosynovitis, rheumatoid arthritis (RA), osteoarthritis, skier's and gamekeeper's thumb (ulnar collateral ligament [UCL] injury), scaphoid fracture, and hypertonicity. For people who have de Quervain tenosynovitis, a forearm-based thumb orthosis provides rest, support, and protection of the tendons that course along the radial side of the wrist into the thumb joints. The therapist also applies a forearm-based thumb immobilization orthosis to fabricate postoperatively for control of motion in persons with RA after a joint arthrodesis or replacement. With the resulting muscle imbalance from a median nerve injury, the therapist may apply a hand-based thumb immobilization orthosis to keep the thumb web space adequately open. (Refer to Chapter 13 for more information about nerve injury.) In addition, the thumb immobilization orthosis can position the thumb before surgery.[25] The orthosis provides support and positioning after traumatic thumb injuries, such as sprains, joint dislocations, ligament injuries, and scaphoid fractures. Frequently a hand-based thumb immobilization orthosis is applied to persons with skier's or gamekeeper's thumb, which involves the UCL of the thumb MCP joint. For **hypertonicity,** a thumb orthosis sometimes called a *figure-eight thumb wrap* or *thumb loop orthosis* facilitates hand use by decreasing the palm-in-thumb posture or palmar adduction that is often associated with this condition. Therefore, because the thumb orthosis is so commonly prescribed, it is important that therapists become familiar with its application and fabrication.

Functional and Anatomic Considerations for Orthotic Intervention of the Thumb

The thumb is essential for hand functions because of its overall importance to grip, pinch, and fine manipulation. The thumb's exceptional mobility results from the unique shape of its saddle joint (the CMC joint), the arrangement of its ligaments, and its intrinsic musculature.[5,13,53] The thumb provides stability for grip, pinch, and mobility because it opposes the fingers for fine manipulations.[57] Sensory input to the tip of the thumb is important for functional grasp and pinch.

A thorough understanding of the anatomy and functional movements of the thumb is necessary before the therapist attempts to fabricate a thumb orthosis. The most crucial aspect of the thumb immobilization orthotic design is the position of the CMC joint.[57] Positioning of the thumb in a thumb post allows for palmar abduction and some opposition, which are critical motions for functional prehension. See Chapter 4 for a review of the anatomy and functional movements of the thumb.

Features of the Thumb Immobilization Orthosis

The thumb immobilization orthosis prevents motion of one, two, or all of the thumb joints.[23] The orthosis has numerous design variations. It can be a volar (Figure 8-1), dorsal (Figure 8-2), or radial gutter (Figure 8-3) depending on the person's condition and purpose of the orthosis. The orthosis may be hand based or wrist based, depending on the person's diagnosis, the anatomic structures involved, and the associated pain at the wrist. If the wrist is included, the wrist position varies according to the diagnosis. For example, with de Quervain tenosynovitis, the wrist is commonly positioned in 15 degrees of extension to take the pressure off of the tendons.[9]

The orthotic components fabricated in the final product vary according to the thumb joints that are included. The final orthotic product is formed based on the therapeutic goals for the client. The therapist must have a good understanding of the purpose and the fabrication process for the various orthotic components. Central to most thumb immobilization orthoses are three components: (1) the opponens bar, (2) C bar, and (3) thumb post (Figure 8-4).[23] The opponens bar and C bar position the thumb, usually in some degree of palmar abduction. The thumb post, which is an extension of the C bar, immobilizes the MCP only or both the MCP and IP joints.

The position of the thumb in an orthosis varies from palmar abduction to radial abduction, depending on the person's diagnosis. With some conditions, such as arthritis, the therapist facilitates prehension by stabilizing the thumb CMC joint in palmar abduction and opposition. Certain diagnostic protocols—such as those for extensor pollicis longus (EPL) repairs, tendon transfers for thumb extension, and extensor tenolysis of the thumb—require the thumb to have an extension and a radial abducted position.[10] The thumb immobilization orthosis may do one of the following:

* Stabilize only the CMC joint
* Include the CMC and MCP joints
* Encompass all three (CMC, MCP, and IP) joints

The physician's order may specify which thumb joints to immobilize in the orthosis. In some situations, the therapist may be responsible for determining which joints the orthosis should stabilize. The therapist uses diagnostic protocols and an assessment of the person's pain to make this decision. When the therapist deems it necessary to limit thumb motion and to protect the thumb, the IP may be immobilized. Certain diagnostic protocols (such as those for thumb replantations, tendon transfers, and tendon repairs) often require the inclusion of the IP joint in the orthosis.[51] Overall the therapist should fabricate an orthosis that is the most supportive and least restrictive in movement.

Diagnostic Indications

Therapists fabricate thumb immobilization orthoses in general and specialized hand therapy practices. Specific diagnostic conditions that require a thumb immobilization

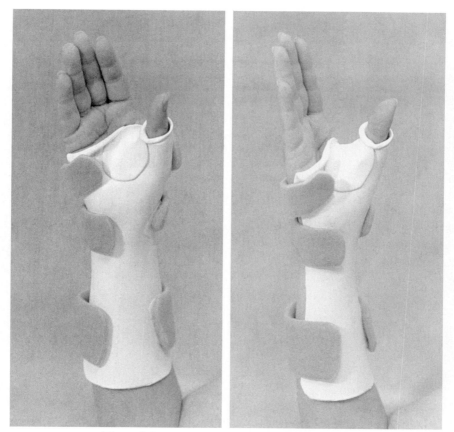

Figure 8-1 A volar thumb immobilization orthosis.

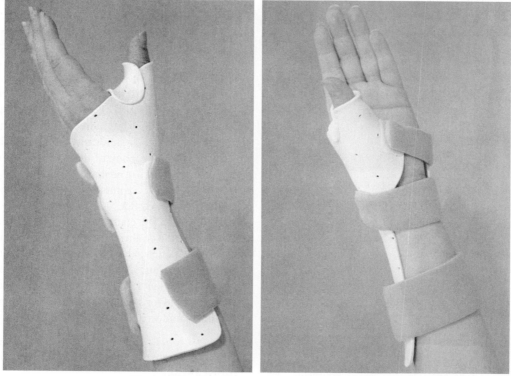

Figure 8-2 A dorsal thumb immobilization orthosis.

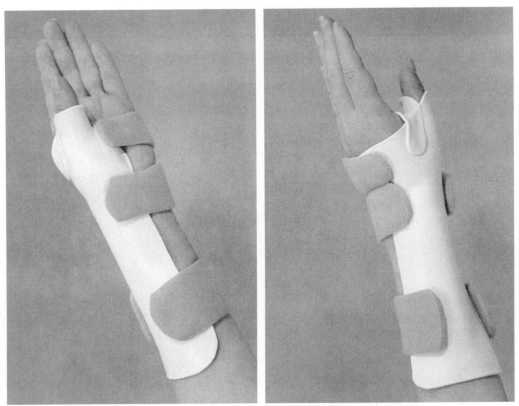

Figure 8-3 A radial gutter thumb immobilization orthosis.

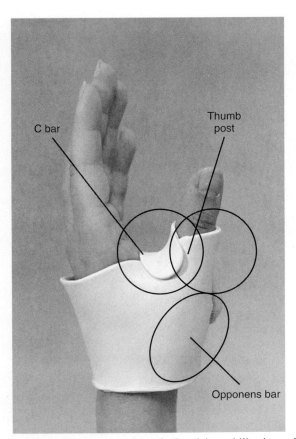

Figure 8-4 The three components of a thumb immobilization orthosis. The opponens bar in conjunction with a C bar and a thumb post.

orthosis include, but are not limited to, the following: scaphoid fractures, stable fractures of the proximal phalanx of the first metacarpal, tendon transfers, radial or UCL strains, repair of MCP joint collateral ligaments, RA, osteoarthritis, de Quervain tenosynovitis, and median nerve injuries. Other conditions include MCP joint dislocations, capsular tightness of the MCP and IP joints after trauma, post-traumatic adduction contracture, extrinsic flexor or extensor muscle contracture, flexor pollicis longus (FPL) repair, uncomplicated EPL repairs, distal radius fractures, hypertonicity, and congenital adduction deformity of the thumb.

Intervention for many of these conditions may require the expertise of experienced hand therapists. In general clinical practice, therapists commonly treat persons who have de Quervain tenosynovitis, RA, osteoarthritis, fractures, and ligament injuries. (Table 8-1 contains guidelines for these hand conditions.) The novice therapist should keep in mind that physicians and experienced therapists may have their own guidelines for positioning and orthotic wearing schedules. The therapist should also be aware that thumb palmar abduction may be uncomfortable for some persons. Therefore, the thumb may be positioned midway between radial and palmar abduction.

Orthotic Intervention for de Quervain Tenosynovitis

De Quervain tenosynovitis, which results from repetitive thumb motions and wrist ulnar deviation, is a form of

HAND CONDITION	TYPE OF ORTHOSIS, POSITION	WEARING SCHEDULE
Soft Tissue Inflammation		
De Quervain tenosynovitis	During an acute flare-up, the therapist provides a thumb immobilization orthosis (wrist extension, thumb CMC palmar abduction immobilization orthosis, [ASHT 1992]). Orthosis can be long forearm-based or a radial gutter orthosis; the wrist is in 15 degrees of extension, the thumb CMC joint is palmarly abducted 40 to 45 degrees, and the thumb MCP is positioned in neutral. Other positioning options are discussed in the chapter.	This person wears the orthosis during the night and as needed in the day to avoid pain and rest the tendons. The orthosis is removed for pain free occupations during the day to help remodel and nourish collagen formation.
Arthritis		
Rheumatoid arthritis: Periods of pain and inflammation in the thumb joints	The therapist provides a forearm-based thumb immobilization orthosis (wrist extension, thumb CMC palmar abduction, and MCP flexion immobilization orthosis). The wrist is in 20 to 30 degrees of extension; the thumb CMC joint is either palmarly abducted 45 degrees, or midway between radial and palmar abduction, depending on person's tolerance; and the MCP joint (if included) is in 5 degrees of flexion. Other specific orthoses for arthritic deformities are discussed in the chapter.	The person wears the orthosis continuously during periods of pain and inflammation with removal for exercise and hygiene. The therapist adjusts the wearing schedule according to the person's pain and inflammation levels.
Osteoarthritis		
CMC joint of the thumb	Orthotic approaches are individualized because there is no one recommended approach. Options include a hand-based thumb immobilization orthosis with the MCP joint immobilized or free, depending on the protocol. The thumb CMC joint is palmarly abducted to a position that the person can tolerate. Or, a hand-based orthosis that frees the thumb MCP joint for motion and stabilizes the first CMC joint in extension. A forearm-based orthosis can be provided for nighttime wear with scaphotrapezial joint involvement, or if the person requires more support.[14]	The person wears the orthosis continuously during an acute flare-up with removal for ROM and hygiene. Once pain has decreased, the orthosis can be selectively worn during activities to help position and stabilize the thumb.
Traumatic Injuries of the Thumb		
Skier's/ Gamekeeper's thumb (UCL injury)	The therapist provides a hand-based thumb orthosis (MCP radial and ulnar deviation restriction orthosis) (ASHT, 1992). The MCP joint is immobilized, the thumb CMC joint is palmarly abducted 40 degrees, and the MCP joint is in neutral. The thumb post for the hand-based orthosis can position the MCP joint in slight ulnar deviation to take the stress off the UCL. (It is important to position the thumb CMC joint in a position of comfort and may not be exactly in the suggested degrees.)	• Grade I—The person wears the orthosis continuously for 3 to 4 weeks with removal for hygiene. • Grade II—The person wears the orthosis continuously for 4 to 5 weeks except for removal for hygiene. • Grade III—After immobilization in a cast, the person is provided with the thumb immobilization orthosis and follows the same protocol described previously for grade I.
Scaphoid fracture (stable and nondisplaced)	There are many variations of orthotics. One option is that the therapist provides a forearm volar or a dorsal/volar thumb immobilization orthosis (thumb CMC palmar abduction and MCP in 0 to 10 degrees flexion and the wrist in neutral).	The wear schedule varies widely depending on the time after injury, the bone status, the physician preference, and the location of the fracture on the scaphoid. If the person has undergone a long course of casting and the physician is worried about bony union (This is often the case.), initially, the orthosis will be prescribed for continuous wear with removal for hygiene and to check the skin.
Hypertonicity	The therapist provides a thumb loop orthosis or a figure-eight thumb wrap orthosis, which can be customized out of thermoplastic or soft material. A prefabricated orthosis can also be used. With a prefabricated orthosis, a Neoprene strip is wrapped around the thumb web space and the hand to provide radial or palmar abduction while pulling the wrist into extension and radial deviation. Purchased thumb loops are available in sizes to fit premature infants to adults.	The wear schedule varies according to the person's therapeutic needs. The orthosis should be removed and the skin should be carefully monitored at periodic intervals.

CMC, Carpometacarpal; *MCP,* metacarpophalangeal; *ROM,* range of motion; *UCL,* ulnar collateral ligament.

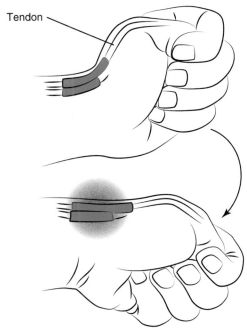

Tendon

Figure 8-5 The Finkelstein test is used to assess the presence of de Quervain tenosynovitis. (From http://www.riversideonline.com/source/images/image_popup/ans7_finkelsteintest.jpg.)

tenosynovitis affecting the abductor pollicis longus (APL) and the extensor pollicis brevis (EPB) in the first dorsal compartment. People whose occupations involve repetitive wrist deviation and thumb motions (such as the home construction tasks of painting, scraping, wall papering, and hammering) are prone to this condition.[27] De Quervain tenosynovitis is the most commonly diagnosed wrist tendonitis in athletes,[42] such as golfers.[33] It may be recognized by pain over the radial styloid, edema in the first dorsal compartment, and positive results from the Finkelstein test (Figure 8-5). The Finkelstein test involves instructing the individual to clench the thumb in a fist and passively deviating in the ulnar direction.[3] A positive test results from pain during this motion (see Figure 8-5).

During the acute phase of this condition, conservative therapeutic management involves immobilization of the thumb and wrist for symptom control[31] to rest the involved tendons.[28] This orthosis is classified by the American Society of Hand Therapists (ASHT) as a wrist extension, thumb CMC palmar abduction, and MCP flexion immobilization orthosis.[2] The orthosis may cover the volar or dorsal forearm or the radial aspect of the forearm and hand. The therapist positions the wrist in 15 degrees of extension, neutral wrist deviation, the thumb midway between palmar and radial abduction (40 to 45 degrees), and the thumb MCP joint in neutral.[9,18] Usually the IP joint is free for functional activities and includes the joint in the orthosis if the person is overusing the thumb or fights the orthosis, causing even more pain. Other recommendations exist for positioning. For example Ilyas and colleagues[28] recommend

conservative intervention by positioning the thumb in 30 degrees of abduction and 30 degrees of MCP flexion. Ultimately the position chosen for the thumb is the one that best relieves the person's symptoms.

Radial gutter or forearm-based thumb orthoses are worn during the night and as needed in the day to avoid pain and rest the tendons. The orthosis is removed for occupations that are pain free during the day in order to help remodel and nourish collagen formation.[18] A prefabricated orthosis is recommend after the person's pain subsides[31] for work and sports activities,[23] or if the person does not want to wear a custom orthosis.[6] Postsurgical management of de Quervain tenosynovitis also involves orthotic intervention, usually for 7 to 10 days.[42]

Few studies have considered the efficacy of thumb orthotic intervention for de Quervain tenosynovitis and results have been variable (Table 8-2). Lane and colleagues[30] studied 300 subjects and compared orthotic intervention with oral nonsteroidal anti-inflammatory drugs (NSAIDs) and steroid injections over a 2- to 4-week time period. Subjects were positioned in a custom thumb immobilization orthosis with the wrist in neutral and the thumb in 30 degrees between palmar and radial abduction. Subjects were placed in three groups based on symptoms (minimal, mild, moderate/severe). Subjects who had mild symptoms responded well to orthotic intervention with NSAIDs. Limitations of this study included no control group for the mild symptom group, small numbers in the mild group, the subjective nature of classifying subjects, and no mention of an orthotic wearing schedule.

Weiss and colleagues[54] (n = 93) compared orthotic intervention to steroid injection or combined in treatment with steroid injections. They did not find strong benefits for thumb orthotic intervention. Witt and colleagues[59] (n = 95) also studied the provision of a long thumb immobilization orthosis including the wrist (which was worn continuously for 3 weeks, along with steroid injection) and had a good success rate. Avci and colleagues[4] focused their research on conservative treatment of 19 pregnant women with de Quervain tenosynovitis. One group received cortisone injections and the other group received thumb orthoses. The group receiving cortisone injections had complete pain relief compared to partial relief from the orthotic wearing group. The orthotic wearing group experienced pain relief only when wearing the orthosis. Finally, the researchers pointed out that pregnancy-related de Quervain disease is self-limiting (with cessation of symptoms after breast feeding is terminated).

Richie and Briner[44] reviewed the literature to evaluate the evidence of treatment options for de Quervain tenosynovitis. They considered seven descriptive studies (n = 459 wrists) comparing effective treatments without control groups. They found the highest success rate for intervention of 83% for injection alone, followed by 61% for injection and orthotic intervention together, 14% for orthotic intervention alone, and 9% for rest or NSAIDs.[44] The authors concluded

Table 8-2 Evidence-Based Practice about Thumb Orthotic Intervention

AUTHOR'S CITATION	DESIGN	NUMBER OF PARTICIPANTS	DESCRIPTION	RESULTS	LIMITATIONS
Carpometacarpal Arthritis					
Egan MY, Brousseau L: Splinting for osteoarthritis of the carpometacarpal joint: a review of the evidence, Am J Occup Ther 61:70-78, 2007.	The studies in the review included: a randomized control trial, a pre-posttest, a retrospective cohort study, and a post-test study.	258 participants in total of all studies	This systematic review was to provide evidence-based recommendations to occupational therapists for CMC osteoarthritis orthotic intervention. Inclusion criteria included either experimental or observational studies that examined the effects of osteoarthritis orthotic intervention. Seven of sixteen articles met the final inclusion criteria. Five of nine articles were theoretical discussions, two were case reports, and one was a systematic review that contained three of the studies.	Overall the authors concluded that some evidence for CMC osteoarthritis orthotic intervention may be effective for pain reduction and that there is not one orthosis recommendation for the condition. This suggests a client-centered approach with orthosis provision.	Results are inconclusive, and further research is warranted
Wajon A, Ada L: No difference between two splint and exercise regimens for people with osteoarthritis of the thumb: a randomised controlled trial, Aust J Physiother 51(4), 245-249, 2005.	Randomized controlled clinical trial	40 participants	Over a 6-week period two orthotic and exercise approaches for patients with trapeziometacarpal (TM) osteoarthritis were compared. The experimental group received a thumb strap orthosis with abduction exercises. The control group received a short opponens orthosis with pinch exercises.	Assessment of pain, strength, and hand function showed no significant difference in improvement. Both groups demonstrated improvement in pain, strength, and hand function measures.	Positive results may have occurred due to other factors than interventions.
Day CS, Gelberman R, Patel AA, et al: Basal joint osteoarthritis of the thumb: a prospective trial of steroid injection and splinting, J Hand Surg 49:247-251, 2004.	Prospective study	30 clients (30 thumbs)	This study evaluated the effectiveness of a single steroid injection and the use of a thumb spica orthosis for individuals with osteoarthritis in stages 1 to 4 and who had trapeziometacarpal (TM) pain. The participants were asked to answer the DASH questionnaire and rated their pain level initially, at 6 weeks and at 18 to 31 weeks after the intervention.	Thirteen of the 30 clients experienced improvement in pain up to 4 weeks following the injection. The remaining 17 clients did not experience pain relief. Of the 13 clients who experienced pain relief, 12 demonstrated increased function and decreased pain. Pain relief and increased function lasted throughout the final follow-up (an average of 21 months). DASH ratings increased. Clients showing the most improvement were in the early stages of TM osteoarthritis (Eaton stages 1, 2, and 3). Clients who did not experience pain relief had the option of surgery.	It is difficult to determine whether the steroid injection or the orthotic intervention was the more effective method in decreasing pain of individuals. Seven of the 30 clients declined follow-up. There was speculation that the injection did not accurately get into the TM joint.

Continued

Table 8-2   Evidence-Based Practice about Thumb Orthotic Intervention—cont'd

AUTHOR'S CITATION	DESIGN	NUMBER OF PARTICIPANTS	DESCRIPTION	RESULTS	LIMITATIONS
Berggren M, Joost-Davidsson A, Lindstrand J, et al: Reduction in the need for operation after conservative treatment of osteoarthritis of the first carpometacarpal joint: a seven year prospective study, *Scand J Plast Reconstr Hand Surg* 35:415-417, 2001.	Prospective longitudinal-study	33 clients randomized into three groups	A hand therapist met with each participant to discuss avoidance of loading the joint through orthoses or accessories (adaptive equipment) and modification of the work environment. • Group 1 received technical accessories (ergonomically-designed assistive devices). • Group 2 received adaptive equipment and a "semistable" orthosis. • Group 3 received adaptive equipment and a "non-stabilizing" leather orthosis. Groups were advised on adapting ADLs to reduce pain and decrease the need for surgery. A hand therapist treated each subject for three sessions over a 7-month period. Adjustments were made to the adaptive equipment or orthoses as needed. A surgeon assessed all subjects at the end of 7 months to determine the need for surgery. The surgeon acted as a blind reviewer.	Of the 33 clients, 23 (70%) avoided surgery. Orthoses were successful to avoid adduction contracture. After a reassessment 7 years later, only two clients required surgery. The authors recommended a 6-month period of conservative treatment before determining a client's need for surgery.	A significant difference in age between clients electing to have surgery (mean age of 59) and those declining surgery (mean age of 65) was present. Older participants may be less likely to elect surgery if their lifestyle does not require the same demands as younger individuals. The mean age of participants in this study was 63, and this may have played a role in the number of participants choosing to have surgery at the conclusion of the study. Treatment for CMC osteoarthritis only included using the same type of orthosis (long or short) in this study with no other intervention options.
Weiss S, LaStayo P, Mills A, et al: Prospective analysis of splinting the first carpometacarpal joint: an objective, subjective and radiographic assessment, *J Hand Ther* 13(3):218-226, 2000.	Randomized control trial	26 hands	Researchers gathered the objective and subjective responses of patients with CMC osteoarthritis who wore short and long opponens orthoses. Radiographic changes associated with wearing of the orthoses were collected. Participants were randomly selected to wear the long and short orthosis. Participants wore the orthoses for 1 week. The function of their hands were documented using 22 ADLs. Participants rated orthosis satisfaction and pain levels on visual analog scales. Participants alternated long or short orthoses after 1 week of wear. The same measures were repeated following week 2. On the final visit, tip pinches were evaluated, and x-rays were taken to assess subluxation.	Subluxation was reduced with both orthoses at the first CMC joint in patients with grades 1 and 2 osteoarthritis. The majority of the patients chose the short orthosis when asked which orthosis they preferred. Pinch strength and pain levels did not improve with either orthosis. Results showed that orthoses did not increase pinch strength or affect pain levels associated with the performance of pinch strength measurements. This study supports that patients with CMC osteoarthritis receive pain relief with orthotic intervention.	

Swigart CR, Eaton RG, Glickel SZ, et al: Splinting in the treatment of arthritis of the first carpometacarpal joint, *J Hand Surg* 24:86-91, 1999.	Retrospective study	114 clients (130 thumbs)	The purpose of the study was to determine the effectiveness of an orthotic intervention protocol for CMC arthritis and its effect on daily activities. Clients with pain and disability associated with CMC arthritis were treated with a long opponens orthosis for 3 to 4 weeks followed by a 3- to 4-week weaning period. The orthosis was designed to eliminate wrist movement, but not to correct any previous deformities. Through a survey, clients self-reported their percentage of perceived improvement in symptoms. Clients choose from 0%, 25%, 50%, 75%, or 100% improvement immediately after the orthosis was worn and 6 months thereafter. Clients were categorized into two groups, A and B, depending on the extent of joint disease present. Group A (57 thumbs) were in stage 1 or 2 of the disease. Group B (69 thumbs) were in stage 3 or 4. Four thumbs were excluded from the study.	Seventy-four of 85 clients responded to the survey. Fifty-three thumbs (67%) experienced some relief with orthotic intervention. Those who experienced relief rated their improvement at 60% initially and 59% 6 months later. Group A (stage 1 and 2) showed greater improvement than Group B, supporting the researchers' hypothesis that conservative treatment (orthotic intervention) is most effective early in the disease process. 22% of clients in Group A who failed to experience improvements elected to have surgery. 61% in Group B elected to have CMC surgery. Many clients who did not experience pain reduction elected not to have surgery and chose to modify their activities to reduce stress on the thumb.	Similar to many retrospective studies, a relatively low response rate (33%) occurred. With any self-report design, there is a potential for misperception and personal bias in the answers.

de Quervain Tenosynovitis

Peters-Veluthamaningal C, van der Windt DA, Winters JC, et al: Corticosteroid injection for de Quervain's tenosynovitis, *Cochrane Database Syst Rev* 8(3):CD005616, 2009.	Systematic review: Two reviewers independently extracted all data from randomized controlled trials. The reviewers assessed each trial for: 1. Randomization 2. Concealment of allocation 3. Blinding of outcome assessor, care provider, and patient 4. Reporting of withdrawals and drop-outs	One study with 18 adults	The objective of this review was to consider efficacy and safety of corticosteroid injections for treatment of de Quervain tenosynovitis in adults. The authors identified five studies. Four studies were excluded. Participants included 19 wrists in 18 pregnant or lactating women. One group received one steroid injection of methylprednisolone and bupivacaine, and the other group received a thumb spica orthosis. All participants in the steroid injection group achieved complete relief of pain, whereas none of the participants in the thumb spica orthosis group had complete relief of pain, 1 to 6 days after intervention.	The study showed uncertainty of the effectiveness of corticosteriod injections in reducing pain because of the very low quality of evidence.	Sample included a small specific group of lactating or pregnant women; therefore the generalizability is limited. Study was short-term over 6 days. Therefore, the effectiveness of sole injections in treating de Quervain tenosynovitis is not reliable.

Continued

Table 8-2 Evidence-Based Practice about Thumb Orthotic Intervention—cont'd

AUTHOR'S CITATION	DESIGN	NUMBER OF PARTICIPANTS	DESCRIPTION	RESULTS	LIMITATIONS
	5. Similarity of groups at baseline regarding the most important prognostic indicators 6. Specification of eligibility criteria 7. Availability of point estimates and measures of variability of primary outcome measures 8. Use of intention-to-treat analysis Each criterion was rated as adequate, inadequate, or unclear.				
Richie CA 3rd, Briner WW Jr: Corticosteroid injection for treatment of de Quervain's tenosynovitis: a pooled quantitative literature evaluation, *J Am Board Fam Pract* 16(2):102-106, 2003.	Systematic review	Seven descriptive studies of de Quervain tenosynovitis with 459 wrists	Criteria for inclusion in the review were: 1. Radial wrist pain 2. First dorsal wrist extensor compartment tenderness 3. Positive Finkelstein test	83% percent pain relief with injection alone group. Other modalities resulting in pain relief were: 61% for injection and orthotic intervention; 14% for orthotic intervention only, and 0% for rest or NSAIDs.	The effects of orthotic intervention alone were not examined. The specific studies selected were not described in detail or in terms of limitations.

| Lane LB, Boretz RS, Stuchin SA: Treatment of de Quervain's disease: role of conservative management, *J Hand Surg* 26:256-260, 2001. | Retrospective study | 319 wrists in 300 clients | The purpose of the study was to compare two methods used to treat de Quervain disease including radial gutter thumb spica orthoses with NSAIDs and steroid injections. Records of 300 clients with symptoms of de Quervain disease between 1980 through 1986 were reviewed. Participants were followed up through a physical exam, telephone call, or written questionnaire. Clients were classified into three groups:
• Group 1 (n=17) had minimal symptoms (discomfort overall the radial side of the wrist during a few ADLs and no pain at rest).
• Group 2 (n=45) had pain over the radial side of the wrist and mild interference with ADLs.
• Group 3 (n=257) had moderate to severe tenderness, a positive Finkelstein test, and swelling. Client improvement was categorized as having complete resolution of symptoms, having improvement, or having no improvement of symptoms. If symptoms were not relieved, the treatment was determined to be unsuccessful, and they were offered a steroid injection. Clients receiving steroid injection(s) were categorized in the steroid group. | Fifteen of the 17 clients in Group 1 reported complete symptom relief with orthotic intervention and NSAID treatment. In Group 2, 20 of 45 clients refused steroid injections and were treated with NSAIDs and orthoses. No one received surgery from Group 2. In Group 3, two of eight clients were treated with orthoses and NSAIDs and experienced symptom improvement. One hundred-eighty-nine of the 249 wrists had complete symptom relief, and 17 had improvement with injections. The researchers concluded that orthotic intervention and NSAID treatment is effective for a small number of persons with de Quervain disease in the early stages. Efficacy of steroid injection for clients with de Quervain disease for whom orthotic intervention and NSAID treatment is not effective. | It is difficult to distinguish between minimal, mild, moderate symptoms of de Quervain disease. Orthotic intervention was not tested alone as a treatment option. There was not a control group for Group 1. |

Continued

Table 8-2 Evidence-Based Practice about Thumb Orthotic Intervention—cont'd

AUTHOR'S CITATION	DESIGN	NUMBER OF PARTICIPANTS	DESCRIPTION	RESULTS	LIMITATIONS
Weiss AP, Akelman E, Tabatabai M: Treatment of de Quervain's disease, *J Hand Surg Am* 19(4):595-598, 1994.	Single group pre-test, post-test design	87 patients with 93 wrists were included in the study with an average follow-up examination of 13 months.	This study compared the use of a mixed steroid/lidocaine injection alone, an immobilization orthosis alone, and the simultaneous use of both an injection and orthosis in improving symptoms in de Quervain tenosynovitis. The entire group of 87 patients (93 wrists) were analyzed twice: First with patients' symptomatic response to injection, followed by an outcome parameter using the need for surgical release to define failure. The relief of symptoms in participants was graded as complete resolution of symptoms, improvement in symptoms, or no improvement in symptoms. If no relief was seen at initial follow-up, surgical release was offered.	Complete relief of symptoms was noted in 28 of 42 wrists receiving an injection alone, 8 of 14 wrists receiving both an injection and orthosis, and 7 of 37 wrists receiving an orthosis alone. No significant difference was noted between the injection alone and injection with orthotic groups. A significant difference was seen between the injection alone and orthosis alone groups and the injection/orthosis and orthois alone groups. When the need for operative release was used as an outcome result for treatment failure, the injection alone and orthosis alone groups demonstrated significance. No additional benefits were seen by the addition of orthotic immobilization for treatment of de Quervain disease. Treatment by injection of a mixed solution of steroid and lidocaine was found to have the best prognosis for improvement in symptoms, the least cost, and little chance of recurrence if improvement is complete and rapid.	No limitations in study design or method were noted. The description of the patient's severity of symptoms or condition was not taken into account. Therefore, using surgery as "failure" may be a limitation. Two different physicians treated the participants, which may have caused a bias in the results.

| Sillem H, Back-man CL, Miller WC, et al: Comparison of two carpometacarpal stabilizing splints for individuals with osteoarthritis, *J Hand Ther* 24(3):216-226, 2011. | Random controlled trial | "Fifty-six participants were assigned randomly to splint order in a two-phase, four-week crossover trial" (p. 216). | "The purpose of the study was to compare the effect of two different splints ([h]ybrid-thermoplastic and [N]eoprene splint and a prefabricated splint) on hand function, pain, and hand strength in adults with CMC OA" (p. 216). | The primary outcome of hand function was assessed using the Australian Canadian Hand Osteoarthritis Hand Index. Differences between the two orthoses were not statistically significant for effect on hand function and grip and pinch strength. However, the hybrid orthosis showed a greater average reduction in pain scores. Both orthoses demonstrated modest improvements in hand function. The prefabricated orthosis was the preferred orthosis, although the hybrid orthosis had a significant greater reduction with pain. The results did show a significant improvement with function and pain reduction with the hybrid orthosis on the dominant hand. This reinforces the client-centered approach to orthotic intervention. | "The therapists were not blinded to the splinting intervention or outcome measures, as they were required to fabricate and fit each splint." There is a possibility of bias "if therapists had a strong preference for one splint or were swayed by participant comments" (p. 223). Any other treatment intervention was not monitored. "The population in this study was a homogenous group with regard to their baseline characteristics, being predominantly females in their 60s" (p. 233). The severity of participants' osteoarthritis was not assessed. Because of communication with subjects at 3 months, some had stopped using the orthoses so long-term effect could not be ascertained. |

ADL, Activity of daily living; *CMC,* carpometacarpal; *DASH,* Disabilities of the Arm, Shoulder, and Hand; *NSAID,* nonsteroidal anti-inflammatory drug.

that the combination of injection and orthotic intervention resulted in a higher percentage of treatment failure (39%) compared to treatment failure of solely providing injections (17%). These authors did not discuss the limitations of the reviewed studies. More research needs to be completed to determine the efficacy of thumb orthotic intervention with de Quervain tenosynovitis. Therapists should review these studies as they provide information about the effectiveness of physician treatments, such as steroid injections, that their clients may receive.

Orthotic Intervention for Rheumatoid Arthritis

Rheumatoid arthritis (RA) often affects the thumb joints, particularly the MCP and CMC joints. Orthotic intervention for RA can reduce pain, slow deformity, and stabilize the thumb joints.[40] One perspective with orthotic intervention is to consider three stages of the disease. In each stage, a different orthotic approach is used even though the therapist may apply the same thumb immobilization orthosis.

The first stage involves an inflammatory process. The goal of orthotic intervention at this stage is to rest the joints and reduce inflammation. The person wears the thumb immobilization orthosis continuously during periods of inflammation and periodically thereafter for pain control as necessary. When the disease progresses in the second stage, the hand requires mechanical support because the joints are less stable and are painful with use. The person wears a thumb immobilization orthosis for support while doing daily activities and perhaps at night for pain relief. In the third stage, pain is usually not a factor, but the joints may be grossly deformed and unstable. In lieu of surgical stabilization, a thumb immobilization orthosis may provide support to increase function during certain activities. At this stage, orthotic intervention is rarely helpful for the person at night unless to help manage pain.[16] Another intervention approach is to provide the person who has arthritis with a rigid and a soft orthosis along with education for the benefits and activity usages of each type.[46]

Common thumb deformities from the arthritic process are boutonnière deformity (type I, MCP joint flexion and IP joint extension) and swan neck deformity (type 3, MCP extension or hyperextension and IP flexion).[13,38] Boutonnière deformity is believed to be the most common type of thumb deformity and is identified by MCP joint flexion and IP joint in hyperextension.[48] During the beginning stages of boutonnière deformity a circumferential Neoprene orthosis may be applied to support the MCP joint with the IP joint free to move.[13] To address progression of MCP joint deformity, Colditz[13] suggested a carefully fabricated thermoplastic orthosis to stabilize the joint to eliminate volar subluxation and to allow for CMC motion (Figure 8-6).

A swan neck deformity is identified by proximal interphalangeal (PIP) hyperextension and distal interphalangeal (DIP) flexion.[10] For early stages of swan neck deformity, a small custom-fitted dorsal thermoplastic orthosis over

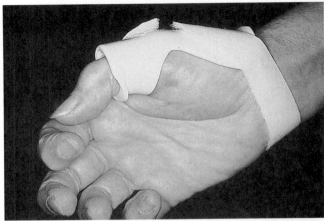

Figure 8-6 This orthosis stabilizes the metacarpophalangeal (MCP) joint. (From Colditz JC: Anatomic considerations for splinting the thumb. In Mackin EJ, Callahan AD, Skirven TM, et al., editors: *Rehabilitation of the hand and upper extremity,* ed 5, St Louis, 2002 Mosby, pp. 1858-1874.)

the MCP joint prevents MCP hyperextension.[13] Later dorsal and radial subluxation at the CMC joint causes CMC joint adduction, MCP hyperextension, and IP flexion.[13] For this deformity, Colditz[13] suggests fabricating a hand-based thumb immobilization orthosis that blocks MCP hyperextension (Figure 8-7). With RA, laxity of the UCL at the IP and MCP joint can also develop. Figure 8-8 shows a functional orthosis, which can also be used with RA or osteoarthritis for lateral instability of the thumb IP joint. Prefabricated options are also available for both boutonnière and swan neck deformities.

One approach to orthotic intervention for a hand with arthritis is to immobilize the thumb in a forearm-based, thumb immobilization orthosis with the wrist in 20 to 30 degrees of extension, the CMC joint in 45 degrees of palmar abduction (if tolerated), and the MCP joint in 0 to 5 degrees of flexion.[51] This orthosis is classified by ASHT as a wrist extension, thumb CMC palmar abduction and MCP extension immobilization orthosis.[2] Resting the hand in this position is extremely beneficial during periods of inflammation, or if the thumb is unstable at the CMC joint.[32] Incorporating the wrist in a forearm-based thumb orthosis is appropriate when the client's wrist is painful or with arthritic involvement.

When fabricating an orthosis on a person who has RA, be aware that the person may have fragile skin. Monitor all areas for potential skin breakdown, including the ulnar head, Lister tubercle, the radial styloid along the radial border, the CMC joint of the thumb, and the scaphoid and pisiform bones on the volar surface of the wrist.[20] Padding the orthosis for comfort to prevent skin irritation may be necessary.

The selected material should be easily adjustable to accommodate changes in swelling and repositioning as the disease progresses. Asking persons about their swelling

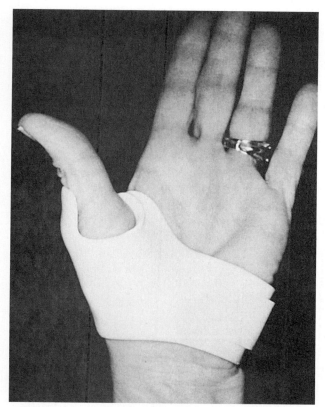

Figure 8-7 This orthosis, which blocks metacarpophalangeal (MCP) hyperextension, is applied for advanced swan neck deformity. (From Colditz JC: Anatomic considerations for splinting the thumb. In Mackin EJ, Callahan AD, Skirven TM, et al., editors: *Rehabilitation of the hand and upper extremity,* ed 5, 2002, St Louis: Mosby, pp. 1858-1874.)

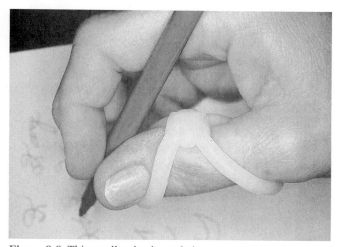

Figure 8-8 This small orthosis can help a person with arthritis who has lateral instability of the thumb interphalangeal (IP) joint. (From Colditz JC: Anatomic considerations for splinting the thumb. In Mackin EJ, Callahan AD, Skirven TM, et al., editors: *Rehabilitation of the hand and upper extremity,* ed 5, St Louis, 2002, Mosby, pp. 1858-1874.)

patterns is important because orthoses fabricated during the day must allow enough room for nocturnal swelling. Thermoplastic material less than 1/8-inch thick is best for small hand orthoses. Orthoses fabricated from heavier thermoplastic material have the potential to irritate other joints.[35] Carefully evaluate all hand orthoses for potential stress on other joints, and instruct persons to wear the orthoses at night, periodically during the day, and during stressful daily activities. However, always tailor any orthotic wearing regimen for each person's therapeutic needs.

Orthoses for Carpometacarpal Osteoarthritis

CMC joint arthritis can occur with osteoarthritis or RA. CMC joint arthritis from **osteoarthritis** is a common thumb condition, affecting 20% of men and women over 40.[35,47,62] Pain from osteoarthritis at the base of the thumb interferes with the person's ability to engage in normal functional activities, because the CMC joint is the most critical joint of the thumb for function.[12,39] Precipitating factors include hypermobility, anatomical predisposition, repetitive grasping, pinching, use of vibratory tools, post-menopausal, and having a family history of the condition.[35,40,58]

CMC arthritis occurs with the trapeziometacarpal joint (basal joint) and sometimes the scaphotrapezial joint. Both joints impact the mobility of the thumb.[40] Over time, the dorsal aspect of the CMC joint is stressed by repetitive pinching and the strong muscle pull of the adductor pollicis muscle and the short intrinsic thumb muscles. Altogether, these forces may cause the first CMC joint to sublux dorsally and radially. This typically results in the first metacarpal losing extension and becoming adducted. The MCP joint hyperextends to accommodate grasp.[16,35,46]

Orthoses help people with CMC arthritis manage pain, preserve their first web space, protect their joints, and provide stability for the intrinsic weakness of the capsular structures. During the early stages of CMC arthritis, orthoses position the hand to prevent the thumb adduction deformity of the metacarpal head and the "dorsoradial subluxation of the metacarpal base on the trapezium."[40] Orthoses stabilize the thumb so that people can perform occupations.[40] Static orthoses are recommended for hypermobile or unstable joints but not for fixed joints.[39]

Many orthotic options exist for people who have CMC osteoarthritis. Orthotic designs range from forearm orthoses (with the CMC and MCP joints included) to hand-based orthoses (with the CMC and MCP joints included, or only the CMC joint included). With any selected design, the thumb is generally positioned in palmar abduction.[39] Based on cadaver research, people with a hypermobile MCP joint who are positioned with the thumb in 30 degrees of MCP flexion may experience reduced pressure on the palmar part of the trapeziometacarpal joint, an area prone to deterioration.[37] Poole and Pellegrini[40] recommend that the thumb be positioned in palmar abduction and 30 degrees MCP

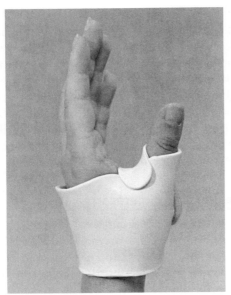

Figure 8-9 A hand-based thumb immobilization orthosis (thumb carpometacarpal [CMC] palmar abduction immobilization orthosis).

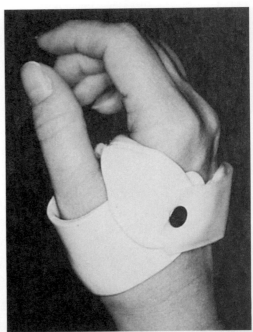

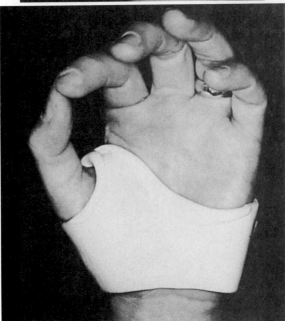

Figure 8-10 An orthosis for rheumatoid arthritis (RA) or osteoarthritis that stabilizes only the carpometacarpal (CMC) joint. (From Colditz JC: Anatomic considerations for splinting the thumb. In Mackin EJ, Callahan AD, Skirven TM, et al., editors: *Rehabilitation of the hand and upper extremity,* ed 5, St Louis, 2002, Mosby, pp.1858-1874.)

flexion. They postulate that the 30 degrees of flexion benefits the position of the trapeziometacarpal joint allowing increased mobility for people in the earlier stages of the disease (Stages I and II). From a review of research evidence, no one orthotic approach was better than another. There is fair evidence that application of orthoses decreases pain and increases function.[22]

Melvin[35] suggested fabricating a dorsal hand-based thumb immobilization orthosis (thumb CMC palmar abduction immobilization orthosis; Figure 8-9)[2] with the primary therapeutic goal of restricting the mobility of the thumb joints to decrease pain and inflammation. The dorsal orthosis stabilizes the CMC and MCP joints in the maximal amount of palmar abduction that is comfortable for the person and allows for a functional pinch. Orthotic intervention of both joints in a thumb post stabilizes the CMC joint in abduction so that the base of the MCP is stabilized. With the orthosis on, the person should continue to perform complete functional tasks, such as writing, comfortably. This thumb immobilization orthosis may be fabricated from a thin (1/16-inch for a frail person or 3/32-inch) conforming thermoplastic material.

Another orthotic option for CMC osteoarthritis designed by Colditz[15] is a hand-based orthosis that allows for free motion of the thumb MCP joint and stabilizes the CMC joint to manage pain (Figure 8-10). The wrist is not included in the orthotic design to allow for functional wrist motions (Figure 8-11). Colditz suggested an initial full-time wear of 2 to 3 weeks with removal for hygiene. Afterward, the orthosis should be worn during painful functional activities.[15]

Therapists should fabricate this hand-based orthosis only on hands that have "a healthy MCP joint" because the MCP joint may sustain additional flexion pressure due to the controlled flexion position of the CMC joint.[36] Therapists must be attentive to wear on the MCP joint.[39] Prefabricated orthoses can also be considered for CMC osteoarthritis. However, prefabricated orthoses should be used with caution, because positioning the thumb in abduction within the orthosis can increase MCP joint extension, which can worsen a possible deformity.[6] In a comparison study of a prefabricated thumb orthosis and a hybrid thumb orthosis made from thermoplastic and Neoprene material, the hybrid orthosis reduced pain to a statistically significant degree.[47]

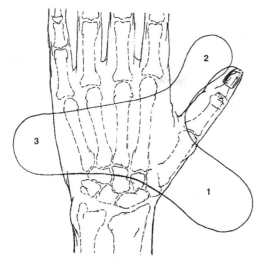

Figure 8-11 A pattern for a thumb carpometacarpal (CMC) immobilization orthosis. (From Colditz JC: The biomechanics of a thumb carpometacarpal immobilization splint: design and fitting, *J Hand Ther* 13(3):228-235, 2000.)

Given the variety of orthotic options available, therapists must critically analyze which orthosis to provide (forearm based or hand based) and which thumb joints to immobilize. Critical thinking considerations include presence of pain, need for stability, work, and functional demands. Researchers offer some guidance. Weiss and colleagues[55] compared providing a long thumb immobilization orthosis with the MCP joint included to a hand-based orthosis with only the CMC joint included. In this 2-week study (n = 26), both orthoses were applied to individuals in grades 1 through 4 of CMC osteoarthritis as rated by Eaton and Littler.[21] Both orthoses were found to be effective for pain control with all grades of the disease. However, the orthoses were only effective in reducing subluxation of the CMC joint for subjects in the earlier stages (grades 1 and 2) of the disease. Subjects in the later stages of the disease (grades 3 and 4) preferred the short orthosis and reported pain relief with orthotic wear. Subjects in grades 1 and 2 slightly preferred the long orthosis (56%). Neither orthosis increased pinch strength nor changed pain levels when completing pinch strength measurements. Activities of daily living (ADLs) improved with the short orthosis (93%) compared to (44%) with the long orthosis. Subjects reported that ADLs were more difficult to complete with the long orthosis.[55]

Swigart and colleagues[49] (n = 114) retrospectively researched the application of a custom long thumb immobilization orthosis with CMC osteoarthritis and found it to be a beneficial conservative treatment. Overall, subjects (regardless of disease stage) benefited from orthotic intervention (with a "60% improvement rate after orthotic intervention and 59% 6 months later"[49]). Some subjects were not able to tolerate the long orthosis because it felt too confining and uncomfortable. Day and colleagues[19] studied orthotic intervention and steroid injections for people with thumb osteoarthritis and found that people in the earlier stages of the disease showed improvement with conservative measures.

Orthoses for Carpometacarpal Rheumatoid Arthritis

Some persons with RA affecting the CMC joint benefit from a hand-based thumb immobilization orthosis (thumb CMC palmar abduction immobilization orthosis),[2] as shown in Figure 8-9.[14,35] If tolerated, position the thumb in enough palmar abduction for functional activities. With a hand-based thumb immobilization orthosis, if the IP joint is painful and inflamed, incorporate the IP joint into the orthosis. However, putting any material (especially plastic) over the thumb pad virtually eliminates thumb and hand function. The person wears this orthosis constantly for a minimum of 2 to 3 weeks with removal for hygiene and exercise. The wearing schedule is adjusted according to the person's pain and inflammation levels.

On the other hand, some therapists stabilize the thumb CMC joint alone with a short hand-based orthosis that is properly molded and positioned (see Figures 8-10 and 8-11). This orthosis works effectively on people who have CMC joint subluxation resulting in adduction of the first MCP joint and anyone with CMC arthritis who can tolerate wearing a rigid orthosis. This orthosis can be also used for CMC osteoarthritis.[13,15]

Often when a physician refers a person who has RA for orthotic intervention, deformities have already developed. If the therapist attempts to place the person's joints in the ideal position of 40 to 45 degrees of palmar abduction, excessive stress on the joints may result. The therapist should always fabricate for a hand affected by arthritis in a position of comfort.[14]

Orthoses for Ulnar Collateral Ligament Injury

A common thumb condition resulting in injury to the **ulnar collateral ligament (UCL)** at the MCP joint of the thumb is known as **skier's thumb** (acute injury) or **gamekeeper's thumb** (chronic injury).[18,29] *Gamekeeper's thumb* was the original name of the injury because gamekeepers stressed this joint when they killed birds by twisting their necks.[13]

The UCL helps stabilize the thumb by resisting radial stresses across the MCP joint.[58] The UCL can be injured if the thumb is forcibly abducted or hyperextended. This can occur from falling with an outstretched hand and the thumb in abduction, such as during skiing.[58] It can also occur from basketball, gymnastics, rugby, volleyball, hockey, and football.[23]

Treatment protocols depend on the extent of ligamental tear. There are protocols that involve immediate postoperative motion, and thus duration of casting postoperatively varies widely. Injuries are classified by the physician as grade I, II, or III.[60] The following is one of many suggested orthotic intervention protocols for each grade of injury. This orthotic intervention protocol is accompanied by hand therapy.[60] Grade I injuries, or those involving microscopic tears with no loss of ligament integrity, are positioned in a hand-based thumb immobilization orthosis with the CMC joint of the thumb in approximately 40 degrees of palmar abduction (or in the most comfortable amount of palmar abduction).[9] Some therapists position the thumb post for the hand-based orthosis so that the MCP joint is in slight ulnar deviation to take the stress off the UCL.[18]

This orthosis is also called a *thumb MCP radial and ulnar deviation restriction orthosis*.[2] The purpose of this orthosis is to provide rest and protection during the healing phase. The person wears the orthosis continuously for 2 to 3 weeks with removal for hygiene purposes. Grade II injuries involve a partial ligament tear, but the overall integrity of the ligament remains intact. The orthotic intervention protocol is the same as for grade I injuries, except that the thumb immobilization orthosis is worn for a longer time period (up to 4 or 5 weeks). Grade III injuries involve a completely torn ligament and usually require surgery.

After the person is casted, the cast is replaced by a thumb immobilization orthosis with the same protocol as described for grade I injuries. There is some evidence that a complete rupture may be managed conservatively with a thumb immobilization orthosis.[29] If the UCL is still in an anatomic position, a thumb immobilization orthosis fabricated with the thumb in neutral with respect to flexion/extension and in maximum tolerated ulnar deviation worn consistently will hopefully heal the tear. The positioning will approximate the ends of the UCL and allow it to scar together. The physician and the therapist must assess whether the person is reliable enough to follow through with the orthosis. If there is any doubt, the person should be casted so that ligament protection is ensured.[46]

A unique "hybrid" orthosis was designed for athletes with a UCL injury who require orthotic intervention for protection during sports activities.[24] This orthotic design is a custom-made circumferential thermoplastic orthosis molded around the MCP joint, which is held in place by a fabricated Neoprene wrap. The advantage of this orthotic design is that it provides MCP stability with the thermoplastic insert and allows for movement of other joints because of the Neoprene stretch. In addition, this orthosis helps control pain and allows for activities involving grip and pinch (Figure 8-12). Therapists could either fabricate both parts of this orthosis or fabricate the circumferential orthosis and purchase a prefabricated Neoprene thumb wrap. For those who return to skiing soon after a UCL injury, researchers suggest fabricating a small thermoplastic orthosis held in place with tape inside a ski glove.[1] Finally, as with any therapeutic intervention, success is dependent on many factors (such as carefully following therapeutic protocols and good surgery techniques).

A radial collateral ligament (RCL) injury (or "golfer's thumb") is an injury that occurs less commonly than UCL injury[8] and requires a hand-based thumb immobilization orthosis. The orthosis is almost the same as for a UCL injury,

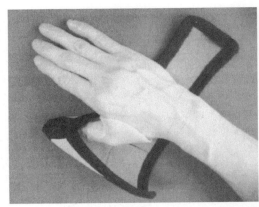

Figure 8-12 A protective orthosis for an ulnar collateral ligament (UCL) injury that combines a custom-made circumferential thermoplastic orthosis molded around the metacarpophalangeal (MCP) joint, which is held in place by a fabricated Neoprene wrap. (From Ford M, McKee P, Szilagyi M: A hybrid thermoplastic and neoprene thumb metacarpophalangeal joint orthosis, *J Hand Ther* 17(1):64-68, 2004.)

except that the thumb is positioned in maximal comfortable radial deviation at the MCP joint. This orthosis is intended to protect the RCL from ulnar stress and alleviate pressure to the healing ligament.[50] The golfer who has injured a thumb and wants to return to the sport may find it difficult to play in a rigid orthosis. Rather than wearing a rigid orthosis during play, the person can be weaned from the orthosis in the same time as required for a UCL injury. The client learns how to wrap the thumb, which will be necessary for at least 1 year post injury,[46] or purchases a soft prefabricated orthosis.

Orthotic Interventions for Scaphoid Fractures

Fracture of the scaphoid bone is the second most common wrist fracture.[7] Similar to Colles fracture, **scaphoid fractures** usually occur because of a fall on an outstretched hand with the wrist dorsiflexed more than 90 degrees[26] and are a consequence of strong forces to the wrist.[17] Scaphoid fractures occur with impact sports, such as basketball, football, and soccer.[26,45,56] Clinically, persons who have a scaphoid fracture present with painful wrist movements and tenderness on palpation of the scaphoid in the anatomical snuffbox between the EPL and the EPB.[7]

Physicians cast the arm and, after the immobilization stage, the hand may be positioned in an orthosis. There are many variations of orthotic options. One option is a volar forearm-based thumb immobilization orthosis[16] or a dorsal/volar forearm thumb immobilization orthosis. The thumb CMC joint is in palmar abduction, the MCP joint is in 0 to 10 degrees flexion, and the wrist is in neutral.

Some clients (especially those in noncontact competitive sports) may benefit from a combination dorsal/volar thumb orthosis for added stability, protection, and pain and edema control (Figure 8-13).[23] Therapists should educate clients that proximal scaphoid fractures take longer to heal, sometimes up to months, because of a poor vascular supply.[23,43]

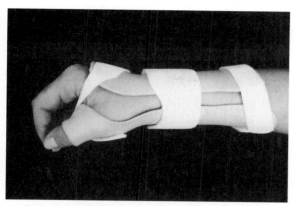

Figure 8-13 This combination volar and dorsal orthosis adds stability to the healing scaphoid fracture. (From Fess EE, Gettle KS, Philips CA, et al: *Hand and upper extremity splinting: principles and methods*, ed 3, St Louis, 2005, Elsevier Mosby.)

For people who play sports and have a healing scaphoid fracture, a soft commercial thumb immobilization orthosis may also be recommended as a protective measure.[26]

Fabrication of a Thumb Immobilization Orthosis

There are many approaches to fabrication of a thumb immobilization orthosis. Figure 8-14 shows a pattern that can be used for either a volar or dorsal thumb immobilization orthosis. The thumb immobilization orthosis radial design[2] provides support on the radial side of the hand while stabilizing the thumb. This design allows some wrist flexion and extension but limits deviation.[35] The therapist usually places the thumb in a palmar abducted position so that the thumb pad can contact the index pad. The therapist leaves the IP joint free for functional movement but can adapt the orthotic pattern to include the IP joint if more support becomes necessary. The thumb can be placed in a position of comfort (i.e., out of the functional plane) if the client does not tolerate the thumb placed in the functional position or when the physician does not want the thumb to incur any stress.

Figure 8-15 shows a detailed radial gutter thumb immobilization pattern that excludes the IP joint. (See Figure 8-3 for a picture of the completed orthotic product.)

1. Position the forearm and hand palm down on a piece of paper. The fingers should be in a natural resting position and slightly abducted; the wrist should be neutral with respect to deviation. Draw an outline of the hand and forearm to the elbow. As you gain experience with pattern drawing, you will not need to draw the entire hand and forearm outline. The experienced therapist can estimate the placement of key points on the pattern.
2. While the person's hand is on the paper, mark an A at the radial styloid and a B at the ulnar styloid. Mark the second and fifth metacarpal heads C and D, respectively. Mark the IP joint of the thumb E, and mark the olecranon process of the elbow F. Then remove the person's hand from the paper pattern.

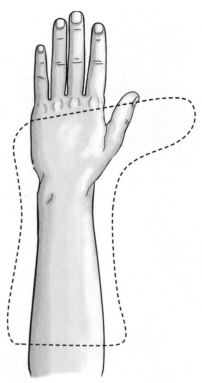

Figure 8-14 A detailed pattern for either a volar or a dorsal thumb immobilization orthosis or hand-based thumb immobilization orthosis.

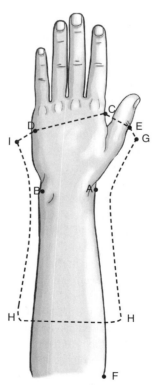

Figure 8-15 A detailed pattern for a radial gutter thumb immobilization orthosis.

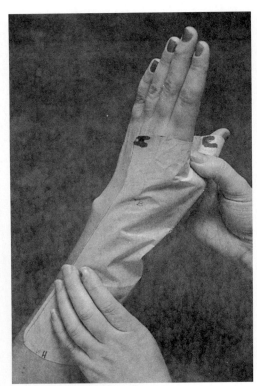

Figure 8-16 To ensure proper fit, place the paper pattern on the person.

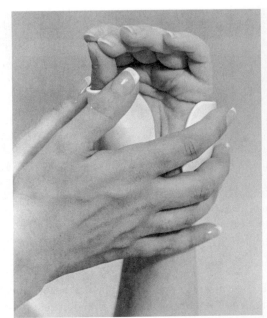

Figure 8-17 Have person lightly touch the thumb tip to the pads of the index and middle fingers to position the thumb in palmar abduction.

3. Place an X two-thirds the length of the forearm on each side. Place another X on each side of the pattern approximately 1 to 1½ inches outside and parallel to the two X markings for the appropriate width of the orthosis. Mark these two Xs H.

4. Draw an angled line connecting the second and fifth metacarpal heads (C to D). Extend this line approximately 1 to 1½ inches to the ulnar side of the hand, and mark it I.

5. Connect C to E. Extend this line approximately ½ to 1 inch. Mark the end of the line G.

6. Draw a line from G down the radial side of the forearm, making sure the line follows the increasing size of the forearm. To ensure that the orthosis is two-thirds the length of the forearm, end the line at H.

7. Begin a line from I, and extend it down the ulnar side of the forearm, making certain that the line follows the increasing size of the forearm. End the line at H.

8. For the proximal edge of the orthosis, draw a straight line that connects both Hs.

9. Make sure the orthotic pattern lines are rounded at G, I, and the two Hs to prevent any injury or discomfort.

10. Cut out the pattern.

11. Place the pattern on the person (Figure 8-16). Make certain the orthosis' edges end mid-forearm on the volar and dorsal surfaces of the person's hand and forearm. Check that the orthosis is two-thirds the forearm length and one-half the forearm circumference. Check the thumb position, and make any necessary adjustments (e.g., additions, deletions) on the pattern.

12. Carefully trace with a pencil the thumb immobilization pattern on a sheet of thermoplastic material.

13. Heat the thermoplastic material.

14. Cut the pattern out of the thermoplastic material.

15. Reheat the material, mold the form onto the person's hand, and make necessary adjustments. Make sure the thumb is correctly positioned as the material hardens by having the person lightly touch the thumb tip to the pads of the index or middle fingers. Another approach is to provide light pressure over the plastic of the thumb MCP joint to align it in palmar abduction (Figure 8-17 and Figure 8-18).

16. Add three 2-inch straps (one at the wrist joint, one toward the proximal end of the forearm trough, and one across the dorsal aspect of the hand) connecting the hypothenar bar to the metacarpal bar.

Fabrication of a Dorsal Hand-Based Thumb Immobilization Orthosis

Hand-based thumb immobilization orthoses can be fabricated for people who have the following diagnoses: low median nerve injury, UCL or RCL injury of the MCP joint, CMC arthritis, and the potential for a first web space contracture. Each of these diagnoses may require placement of the thumb post in a different degree of abduction, based on protocols and comfort of the patient. With this orthosis, the IP joint is usually left free for functional movement, unless there is extreme pain in that joint. However, if the IP joint is left free (especially during rigorous activity) it too can become vulnerable to stresses. This hand-based orthotic design is most appropriate for stabilizing the MCP joint because the

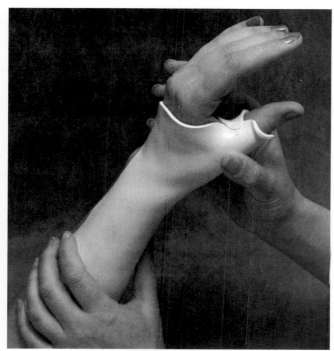

Figure 8-18 Although the actual movement comes from the car-pometacarpal (CMC) joint, provide light pressure on the thumb metacarpophalangeal (MCP) joint to position the thumb correctly in palmar abduction.

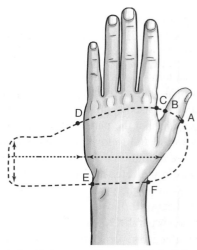

Figure 8-19 A detailed pattern for a hand-based thumb immobilization orthosis.

position of the CMC is irrelevant. Finally, because this hand-based orthotic design incorporates the dorsal aspect of the palm, the therapist may need to add padding since the dorsal skin has a minimal subcutaneous layer and the boniness of the dorsal palm can cause skin breakdown.

Figure 8-19 shows a detailed hand-based dorsal thumb immobilization pattern. (See Figure 8-9 for a picture of the completed orthotic product.)

1. Position the person's forearm and hand palm down on a piece of paper. Ensure that the client's thumb is radially abducted. The fingers should be in a natural resting position and slightly abducted. Draw an outline of the hand, including the wrist and a couple of inches of the forearm.
2. While the person's hand is on the paper, mark the IP joint of the thumb on both sides, and label it A (radial side of thumb) and B (ulnar side of the thumb), respectively. Then mark the second and fifth metacarpal heads C and D, respectively. Mark the wrist joint on the ulnar side of the hand E, and mark F on the radial side of the wrist. Remove the hand from the pattern.
3. Start in the web space. Draw an angled line connecting the marks of the second and fifth metacarpal heads (D to C). Then connect C to B and B to A. Curve the line around and angle it down to F. Connect F to E. Then extend the line out from E approximately equal to the length of the pattern on the hand. Go up vertically, curve the line around, and connect it to D. Make sure that all edges on this pattern are rounded.

4. Cut out the pattern, check fit, and make any adjustments. Make sure the pattern allows enough room for an adequately fitting thumb post.
5. Position the person's upper extremity with the elbow resting on the table and the forearm in a neutral position.
6. Trace the pattern onto a sheet of thermoplastic material.
7. Heat the thermoplastic material.
8. Cut the pattern out of the thermoplastic material.
9. Measure the CMC joint with a small goniometer to make sure it is in the correct position.
10. Reheat the thermoplastic material.
11. Mold the orthosis onto the person's hand. First form the thumb post around the thenar area. Make sure the thumb is correctly positioned as the material hardens. Allowances are made in the circumference of the thumb post to ensure that the client can move the thumb. This is particularly important when fabricating an orthosis from thermoplastic material that shrinks or has memory. Roll the volar part of the thumb post proximal to the thumb IP crease to allow adequate IP flexion. Then form the orthosis across the dorsal side of the hand from the thumb (radial side) to the ulnar side. Curving around the ulnar side, fit the thermoplastic material proximal to the distal palmar crease on the volar side of the hand. There will be just enough room between the thumb post and the end of the orthosis on the ulnar side to add a strap across the palm. Make sure the proximal end of the orthosis is flared to prevent skin breakdown.
12. After the thermoplastic material has hardened, check that the person can perform IP thumb flexion without impingement by the thumb post and that he or she can perform all wrist movements without interference by the proximal end of the orthosis. Make adjustments as necessary.
13. Add one strap across the palm.

Orthotic Intervention Pattern for Volar Forearm-Based Orthosis, Radial Gutter and/or a Dorsal Hand-Based Thumb Immobilization Orthosis

This orthotic pattern is versatile because it can be used for the fabrication of three different thumb orthoses (Figure 8-20). With a volar-based thumb immobilization orthosis for a proper fit, ensure that the pattern is fitted proximal to the distal palmar crease and follows the curves of the forearm. For a hand-based thumb immobilization orthosis, the dotted line on the pattern indicates the proximal end of the orthosis, which fits distal to the wrist joint. With this hand-based thumb immobilization orthosis, the section of the orthotic pattern that extends parallel to the ulnar side of the hand may need to be lengthened in order to fit around to the palmar (volar) side of the hand. For the radial gutter thumb immobilization orthosis, fit the pattern mid-forearm. Review the instructions earlier in the chapter for tips on general fabrication of radial gutter and dorsal hand-based thumb immobilization orthoses. For any of the three types of thumb orthoses, carefully check the pattern on the client before cutting out the thermoplastic material. The portion of the pattern that will cover the thenar eminence may need to be enlarged to fit the person's hand. In addition, to fit the thumb post pull the section that has a star drawn on it over the first web space and the section with a triangle on it around to the palmar (volar) aspect of the hand where it meets the "star" section.

Technical Tips for Proper Fit

1. Before molding the orthosis, place the person's elbow on a tabletop, positioned in 90 degrees of flexion and the forearm in a neutral position. Position the thumb and wrist according to diagnostic indications.

2. Monitor joint positions by measuring during and after orthotic fabrication. Place the thumb in as close to a palmar abduction position as is comfortable for the person. The best way to position the thumb in palmar abduction for fabrication of an orthosis is to have the person lightly touch the thumb tip to the pad of the index or middle finger. However, there will be some persons (for example, a person who has RA) who will find the thumb post more comfortable between radial and palmar abduction.

3. Follow the natural curves of the longitudinal, distal, and proximal arches. Ensure the orthosis completely covers the thenar eminence. Be especially careful to check that the index finger has full flexion because of its close proximity to the opponens bar, C bar, and thumb post and if necessary carefully roll the area just proximal to the proximal palmar crease.

4. With a volar forearm orthosis check that the distal end of the orthosis is positioned just proximal to the distal palmar crease and that it does not interfere with finger flexion. Also check that the forearm part of the orthosis is ½ the circumference of the forearm.

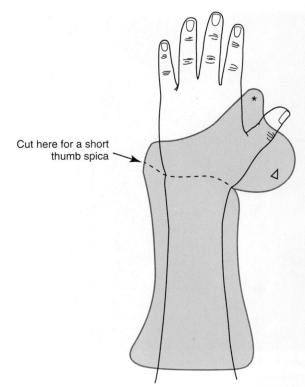

Figure 8-20 Pattern for a volar forearm-based orthosis, radial gutter orthoses, and/or a dorsal hand-based thumb immobilization orthosis.

Cut here for a short thumb spica

5. For a radial gutter orthosis check that the forearm trough is correctly placed in mid-forearm (i.e., place a goniometer with the axis at mid-wrist, one arm extending between the third and fourth digits, and the other arm pointing toward the mid-forearm).

6. When molding the thumb post, overlap the thermoplastic material into the thumb web space (Figure 8-21). Be certain the thumb IP joint remains in extension during molding to facilitate later orthotic application and removal. Be extremely careful in making adjustments with a heat gun on the thumb post, or the result may be an inappropriate fit.

7. When applying thermoplastic material that shrinks during cooling and because the thumb is circumferential in shape, allowances must be made to ensure easy application and removal of the orthosis. The orthosis must provide enough support to the thumb in the thumb post. The thumb must not move excessively. There are several options to address the correct size of the thumb post. One is to have the person make very small thumb circles as the plastic cools, because this motion allows for some extra room.[46] Another option is to gently flare the thumb post with a narrow pencil[34] or popsicle stick.

8. Before the orthosis is completely cool, remove the orthosis from the thumb to ensure that the orthosis can be easily doffed and donned.

9. A thumb post can be fabricated with overlapping material that does not bond. This design method allows for adjustment to expand or contract the thumb post with Velcro straps that secure the post.[46]

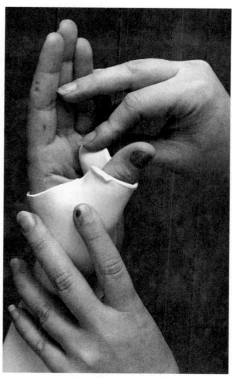

Figure 8-21 Overlap the extra thermoplastic material into the thumb web space.

10. For a thumb immobilization orthosis that allows IP mobility, make sure the distal end of the thumb post on the volar surface has been rolled to allow full IP flexion, yet remains high enough for full support (Figure 8-22). When fabricating the thumb post, place the thermoplastic material slightly over the IP joint and while stabilizing the thumb MCP joint have the person slowly flex the IP joint. Roll the distal end of the thumb post on the volar side to allow for full IP excursion. This technique results in a thumb post that is high enough for adequate support, while not interfering with IP mobility.

11. Check that the distal end of the thumb post is just proximal to the IP joint and has not migrated lower. Make sure that the orthosis does not interfere with functional hand movements.

Patient Safety Tips and Precautions for Fabrication of Thumb Orthoses

The cautious therapist checks for areas of skin pressure over the distal ulna, the superficial branch of the radial nerve at the radial styloid, and the volar and dorsal surfaces of the thumb MCP joint. Specific precautions for the molding of the orthosis include the following:

• If the thumb post extends too far distally on the volar surface of the IP joint, the result is restriction of the IP joint flexion and a likely area for skin irritation.
• Because of its close proximity to the opponens bar, C bar, and thumb post, the radial base of the first metacarpal and first web space has a potential for skin irritation.

• With a radial gutter orthosis, monitor the orthosis for a pressure area at the midline of the forearm on the volar and dorsal surfaces. Pull the sides of the forearm trough apart if it is too tight.
• Be careful to fabricate an orthosis that is supportive to the thumb's joints and is not too constrictive. Providing enough support allows the orthosis to meet therapeutic goals. Constriction results in decreased circulation and possible skin breakdown. Make allowances for edema when fabricating the thumb post.
• If using a thermoplastic material that has memory properties, be aware that the material shrinks when cooling. Therefore, the thumb post opening must remain large enough for comfortable application and removal of the orthosis. Refer to technical tips for suggestions on fabricating the thumb post.

Impact on Occupations

Having a workable thumb for grasp and pinch is paramount for functional activities. Research findings support the thumb's functional importance. Swigart and colleagues[49] established that people with CMC arthritis had decreased involvement in crafts and changed their athletic involvement. With gamekeeper's thumb, lack of thenar strength and adequate pinch can impact daily functional activities, such as turning a key or opening a jar.[63]

Even with the stability provided by an orthosis, some people may find it more difficult to perform meaningful occupations. For example, Weiss and colleagues[55] found in their study (n = 25) that with some subjects, the long thumb immobilization orthosis inhibited function and was more than necessary to meet therapeutic goals. Therefore, the goal of orthotic intervention is to improve function for meaningful activities. It is intended that with the benefits of orthotic wear and a therapeutic program the person will return to functional and meaningful activities.[63]

Prefabricated Orthoses

Deciding to provide a client with a prefabricated thumb orthosis requires careful reflection. Therapists should critically consider the condition for which the orthosis is being provided, materials that the orthosis is made out of, the design of the orthosis, and comfort factors. Therapists should remember that because prefabricated thumb orthoses are made for a mass population, the thumb positioning is often in some degree of radial abduction, which may or may not be the correct position for the patient. Furthermore, therapists should review the literature to determine whether a custom thumb orthosis is preferable over a prefabricated thumb orthosis to treat a condition.

Conditions

Prefabricated thumb orthoses are manufactured for a variety of conditions, including arthritis, thumb MCP collateral ligament injuries, de Quervain tenosynovitis, and hypertonicity. Orthotic types and positions for all these conditions have been discussed in this chapter (see Table 8-1).

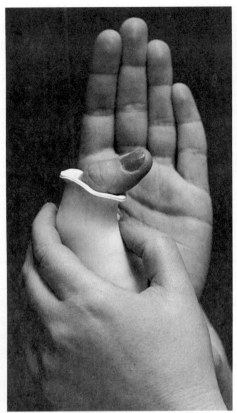

Figure 8-22 Roll the distal end of the thumb post to allow full interphalangeal (IP) flexion.

Materials

Therapists should be aware of the characteristics of the wide variety of materials available for prefabricated thumb orthoses. Material firmness varies from soft to rigid. Soft materials are often used with thumb orthotic intervention because they can be easier to apply and provide a more comfortable fit for a client with a painful and edematous thumb IP joint than a rigid orthosis. Neoprene is a commonly used soft material for prefabricated orthoses. It has the advantage of providing hugging support with flexibility for function, but it has the disadvantage of retaining moisture next to the skin increasing the possibility of skin breakdown. Another soft material used in prefabricated orthoses is leather. Leather orthoses absorb perspiration and are pliable; however, they often become odiferous and soiled. Some orthoses are lined with moisture wicking material or are fabricated from perforated material to address this issue. Examples of prefabricated orthoses made from rigid materials are those fabricated out of thermoplastic, vinyl, or adjustable polypropylene materials.

An awareness of the orthosis' function, condition for which it is being used, and the client's occupational demands help therapists critically determine the degree of material firmness to use. A prefabricated orthosis made from a rigid material might be very appropriate for a client engaged in sports, heavier work activities, or for any condition that requires a higher amount of support and protection. Finally, people who are allergic to latex require orthoses be made from latex-free materials.

Design and Comfort

Similar to custom fabricated thumb orthoses, prefabricated orthoses are either hand-based or forearm-based. The hand-based thumb immobilization designs provide support to the thumb joints through the circumferential thumb post component, thermoplastic material, or optional stays. The forearm-based immobilization designs derive some of their support from a longer lever arm. Prefabricated forearm-based orthoses contain many features which should be critically considered for client usage. Examples of these features are adjustable or additional straps and adjustable thumb stays to provide optimal support and fit. Some designs for both the forearm- and hand-based orthoses are hybrid designs. These orthoses usually have a softer outer layer with removable and adjustable inserts made out of thermoplastic material to customize the fit.

Another consideration is the comfort of the prefabricated thumb orthosis. Factors to think about are adjustability, temperature, bulkiness, and padding of the possible orthotic selection. When adjusting the orthosis therapists should take into account the number and location of strap and types of strapping material to obtain an appropriate fit. For example, with a long thumb orthosis the therapist should consider whether the wrist straps provide adequate support. With temperature the type of thermoplastic material that is used for the prefabricated orthosis is taken into account as some materials are more breathable than others. Thumb orthoses made from Neoprene or other soft materials are usually more breathable than rigid thermoplastic materials. A prefabricated orthosis made from a breathable material might be a consideration for a person living or working in a hot environment. A person with arthritis might prefer a thumb orthosis that provides warmth. Padding may be an essential consideration with a person who has a tendency toward skin breakdown. Thumb immobilization orthoses may chafe the web space, so the therapist must monitor for fit and consider padding in that area. Some prefabricated thumb immobilization designs include added features, such as a gel pad for scar control or leather for added durability. Figure 8-23 outlines prefabricated thumb orthotic options.

Summary

Thumb orthotic intervention is commonly provided in clinical practice. Applying a critical analysis approach helps to determine the most optimal thumb orthotic intervention. It behooves therapists to be aware of the variety of orthoses (whether custom fabricated or prefabricated) to provide clients with orthoses that address specific conditions and occupational needs.

Review Questions

1. What are the general reasons for provision of a thumb immobilization orthosis?
2. What are three common conditions that require thumb immobilization orthoses?
3. What are some clinical indications for including the thumb IP joint in a thumb immobilization orthosis?

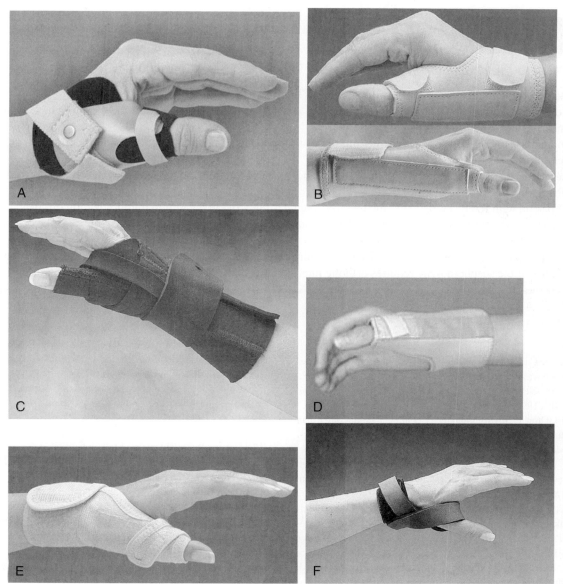

Figure 8-23 **A,** This thermoplastic orthosis supports the metacarpophalangeal (MCP) and carpometacarpal (CMC) joints. **B,** Thumb orthosis is made from leather. **C,** This Comfort Cool Wrist and Thumb CMC Restriction Orthosis is made out of perforated Neoprene, which keeps the extremity cool. It has additional strapping at the wrist to allow for extra support. **D,** This Rolyan Preferred First thumb orthosis can be used with a person who has arthritis because it contains extra layers to help wick moisture from the skin, retain body warmth, and provide heat. **E,** This Roylan Gel Shell thumb spica orthosis contains a gel shell Rolyan pad that helps with scar formation and hypersensitivity. It also contains a moldable thermoplastic stay that can be adjusted along the radial side of the hand. **F,** This Rolyan thumb loop is latex free and positions the thumb to decrease tone and facilitate function. These thumb orthoses for boutonnière deformity **(G)** and swan neck deformity **(H)** are comfortable for long-term wear. (**A,** ThumSaver MP; courtesy of 3-Point Products, Stevensville, MD. **B,** Collum CMC Thumb Brace; courtesy of Adaptive Abilities, Oroville, WA. **C-F,** Courtesy of Sammons Preston Rolyan, Bollington, IL. **G** and **H,** Courtesy of Silver Ring Splint Company http://www.silverringsplint.com/our-splints/siris-swan-neck-splint/ will need permission.)

4. What is an appropriate wearing schedule for a person with RA who wears a thumb immobilization orthosis?
5. What is the suggested position for a thumb orthosis for a person who has CMC joint arthritis? What joints are stabilized?
6. Which type of thumb immobilization orthosis should a therapist fabricate for a person who has de Quervain tenosynovitis?

7. What does the research evidence for orthotic intervention of de Quervain tenosynovitis indicate?
8. Which type of thumb immobilization orthosis should be fabricated for an injury of the thumb UCL?
9. What is the orthotic wearing schedule for each grade of an UCL injury?

SELF-QUIZ 8-1*

Please circle either true (T) or false (F).

1. T F One purpose of a thumb immobilization orthosis is to protect the thumb.
2. T F A therapist should apply a thumb immobilization orthosis to a client only during the chronic phase of de Quervain tenosynovitis.
3. T F Fabricating either a long forearm thumb immobilization orthosis or a radial gutter thumb immobilization orthosis is best for a person who has de Quervain tenosynovitis.
4. T F Thermoplastic material more than ⅛-inch thick is best used for an orthosis for a person who has RA because this material adds more support.
5. T F If a person with RA has wrist pain, the therapist includes the wrist in the thumb immobilization orthosis.
6. T F Orthotic intervention for grade I ulnar collateral thumb injuries may require that the person wear the orthosis continuously for 2 to 3 weeks with removal only for hygiene.
7. T F The main purpose of orthotic intervention for an ulnar collateral thumb injury is to keep the web space open.
8. T F Fracture of the scaphoid bone requires orthotic intervention in a hand-based thumb immobilization orthosis.

*See Appendix A for the answer key.

References

1. Alexy C, De Carlo M: Rehabilitation and use of protective devices in hand and wrist injuries, *Clin Sports Med* 17(3):635–655, 1998.
2. American Society of Hand Therapists: *Splint classification system*, Garner, NC, 1992, American Society of Hand Therapists.
3. Andréu J, Otón T, Silva-Fernández L, et al.: Hand pain other than carpal tunnel syndrome (CTS): the role of occupational factors, *Best Pract Res Clin Rheumatol* 25(1):31–42, 2011.
4. Avci S, Yilmaz C, Sayli U: Comparison of nonsurgical treatment measures for de Quervain's disease of pregnancy and lactation, *J Hand Surg Am* 27(2):322–324, 2002.
5. Belkin J, English C: Hand splinting: principles, practice, and decision making. In Pedretti LW, editor: *Occupational therapy: practice skills for physical dysfunction*, ed 4, St Louis, 1996, Mosby, pp 319–343.
6. Biese J: Short splints: indications and techniques. In Mackin EJ, Callahan AD, Skirven TM, et al.: *Rehabilitation of the hand and upper extremity*, ed 5, St Louis, 2002, Mosby, pp 1846–1857.
7. Cailliet R: *Hand pain and impairment*, Philadelphia, 1994, FA Davis.
8. Campbell PJ, Wilson RL: Management of joint injuries and intraarticular fractures. In Mackin EJ, Callahan AD, Skirven TM, et al.: *Rehabilitation of the hand and upper extremity*, ed 5, St Louis, 2002, Mosby, pp 396–411.
9. Cannon NM: *Diagnosis and treatment manual for physicians and therapists*, ed 4, Indianapolis, 2001, The Hand Rehabilitation Center of Indiana.
10. Cannon NM: *Fundamentals of hand therapy: clinical reasoning and treatment guidelines for common diagnoses of the upper extremity*, Philadelphia, 2007, Elsevier.
11. Cannon NM, Foltz RW, Koepfer JM, et al.: *Manual of hand splinting*, New York, 1985, Churchill Livingstone.
12. Chaisson C, McAlindon TS: Osteoarthritis of the hand: clinical features and management, *J Musculoskelet Med* 14:66–68, 1997. 71–74, 77.
13. Colditz JC: Anatomic considerations for splinting the thumb. In Mackin EJ, Callahan AD, Skirven TM, et al.: *Rehabilitation of the hand and upper extremity*, ed 5, St Louis, 2002, Mosby, pp 1858–1874.
14. Colditz JC: Arthritis. In Malick MH, Kasch MC, editors: *Manual on management of specific hand problems*, Pittsburgh, 1984, AREN Publications, pp 112–136.
15. Colditz JC: The biomechanics of a thumb carpometacarpal immobilization splint: design and fitting, *J Hand Ther* 13(3):228–235, 2000.
16. Colditz JC: *Personal communication*, April 1995.
17. Cooney WP: III: Scaphoid fractures: current treatments and techniques, *Instructional Course Lectures* 52:197–208, 2003.
18. Cooper C: *Personal communication*, June 2012.
19. Day CS, Gelberman R, Patel AA, et al.: Basal joint osteoarthritis of the thumb: a prospective trial of steroid injection and splinting, *J Hand Surg Am* 29(2):247–251, 2004.
20. Dell PC, Dell RB: Management of rheumatoid arthritis of the wrist, *J Hand Ther* 9(2):157–164, 1996.
21. Eaton RG, Littler W: Ligament reconstruction for the painful thumb carpometacarpal joint, *J Bone Joint Surg Am* 55:1655–1666, 1973.
22. Egan MY, Brousseau L: Splinting for osteoarthritis of the carpometacarpal joint: a review of the evidence, *Am J Occup Ther* 61:70–78, 2007.
23. Fess EE, Gettle KS, Philips CA, et al.: *Hand splinting principles and methods*, ed 3, St Louis, 2005, Elsevier/Mosby.
24. Ford M, McKee P, Szilagyi M: A hybrid thermoplastic and neoprene thumb metacarpophalangeal joint orthosis, *J Hand Ther* 17(1):64–68, 2004.
25. Geisser RW: Splinting the rheumatoid arthritic hand. In Ziegler EM, editor: *Current concepts in orthosis*, Germantown, WI, 1984, Rolyan Medical Products, pp 29–49.
26. Geissler WB: Carpal fractures in athletes, *Clin Sports Med* 20(1):167–188, 2001.
27. Idler RS: Helping the patient who has wrist or hand tenosynovitis. Part 2: managing trigger finger and de Quervain's disease, *J Musculoskelet Med* 14:62–65, 1997. 68, 74–75.
28. Ilyas AM, Ast M, Schaffer A, et al.: De Quervain tenosynovitis of the wrist, *J Am Acad Orthop Surg* 15(12):757–764, 2007.
29. Landsman JC, Seitz WH, Froimson AI, et al.: Splint immobilization of gamekeeper's thumb, *Orthopedics* 18(12):1161–1165, 1995.

30. Lane LB, Boretz RS, Stuchin SA: Treatment of de Quervain's disease: role of conservative management, *J Hand Surg Br* 26(3):258–260, 2001.

31. Lee MP, Nasser-Sharif S, Zelouf DS: Surgeon's and therapist's management of tendonopathies in the hand and wrist. In Mackin EJ, Callahan AD, Skirven TM, et al.: *Rehabilitation of the hand and upper extremity*, ed 5, St Louis, 2002, Mosby, pp 931–953.

32. Marx H: Rheumatoid arthritis. In Stanley BG, Tribuzi SM, editors: *Concepts in hand rehabilitation*, Philadelphia, 1992, FA Davis, pp 395–418.

33. McCarroll JR: Overuse injuries of the upper extremity in golf, *Clin Sports Med* 20(3):469–479, 2001.

34. McKee P, Morgan L: *Orthotics and rehabilitation: splinting the hand and body*, Philadelphia, 1998, FA Davis.

35. Melvin JL: *Rheumatic disease in the adult and child*, ed 3, Philadelphia, 1989, FA Davis.

36. Melvin JL: Therapist's management of osteoarthritis in the hand. In Mackin EJ, Callahan AD, Skirven TM, et al.: *Rehabilitation of the hand and upper extremity*, ed 5, St Louis, 2002, Mosby, pp 1646–1663.

37. Moulton MJ, Parentis MA, Kelly MJ, et al.: Influence of metacarpophalangeal joint position on basal joint-loading in the thumb, *J Bone Joint Surg Am* 83(5):709–716, 2001.

38. Nalebuff EA: Diagnosis, classification and management of rheumatoid thumb deformities, *Bull Hosp Joint Dis* 29(2):119–137, 1968.

39. Neumann DA, Bielefeld T: The carpometacarpal joint of the thumb: stability, deformity, and therapeutic intervention, *J Orthop Sports Phys Ther* 33(7):386–399, 2003.

40. Ouellette E: The rheumatoid hand: orthotics as preventive, *Semin Arthritis Rheum* 21(2):65–72, 1991.

41. Poole JU, Pellegrini VD Jr: Arthritis of the thumb basal joint complex, *J Hand Ther* 13(2):91–107, 2000.

42. Rettig AC: Wrist and hand overuse syndromes, *Clin Sports Med* 20(3):591–611, 2001.

43. Rettig ME, Dassa GL, Raskin KB, et al.: Wrist fractures in the athlete: distal radius and carpal fractures, *Clin Sports Med* 17(3):469–489, 1998.

44. Richie 3rd CA, Briner WW Jr: Cortisosteroid infection for treatment of de Quervain's tenosynovities: a pooled quantitative literature evaluation, *J Am Board Fam Pract* 16(2):102–106, 2003.

45. Riester JN, Baker BE, Mosher JF, et al.: A review of scaphoid fracture healing in competitive athletes, *Am J Sports Med* 13(3):159–161, 1985.

46. Schultz-Johnson K: *Personal communication*, June 2006.

47. Sillem H, Backman CL, Miller WC, et al.: Comparison of two carpometacarpal stabilizing splints for individuals with osteoarthritis, *J Hand Ther* 24(3):216–226, 2011.

48. Skirven T, Osterman A, Fedorczyk J, et al.: *Rehabilitation of the hand and upper extremity*, ed 6, Philadelphia, 2011, Elsevier Mosby.

49. Swigart CR, Eaton RG, Glickel SZ, et al.: Splinting in the treatment of arthritis of the first carpometacarpal joint, *J Hand Surg Am* 24(1):86–91, 1999.

50. Tang P: Collateral ligament injuries of the thumb metacarpophalangeal joint, *J Am Acad Orthop Surg* 19(5):287–296, 2011.

51. Tenney CG, Lisak JM: *Atlas of hand splinting*, Boston/Toronto, 1986, Little, Brown & Co.

52. Tubiana R, Thomine JM, Mackin E: *Examination of the hand and wrist*, St Louis, 1996, Mosby.

53. Van Heest AE, Kallemeier P: Thumb carpal metacarpal arthritis, *J Am Acad Orthop Surg* 16(31):140–151, 2008.

54. Weiss AP, Akelman E, Tabatabai M: Treatment of de Quervain's disease, *J Hand Surg Am* 19(4):595–598, 1994.

55. Weiss S, LaStayo P, Mills A, et al.: Prospective analysis of splinting the first carpometacarpal joint: an objective, subjective and radiographic assessment, *J Hand Ther* 13(3):218–226, 2000.

56. Werner SL, Plancher KD: Biomechanics of wrist injuries in sports, *Clin Sports Med* 17(3):407–420, 1998.

57. Wilton JC: *Hand splinting: principles of design and fabrication*, London, 1997, WB Saunders.

58. Winzeler S, Rosenstein BD: Occupational injury and illness of the thumb, *AAOHN J* 44(10):487–492, 1996.

59. Witt J, Pess G, Gelberman RH: Treatment of de Quervain tenosynovitis: a prospective study of the results of injection of steroids and immobilization in a splint, *J Bone Joint Surg Am* 73(2):219–222, 1991.

60. Wright HH, Rettig AC: Management of common sports injuries. In Hunter JM, Mackin EJ, Callahan AD, editors: *Rehabilitation of the hand*, ed 4, St Louis, 1995, Mosby, pp 1809–1838.

61. Yao J, Park M: Early treatment of degenerative arthritis of the thumb carpometacarpal joint, *Hand Clinics* 24(3):251–261, 2008.

62. Zelouf DS, Posner MA: Hand and wrist disorders: how to manage pain and improve function, *Geriatrics* 50(3):22–26, 1995. 29–31.

63. Zeman C, Hunter RE, Freeman JR, Purnell ML, Mastrangelo J: Acute skier's thumb repaired with a proximal phalanx suture anchor, *Am J Sports Med* 26(5):644–650, 1998.

APPENDIX 8-2   **LABORATORY EXERCISES**

Laboratory Exercise 8-1

These components are in various types of thumb immobilization orthoses. They are also part of other orthoses, such as the wrist cock-up and resting hand orthosis. Label the orthotic components shown in the following figure.

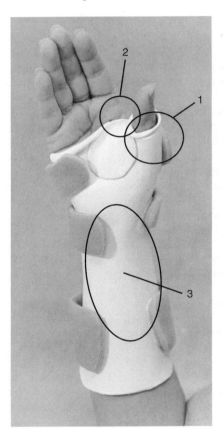

1. _____
2. _____
3. _____

Laboratory Exercise 8-2

1. Practice making a pattern for a radial gutter thumb immobilization orthosis on another person. Use the detailed instructions on the previous pages to draw the pattern. Make necessary adjustments to the pattern after cutting it out.
2. Practice drawing a pattern for a radial gutter thumb immobilization orthosis on the following outlines of the hands without using detailed instructions. Label the landmarks.

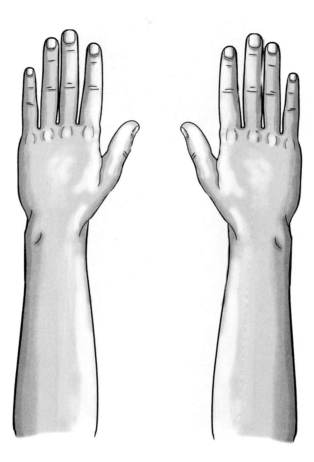

Laboratory Exercise 8-3*

The following illustration shows a thumb immobilization orthosis for a 35-year-old woman working as an administrative assistant (secretary). She has a long history of rheumatoid arthritis (RA). Her physician ordered a thumb immobilization orthosis after she complained of thumb metacarpophalangeal (MCP) joint pain and inflammation. Keeping in mind the diagnostic protocols for thumb immobilization orthotic intervention, identify two problems with the illustrated orthosis.

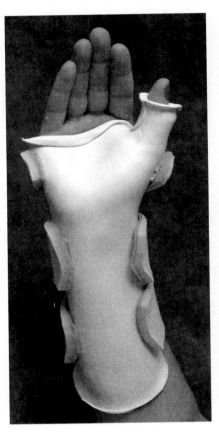

1. List two problems with this orthosis.
    a. _____
    b. _____
2. What problems might result from continual orthotic wear?
    _____
    _____
    _____

Laboratory Exercise 8-4

On a partner, practice fabricating a radial gutter or a volar forearm-based thumb immobilization orthosis that does not immobilize the thumb interphalangeal (IP) joint. Before starting, use a goniometer to ensure that the wrist is in 15 degrees of extension, the carpometacarpal (CMC) joint of the thumb in 45 degrees of palmar abduction, and the MCP joint of the thumb in 5 to 10 degrees of flexion. Check the finished product to ensure that full finger flexion and thumb IP flexion are possible after you fit the orthosis, and make all adjustments. Use Form 8-1 as a check-off sheet for a self-evaluation of the thumb immobilization orthosis. Use Grading Sheet 8-1 as a classroom grading sheet.

APPENDIX 8-3 FORM AND GRADING SHEET

FORM 8-1* Thumb immobilization orthosis

Name: _____

Date: _____

Type of thumb immobilization orthosis:

Volar ○   Dorsal ○   Radial gutter ○   Hand based ○

Thumb joint position: _____

After the person wears the orthosis for 30 minutes, answer the following questions. (Mark NA for non-applicable situations.)

Evaluation Areas				**Comments**

Design

1. The wrist position is at the correct angle.	Yes ○	No ○	NA ○	
2. The thumb position is at the correct angle.	Yes ○	No ○	NA ○	
3. The thenar eminence is not restricted or flattened.	Yes ○	No ○	NA ○	
4. The thumb post provides adequate support and is not constrictive.	Yes ○	No ○	NA ○	
5. The orthosis is two-thirds the length of the forearm.	Yes ○	No ○	NA ○	
6. The orthosis is one-half the width of the forearm.	Yes ○	No ○	NA ○	

Function

1. The orthosis allows full thumb interphalangeal (IP) flexion.	Yes ○	No ○	NA ○	
2. The orthosis allows full metacarpophalangeal (MCP) joint flexion of the fingers.	Yes ○	No ○	NA ○	
3. The orthosis provides wrist support that allows functional activities.	Yes ○	No ○	NA ○	

Straps

1. The straps avoid bony prominences.	Yes ○	No ○	NA ○	
2. The straps are secure and rounded.	Yes ○	No ○	NA ○	

Comfort

1. The edges are smooth with rounded corners.	Yes ○	No ○	NA ○	
2. The proximal end is flared.	Yes ○	No ○	NA ○	
3. The orthosis does not cause impingements or pressure sores.	Yes ○	No ○	NA ○	

Cosmetic Appearance

1. The orthosis is free of fingerprints, dirt, and pencil and pen marks.	Yes ○	No ○	NA ○	
2. The orthosis is smooth and free of buckles.	Yes ○	No ○	NA ○	

Therapeutic Regimen

1. The person has been instructed in a wearing schedule.	Yes ○	No ○	NA ○	
2. The person has been provided orthotic precautions.	Yes ○	No ○	NA ○	
3. The person demonstrates understanding of the education.	Yes ○	No ○	NA ○	
4. Client or caregiver knows how to clean the orthosis.	Yes ○	No ○	NA ○	

FORM 8-1 Thumb immobilization orthosis—cont'd

Discuss possible orthotic adjustments or changes you should make based on the self-evaluation. (What would you do differently next time?)

_____

_____

_____

_____

_____

_____

_____

_____

_____

Discuss possible areas to improve with clinical safety when fabricating the orthosis.

_____

_____

_____

_____

_____

*See Appendix B for a perforated copy of this form.

Grading Sheet 8-1*

Thumb Immobilization Orthosis

Name: _____

Date: _____

Type of thumb immobilization orthosis:

Volar ○   Dorsal ○   Radial gutter ○   Hand based ○

Thumb joint position: _____

Grade: _____

1 = Beyond improvement, not acceptable

2 = Requires maximal improvement

3 = Requires moderate improvement

4 = Requires minimal improvement

5 = Requires no improvement

Evaluation Areas

Design

1. The wrist position is at the correct angle.	1	2	3	4	5
2. The thumb position is at the correct angle.	1	2	3	4	5
3. The thenar eminence is not restricted or flattened.	1	2	3	4	5
4. The thumb post provides adequate support and is not constrictive.	1	2	3	4	5
5. The orthosis is two-thirds the length of the forearm.	1	2	3	4	5
6. The orthosis is one-half the width of the forearm.	1	2	3	4	5

Function

1. The orthosis allows full thumb motion.	1	2	3	4	5
2. The orthosis allows full metacarpophalangeal (MCP) joint flexion of the fingers.	1	2	3	4	5
3. The orthosis provides wrist support that allows functional activities.	1	2	3	4	5

Straps

1. The straps avoid bony prominences.	1	2	3	4	5
2. The straps are secure and rounded.	1	2	3	4	5

Comfort

1. The edges are smooth with rounded corners.	1	2	3	4	5
2. The proximal end is flared.	1	2	3	4	5
3. The orthosis does not cause impingements or pressure sores.	1	2	3	4	5

Cosmetic Appearance

1. The orthosis is free of fingerprints, dirt, and pencil and pen marks.	1	2	3	4	5
2. The thermoplastic material is not buckled.	1	2	3	4	5

Comments:

_____

_____

_____

_____

_____

*See Appendix C for a perforated copy of this sheet.

APPENDIX 8-1   CASE STUDIES

CASE STUDY 8-1*

Read the following scenario, and use your clinical reasoning skills to answer the questions based on information in this chapter.

Jack, a 10-year-old male, was skiing with his family on vacation. During one run on the bunny hill, he fell in a snow drift beside a tree with an outstretched right dominant hand and his thumb positioned in abduction. His thumb became painful and edematous. The physician diagnosed a partial tear of the ulnar collateral ligament (UCL; grade II) and casted the forearm, wrist, and thumb. After the cast is removed, a referral to therapy indicates the need for a thumb orthosis.

1. What type of orthosis should be selected? How should the thumb be positioned?

2. What is the purpose of the orthosis?

3. List three patient precautions to be aware of when creating this thumb immobilization orthosis.

4. What considerations should be made due to the patient's age?

5. What is the suggested wearing schedule?

6. Before the 4th- to 5th-week healing period is over, Jack's physician releases him to resume skiing. Jack is looking forward to skiing again. Jack's physician ordered the fabrication of an orthosis to wear while skiing. What type of orthosis might the therapist fabricate?

*See Appendix A for the answer key.

CASE STUDY 8-2*

Read the following scenario, and use your clinical reasoning skills to answer the questions based on information in this chapter.

Margaret, a 58-year-old woman employed as a librarian, went to her physician complaining of thumb pain at the carpometacarpal (CMC) joint. She experiences pain while completing her activities of daily living (ADLs). This pain had occurred for less than 1 year. She was particularly concerned that the pain was being exacerbated by her job demands of manipulating, lifting, and carrying books. At home she was having difficulty with many of her ADLs and was concerned about not being able to knit or cross-stitch. Clinical examination revealed no additional pain or symptoms in the wrist, fingers, or other joints of the thumb. Margaret was diagnosed with osteoarthritis of the CMC joint. Her physician ordered therapy and fabrication of a thumb orthosis. The order was not specific and did not state which joints should be stabilized in the orthosis. No orthotic design was mentioned.

1. What type of orthosis might the therapist fabricate? Which thumb joints should be stabilized?

   _____
   _____
   _____

2. What is the purpose of the orthosis?

   _____
   _____

3. What is the suggested wearing schedule?

   _____
   _____
   _____

4. What factors must be considered when determining whether to provide a custom-made or a prefabricated orthosis?

   _____
   _____
   _____

5. Margaret discontinued therapy, and 3 years later her symptoms worsened due to continuing her hobby of needlework and her work and home demands. She presented with pain in her wrist and the thumb metacarpophalangeal (MCP) joint due to progression of the osteoarthritis. Describe an orthosis that the therapist might consider fabricating.

   _____
   _____
   _____

6. What position should the therapist place the thumb in the thumb post?

   _____
   _____

*See Appendix A for the answer key.

CHAPTER 9

Hand Immobilization Orthoses

Brenda M. Coppard

Key Terms

antideformity position
complex regional pain syndrome (CRPS)
Dupuytren contracture
functional position

Chapter Objectives

1. List diagnoses that benefit from resting hand orthoses (hand immobilization orthoses).
2. Describe the functional or mid-joint position of the wrist, thumb, and digits.
3. Describe the antideformity or intrinsic-plus position of the wrist, thumb, and digits.
4. List the purposes of a resting hand orthosis (hand immobilization orthosis).
5. Identify the components of a resting hand orthosis (hand immobilization orthosis).
6. Explain the precautions to consider when fabricating a resting hand orthosis (hand immobilization orthosis).
7. Determine a resting hand (hand immobilization) orthotic-wearing schedule for different diagnostic indications.
8. Describe orthotic cleaning techniques that address infection control.
9. Apply knowledge about the application of the resting hand orthosis (hand immobilization orthosis) to a case study.
10. Use clinical judgment to evaluate a fabricated resting hand orthosis (hand immobilization orthosis).

Rosa is a 53-year-old female who has rheumatoid arthritis. Recently she experienced an exacerbation of her condition. She found it difficult to manage her job, household, and activities of daily living due to pain and stiffness. Upon a referral to the therapy clinic, Rosa was asked if she had worn any orthoses in the past to rest her hands during periods of exacerbation.

Physicians commonly order resting hand orthoses, also known as *hand immobilization orthoses*[1] or *resting hand orthoses*. A resting hand orthosis is a static orthosis that immobilizes the fingers and wrist. The thumb may or may not be immobilized by the orthosis. Therapists fabricate custom resting hand orthoses or purchase them commercially. Some of the commercially available resting hand orthoses are prefabricated, premolded, and ready to wear. Table 9-1 outlines prefabricated orthoses for the wrist and hand. Others are available as precut resting hand orthotic kits that include the precut thermoplastic material and strapping mechanism. Each of these orthoses has advantages and disadvantages.

Premolded Hand Orthoses

Therapists order premolded commercial orthoses according to hand size (i.e., small, medium, large, and extra large) for the right or left hand. An advantage of premade orthoses is their quick application (usually only straps require adjusting). There is an advantage to ordering a premolded resting hand orthosis made from perforated material. The premolded orthosis has perforations only in the body of the orthosis. The edges are smooth because there are no perforations near the edges of the orthosis. However, if the perforated premolded or precut orthosis must be trimmed through the perforations, a rough edge may result. Perforations at the edges of orthoses are undesirable because of the discomfort they often create.

A disadvantage of the commercial orthosis is a less-than-ideal fit for each person. With premolded orthoses, the therapist has little control over positioning joints into particular therapeutic angles, which may be different from the angles already incorporated into the orthotic design. The orthoses must be ordered for application on the right or left extremity, whereas the precut orthosis is universal for the right or left hand.

Table 9-1   Examples of Wrist/Hand Orthoses

THERAPEUTIC OBJECTIVE	DESCRIPTION	
Resting hand orthoses immobilize the wrist, thumb, and metacarpophalangeal (MCP) joints to provide rest and reduce inflammation. The proximal interphalangeal (PIP) and distal interphalangeal (DIP) joints are free to move for functional tasks.	Similar to the resting hand orthotic design, orthoses can provide rest to the wrist, thumb, and MCP joints (Figure 9-1). Padding and strapping systems can help control deviation of the wrist and MCPs. Orthoses are available in different sizes for the right and left hands.	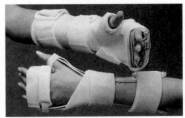 **Figure 9-1** This orthosis is based on a resting hand design and is often used for individuals with rheumatoid arthritis (RA). (Rolyan Arthritis Mitt splint; courtesy of Rehabilitation Division of Smith & Nephew, Germantown, WI.)
Designed to optimally position the hand in an intrinsic-plus position after a burn injury.	Burn resting hand orthoses typically position the wrist in 20 to 30 degrees of extension, the MCP joints in 60 to 80 degrees of flexion, the PIP and DIP joints in full extension, and the thumb midway between radial and palmar abduction (Figure 9-2).	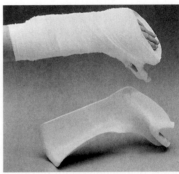 **Figure 9-2** This resting hand orthosis positions the hand in an antideformity position for individuals with hand burns. (Rolyan Burn splint; courtesy of Rehabilitation Division of Smith & Nephew, Germantown, WI.)
Several orthoses are designed to manage spasticity.	Ball orthoses implement a reflex-inhibiting posture by positioning the wrist in neutral (or slight extension) and the fingers in extension and abduction. Cone orthoses combine a hand cone and a forearm trough, which maintains the wrist in neutral, inhibits the long finger flexors, and maintains the web space (Figure 9-3). A resting hand orthosis positioning the hand in a functional position is advocated for spasticity (Figure 9-4).	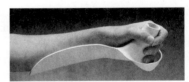 **Figure 9-3** This cone orthosis is often used to help manage tone abnormalities. (Preformed Anti-Spasticity Hand Splint; courtesy of North Coast Medical, Inc., Morgan Hill, CA.) 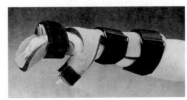 **Figure 9-4** This resting hand orthosis is fabricated of soft materials and includes a dorsal forearm base design. (Progress Dorsal Anti-Spasticity splint; courtesy of North Coast Medical, Inc., Morgan Hill, CA.)

Precut Orthotic Kits

A resting hand orthotic kit typically contains strapping materials and precut thermoplastic material in the shape of a resting hand orthosis. Kits are available according to hand size (i.e., small, medium, large, and extra large). An advantage of using a kit is the time the therapist saves by the elimination of pattern making and cutting of thermoplastic material. Similar to premolded orthoses, precuts from perforated materials contain perforations in only the body of the orthosis. Precuts are interchangeable for right or left extremity application. The therapist has control over joint positioning. A disadvantage is that the pattern is not customized to the person. Therefore, the precut orthosis may require many adjustments to obtain a proper fit.

Customized Orthoses

A therapist can customize a resting hand orthosis by making a pattern and fabricating the orthosis from thermoplastic material. The advantage is an exact fit for the person, which increases the orthosis' support and comfort. The therapist also has control over joint positioning. A disadvantage is that customization may require more of the therapist's time to complete the orthosis and may be more costly. In addition, when a resting hand orthosis pattern is cut out of perforated thermoplastic material, it is difficult to obtain smooth edges because of the likelihood of needing to cut through the perforations (which causes a rough edge). Commercially-available products, such as the Rolyan Aquaplast UltraThin Edging Material, can be applied over the rough edges to create a smooth-edged reinforcement on orthoses fabricated from Aquaplast materials.[38]

Therapists must make informed decisions about whether they will fabricate or purchase an orthosis. Many products are advertised to save time and to be effective, but few studies compare orthotic materials when used by therapists with the same level of experience.[20] Lau[20] compared the fabrication of a resting hand orthosis with use of a precut orthosis; he compared the QuickCast (fiberglass material) with Ezeform

thermoplastic material. The study employed second-year occupational therapy students as orthotic-makers and first-year occupational therapy students as their clients.

The clients responded to a questionnaire addressing comfort, weight, and aesthetics. The orthotic makers also responded to a questionnaire asking about measuring fit, edges, strap application, aesthetics, safety, and ease of positioning. The analysis of timed trials revealed no significant difference in time required for fabricating the precut Quick-Cast and the Ezeform thermoplastic material. The thermoplastic material was rated safer than the fiberglass material. Because of the small sample, these results should be cautiously interpreted, and further studies are warranted.

Purpose of the Resting Hand Orthosis

The resting hand has three purposes: to immobilize, to position in functional alignment, and to retard further deformity.[22,47] When inflammation and pain are present in the hand, the joints and surrounding structures become swollen and result in improper hand alignment. Rest through immobilization reduces symptoms. The therapist may provide an orthosis for a person with arthritis who has early signs of ulnar drift by placing the hand in a comfortable neutral position with the joints in mid-position. The resting hand orthosis may retard further deformity for some persons. Joints that are receptive to proper positioning may allow for optimal maintenance of range of motion (ROM).[47]

Components of the Resting Hand Orthosis

The therapist must know the orthosis' components to make adjustments for a correct fit. Four main components comprise the resting hand orthosis: the forearm trough, the pan, the thumb trough, and the C bar (Figure 9-5).[13]

Forearm troughs can be volar or dorsal based. The volar based forearm trough at the proximal portion of the orthosis supports the weight of the forearm. Dorsally based forearm

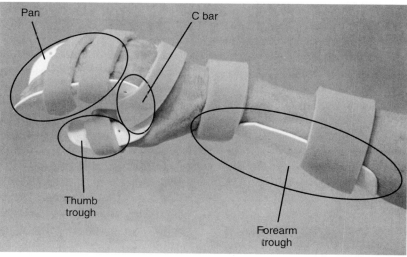

Figure 9-5 The components of a resting hand orthosis are the forearm trough, pan, thumb trough, and C bar.

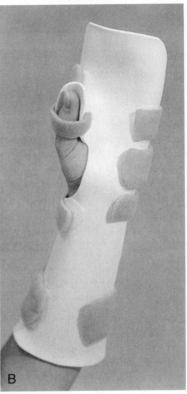

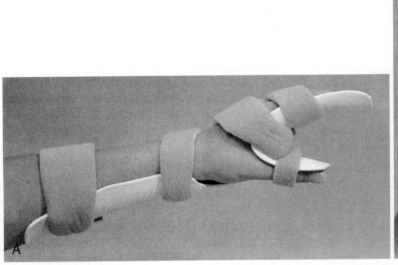

Figure 9-6 Volar-based resting hand orthosis. **A,** Side view. **B,** Volar view.

troughs are located on the dorsum of the forearm. The therapist applies biomechanical principles to make the trough about two-thirds the length of the forearm to distribute pressure of the hand and to allow elbow flexion when appropriate. The width is one-half the circumference of the forearm. The proximal end of the trough is flared or rolled to avoid a pressure area.

When a great amount of forearm support is desired, a volar based forearm trough is the best design (Figure 9-6). When the volar surface of the forearm must be avoided because of sutures, sores, rashes, or intravenous needles, a dorsally based forearm trough design is frequently used (Figure 9-7). Dorsally based troughs are a beneficial design for applying a resting hand orthosis to a person with hypertonicity. The forearm trough is used as a lever to extend the wrist in addition to extending the fingers.

The pan of the orthosis supports the fingers and the palm. The therapist conforms the pan to the arches of the hand, thus helping to maintain such hand functions as grasping and cupping motions. The pan should be wide enough to house the width of the index, middle, ring, and little fingers when they are in a slightly abducted position. The sides of the pan should be curved so that they measure approximately ½ inch in height. The curved sides add strength to the pan and ensure that the fingers do not slide radially or ulnarly off the sides of the pan. However, if the pan's edges are too high, the positioning strap bridges over the fingers and fails to anchor them properly.

The thumb trough supports the thumb and should extend approximately ½ inch beyond the end of the thumb. This extension allows the entire thumb to rest in the trough. The width and depth of the thumb trough should be one-half the circumference of the thumb, which typically should be in a palmarly abducted position. The therapist should attempt to position the carpometacarpal (CMC) joint in 40 to 45 degrees of palmar abduction[42] and extend the thumb's interphalangeal (IP) and metacarpal joints.

The C bar keeps the web space of the thumb positioned in palmar abduction. If the web space tightens, it inhibits cylindrical grasp and prevents the thumb from fully opposing the other digits. From the radial side of the orthosis, the thumb, the web space, and the digits should resemble a C (see Figure 9-6).

Resting Hand Orthosis Positions

Generally, two types of positioning are accomplished by a resting hand orthosis: a functional (mid-joint) position and an antideformity (intrinsic-plus) position. Diagnostic indication determines the general position used.

Functional Position

To relieve stress on the wrist and hand joints, the resting hand orthosis positions the hand in a functional or mid-joint position (Figure 9-8). According to Lau[20] "The exact specifications of the functional position of the hand in a resting hand orthosis and the recommended joint positions vary." One **functional position** that we suggest places the wrist in

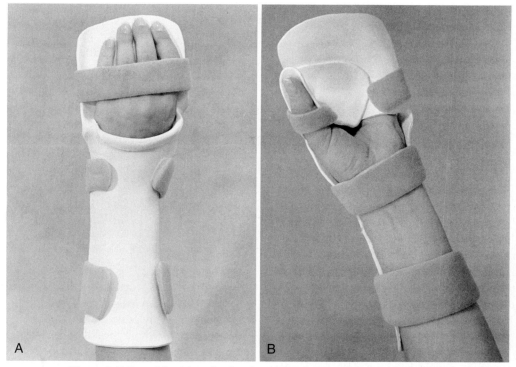

Figure 9-7 Dorsal-based resting hand orthosis. **A,** Dorsal view. **B,** Volar view.

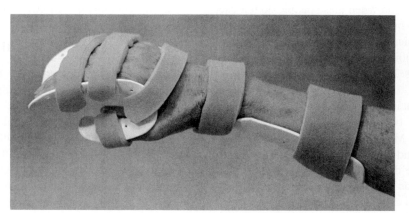

Figure 9-8 A resting hand orthosis with the hand in a functional (mid-joint) position.

20 to 30 degrees of extension, the thumb in 45 degrees of palmar abduction, the metacarpophalangeal (MCP) joints in 35 to 45 degrees of flexion, and all proximal interphalangeal (PIP) and distal interphalangeal (DIP) joints in slight flexion.

Antideformity Position

The antideformity (also known as protected or safe) position is often used to place the hand in such a fashion as to maintain a tension/distraction of anatomic structures to avoid contracture and promote function. The **antideformity position** places the wrist in 15 to 20 degrees of extension, the thumb midway between radial and palmar abduction, the thumb IP joint in full extension, the MCPs at 60 to 70 degrees of flexion, and the PIPs and DIPs in full extension (Figure 9-9).[44]

Diagnostic Indications

Several diagnostic categories may warrant the provision of a resting hand orthosis. Persons who require resting hand orthoses commonly have arthritis;[2,9,31] postoperative Dupuytren contracture release;[10,34] burn injuries to the hand, tendinitis, hemiplegic hand;[33] hypertonic hand and wrist;[28] and tenosynovitis.[36] Table 9-2 lists evidence associated with hand orthoses related to a variety of diagnostic conditions.

The resting hand orthosis maintains the hand in a functional or antideformity position, preserves a balance between extrinsic and intrinsic muscles, and provides localized rest to the tissues of the fingers, thumb, and wrist.[42] Although hand immobilization orthoses are commonly used, a paucity of literature exists on their efficacy. Thus, it is a ripe area for future research. Therapists should consider the resting hand

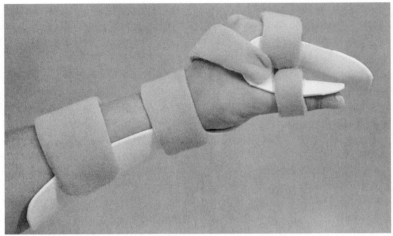

Figure 9-9 A resting hand orthosis with the hand in an antideformity (intrinsic-plus) position.

orthosis as a legitimate intervention for appropriate conditions despite the lack of evidence.

Rheumatoid Arthritis

Therapists often provide resting hand orthoses for people with rheumatoid arthritis (RA) during periods of acute inflammation and pain[3,47] and when these people do not use their hands for activities but require support and immobilization.[21] The biomechanical rationale for orthotic intervention of acutely inflamed joints is to reduce pain by relieving stress and muscle spasms. However, it may not additionally prevent deformity.[3,11]

Typical joint placement in an orthosis for a person with RA is to position the wrist in 10 degrees of extension, the thumb in palmar abduction, the MCP joints in 35 to 45 degrees of flexion, and all the PIP and DIP joints in slight flexion.[30] For a person who has severe deformities or exacerbations from arthritis, the resting hand orthosis may also position the wrist at neutral or slight extension and 5 to 10 degrees of ulnar deviation.[14,23] The thumb may be positioned midway between radial and palmar abduction to increase comfort. These joint angles are ideal. Therapists use clinical judgment to determine what joint angles are positions of comfort for orthotic intervention.

Note that wrist extension varies from the typical 30 degrees of extension. When the wrist is in slight extension, the carpal tunnel is open—as opposed to being narrowed, with 30 degrees of extension.[30] Finger spacers may be used in the pan to provide comfort and to prevent finger slippage in the orthosis.[30] Melvin[30] cautions that finger spacers should not be used to passively correct ulnar deformity because of the risk for pressure areas. In addition, once the orthosis is removed there is no evidence that orthotic wear alters the deformity. However, it may prevent further deformity.

Acute Rheumatoid Arthritis

In persons who have RA, the use of orthoses for purposes of rest during pain and inflammation is controversial.[9] Periods of rest (3 weeks or less) seem to be beneficial, but longer periods may cause loss of motion.[31] Phillips[32] recommends that persons with acute exacerbations wear orthoses full-time except for short periods of gentle ROM exercise and hygiene. Biese[3] recommends that persons wear orthoses at night and part-time during the day. In addition, persons may find it beneficial to wear orthoses at night for several weeks after the acute inflammation subsides.[4]

Chronic Rheumatoid Arthritis

When providing an orthosis for a joint with chronic RA, the rationale is often based on biomechanical factors. According to Falconer,[11] "Theoretically, by realigning and redistributing the damaging internal and external forces acting on the joint, the orthosis may help to prevent deformity…or improve joint function and functional use of the extremity." Therapists who provide orthoses to persons with chronic RA should be aware that prolonged use of a resting hand orthosis may also be harmful.[11] Studies on animals indicate that immobilization leads to decreased bone mass and strength, degeneration of cartilage, increase in joint capsule adhesions, weakness in tendon and ligament strength, and muscle atrophy.[11]

In addition to orthotic intervention, persons with RA benefit from a combination of management of inflammation, education in joint protection, muscle strengthening, ROM maintenance, and pain reduction.[11,32] Persons in late stages of RA who have skeletal collapse and deformity may benefit from the support of an orthosis during activities and at nighttime.[3,5]

Compliance of persons with RA in wearing resting hand orthoses has been estimated at approximately 50%.[12] The degree to which a person's compliance with an orthotic-wearing schedule affects the disease outcome is unknown. However, research indicates that some persons with RA who wore their orthoses only at times of symptom exacerbation did not demonstrate negative outcomes in relation to ROM or deformities.[12]

Wearing schedules for resting hand orthoses vary depending on the diagnostic condition, orthotic purpose, and

Table 9-2 Evidence-Based Practice Related to Wrist Hand Orthoses

AUTHOR'S CITATION	DESIGN	NUMBER OF PARTICIPANTS	DESCRIPTION	RESULTS	LIMITATIONS
Arthritis					
Adams J, Burridge J, Mullee M, et al: The clinical effectiveness of static resting splints in early rheumatoid arthritis: a randomized controlled trial, *Rheumatology* 47, 1548-1553, 2008.	Prospective, randomized controlled trial	80	The purpose of this study was to determine the effectiveness of using static resting orthoses for patients with early stages of RA. All participants received occupational therapy treatment for their RA symptoms, including education on joint protection and hand and wrist exercises. The orthosis group was also provided with resting hand orthoses that positioned the hand in an intrinsic plus position to wear during periods of no activity.	No significant differences were noted in grip strength, MCP ulnar deviation, or pain level. One key area of difference was the patients' reported experience of morning stiffness. The orthosis group had a significantly lower number of patients reporting morning stiffness.	Limitations of this study include the fact that early stages of RA can cause difficulty with establishing effectiveness of an intervention, due to the likelihood that a condition was poorly controlled. Medication was considered in the results, but a second limitation is that it may have had a significant role in condition management between groups. The duration of the study may not have been long enough. Finally, there may be a better design for the orthoses used in the intervention.
Feinberg J, Brandt KD: Use of resting splints by patients with rheumatoid arthritis, *Am J Occup Ther* 35(3):173-178, 1981.	Retrospective study	50	50 patients with RA who had previously used an orthosis were identified for follow-up visits. The patients were identified as "compliant," meaning that they wore the orthosis 50% of the time or more, or "noncompliant," indicating they wore the orthosis less than 50% of the time. Factors that were addressed in this study included the effect of the orthosis on adherence to an orthosis-wearing schedule, as well as amounts of pain, morning stiffness, and ROM.	31 out of 50 participants were deemed compliant, wearing their orthosis 50% or more of the time recommended by the therapist. Greatest compliance was found to be in patients between the ages of 40 and 70, as well as individuals who had been diagnosed with RA for 2 years or less. Overall most patients felt some benefit from wearing the orthoses, particularly during the initial phase of orthosis use. Long-term use of orthoses for pain management varied, depending on the patient's symptoms of RA.	Limitations for this study include the fact that orthoses were not of uniform design; they had been modified for the comfort of each patient. Additionally, there was a wide range of time from initial fitting of orthoses to the follow-up appointment (between 3 months and 34 months). A final limitation that may have affected results of this study was that there was a wide range of time since the patient had been diagnosed with RA.

Table 9-2 Evidence-Based Practice Related to Wrist Hand Orthoses—cont'd

AUTHOR'S CITATION	DESIGN	NUMBER OF PARTICIPANTS	DESCRIPTION	RESULTS	LIMITATIONS
Dupuytren Contracture					
Jerosch-Herold C, Shepstone L, Choinowski AJ, et al: Night-time splinting after fasciectomy or dermofasciectomy for Dupuytren's contracture: a pragmatic, multi-centre, randomized controlled trial, *BMC Musculoskelet Disord* 12:136-144, 2011.	Prospective study	154	The purpose of this study was to evaluate the effectiveness of a night orthosis on function, finger extension, and patient satisfaction. Patients from five regional hospitals were randomized to receive hand therapy only or hand therapy plus using an orthosis at night.	This study found that there was no statistically significant difference in the recovery of patients who received the orthosis to use at nighttime and the patients who received hand therapy only.	Limitations of this study include the fact that the primary measure of outcome was based on patient report, and neither the patients nor the researchers assessing secondary outcomes were blinded.
Tone Reduction					
McPherson JJ, Kreimeyer D, Aalderks M, et al: A comparison of dorsal and volar resting hand splints in the reduction of hypertonus, *Am J Occup Ther* 36(10): 664-670, 1982.	Prospective study	10	The purpose of this study was to compare the effectiveness of dorsal and volar based resting hand orthoses on reducing abnormal muscle tone. All participants had hypertonus wrist flexors, as sequelae of either a cerebrovascular accident, traumatic brain injury, or cerebral palsy.	This study found that both the dorsal and volar based resting hand orthoses were effective in reducing the amount of hypertonus. The group who wore the dorsal orthoses experienced a reduction of hypertonus equal to 7.25 lbs of pull, and the volar based orthoses resulted in a reduction of hypertonus equal to 7.0 lbs of pull. This difference in reduction of hypertonus is not statistically significant.	Limitations of this study include the small sample size, and the use of a measurement technique that does not "measure the hyper-reflexive status of the neuromuscular spindle" (p. 668).

Constraint Induced Movement Therapy

Uswatte G, Taub E, Morris D, et al: Contribution of the shaping and restraint components of Constraint-Induced Movement therapy to treatment outcome, *NeuroRehabilitation* 21(2):147-156, 2006.

17

Prospective study

The purpose of this study was to examine how various types of training (task-practice) and restraint (sling, half-glove, no restraint) affected outcomes of occupational therapy treatment. Participants were divided into four groups (sling & task practice, sling & shaping, half-glove & shaping, shaping only). Participants in the sling group had their less-affected arm placed in a resting hand orthosis/sling during the waking hours.

Results indicate that participants from all groups improved use of the more-impaired arm and experienced a reduction in time to complete bilateral tasks as a result of task training and restraint intervention. Immediately post treatment, no significant difference in assessment results was detected between the four groups. Two years following treatment, the sling & task participants demonstrated larger gains in assessment results as compared to the remaining groups.

After post-treatment assessment, different training intensity was given to the half-glove & shaping group than was given to the sling & shaping group. This may have altered the results of the 2-year follow-up assessment. A second limitation is that task-practice contains some important aspects of shaping. A third limitation is that the level of compliance with wearing the restraints was measured by self-report of the participants. Finally, the sample sizes of the groups in this study were small.

MCP, Metacarpophalangeal; *RA,* rheumatoid arthritis; *ROM,* range of motion.

physician order (Table 9-3). Persons with RA often wear resting hand orthoses at night. A person who has RA may also wear a resting hand orthosis during the day for additional rest but should remove the orthosis at least once each day for hygiene and appropriate exercises. A person who has bilateral hand orthoses may choose to wear alternate orthoses each night.

Hand Burns

For persons who have hand burns, therapists do not position the person in the functional position. Instead, the therapist places the hand in the intrinsic-plus or antideformity position (see Figure 9-9). Richard and colleagues[36] conducted an in-depth literature review to find a standard dorsal hand burn

Table 9-3 Conditions That Require a Resting Hand Orthosis

DIAGNOSIS	SUGGESTED WEARING SCHEDULE	POSITION
Rheumatoid Arthritis		
Acute exacerbation*	Fitted to maintain as close to a functional (mid-joint) position as possible until exacerbation is over. Removed for hygiene and exercise purposes, and worn during the day and at nighttime as necessary. Finger deformities must be taken into consideration if present.	• Wrist: Neutral or 20 to 30 degrees of extension depending on person's tolerance, 15 to 20 degrees of meta-carpophalangeal (MCP) flexion, and 5 to 10 degrees of ulnar deviation • Thumb: Position of comfort in between radial and palmar abduction
Hand Burns		
Dorsal or volar hand burns*	Generally, worn immediately after the burn injury. Continuously worn until healing begins, and removed for dressing changes, hygiene, and exercises.	• Wrist: Volar or circumferential burn (30 to 40 degrees of extension), dorsal burn (0 degrees = neutral) • MCPs: Flexion of 70 to 90 degrees • Proximal interphalangeal (PIP) and distal interphalangeal (DIP): Full extension • Thumb: Palmar abduction and extension
Acute phase	Initially, worn at all times except for therapy. Monitor fit for fluctuations in bandage bulk and edema. As range of motion (ROM) improves, decrease wearing time to allow for participation in activities.	Position as close to the previously indicated position as possible.
Skin graft phase	Worn after skin graft at all times for 5 days or with physician's order for removal.	Position as close to antideformity position as possible.
Rehabilitation phase	Orthosis worn during nighttime to maintain ROM. Wear should be limited during daytime to allow for participation in activities.	Position joints to oppose deforming forces.
Dupuytren disease contractures*	Worn after surgery and removed for hygiene and exercise. Worn at nighttime.	• Wrist: Neutral or slight extension • MCP, PIP, and DIPs: Full extension
Trauma		
Crush injuries of the hand	Fitted after the injury to reduce pain and edema and to prevent shortening of critical tissue and contracture formation. Worn at nighttime, and possibly worn as necessary during painful periods.	• Wrist: Extension of 0 to 30 degrees • MCPs: Extension of 60 to 80 degrees • PIP and DIPs: Full extension • Thumb: Palmar abduction and extension
Complex regional pain syndrome (CRPS)	Orthosis is worn at all times, initially with removal for therapy, hygiene, and activities of daily living (ADLs; if possible). Person should be weaned from orthosis with pain reduction and improved motion.	Adjust to a position of comfort with the ideal position being: • Wrist: 20 degrees of extension, thumb in palmar abduction • MCPs: 70 degrees of flexion • PIPs: 0 to 10 degrees of extension

*Diagnosis may require additional types of orthotic intervention.

orthotic design. The literature cited 43 orthoses to position the dorsally burned hand joints. Twenty-six of these orthoses were labelled as antideformity orthoses, and 17 were identified as having a position of function. Thus, a wide range of orthotic designs exists for dorsal hand burns.[36]

Positioning may vary, depending on the surface of the hand that is burned. In general, the goal of providing an orthosis in the antideformity position is to prevent deformity by keeping structures whose length allows motion from shortening. These structures are the collateral ligaments of the MCPs, the volar plates of the IPs, and the wrist capsule and ligaments. The dorsal skin of the hand maintains its length in the antideformity position. The thumb web space is also vulnerable to remodeling in a shortened form in the presence of inflammation and in a situation in which tension of the structure is absent.

The antideformity position for a palmar or circumferential burn places the wrist in 30 to 40 degrees of extension and 0 degrees (i.e., neutral) for a dorsal hand burn. For dorsal and volar burns, the therapist should flex the MCPs into 70 to 90 degrees, fully extend the PIP joints and DIP joints, and palmarly abduct the thumb to the index and middle fingers with the thumb IP joint extended.[37] After a burn injury, the thumb web space is at risk for developing an adduction contracture.[43] Therefore, palmar abduction of the thumb is the position of choice for the thumb CMC joint.

These joint angles are ideal. Some persons with burns may not initially tolerate these joint positions. When tolerable, the resting hand orthosis for the person who has hand burns can be adjusted more closely to the ideal position. As healing occurs, the orthosis is modified to maintain the palmar arches of the hand.[39] Stages of burn recovery should be considered with orthotic intervention. The phases of recovery are emergent, acute, skin grafting, and rehabilitation.

Emergent Phase

The emergent phase is the first 24 to 72 postburn hours.[44] From 8 to 12 hours after the burn, dorsal edema occurs and encourages wrist flexion, MCP joint hyperextension, and IP joint flexion.[8,44] Edema peaks up to 36 hours after the burn injury and begins to dissipate after 1 or 2 days. Usually the edema is resolved by 7 to 10 days after injury; however, destruction of the dorsal veins or lymphatic vessels may result in chronic edema.[44] Static orthosis intervention is initiated during the emergent phase to support the hand and maintain the length of vulnerable structures.[8] Positioning to counteract the forces of edema includes placing the wrist in 15 to 20 degrees of extension, the MCP joints in 90 degrees of flexion, and the PIP and DIP joints in full extension with the thumb positioned midway between palmar and radial abduction and with the IP joint slightly flexed.[44]

For children with dorsal hand burns, during the emergent phase, the MCP joints may not need to be flexed as far as 60 to 70 degrees. deLinde and Knothe[7] suggested that for children under the age of 3 therapists may not need to use an orthosis, unless it is determined that the wrist requires support. If a child is age 3 or older, orthotic intervention should be considered. Young children who have burned hands may not need orthoses because the bulky dressings applied to the burned hand may provide adequate support.

A prefabricated resting hand orthosis in an antideformity position can be applied if a therapist cannot immediately construct a custom-made orthosis.[8] deLinde and Miles[8] suggested that prefabricated orthoses may be appropriate for superficial burns with edema for the first 3 to 5 days. For full-thickness burns with excessive edema, custom-made orthoses are necessary.[8] An orthosis applied in the first 72 hours after a burn may not fit the person 2 hours after application because of the significant edema that usually follows a burn injury.

The therapist closely monitors the person to make necessary adjustments to the orthosis. When fabricating a custom orthosis for a person with excessive edema, a therapist avoids forcing wrist and hand joints into the ideal position and risking ischemia from damaged capillaries.[8] With edema reduction, serial orthotic intervention may be necessary as ROM is gained toward the ideal position. Serial resting hand orthoses for persons with burns should conform to the person, rather than conforming persons to the orthoses.[8]

Persons with hand burns have bandages covering burn sites. According to Richard and colleagues,[35] "As layers of bandage around the hand increase, accommodation for the increased bandage thickness must be accounted for in the [orthotic] design, if it is to fit correctly." To correct for bandage thickness, the orthosis' bend corresponding to MCP flexion in the pan is formed more proximally.[35]

The initial orthotic provision for a person with hand burns is applied with gauze rather than straps. The gauze reduces the risk of compromising circulation. Orthoses on adults are removed for exercise, hygiene, and appropriate functional tasks. For children, orthoses are removed for exercise, hygiene, and play activities.[8]

Acute Phase

The acute phase begins after the emergent phase and lasts until wound closure.[8] Once edema begins to decrease, serial adjustments are made to the orthosis. Therefore, it is advantageous to use thermoplastic material with memory properties. During the acute phase, therapists monitor the direction of deforming forces and make adjustments in the existing orthosis or design an additional orthosis to "orient the collagen being deposited during the early stages of wound healing as well as maintain joint alignment."[7]

Healing wounds are also monitored, and orthoses are evaluated for fit and for correct donning and doffing. As ROM is improved, the person decreases wearing of the orthosis during the day. If the person is unwilling or uncooperative in participating in self-care and supervised activities, the orthosis is worn continuously to prevent contractures. It is important for persons to wear orthoses at nighttime.

Skin Graft Phase

Before a skin graft, it is crucial to obtain full ROM. After the skin graft, the site needs to be immobilized for 3 to 5 days postoperatively.[8,44] Usually an antideformity position resting hand orthosis is appropriate. The orthosis may have to be applied in the operating room or bedside to ensure immobilization of the graft.

Rehabilitation Phase

The rehabilitation phase occurs after wound closure or graft adherence until scar maturation.[8] Throughout the person's rehabilitation after a burn, orthoses may be donned over an extremity covered with a pressure garment. Orthoses may be used in conjunction with materials that manage scar formation, including silicone gel sheeting or elastomer/elastomer putty inserts. During the rehabilitation phase, static and dynamic orthotic intervention may be needed. Plaster or synthetic material casting may also be considered.[7]

Persons commonly wear resting hand orthoses during the healing stages of burns. After wounds heal, persons may wear day orthoses with pressure garments or elastomer molds to increase ROM and to control scarring. In addition to daytime orthoses, it is important for the person to wear a resting hand orthosis at night to maintain maximum elongation of the healing skin and provide rest and functional alignment.

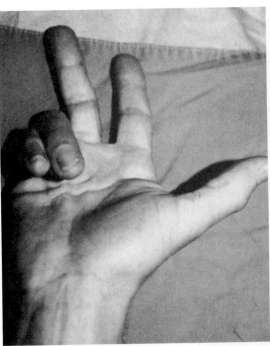

Figure 9-10 Dupuytren contracture of the palm and little finger. Note the nodules and cord. (From Hurst: Dupuytren's disease: surgical management. In Skirven TM, Osterman AL, Fedorczyk JM, et al., editors: *Rehabilitation of the hand and upper extremity,* ed 6, St Louis, 2011, Mosby, p. 267.)

Dupuytren Disease

Dupuytren disease is a benign fibromatosis characterized by the formation of finger flexion contracture(s) with a thickened band of palmar and digital fascia.[16,24] Palpable nodules first develop in the distal palmar crease, usually in line with the finger(s). Slowly the condition matures into a longitudinal cord that is readily distinguishable from a tendon (Figure 9-10).[16,24] In addition, pain and decreased ROM are the primary symptoms that often lead to impaired functional performance.[17] Dupuytren contractures are common and often severe in persons of Northern European origin. However, this disorder is present in most ethnic groups.[24] Epilepsy, diabetes mellitus, smoking, AIDS, vascular disorders, and alcoholism are associated with Dupuytren contracture.[16,17,24,41] Persons with Dupuytren diathesis (a more aggressive form of the disease) often have a family history of the disease, bilateral involvement, lesions (e.g., plantar fibromatosis), male gender with onset usually younger than 50 years.[15]

When a **Dupuytren contracture** is apparent, stretching or orthotic intervention that positions joints in extension does not delay the progression of the contracture.[16,24] Surgery is performed to release contractures. Although surgery does not cure the disease, it is often indicated in the presence of painful nodules; uncomfortable induration; and MCP, PIP, or DIP joint contractures.[16,25] Surgical procedures to treat Dupuytren disease include fasciotomy, regional fasciectomy, and dermofasciectomy.[16,25,34] Fasciectomies options

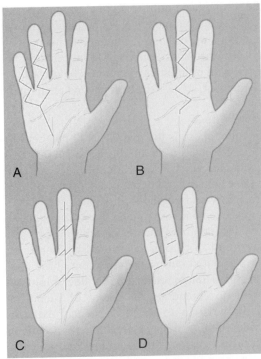

Figure 9-11 Four basic skin incision patterns for Dupuytren fasciectomy. **A,** Zigzag. **B,** Littler-Brunner. **C,** Longitudinal. **D,** Transverse (open palm technique). (From Hurst: Dupuytren's disease: surgical management. In Skirven TM, Osterman AL, Fedorczyk JM, et al., editors: *Rehabilitation of the hand and upper extremity,* ed 6, St Louis, 2011, Mosby, p. 273.)

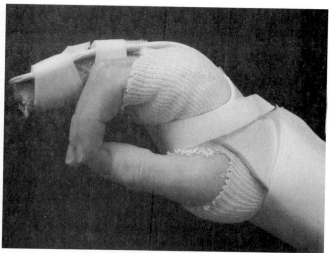

Figure 9-12 Dorsal static protective orthosis for immediate wear post fasciectomy. The design allows for flexion, but not metacarpophalangeal (MCP) joint extension, in a controlled range preventing neurovascular and wound tension. The person exercises within the orthosis, strapping the interphalangeal (IP) joints to the dorsal hood between exercise sessions. (From Evans: Therapeutic management of Dupuytren's contracture. In Skirven TM, Osterman AL, Fedorczyk JM, et al., editors: *Rehabilitation of the hand and upper extremity*, ed 6, St Louis, 2011, Mosby, p. 283.)

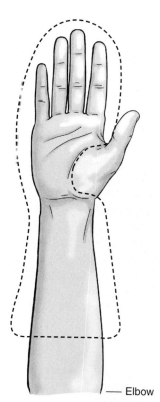

— Elbow

Figure 9-13 A pattern for a resting hand orthosis after surgical release of Dupuytren contracture. Note that the thumb is not incorporated into the orthotic design.

include: open, closed, needle, and enzymatic (experimental).[16] Four incision patterns are used for Dupuytren fasciectomies (Figure 9-11). The incision patterns include: A) zigzag plasty, B) Littler-Brunner, C) Z-plasty, or D) transverse incisions. Most Dupuytren surgeries are completed in an ambulatory or day surgery setting.[16]

With longitudinal follow up, recurrence after surgery is likely 100%.[27] Intermediate results of surgery may vary, depending on the affected joint.[24] For example, the MCP joint has a single fascial cord that is relatively easy to release. The PIP joint has four fascial cords that are difficult to release. In addition, the soft tissue around the PIP joint may contract and pull the joint into flexion, and components of the extensor mechanism may adhere to surrounding structures. The PIP joint of the little finger is the most difficult to correct. Flexion contractures at the DIP joint are uncommon but are difficult to correct for the same reasons as the PIP joint contracture. Contractures of the web spaces may be present, limiting the motion of adjacent fingers. Web space contractures may also result in poor hygiene between the fingers.

Therapy and orthotic intervention begins 24 hours after surgery.[10] Postoperative orthotic intervention may include the fabrication of a dorsal static protective orthosis (Figure 9-12).[10] The dorsal static protective orthosis positions the wrist at neutral, the MCP joints at 35 to 45 degrees of flexion, and the IP joints in relaxed extension.[10] Note that the digits receiving surgery release are the only digits included in the orthosis. The thumb is positioned in mild abduction if the first web space was a surgical site, resting hand orthosis,

or a dorsal forearm-based static extension orthosis. Some therapists and physicians prefer a resting hand orthosis post Dupuytren release, the wrist is placed in a neutral or slightly flexed position. The MCP, PIP, and DIP joints are positioned in full extension. If the thumb is involved, it is incorporated into the orthosis. However, the uninvolved thumb usually does not need to be immobilized in the orthosis. Therefore, the orthosis will not have a thumb trough component (Figure 9-13). The thumb may be incorporated into the orthosis, particularly when the adjacent index finger has been released from a contracture. Note that the dorsal static protective orthosis is a no-tension approach to orthotic intervention. The protective orthosis is worn for 3 weeks. Daytime wear is discontinued. Then, a volar hand based extension orthosis (Figure 9-14) with straps positioned over the MCP and PIP joints to maintain or improve extension is provided, and the person wears this orthosis during nighttime.[10]

Generally, after a surgical release of a Dupuytren contracture, the person wears the initial orthosis continuously during both day and night with removal for hygiene and exercise. The orthosis is worn until the wounds completely heal. Orthoses are worn longer in the presence of a PIP contracture release. As the risk of losing ROM dissipates, the person may be weaned from orthotic use.

Therapists working with persons who undergo a Dupuytren release must be aware of possible complications. Complications include excessive inflammation, wound infection,

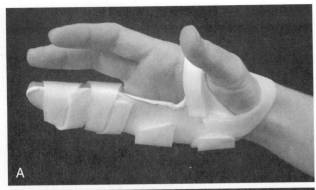

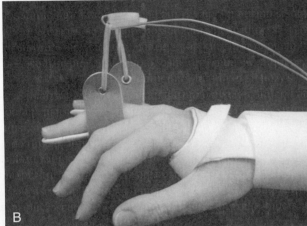

Figure 9-14 A volar hand based extension orthosis with straps over the metacarpophalangeal (MCP) and proximal interphalangeal (PIP) joints is used to maintain or improve extension. (From Evans: Therapeutic management of Dupuytren's contracture. In Skirven TM, Osterman AL, Fedorczyk JM, et al., editors: *Rehabilitation of the hand and upper extremity,* ed 6, St Louis, 2011, Mosby, p. 284.)

abnormal scar formation, joint contractures, stiffness, pain, and complex regional pain syndrome.[10,34] Occasionally in severe cases with complications, mobilization orthoses can be used when MCP and PIP joint extension are unsatisfactory and when the use of multiple digit static orthoses are difficult for the person to don independently.[10]

Complex Regional Pain Syndrome (Reflex Sympathetic Dystrophy)

Complex regional pain syndrome (CRPS) is a term that describes post-traumatic pain that manifests by "inappropriate automatic activity and impaired extremity function."[18] Typical symptoms include the following[18]:

- Pain: Out of proportional intensity to the injury, often described as throbbing, burning, cutting, searing, and shooting
- Skin color changes: Blotchy, purple, pale, or red
- Skin temperature changes: Warmer or cooler compared to contralateral side
- Skin texture changes: Thin, shiny, and sometimes excessively sweaty

- Swelling and stiffness
- Decreased ability to move the affected body part

There are two types of CRPS. CRPS I is usually triggered by tissue injury. The term applies to all persons with the symptoms listed previously, but with no underlying peripheral nerve injury. CRPS II is associated with the symptoms in the presence of a peripheral nerve injury.

The goal of rehabilitation for persons with CRPS is to eliminate one of the three etiologic factors: pain, diathesis, and abnormal sympathetic reflex.[19,46] This is accomplished by minimizing ROM and strength losses, managing edema, and providing pain management so that the therapist is able to maximize function and provide activities of daily living (ADLs) and instrumental activities of daily living (IADLs) training for independence. The physician may be able to intervene with medications and nerve blocks.

As part of a comprehensive therapy regimen for CRPS, a resting hand orthosis may initially provide rest to the hand, reduce pain, and relieve muscle spasm.[19,46] Orthotic intervention during the presence of CRPS should be of a low force that does not exacerbate the pain or irritate the tissues.[45] Walsh and Muntzer[45] recommend that the resting hand orthosis position for the person be in 20 degrees of wrist extension, palmar abduction of the thumb, 70 degrees of MCP joint flexion, and 0 to 10 degrees of PIP joint extension. This is an ideal position, which persons with CRPS may not tolerate. Above all, therapists working with persons who have CRPS should avoid causing pain. Therefore, they should be positioned in a position of comfort. Orthoses other than a resting hand orthosis may also be appropriate for this diagnostic population. (See Chapter 7 for a discussion of wrist orthotic intervention for CRPS.)

Resting hand orthoses provided to persons with CRPS are initially to be worn at all times with removal for therapy, hygiene, and (if possible) ADLs. As pain reduction and motion improvement occur, the amount of time that the person wears the orthosis is decreased.

Hand Crush Injury

To provide an orthosis for a crushed hand, position the wrist in 0 to 30 degrees of extension, the MCPs in 60 to 80 degrees of flexion, the PIPs and DIPs in full extension, and the thumb in palmar abduction and extension.[6] Placing a crushed hand into this position provides rest to the injured tissue and decreases pain, edema, and inflammation.[40]

Other Conditions

Resting hand orthoses are appropriate "for protecting tendons, joints, capsular and ligamentous structures."[21] These diagnoses usually require the expertise of experienced therapists and may warrant different orthoses for daytime wear and resting hand orthoses for nighttime use. (See Chapter 13 for orthotic interventions for nerve injuries.)

Table 9-4 Conditions That Require a Resting Hand Splint		
HAND CONDITION	SUGGESTED WEARING SCHEDULE	POSITION
Rheumatoid Arthrities		
Acute exacerbation*	Fitted to maintain as close to a functional (mid-joint) position as possible until exacerbation is over. Removed for hygiene and exercise purposes, and worn during the day at nighttime as necessary. Finger deformities must be taken into consideration if present.	Wrist: neutral or 20 to 30 degrees of extension depending on person's tolerance, 15 to 20 degrees of metacarpophalangeal (MCP) flexion, and 5 to 10 degrees of ulnar deviation. Thumb: position of comfort in between radial and palmar abduction.
Hand Burns		
Dorsal or volar hand burns*	Generally, worn immediately after the burn injury. Continuously worn until healing begins, and removed for dressing changes, hygiene, and exercises.	Wrist: volar or circumferential burn (30 to 40 degrees of extension), dorsal burn (0 degrees = neutral). MCPs: flexion of 70 to 90 degrees. proximal interphalangeal (DIP): full extension. Thumb: palmar abduction and extension. Splint as close to the previously indicated position as possible.
Acute phase	Initially, worn at all times except for fluctuations in bandage bulk and edema. As range of motion (ROM) improves, decrease wearing time to allow for participation in activities.	
Skin graft phase	Worn after skin graft at all times for 5 days or with physician's order for removal.	Position as close to antideformity position as possible
Rehabilitation phase	Splint worn during nighttime to maintain ROM. Splint wear should be limited during daytime to allow for participation in activities.	Position joints to oppose deforming forces
Dupuytren's Disease		
Contractures*	Worn after surgery and removed for hygiene and exercise. Worn at nighttime.	Wrist: neutral or slight extension. MCP, PIP, and DIPs: full extension.
Trauma		
Crush injuries of the hand	Fitted after the injury to reduce pain and edema and to prevent shortening of critical tissue and contracture formation. Worn at nighttime, and possibly worn as necessary during painful periods.	Wrist: extension of 0 to 30 degrees. MCPs: of 60 to 80 degrees. PIP and DIPs: full extension. Thumb: palmar abduction and extension.
Complex regional pain syndrome	Splint is worn at all times, initially with removal for therapy, hygiene, and activities of daily living (if possible). Person should be weaned from splint with pain reduction and improved motion.	Splint in position of comfort with the ideal position being wrist: 20 degrees of extension, thumb in palmar abduction. MCPs: 70 degrees of flexion. PIPs: 0 to 10 degrees of extension.

*Diagnosis may require additional types of splinting.

Therapists sometimes use resting hand orthoses to treat persons who experience a stroke and who are at risk for developing contractures because of increased tone or spasticity.[22] (See Chapter 14 for more information on orthotic intervention for a person who has an extremity with increased tone or spasticity.) Table 9-4 lists common hand conditions that may require a resting hand orthosis and includes information regarding suggested hand positioning and orthotic-wearing schedules. Beginning therapists should remember that these are general guidelines, and physicians and experienced therapists may have their own specific protocols for orthotic positioning and wearing.

Fabrication of a Resting Hand Orthosis

Beginning orthotic makers may learn to fabricate orthotic patterns by following detailed written instructions and by looking at pictures of orthotic patterns. As beginners gain more experience, they will easily draw orthotic patterns without having to follow detailed instructions or pictures. Steps for fabricating a resting hand orthosis can be found in the following Procedure. The therapist must also be sure to teach the wearer or caregiver to clean the orthosis when open wounds with exudate are present (Box 9-1).

Box 9-1   Cleaning Techniques for Orthoses to Control Infection

During Orthotic Fabrication
1. After cutting a pattern from the thermoplastic material, reimmerse the plastic in hot water.
2. Remove and spray with quaternary ammonia cleaning solution.
3. Place the orthosis between two clean cloths to maintain heat and reduce the microorganism contamination from handling the material.
4. Use gloves when molding the orthosis to the person. Latex gloves are recommended. Vinyl gloves adhere to the plastic.

Donning an Orthosis in the Operating Room
Follow steps 1 through 4.
5. Clean the orthosis after the fit evaluation is completed, and place in a clean cloth during transportation.
6. Transport the orthosis only when the person receiving the orthosis is in the operating room.
7. Keep the orthosis in clean cloth until it is needed in the operating room. The orthosis in the cloth should be kept off of sterile surfaces in the operating room.
8. When the person leaves the operating room, all orthoses should be taken with him or her to the appropriate recovery room.

Data from Wright MP, Taddonio TE, Prasad JK, et al: The microbiology and cleaning of thermoplastic splints in burn care, *J Burn Care & Rehabil* 10(1):79-83, 1989.

PROCEDURE   for Fabrication of a Resting Hand Orthosis

The first step in the fabrication of a resting hand orthosis is drawing a pattern similar to that shown in Figure 9-15, A.
1. Place the person's hand flat and palm down, with the fingers slightly abducted, on a paper towel. Trace the outline of the upper extremity from one side of the elbow to the other.
2. While the person's hand is on the piece of paper, mark the following areas: (1) the radial styloid A and the ulnar styloid B, (2) the CMC joint of the thumb C, (3) the apex of the thumb web space D, (4) the web space between the second and third digits E, and (5) the olecranon process of the elbow F.
3. Remove the person's hand from the piece of paper. Draw a line across, indicating two-thirds of the length of the forearm. Then label this line G. After doing this, extend line G about 1 to 1½ inches beyond each side of the outline of the arm. Then mark an H about 1 inch from the outline to the radial side of A. Mark an I about 1 inch from the outline to the ulnar side of B.
4. Draw a dotted vertical line from the web space of the second and third digits (E) proximally down the palm about 3 inches. Draw a dotted horizontal line from the bottom of the thumb web space (D) toward the ulnar side of the hand until the line intersects the dotted vertical line. Mark a J at the intersection of these two dotted lines. Mark an N about 1 inch from the outline to the radial side of D.
5. Draw a solid vertical line from J toward the wrist. Then curve this line so that it meets C on the pattern (see Figure 9-15, A). This part of the pattern is known as *the thumb trough*. After reaching C, curve the line upward until it reaches halfway between N and D.
6. Mark a K about 1 inch to the radial side of the index finger's PIP joint. Mark an L 1 inch from the top of the outline of the middle finger. Mark an M about 1 inch to the ulnar side of the little finger's PIP joint.
7. Draw the line that ends to the side of N through K, and extend the line upward and around the corner through L. From L, round the corner to connect the line with M, and then pass it through I. Continue drawing the line, and connect it with the end of G. Connect the radial

end of G to pass through H. From H, extend the line toward C. Curve the line so that it connects to C (see Figure 9-15, A).
8. Cut out the pattern. Cut the solid lines of the thumb trough also. Do not cut the dotted lines.
9. Place the pattern on the person in the appropriate joint placement. Check the length of the pan, thumb trough, and forearm trough. Assess the fit of the C bar by forming the paper towel in the thumb web space. Make necessary adjustments (e.g., additions, deletions) on the pattern.
10. With a pencil, trace the pattern onto the sheet of thermoplastic material.
11. Heat the thermoplastic material.
12. Cut the pattern out of the thermoplastic material, and reheat it. Before placing the material on the person, think about the strategy that you will employ during the molding process.
13. Instruct the person to rest the elbow on the table. The arm should be vertical and the hand relaxed. Although some thermoplastic materials in the vertical position may stretch during the molding process, the vertical position allows the best control of the wrist position. Mold the plastic form onto the person's hand and make necessary adjustments. Cold water or vapocoolant spray can be used to hasten the cooling time. However, this is not appropriate for persons with open wounds, such as burns.
14. Add straps to the pan, the thumb trough, and the forearm trough (see Figure 9-15, B). One pan strap is located across the PIP joints; the other is just proximal to the MCP joints. The strap across the thumb lies proximal to the IP joint. The forearm has two straps: one courses across the wrist, and one is located across the proximal forearm trough. (See also Laboratory Exercise 9-1.)

TECHNICAL TIPS for a Proper Fit

- For persons who have fleshier forearms, the pattern requires an allowance of more than 1 inch on each side. To be accurate, the therapist could measure

PROCEDURE   for Fabrication of a Resting Hand Orthosis—cont'd

the circumference of the person's forearm at several locations and make the pattern corresponding to the location of the measurements one-half of these measurements.

- Check the pattern carefully to determine fit, particularly the length of the pan, thumb trough, and forearm trough and the conformity of the C bar. Moistening the paper towel pattern allows detailed assessment of pattern fit.
- Select a thermoplastic material with strength or rigidity. Avoid materials with excessive stretch characteristics. The orthotic material must be strong enough to support the entire hand, wrist, and forearm. A thermoplastic material with memory can be reheated several times and is beneficial if the orthosis requires serial adjustments. To make an orthosis more lightweight, select a thermoplastic material that is perforated or is thinner than ⅛ inch, especially to manage conditions such as RA.
- Make sure the orthosis supports the wrist area well. If the thumb trough is cut beyond the radial styloid, the wrist support is compromised.
- Measure the person's joints with a goniometer when possible to ensure a correct therapeutic position before applying the thermoplastic material. Be cautious of positioning the wrist in too much ulnar or radial deviation.
- When applying the straps, be sure the hand and forearm securely fit into the orthosis. For maximal joint control, place straps across the PIPs, thumb IP, palm, wrist, and proximal forearm. Additional straps

may be necessary, particularly for persons who have hypertonicity.

- Contour the orthotic pan to the hand to preserve the hand's arches. The pan should be wide enough to comfortably support the width of the index, middle, ring, and little fingers.
- Make sure the C bar conforms to the thumb web space (see Figure 9-15, C). The therapist may find it helpful to stretch the edge of the C bar and then conform it to the web space. Cut any extra material from the C bar as necessary.
- Verify that the thumb trough is long enough and wide enough. Stretch or trim the thumb trough as necessary.
- For fabrication of a dorsally based resting hand orthosis, the pattern remains the same—with the addition of a slit cut at the level of the MCP joints in the pan portion of the orthosis. The slit begins and ends about 1 inch from the ulnar and radial sides of the pan, as shown in Figure 9-15, D. When the orthosis is placed on the person, the person inserts the hand through the slit in such a way so that the fingers rest on top of the pan portion and the forearm trough rests on the dorsal surface of the forearm. The edges of the slit require rolling or slight flaring away from the surface of the skin to prevent pressure areas. In addition, the thumb trough is a separate piece and must be attached to the pan and wrist portion of the orthosis. Thus, material with bonding or self-adherence characteristics is important. (See also Laboratory Exercise 9-2.)

Precautions for a Resting Hand Orthosis

The therapist should take precautions when applying an orthosis to a person. If the diagnosis permits, the therapist should instruct the person to remove the orthosis for an ROM schedule to prevent stiffness and control edema.

- The therapist should monitor the person for pressure areas from the orthosis. With burns and other conditions resulting in open wounds, the therapist should make adjustments frequently as bandage bulk changes.
- To prevent infection, the therapist must teach the person or caregiver to clean the orthosis when open wounds with exudate are present. After removing the orthosis, the person or caregiver can clean it with warm soapy water, hydrogen peroxide, or rubbing alcohol and dry it with a clean cloth (see Box 9-1). Rubbing alcohol may be the most effective for removing skin cells, perspiration, dirt, and exudate.
- For a resting hand orthosis for a person in an intensive care unit (ICU), supplies and tools should be kept as sterile as possible. Careful planning about supply needs before going into the unit helps prevent repetitious trips. Enlist the help of a second person, aide, or therapist to assist with the orthotic process. The therapist working

in a sterile environment follows the facility's protocol on universal precautions and body substance procedures. Prepackaged sterilized equipment can be used for orthotic provision. Alternatively, any equipment that can withstand the heat from an autoclave can be used.

- Depending on facility regulations, various actions may be taken to ensure optimal wear and care of an orthosis. The therapist should consider hanging a wearing schedule in the person's room. This precaution is especially helpful if others are involved in applying and removing the orthosis. A photograph of the person wearing the orthosis posted in the room or in the person's care plan in the chart may help with correct orthotic application. The therapist informs nursing staff members of the wearing schedule and care instruction.
- After providing an orthosis to a person in the ICU, the therapist should follow up at least once after the orthosis' application regarding the fit and the person's tolerance of the orthosis. Orthoses on persons with burns require frequent adjustments. As the person recovers, the orthotic design may change several times.
- A person who has RA may benefit from an orthosis made from thinner thermoplastic (less than ⅛ inch). This type of orthosis reduces the weight over affected joints.[29]

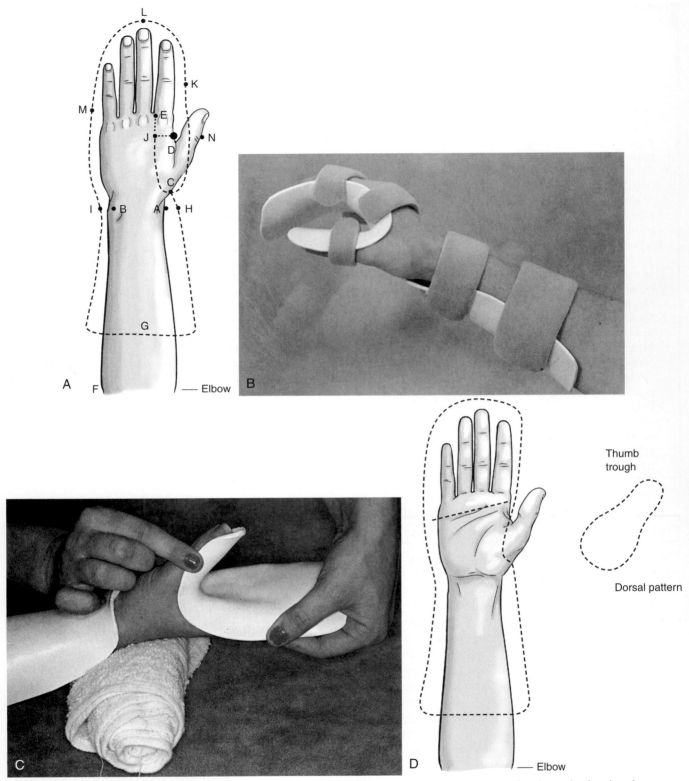

Figure 9-15 Fabrication of a resting hand orthosis. **A,** Detailed pattern. **B,** Strap placement. **C,** C bar conformity to the thumb web space on a resting hand orthosis. **D,** Pattern for a dorsal-based resting hand orthosis.

Review Questions

1. What are four common diagnostic conditions in which a therapist may provide a resting hand orthosis for intervention?

2. In what position should the therapist place the wrist, MCPs, and thumb for a functional resting hand orthosis?

3. For a person with RA who needs a resting hand orthosis, how should the joints be positioned?

4. When might a therapist use a dorsally based resting hand orthosis rather than a volar based orthosis?

5. In what position should the therapist place the wrist, MCPs, and thumb for an antideformity resting hand orthosis?

6. What are the three purposes for using a resting hand orthosis?

7. What are the four main components of a resting hand orthosis?

8. Which equipment must be sterile to make a resting hand orthosis in a burn unit?

References

1. American Society of Hand Therapists: *Splint classification system*, Garner, NC, 1992, American Society of Hand Therapists.

2. Beasley J: Therapist's Examination and conservative management of arthritis of the upper extremity. In Skirven TM, Osterman AL, Fedorczyk JM, et al.: *Rehabilitation of the hand and upper extremity*, ed 6, Philadelphia, PA, 2011, Mosby.

3. Biese J: Therapist's evaluation and conservative management of rheumatoid arthritis in the hand and wrist. In Mackin EJ, Callahan AD, Skirven TM, et al.: *Rehabilitation of the hand: surgery and therapy*, ed 5, St Louis, 2002, Mosby.

4. Boozer J: Splinting the arthritic hand, *J Hand Ther* 6(1):46, 1993.

5. Callinan NJ, Mathiowetz V: Soft versus hard resting hand splints in rheumatoid arthritis: pain relief, preference and compliance, *Am J Occup Ther* 50:347–353, 1996.

6. Colditz 1995

7. deLinde LG, Knothe B: Therapist's management of the burned hand. In Mackin EJ, Callahan AD, Skirven TM, et al.: *Rehabilitation of the hand: surgery and therapy*, ed 5, St Louis, 2002, Mosby.

8. deLinde LG, Miles WK: Remodeling of scar tissue in the burned hand. In Hunter JM, Mackin EJ, Callahan AD, editors: *Rehabilitation of the hand: surgery and therapy*, ed 4, St Louis, 1995, Mosby.

9. Egan M, Brosseau L, Farmer M, et al.: Splints/orthoses in the treatment of rheumatoid arthritis, *Cochrane Database Syst Rev* 1: CD004018, 2003.

10. Evans RB: Therapeutic management of Dupuytren's contracture. In Skirven TM, Osterman AL, Fedorczyk JM, et al.: *Rehabilitation of the hand and upper extremity*, ed 6, Philadelphia, PA, 2011, Mosby.

11. Falconer J: Hand splinting in rheumatoid arthritis, *J Hand Ther* 4(2):81–86, 1991.

12. Feinberg J: Effect of the arthritis health professional on compliance with use of resting hand splints by persons with rheumatoid arthritis, *J Hand Ther* 5(1):17–23, 1992.

13. Fess EE, Philips CA: *Hand splinting principles and methods*, ed 2, St Louis, 1987, Mosby.

14. Geisser RW: Splinting the rheumatoid arthritic hand. In Ziegler EM, editor: *Current concepts in orthotics: a diagnosis-related approach to splinting*, Germantown, WI, 1984, Rolyan Medical Products.

15. Hindocha S, Stanley JK, Watson SJ, et al.: Dupuytren's diathesis revisited: evaluation of prognostic indicators for risk of disease recurrence, *J Hand Surg* 31(10):1626–1634, 2006.

16. Hurst L: Dupuytren's disease: surgical management. In Skirven TM, Osterman AL, Fedorczyk JM, et al, editors: *Rehabilitation of the hand and upper extremity*, ed 6, Philadelphia, PA, 2011, Mosby.

17. Kaye R: Watching for and managing musculoskeletal problems in diabetes, *J Musculoskelet Med* 11(9):25–37, 1994.

18. Koman LA, Li Z, Smith BP, et al.: Complex regional pain syndrome: types I and II. In Mackin EJ, Callahan AD, Skirven TM, et al, editors: *Rehabilitation of the hand: surgery and therapy*, ed 5, St Louis, 2011, Mosby.

19. Lankford LL: Reflex sympathetic dystrophy. In Hunter JM, Mackin EJ, Callahan AD, editors: *Rehabilitation of the hand: surgery and therapy*, ed 4, St Louis, 1995, Mosby.

20. Lau C: Comparison study of QuickCast versus a traditional thermoplastic in the fabrication of a resting hand splint, *J Hand Ther* 11:45–48, 1998.

21. Leonard J: Joint protection for inflammatory disorders. In Hunter JM, Schneider LH, Mackin EJ, et al.: *Rehabilitation of the hand: surgery and therapy*, ed 3, St Louis, 1990, Mosby.

22. Malick MH: *Manual on static hand splinting*, Pittsburgh, 1972, Hamarville Rehabilitation Center.

23. Marx H: Rheumatoid arthritis. In Stanley BG, Tribuzi SM, editors: *Concepts in hand rehabilitation*, Philadelphia, 1992, FA Davis.

24. McFarlane RM: The current status of Dupuytren's disease, *J Hand Ther* 8(3):131–184, 1995.

25. McFarlane RM, MacDermid JC: Dupuytren's disease. In Hunter JM, Mackin EJ, Callahan AD, editors: *Rehabilitation of the hand: surgery and therapy*, ed 4, St Louis, 1995, Mosby.

26. McFarlane RM, MacDermid JC: Dupuytren's disease. In Mackin EJ, Callahan AD, Skirven TM, et al.: *Rehabilitation of the hand: surgery and therapy*, ed 5, St Louis, 2002, Mosby.

27. McGrouther D: Dupuytren's contracture. In Green D, Hotchkiss R, Pederson W, et al.: *Green's operative hand surgery*, ed 5, Edinburgh, 2005, Churchill-Livingstone, pp 159–185.

28. McPherson JJ, Kreimeyer D, Aalderks M, et al.: A comparison of dorsal and volar resting hand splints in the reduction of hypertonus, *Am J Occup Ther* 36(10):664–670, 1982.

29. Melvin JL: *Rheumatic disease: occupational therapy and rehabilitation*, ed 2, Philadelphia, 1982, FA Davis.

30. Melvin JL: *Rheumatic disease in the adult and child: occupational therapy and rehabilitation*, Philadelphia, 1989, FA Davis.

31. Ouellette EA: The rheumatoid hand: orthotics as preventative, *Semin Arthritis Rheum* 21:65–71, 1991.

32. Philips CA: Therapist's management of persons with rheumatoid arthritis. In Hunter JM, Mackin EJ, Callahan AD, editors: *Rehabilitation of the hand: surgery and therapy*, ed 4, St Louis, 1995, Mosby.

33. Pizzi A, Carlucci G, Falsini C, et al.: Application of a volar static splint in poststroke spasticity of the upper limb, *Arch Phys Med Rehabil* 86:1855–1859, 2005.

34. Prosser R, Conolly WB: Complications following surgical treatment for Dupuytren's contracture, *J Hand Ther* 9(4):344–348, 1996.

35. Richard R, Schall S, Staley M, et al.: Hand burn splint fabrication: correction for bandage thickness, *J Burn Care Rehabil* 15(4):369–371, 1994.

36. Richard R, Staley M, Daugherty MB, et al.: The wide variety of designs for dorsal hand burn splints, *J Burn Care Rehabil* 15(3):275–280, 1994.

37. Salisbury RE, Reeves SU, Wright P: Acute care and rehabilitation of the burned hand. In Hunter JM, Schneider LH, Mackin EJ, et al.: *Rehabilitation of the hand: surgery and therapy*, ed 3, St Louis, 1990, Mosby, pp 831–840.

38. Sammons Preston Rolyan: *Hand rehab catalog*, Bolingbrook, IL, 2005, Sammons Preston Rolyan.

39. Skirven TM, Osterman AL, Fedorczyk JM, et al.: *Rehabilitation of the hand and upper extremity*, ed 6, Philadelphia, PA, 2011, Mosby.

40. Stanley BG, Tribuzi SM: *Concepts in hand rehabilitation*, Philadelphia, 1992, FA Davis.

41. Swedler WI, Baak S, Lazarevic MB, et al.: Rheumatic changes in diabetes: Shoulder, arm, and hand, *J Musculoskelet Med* 12(8):45–52, 1995.

42. Tenney CG, Lisak JM: *Atlas of hand splinting*, Boston, 1986, Little, Brown & Co.

43. Torres-Gray D, Johnson J, Mlakar J: Rehabilitation of the burned hand: questionnaire results, *J Burn Care Rehabil* 17(2):161–168, 1996.

44. Tufaro PA, Bondoc SL: Therapist's management of the burned hand. In Skirven TM, Osterman AL, Fedorczyk J, et al.: *Rehabilitation of the hand and upper extremity*, ed 6, Philadelphia, PA, 2011, Mosby.

45. Walsh MT, Muntzer E: Therapist's management of complex regional pain syndrome (reflex sympathetic dystrophy). In Mackin EJ, Callahan AD, Skirven TM, et al.: *Rehabilitation of the hand: surgery and therapy*, ed 5, St Louis, 2002, Mosby.

46. Walsh MT: Therapist's management of complex regional pain syndrome. In Skirven TM, Osterman AL, Fedorczyk J, et al.: *Rehabilitation of the hand and upper extremity*, ed 6, Philadelphia, PA, 2011, Mosby.

47. Ziegler EM: *Current concepts in orthotics: a diagnostic-related approach to splinting*, Germantown, WI, 1984, Rolyan Medical Products.

APPENDIX 9-1   CASE STUDIES

CASE STUDY 9-1*

Read the following scenario, and use your clinical reasoning skills to answer the questions based on information in this chapter.

Juan, a 39-year-old man with bilateral dorsal hand burns, has just been admitted to the intensive care unit (ICU). Juan has second- and third-degree burns resulting from a torch exploding in his hands. He is receiving intravenous pain medication and is not alert. Approximately 14 hours have passed since his admission, and you just received orders to fabricate bilateral hand orthoses.

1. Which type of orthosis is appropriate for dorsal hand burns?
   a. Bilateral resting hand orthoses with the hand in a functional (mid-joint) position
   b. Bilateral resting hand orthoses with the hand in an antideformity (intrinsic-plus) position
   c. Bilateral wrist cock-up orthoses
2. What is the appropriate wrist position?
   a. Neutral
   b. 30 degrees of flexion
   c. 30 degrees of extension
3. What is the appropriate metacarpophalangeal (MCP) position?
   a. 70 to 90 degrees of extension
   b. 70 to 90 degrees of flexion
   c. Full extension
4. What is the appropriate thumb position?
   a. Radial abduction
   b. Palmar abduction
   c. Full flexion
5. Which of the following statements is false regarding the orthosis process for the previous scenario?
   a. The supplies should be sterile.
   b. An extremely stretchable material is necessary to fabricate the orthoses over the bandages.
   c. The therapist should give an orthotic-wearing schedule to the ICU nurse for inclusion in the treatment plan.

*See Appendix A for the answer key to this case study.

CASE STUDY 9-2*

Read the following scenario, and use your clinical reasoning to answer the questions based on information from this chapter and previous chapters.

Ken is a 45-year-old right-hand-dominant man with diabetes mellitus and Dupuytren disease; he underwent an elective surgical procedure to release proximal interphalangeal (PIP) flexion contractures in his right ring and little fingers. The physician used a Z-plasty open palm technique. Ken returns from the surgical suite, and you receive an order to "evaluate, treat, and provide orthosis." Ken is an accountant who is married with a 16-year-old son.

1. What diagnosis in Ken's past medical history is associated with Dupuytren disease?
2. What orthotic designs are appropriate for Ken's condition?
3. What therapeutic position will be used in the orthotic design?
4. What wearing schedule will you give Ken?
5. You notice that Ken's bandage bulk is considerable. How will you design the orthosis to accommodate for bandage thickness? What type of thermoplastic material properties will you choose?
6. How frequently will Ken require therapy?
7. What support systems may Ken require for rehabilitation from this surgery?

*See Appendix A for the answer key to this case study.

APPENDIX 9-2   LABORATORY EXERCISES

Laboratory Exercise 9-1 Making a Hand Orthosis Pattern

1. Practice making a resting hand orthosis pattern on another person. Use the detailed instructions provided to draw the pattern. Cut out the pattern, and make necessary adjustments.
2. Use the outline of the hands following to draw the resting hand orthosis pattern without using the detailed instructions.

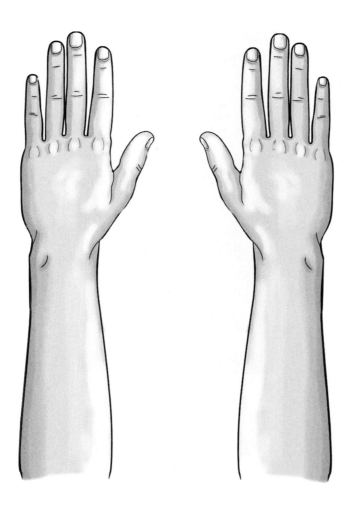

Laboratory Exercise 9-2* Identifying Problems with Orthoses

There are three persons who sustained burns on their hands. Their wounds have healed, and they must wear orthoses at night to prevent contractures. The therapist fabricated the following orthoses. Look at each picture and identify the problem with each.

1. What is the problem with this orthosis?

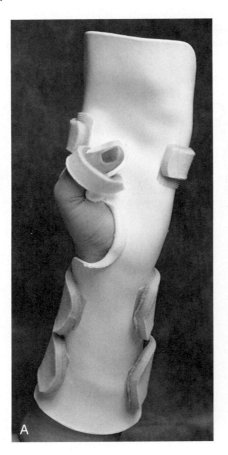

Laboratory Exercise 9-2* Identifying Problems with Orthoses—cont'd

2. What is the problem with this orthosis?

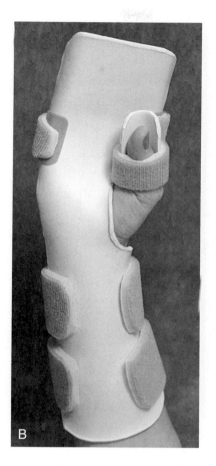

Continued

Laboratory Exercise 9-2* Identifying Problems with Orthoses—cont'd

3. What is the problem with this orthosis?

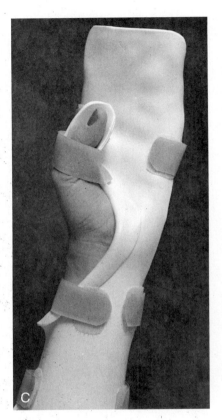

Laboratory Exercise 9-3 Fabricating a Hand Orthosis

Practice fabricating a resting hand orthosis on a partner. Before starting, determine the position in which you should place your partner's hand. Use a goniometer to measure the angles of wrist extension, metacarpophalangeal (MCP) flexion, and thumb palmar abduction to ensure a correct position. After fitting the orthosis and making all adjustments, use Form 9-1 as a self-evaluation check-off sheet. Use Grading Sheet 9-1 as a classroom grading sheet. (Grading Sheet 9-1 may also be used as a self-evaluation sheet.)

FORM 9-1* Resting Hand Orthosis

Name: _____

Date: _____

Position of resting hand orthosis:

Functional position (mid-joint) ○   Antideformity position (intrinsic plus) ○

Answer the following questions after the person wears the orthosis for 30 minutes. (Mark NA for non-applicable situations.)

Evaluation Areas				Comments
Design				
1. The wrist position is at the correct angle.	Yes ○	No ○	NA ○	
2. The metacarpophalangeals (MCPs) are at the correct angle.	Yes ○	No ○	NA ○	
3. The thumb is in the correct position.	Yes ○	No ○	NA ○	
4. The wrist has adequate support.	Yes ○	No ○	NA ○	
5. The pan is wide enough for all the fingers.	Yes ○	No ○	NA ○	
6. The length of the pan and thumb trough is adequate.	Yes ○	No ○	NA ○	
7. The orthosis is two-thirds the length of the forearm.	Yes ○	No ○	NA ○	
8. The orthosis is half the width of the forearm.	Yes ○	No ○	NA ○	
9. Arches of the hand are supported and maintained.	Yes ○	No ○	NA ○	
Function				
1. The orthosis completely immobilizes the wrist, fingers, and thumb.	Yes ○	No ○	NA ○	
2. The orthosis is easy to apply and remove.	Yes ○	No ○	NA ○	
Straps				
1. The straps are rounded.	Yes ○	No ○	NA ○	
2. Straps are placed to adequately secure the hand/arm to the orthosis.	Yes ○	No ○	NA ○	
Comfort				
1. The edges are smooth with rounded corners.	Yes ○	No ○	NA ○	
2. The proximal end is flared.	Yes ○	No ○	NA ○	
3. The orthosis does not cause impingements or pressure areas.	Yes ○	No ○	NA ○	
Cosmetic Appearance				
1. The orthosis is free of fingerprints, dirt, and pencil or pen marks.	Yes ○	No ○	NA ○	
2. The orthosis is smooth and free of buckles.	Yes ○	No ○	NA ○	
Therapeutic Regimen				
1. The person has been instructed in a wearing schedule.	Yes ○	No ○	NA ○	
2. The person has been provided with orthosis precautions.	Yes ○	No ○	NA ○	
3. The person demonstrates understanding of the education.	Yes ○	No ○	NA ○	
4. Client/caregiver knows how to clean the orthosis.	Yes ○	No ○	NA ○	

FORM 9-1* Resting Hand Orthosis—cont'd

Discuss adjustments or changes you would make based on the self-evaluation.

_____

_____

Discuss possible areas to improve with clinical safety when fabricating the orthosis.

_____

_____

GRADING SHEET 9-1*

Resting Hand Orthosis

Name: _____

Date: _____

Position of resting hand orthosis:

Functional position (mid-joint) ○   Antideformity position (intrinsic plus) ○

Grade: _____
1 = Beyond improvement not acceptable
2 = Requires maximal improvement
3 = Requires moderate improvement
4 = Requires minimal improvement
5 = Requires no improvement

Evaluation Areas						**Comments**
Design						
1. The wrist position is at the correct angle.	1	2	3	4	5	
2. The metacarpophalangeals (MCPs) are at the correct angle.	1	2	3	4	5	
3. The thumb is in the correct position	1	2	3	4	5	
4. The wrist has adequate support.	1	2	3	4	5	
5. The pan is wide enough for all the fingers.	1	2	3	4	5	
6. The length of the pan and thumb trough is adequate.	1	2	3	4	5	
7. The orthosis is two-thirds the length of the forearm.	1	2	3	4	5	
8. The orthosis is half the width of the forearm.	1	2	3	4	5	
9. Arches of the hand are supported and maintained.	1	2	3	4	5	
Function						
1. The orthosis completely immobilizes the wrist, fingers, and thumb.	1	2	3	4	5	
2. The orthosis is easy to apply and remove.	1	2	3	4	5	
Straps						
1. The straps are rounded.	1	2	3	4	5	
2. Straps are placed to adequately secure the hand/arm to the orthosis.	1	2	3	4	5	
Comfort						
1. The edges are smooth with rounded corners.	1	2	3	4	5	
2. The proximal end is flared.	1	2	3	4	5	
3. The orthosis does not cause impingements or pressure areas.	1	2	3	4	5	
Cosmetic Appearance						
1. The orthosis is free of fingerprints, dirt, and pencil or pen marks.	1	2	3	4	5	
2. The orthosis is smooth and free of buckles.	1	2	3	4	5	

CHAPTER 10

Elbow and Forearm Immobilization Orthoses

Salvador Bondoc

Key Terms

anterior elbow immobilization orthosis
concomitant injury
cubital tunnel syndrome
distal humerus
elbow instability
Essex-Lopresti fracture
medial and lateral epicondyle
Monteggia fracture
olecranon process
open reduction internal fixation (ORIF)
posterior elbow immobilization orthosis
radial head
"terrible triad" injury
valgus
varus

Chapter Objectives

1. Define anatomic and biomechanical considerations for orthotic intervention of the elbow and forearm.
2. Discuss clinical/diagnostic indications for elbow and forearm immobilization orthoses.
3. Identify the components of elbow immobilization orthoses.
4. Describe the fabrication process for an anterior and posterior elbow orthosis.
5. Review the precautions for elbow and forearm immobilization orthoses.
6. Use clinical reasoning to evaluate a problematic elbow or forearm immobilization orthosis.
7. Use clinical reasoning to evaluate a fabricated elbow or forearm immobilization orthosis.
8. Apply knowledge about the application of elbow or forearm immobilization orthoses to a case study.

Lloyd was playing hockey in a recreation league and fell on his outstretched hand. When he went to the emergency room, he was diagnosed with a dislocation of the ulnohumeral joint. The physician explained to Lloyd that the ulnohumeral joint played an important role in stabilizing the elbow. He subsequently was immobilized in a cast. After the cast was removed, Lloyd had difficulty straightening his elbow joint. He received a referral for occupational therapy. Lloyd wondered what therapy would entail. During his first therapy session, he realized that his stiff elbow was a common complication after an elbow cast removal. He was motivated to regain his motion so that he could play hockey again.

Anatomic and Biomechanical Considerations

The mechanical analogue of the elbow joint is a simple hinge. Yet, the sagittal plane motion of flexion and extension is produced by two articulations with different arthrokinematic properties: the humeroulnar and the humeroradial joints. The humeroulnar articulation consists of the trochlear notch of the proximal ulna and the trochlea of the distal humerus. The humeroradial articulation is formed by the fovea of the proximal radius and the capitellum of the distal humerus. These joint structures share a singular capsule along with the proximal radioulnar joint (PRUJ) and are highly congruent.[16] Although the PRUJ is anatomically linked to the humeroradial and humeroulnar articulations, the motion produced is functionally distinct. The PRUJ along with the distal radioulnar joint at the wrist form a singular longitudinal axis that affords pronation and supination of the forearm.[15] With the high congruence of the joint surfaces, any fracture or dislocation affecting the joint surfaces could lead to loss of available range of motion in either or both extension-flexion and supination-pronation. Furthermore, given the single capsule configuration of the elbow joint complex, prolonged immobilization could further accentuate the loss or restriction in the range of motion in all three elbow joints.

During range of motion assessment, normal elbow flexion produces a soft end feel with the contact of the soft tissues and the volar surfaces of the forearm and arm. Meanwhile, elbow extension produces a hard end feel as the olecranon process of the ulna comes into contact with the olecranon fossa of the distal humerus. The forearm tends to deviate laterally when the forearm is supinated during elbow extension. The **valgus** angulation of the elbow, also known as *the carrying angle,* is 10 to 15 degrees from the longitudinal axis of the humerus and is attributed to the distal expansion of the medial aspect of the trochlea.[16,22] This valgus angle must be considered when applying immobilization or mobilization orthoses to the elbow in extension. In the absence of trauma or underlying pathology, an elbow in excessive valgus position (typically observed with prolonged weight bearing in elbow extension and forearm supination) may lead to a disruption or laxity of the medial collateral ligament.

Throughout the ranges of elbow flexion and extension, the medial and lateral collateral ligament complexes also contribute to the stability of the elbow joint. Elements of the medial collateral ligament complex produce valgus (medial) restraint from maximum extension to 120 degrees of flexion.[24] Meanwhile, the lateral (ulnar) collateral ligament complex remains taut throughout the range of motion and is further accentuated when the elbow undergoes **varus** stress.[20] Given the contribution of the collateral ligament complex to elbow stability, injury to either or both ligaments could also alter elbow alignment and range of motion.

The volar surface of the elbow is filled with soft tissue and features a transverse crease that, depending on a person's muscle mass and elbow joint complex laxity, may lie on a flat or concave surface when the elbow is in full extension. This volar area is bordered by the biceps brachii superiorly, the bellies of the brachioradialis, the common hand extensors laterally, and the common hand flexors medially. The landscape of the dorsal elbow surface is bony. When the elbow is in 90 degrees of flexion, the center points of the **olecranon process** and the **medial and lateral epicondyles** form a triangular configuration. These bony prominences are potential sources of irritation and must be protected during orthotic fabrication and fitting.

Clinical Indications and Common Diagnoses

Immobilization orthoses for the elbow and the forearm are commonly constructed to protect and support healing structures following a traumatic injury to the bones, muscles, ligaments, and related soft tissues. These conditions are managed either conservatively or surgically. Conservative management may involve manipulation or closed reduction prior to immobilization and is often indicated for simple fractures. Surgical interventions vary based on the client's presentation and goals, surgeon's choice, and available resources. The more common surgical fixation procedures involve open reduction with internal fixation using plates and screws and/or wiring. Other surgical procedures used for the elbow include hinged external fixation, arthroplasty (joint replacement), and nerve transposition. In cases of external fixations, an additional elbow immobilization orthosis may be unnecessary.

An elbow immobilization orthosis may be indicated to manage pain and support unstable structures (e.g., arthritis), restrict motion and provide rest (e.g., ulnar nerve entrapment), or to prevent loss of or to improve motion (e.g., elbow stiffness and contractures) through progressive application. Elbow orthoses for the purpose of immobilization may be commercially prefabricated or custom-made. The appropriate choice of orthosis depends on the clinical indication and the preferences of the surgeon, therapist, and client. Table 10-1 provides a summary and comparison of conditions where an elbow immobilization orthosis is indicated.

Elbow Fractures and Dislocation

Traumatic fractures of the elbow may occur to the distal humerus, proximal ulna, proximal radius, or any combination. The incidence of elbow fractures is almost evenly distributed to the aforementioned structures with distal humerus and proximal radius being more common.[14] Fractures are often complicated by **concomitant injury** to surrounding soft tissues, blood vessels, or nerves. More complex forms of elbow fractures involve the articular surfaces and may include joint dislocations. However, joint dislocations may occur from disruptions in soft tissue support without fractures. Complex elbow injuries, if not properly treated, have a poor prognosis with recurrent instability, stiffness, and pain.[12]

Distal Humerus Fractures

Fractures to the **distal humerus** comprise about a third of all elbow fractures.[14] Intra-articular fractures may occur to one or both condyles, because they articulate with the ulna or radius and result from compression forces across the elbow. Extra-articular fractures are typically supracondylar (above the condyles) or transcondylar (across the condyles above the articular surfaces) in nature. These fractures generally result from a fall on an outstretched hand.[10] Conservatively treated simple, nondisplaced fractures or post-surgical elbow fixation of more complex, unstable fractures are immobilized in a long arm cast or posterior elbow orthosis. A posterior elbow orthosis (Figure 10-1) is designed to position the elbow at 90 degrees flexion and forearm in neutral. The duration of orthotic use may depend on the speed of bone and soft tissue healing. In many cases, there is an overlap between immobilization orthoses for healing and mobilization orthoses to prevent or manage soft tissue tightness. Therapists must collaborate with the client's physician to ensure timeliness of intervention.

Proximal Radius Fractures

Proximal radius fractures are the most common of all elbow fractures.[24] In one estimate,[14] at least a third of all elbow

Table 10-1   Conditions That Require an Elbow Immobilization Splint

CONDITION	SUGGESTED WEARING SCHEDULE	TYPE OF SPLINT AND POSITION
Elbow fractures	After removal of the postoperative dressing, the therapist fabricates an elbow immobilization splint. The splint is worn at all times, and removed for exercises and hygiene if permitted.	Posterior angle depends on which structures need to be protected.
Elbow arthroplasty	After removal of the postoperative dressing the therapist fabricates an elbow immobilization splint or fits the client for a brace. The splint is worn at all times, and removed for protected range-of-motion exercises until the joint is stable.	Posterior in 90 degrees of flexion, or Bledsoe brace or Mayo elbow brace in 90 degrees.
Elbow instability	After removal of the postoperative dressing a posterior elbow immobilization splint in 120 degrees of flexion is provided. Therapist-supervised protected range-of-motion exercises are performed until the joint become more stable. The client is not permitted to remove the splint unsupervised.	Posterior in 120 degrees of flexion or brace locked in 120 degrees.
Biceps/triceps repair	Splint is worn at all times and removed for protected range-of-motion exercises.	Posterior elbow splint immobilized in prescribed angle based on structures requiring protection. Splint is usually adjusted to increase the angle of immobilization by 10 to 15 degrees per week at 3 weeks postoperatively.
Cubital tunnel syndrome	A nighttime splint is provided for use while sleeping. Proper positioning during work and leisure activities is reviewed.	Volar splint elbow immobilized in 30 to 45 degrees extension or reverse elbow pad.

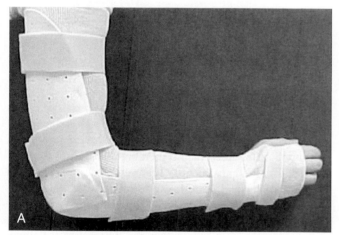

Figure 10-1 Posterior elbow orthosis with elbow in 90 degrees flexion.

fractures occur in the **radial head** and neck. These elbow fractures occur by axial loading on a pronated forearm with the elbow in more than 20 degrees of flexion. The severity of the fracture and the client's contexts determine intervention. Simple or minimally displaced radial head fractures with no evidence of mechanical block are often treated with gentle active mobilization early in the recovery period using a **posterior elbow immobilization orthosis** (see Figure 10-1). This orthosis positions the elbow in 90 degrees of flexion and forearm in neutral for rest and protection. Displaced radial fractures may be treated surgically depending on the presence of mechanical block and the number of fracture segments.[17] Surgeons may elect to use an **open reduction internal fixation (ORIF)** technique or radial head replacement. In either case, clients need to be immobilized with a cast or commercially-available brace immediately following the surgery. Immobilization orthotic provision may continue following cast removal, depending on the client's condition (i.e., rate of healing, joint stability, presence of concomitant collateral ligament injury, and so on) and the surgeon's preference. For clients with ORIFs, the objective is to maintain the stability of the radial fixation by immobilizing the elbow in greater than 90 degrees flexion with the forearm in neutral or pronated position (Figure 10-2). As the client improves, the elbow angle may be adjusted toward extension. For clients with radial head arthroplasties, the choice of immobilization is largely dependent on the integrity of the supportive ligaments and capsule. Some surgeons may opt for commercially-available adjustable hinged braces, such as the Bledsoe brace (Figure 10-3), or a therapist may fabricate a custom hinged elbow device that may be adjusted or locked in the direction of both flexion and extension.

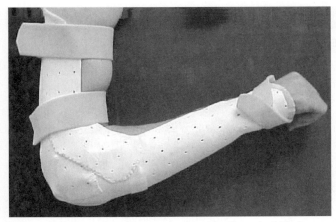

Figure 10-2 Posterior elbow orthosis with elbow in 120 degrees flexion.

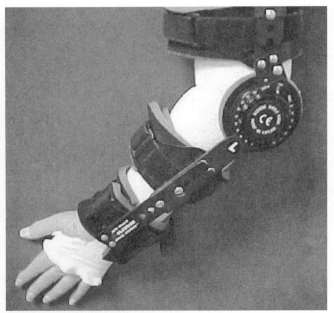

Figure 10-3 Bledsoe brace. (Courtesy of Bledsoe Brace Systems, Grand Prairie, TX.)

Proximal Ulnar Fractures

Most proximal ulnar fractures occur either at the olecranon or the coronoid process. Olecranon fractures typically result from a direct impact or from a hyperextension force.[3] Olecranon fractures are often amenable to ORIF using a plate and screws or tension wiring.[6] Many olecranon fractures involve the triceps either by rupture or avulsion. Following acute management surgically or conservatively (closed reduction), the elbow is braced or dorsally positioned in 30 to 45 degrees flexion to minimize the passive tension on the triceps. Fractures of the coronoid process are more complex and associated with significant instability.[13] (This topic is described later.) Approaches to management are varied[2] and include a more conservative cast immobilization or progressive hinged external fixation for several weeks. In such cases, the purpose of rehabilitative orthotic provision shifts towards mobilization after cast removal due to stiffness.

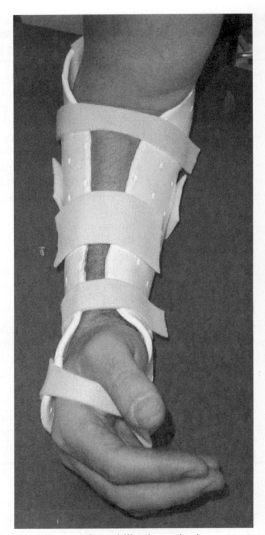

Figure 10-4 Forearm immobilization orthosis, sugar tong type.

Forearm Fractures

Many complex elbow fractures affecting the proximal radius and ulna result in disruption of the proximal and/or distal radioulnar joint(s). Radial head fractures associated with disruption of the interosseous membrane and dislocation of the distal radioulnar joint are also termed **Essex-Lopresti fractures.** Proximal ulnar fractures along with the dislocation of the radial head at the PRUJ are also known as **Monteggia fracture.** The objective of managing these fractures is to restore the joint articulation and kinematics for elbow and forearm mobility. The initial aim of management is to stabilize the forearm by restricting rotation. Restriction may be accomplished through bracing, orthoses, or casting that extends throughout the upper limb proximal to the elbow and distal to the wrist. Examples of the orthoses used to immobilize the forearm and wrist and restrict the elbow include a sugar tong orthosis (Figure 10-4) and a Muenster orthosis. Both examples enable some degree of elbow motion typically within the functional range of 30 to 130 degrees of sagittal motion.

Elbow Dislocations

Dislocations of the elbow are common and may occur with or without fractures. Dislocations without fractures are considered simple, whereas dislocations with fractures (typically of avulsion type) are considered complex. Nearly all elbow dislocations, simple and complex, occur in posterior or posterolateral directions,[5] resulting in joint instability. A common pattern of complex **elbow instability** results from a dislocation of the ulnohumeral joint and injury to the varus and valgus stabilizers of the elbow and the radial head.[11] This injury occurs due to a forceful fall on an outstretched hand. If a coronoid avulsion fracture is involved, the condition is termed a **"terrible triad" injury.**

To prevent instability, simple dislocations are managed in one or more of the following options: (1) cast immobilization, (2) surgical repair of ruptured collateral ligaments, or (3) early mobilization following a reduction or repair procedure. Clients who undergo an early mobilization program with or without ligament repair require supportive orthotic provision during periods of rest. Wolf and Hotchkiss[23] described a conservative approach to manage a post-reduction elbow dislocation to prevent lateral instability using active mobilization within limits of pain and orthotic provision. The immobilization orthosis places the elbow in 100 to 120 degrees of elbow flexion with the forearm in neutral to a fully pronated position. An alternative is a commercially-available hinged brace that stabilizes the elbow while at rest and may be adjusted during exercise.

Biceps Rupture

Distal biceps tendon rupture is uncommon and occurs more frequently to the long head branch within the shoulder. Such injury occurs more often in middle-aged men. The typical mechanism of injury is eccentric loading of the biceps while the elbow is in a flexed position.[18] Conservative management is often indicated for partial tears, using an elbow brace or immobilization orthosis. This orthosis places the elbow in 90 degrees flexion with the forearm in neutral to supination. Post-operative bracing or orthotic provision is indicated for full tears with the forearm in supination. The supinated position is necessary to minimize the mechanical impingement of the distal biceps. Seiler and colleagues[21] observed that 85% of the PRUJ space is occupied by the biceps tendon when the forearm is pronated. They theorized that repetitive pronation contributes to the pathophysiology of the distal biceps rupture through mechanical shearing and hypovascularization. Whether the client's elbow is conservatively or surgically managed, the orthosis or brace is progressively adjusted into extension as gentle exercises are introduced and upgraded over a typical course of tendon healing of 4 to 8 weeks.

Cubital Tunnel Syndrome

Cubital tunnel syndrome is the second most common site of nerve compression in the upper extremity.[1,19] Anatomically,

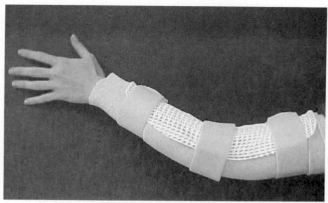

Figure 10-5 Anterior elbow orthosis with elbow in 30 degrees of extension.

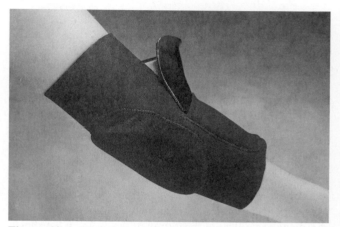

Figure 10-6 Pil-O-Splint. (Courtesy of North Coast Medical, Gilroy, CA.)

the ulnar nerve is susceptible to injury at the elbow secondary to its superficial location situated between the medial epicondyle of the humerus and the olecranon. Injury to the nerve may occur as a result of trauma or prolonged or sustained motion that compresses the nerve over time.[7] Ulnar nerve entrapment following a trauma may arise immediately or gradually due to tethering of the nerve as it courses through a region that may be occupied by edema or adherent scar. Symptoms include pain and paresthesias (numbness, tingling) in the fourth and fifth digits of the hand. In advanced stages, weakness and atrophy of the hypothenar muscles and thumb adductor may be seen (see Chapter 13).

Conservative management focuses on avoiding postures and positions that aggravate the symptoms. Clients are instructed to avoid repetitive or sustained elbow flexion. A nighttime anterior elbow extension orthosis is fabricated with the elbow positioned in 30 to 45 degrees extension (Figure 10-5). If the exposed cubital tunnel region remains irritated, a posterior elbow orthosis with a "belly gutter" to the posteromedial aspect of the elbow may be an option. There are commercially-available soft orthotic devices, such as the Pil-O-Splint (North Coast Medical, Gilroy, CA) (Figure 10-6) and the Comfort Cool ulnar protector (North Coast Medical) (Figure 10-7) that offer additional

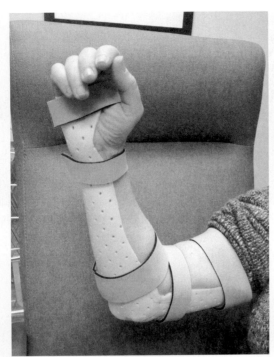

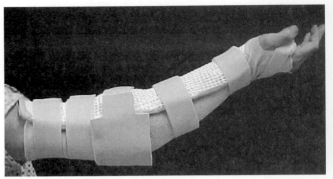

Figure 10-8 A serial static elbow extension orthosis.

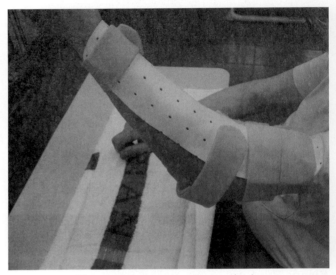

Figure 10-7 Comfort Cool ulnar protector. (Courtesy of North Coast Medical, Gilroy, CA.)

Figure 10-9 Posterior elbow orthosis.

alternatives if a thermoplastic orthotic device is not tolerated by the client. However, management of cubital tunnel syndrome incorporates behavior modification on the part of the client, regardless of the design of the protective orthosis.

Elbow Stiffness

Stiffness is a common consequence of trauma to the elbow joint complex whether managed conservatively or surgically. Elbow stiffness may be a common consequence for clients with osteoarthritis. Elbow stiffness may be classified as intrinsic or extrinsic.[4] Intrinsic elbow stiffness may have intra-articular pathology, such as partial arthrodesis or loss of cartilaginous lining (i.e., osteoarthritis), or may be due to a loss of articular congruency from a less than accurate reduction and fixation after a fracture or dislocation. End range of motion assessment of intrinsic stiffness often yields a "bone-on-bone" end feel. On the other hand, extrinsic elbow stiffness is a result of contractures to the surrounding capsular, ligamentous, and adjacent soft tissue structures including skin, muscle, and tendon. Often times, the elbow is held in mid flexion post-injury. As the body undergoes the phases of healing (i.e., inflammatory response to repair and remodeling), tenacious edema, scarring, pain, and immobilization all contribute to the elbow's propensity to develop contractures of the soft tissues. To address this problem, early intervention is indicated through the controlled active motion and orthotic provision or bracing that provides low-load and prolonged stretch.[8]

There are two general approaches to orthotic provision that incorporate low-load and prolonged stretch to address elbow stiffness: (1) static progressive or serial static orthoses (Figure 10-8), and (2) dynamic orthoses. The mechanism

behind static progressive or serial static orthoses is stress relaxation (i.e., when the tissue is stretched, the load needed to maintain the stretched state decreases and becomes better tolerated). The mechanism behind dynamic orthotic provision is creep where load is constantly applied to cause a change in the viscoelastic properties of tissues.[4] Although both approaches are well supported by evidence, many clients and therapists prefer static progressive orthoses due to better wearing tolerance and adherence.

When there is substantial fibrosis and maturation of scars, extrinsic contractures may be resistant to orthotic provision or bracing and may require open or arthroscopic release. Intrinsic contractures may only respond to rehabilitative management when anatomically possible. To achieve full range of motion of the elbow, tissue release and joint arthroplasty may be necessary.[4]

Features of Elbow Orthoses

Posterior Elbow Orthosis

A posterior elbow orthosis (Figure 10-9) is a common orthotic choice for many acute post-traumatic and post-surgical elbow conditions. The orthosis is easy to wear and offers rest and protection to painful and healing structures.

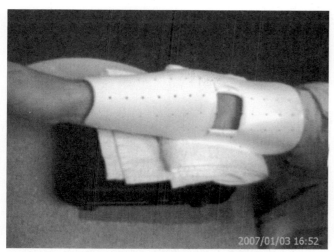

Figure 10-10 Anterior elbow immobilization orthosis.

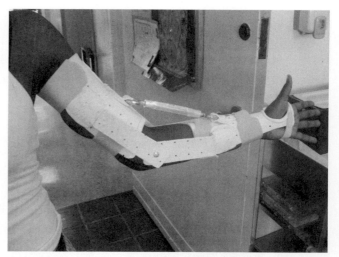

Figure 10-11 Anterior elbow immobilization orthosis with a cubital window.

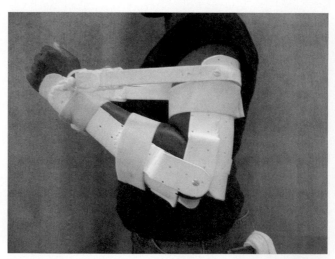

Figure 10-12 Static progressive elbow orthosis with a turnbuckle.

Because of the prominent bony prominences located at the posterior elbow, measures to avoid pressure or provide pressure relief should be built into the orthotic design. Edema, a common consequence of elbow injury and surgery, must also be accommodated into the orthotic design and managed through compression sleeves. Sleeves will keep the skin, which is covered by the orthosis, dry.

Anterior Elbow Orthosis

An anterior elbow orthosis is indicated in situations where there is a posterior wound that cannot tolerate posterior pressure or contact. An anterior elbow orthosis is also used to prevent or correct elbow flexion contractures. Following a contracture release of a stiff elbow, an anterior elbow orthosis is used as a serial static orthosis to slowly gain extension of the elbow over time by remolding the orthosis in increased extension at weekly intervals. In addition, the anterior design is effective in blocking elbow flexion, such as with ulnar nerve compression neuropathies.

For extension contractures of 35 to 30 degrees, an anterior elbow extension orthosis is fabricated for use when the client is at rest (Figure 10-10). As the position of comfort tends to be in flexion, it is recommended to gradually increase the wearing schedule to allow the client to get used to keeping the elbow in extension. During the fabrication process, the orthosis may be molded to create a small space near the cubital fossa. During application, the client may apply additional stretch to the elbow by attempting to fully approximate the cubital fossa against the orthosis. If needed, a design modification of creating a cubital window may provide the client a visual guide (Figure 10-11). As the client's elbow extension increases, the anterior elbow orthosis may be remolded to further provide static stretch until the goal is attained.

Static Progressive Elbow Extension

For extension contractures of greater than 35 degrees, a static progressive elbow orthosis is either fabricated or provided. An

effective design for a static progressive elbow extension orthosis is a custom turnbuckle orthosis (Figure 10-12).[9] This orthosis features a long radial gutter distally, an anterior arm trough proximally, a pair of hinges, and a turnbuckle. The expandable adjustment of the turnbuckle rods affords incremental stretch. It should be noted that fabrication of this static progressive orthosis requires experience, expertise, and time. Simpler alternatives to the turnbuckle orthosis are commercially available, including the Mayo elbow universal brace (Figure 10-13) and the JAS elbow orthosis (Figure 10-14). Both braces are adjustable to the desired range and degree of stretch.

Static Progressive Elbow Flexion

For flexion contracture that prevents a client from achieving greater than 90 degrees of flexion, a custom static progressive elbow flexion orthosis is indicated (Figure 10-15). This orthosis is referred to as the *"come-along" orthosis.* This orthosis features an ulnar gutter distally, a dorsal arm trough proximally, a pair of hinges, and strapping with an embedded series of D-rings. The straps with D-rings may

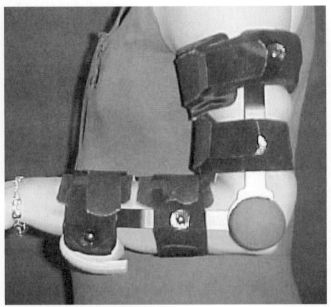

Figure 10-13 Mayo elbow universal brace. (Courtesy of Aircast, Summit, NJ.)

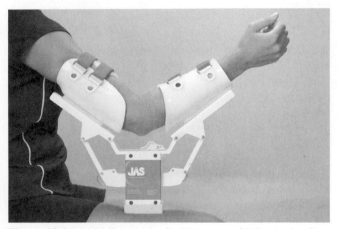

Figure 10-14 JAS elbow orthosis. (Courtesy of Joint Active Systems, Effingham, IL.)

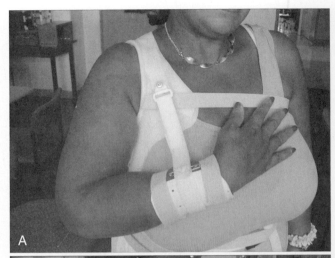

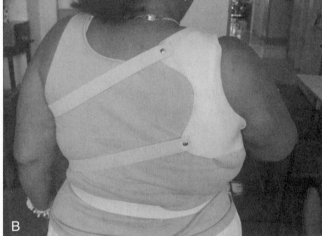

Figure 10-15 Custom, static progressive elbow flexion orthosis, front **(A)** and back **(B).**

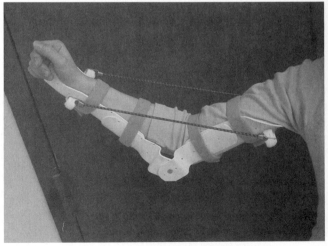

Figure 10-16 Progressive elbow flexion orthosis using bungee cords.

be progressively advanced to provide the requisite flexion stretch. The therapist must assess the onset of ulnar nerve symptoms (e.g., report of numbness and tingling along the ulnar side of the hand and medial forearm) with prolonged elbow flexion. If such symptoms occur, the therapist examines and addresses the potential cause including scar adhesions and edema that may restrict ulnar nerve gliding. An alternative to the use of D-straps is bungee cords (Figure 10-16). However, with bungee cords the therapeutic mechanism changes from static progressive stress relaxation to dynamic orthotic provision creep (see Chapter 12).

For flexion contracture that prevents a client with minimal elbow flexion motion (<90 degrees), a "holster-and-cuff" design is recommended (Figure 10-17). The main biomechanical difference between this orthosis and the static progressive "come-along" orthosis is the length of the proximal moment arm. In a class I lever where the

axis or fulcrum is in the middle of the effort and weight, the mechanical advantage favors the effort with a longer moment arm (Figure 10-18). Again, the fabrication of these static progressive flexion orthoses requires experience, expertise, and time.

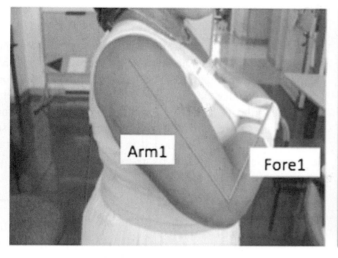
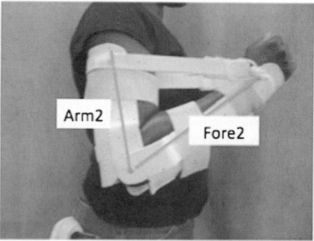

Mechanical Advantate (MA)
MA = Arm 1/Fore1
MA > 1, where Arm1 > Fore1

Mechanical Advantate (MA)
MA = Arm 2/Fore2
MA < 1, where Arm2 < Fore2

Figure 10-17 Holster (A) and cuff (B) design orthosis.

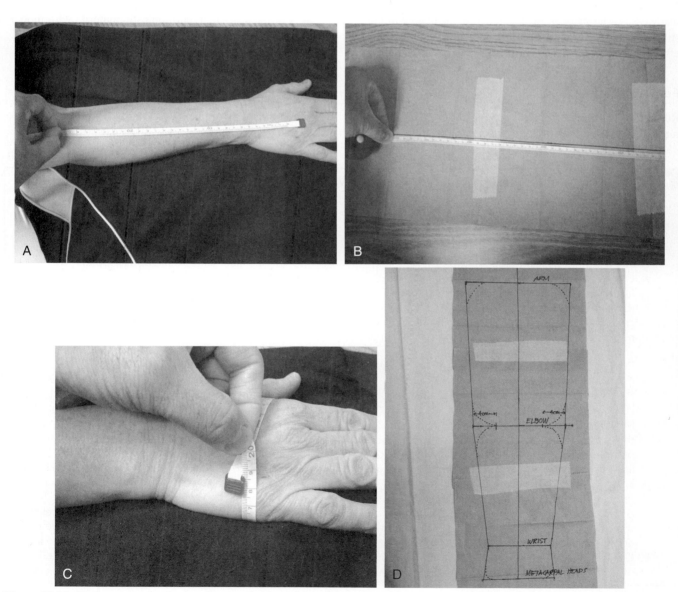

Figure 10-18 Static progressive "come along" orthosis. A, Measurement from distal palmar crease (DPC) to 2 cm distal to axillary fold. B, Drawing line along noted anatomical points. C, Drawing a perpendicular line at DPC. D, Measurements taken at anatomical landmarks.

When the limitations are multi-directional, it may be necessary to fabricate multiple static orthoses for each limitation. The therapist must exercise a depth of reasoning in prioritizing which movement direction should be emphasized. Key considerations include the client's goals, severity of deficit, and response to active interventions, such as exercises, manual therapy and therapeutic activities. It must be noted that for true physiologic change to occur in the contractured tissues, the client must adhere to the wear regiment. Initially, clients are instructed to wear the orthosis for 2-hour intervals, for a total of 6 to 8 hours daily. At first, only short intervals are tolerated. The goal is to develop a tolerance for longer intervals. Clients may also be instructed to adjust the tension, to allow increased motion as tolerated. When more than one orthosis is required, the client may alternate the orthoses during the day, or wear one during the day and the other at night for sleeping. The orthotic regimen is highly individualized and tailored to meet the specific needs and limitations of each client. Off-the-shelf prefabricated static progressive flexion/extension orthoses are currently available and are effective in many cases. The shape of the client's arm, the degree of joint stiffness, and the firmness of joint end feel impact the fit and effectiveness of commercial orthoses.

Forearm Restriction

Restriction of forearm rotation is needed due to shaft fractures of the forearm or fracture-dislocation of the elbow or wrist. An orthosis that is nearly circumferentially positioned to the distal humerus and extending distally to include the wrist provides immobilization to the forearm. Two common designs are a sugar tong (see Figure 10-4) and the Muenster-type orthosis. Both orthoses cover the length of the forearm dorsally and volarly. Note that in providing these orthoses, the wrist is positioned in neutral or near neutral and restricted from sagittal plane movement. The elbow is partially restricted in the sagittal plane.

Fabrication of a Posterior Elbow Immobilization Orthosis

The initial step in the fabrication of an elbow immobilization orthosis is the drawing of a pattern. Elbow orthotic patterns differ from hand patterns in that measurements of the client's arm, elbow, forearm, wrist, and hand are taken and recorded. A pattern is drawn based on the recorded measurements. Tools and materials required to fabricate the orthosis include:

- A perforated ³⁄₁₆-inch thermoplastic material with moderate elasticity, conformability, and bonding
- ⅛-inch polycushion padding
- 1- to 2-inch strap
- 2- or 3-inch stockinette
- Tape measure
- Marker
- Scissors

PROCEDURE **for Fabrication of a Posterior Elbow Immobilization Orthosis**

The following steps describe the fabrication process for a posterior elbow immobilization orthosis in 90 degrees of flexion. The angle of the orthosis is determined by the structures to be protected.

1. Create a pattern by taking the following steps:
   a. Using a tape measure, measure the length of the upper extremity from the distal palmar crease (DPC), along the ulna and up to approximately 2 cm distal to the axillary fold (Figure 10-18, *A*). Take note of the points corresponding to the DPC, ulnar styloid, olecranon process, and proximal arm.
   b. Draw a straight line on the paper using the length determined earlier (see Figure 10-18, *B*). Mark the anatomical points stated earlier along the straight line.
   c. Measure ⅔ of the circumference of the hand at the palmar crease (see Figure 10-18, *C*). Draw a perpendicular line at the DPC point by the straight line referenced in Step 1a. This straight line should bisect the perpendicular line.
   d. Repeat Step 1c on the remaining measurement points: around the wrist by the ulnar styloid, around the elbow by the olecranon, and around the arm above the biceps (see Figure 10-18, *D*).
   e. Cut slits along the olecranon line approximately ⅓ of the width on both sides.

2. Cut the paper pattern from the paper, and measure it on the client in the correct orthotic position. Make sure that the pattern covers the correct length from the DPC to the proximal arm. Ensure the correct girth at the anatomical points identified in Step 1a. Once the pattern is deemed satisfactory, trace it on the thermoplastic material and cut the material (Figure 10-19). If the material is too rigid to be cut, the material may be lightly heated to the point that it may be cut using a pair of scissors. Repetitive heating of the material may cause a loss of rigidity or durability.

3. Position the client for orthotic provision. The ideal position is the client in supine with the shoulder and elbow in 90 degrees of flexion (Figure 10-20). This position takes advantage of gravity to produce an easier and more precise drape of the thermoplastic material. Alternatively, the client may be lying prone with the shoulder abducted in 90 degrees and the forearm dangling over the edge of the plinth/bed.

4. Using disks cut out from polycushion, pad the following bony prominences: olecranon, lateral and medial epicondyles, and the ulnar head at the wrist (Figure 10-21).

5. Cover the padding with a layer of stockinette to prevent it from adhering to the thermoplastic material. If the client has fragile or sensitive skin (e.g., allergic reaction to adhesives), an additional stockinette may be applied prior to sticking the polycushion pads on the bony prominences.

PROCEDURE for Fabrication of a Posterior Elbow Immobilization Orthosis—cont'd

6. The material is heated according to the manufacturer's suggested duration. The material is removed and patted dry.
7. Carefully drape the material over the arm in the proper position described in Step 3. Allow the material to rest on the client's limb before smoothing (Figure 10-22).
8. The overlap between the arm and forearm troughs is pinched and smoothed first (Figure 10-23). Then proceed with ensuring proper drape on the rest of the limb segments. A common error is for the client to extend the elbow slightly during the molding process, causing loss of the flexion angle. Using the non-injured hand, the client supports the limb by the wrist.
9. Once the material has cooled, the padding and stockinette are removed.
10. The elbow seams are smoothed, the edges flared, and the spaces for pressure relief over the bony prominences are further deepened by gently pushing the material (Figure 10-24).
11. An alternative padding using the same thickness may be reinserted to interior of the orthosis.
12. The fit is checked, and adjustments are made as needed.
13. Apply the following straps: proximal upper arm; distal upper arm, proximal to the elbow; proximal forearm; wrist and metacarpals (Figure 10-25).
14. Reapply the orthosis, and recheck the fit (Figure 10-26). If the elbow needs further reinforcement, a small thermoplastic strip may be cut, heated, and applied along corner edges of the elbow.
15. Educate the client in proper donning/doffing, skin checks and precautions, wearing schedule and care of the orthosis.

TECHNICAL TIPS for a Proper Fit

- Select a thermoplastic material that is rigid enough to support the elbow yet conforms well to the arm and joint.
- Align the thermoplastic material along the arm. Make sure to properly position the material before molding.
- An elastic wrap may be used to hold the material in place and free up therapist's hands to support the arm in the correct position. Ensure that the pressure is even throughout the troughs. When using materials that are highly moldable, a wrap may leave unsightly imprints throughout the orthosis.

- Determine that the client has full range of motion of the shoulder and the hand when wearing the orthosis by having the client move in all planes.
- Ensure that the elbow, forearm, and/or wrist joints are in the correct angle during the molding process by checking the joint angles with a goniometer before the material cools.
- Make sure that the orthosis extends as proximal to the axilla as possible, particularly on the lateral side. This position provides adequate support and leverage to properly immobilize the elbow. Make sure the medial side of the proximal portion clears the axilla to prevent irritation.
- If a mistake occurs, it is better to remold the entire orthosis rather than spot heat/fix one area.
- If the material is not rigid enough, reinforce the orthosis with a material that has low memory. Make sure that when adding reinforcements like struts or exoskeletons, the orthosis is actually worn by the client.
- If the client is not adhering to the wear schedule, there is a tendency for the orthosis to curl inward (reducing circumferential opening).
- Use wide straps to properly secure the arm and the forearm in the orthosis. Consider using a figure-eight strap for clients with larger limb girth.

Precautions for Elbow Immobilization Orthoses

- Pad all bony prominences.
- Smooth or flare all edges. For a client with sensitive skin, add moleskin or thin padding as needed. Linings must be monitored for organic grime, dirt, and stains.
- Edema in the elbow is common after injury or surgery. Make sure the client is scheduled for a follow-up visit within several days to modify and adjust the orthosis to accommodate for changes in edema.
- When applying an orthosis over an incision site that is not yet fully closed, make sure to cover the site with non-stick dressing. This protective dressing prevents moisture from transferring to the site from the orthosis.
- Open, draining, or infected wounds should not be covered by orthoses in order to allow for aeration and avoid pressure. Alternative orthoses should be explored.

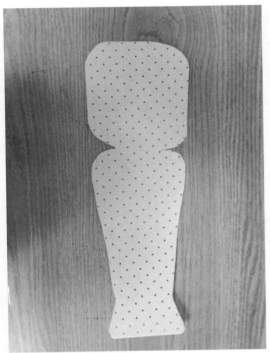

Figure 10-19 Trace pattern and cut out.

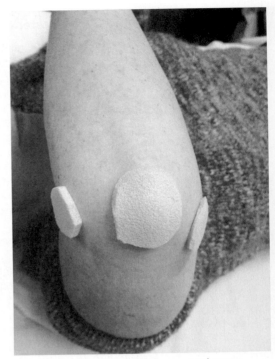

Figure 10-21 Padding bony prominences.

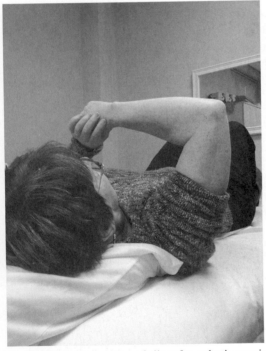

Figure 10-20 Supine position of client for orthotic provision.

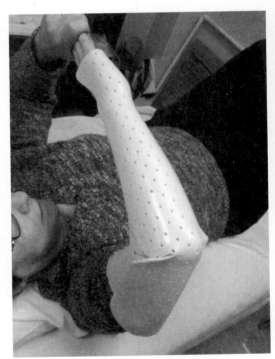

Figure 10-22 Draping material over the arm.

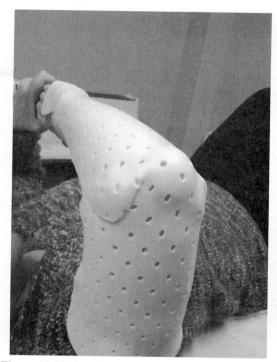

Figure 10-23 Overlapping the arm and forearm troughs.

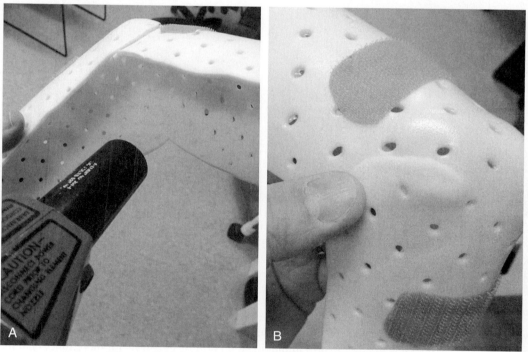

Figure 10-24 Seams are smoothed (**A**) and ends are flared (**B**).

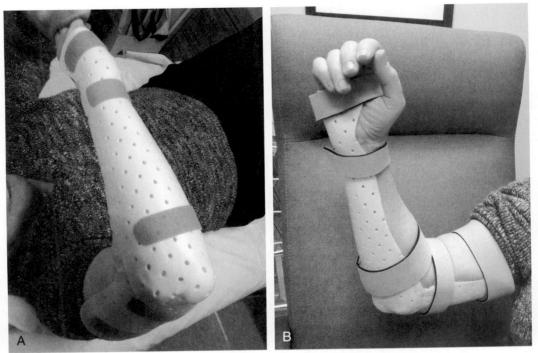

Figure 10-25 **A** and **B**, Strap application.

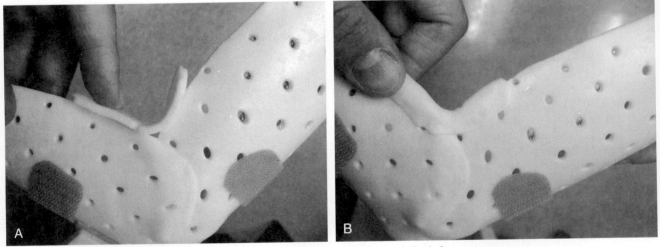

Figure 10-26 **A** and **B**, Rechecking fit for needed reinforcement.

SELF-QUIZ 10-1

Circle either true (T) or false (F).

1. T F Elbow immobilization orthoses can be posterior or anterior.
2. T F It is better that the wrist be left free in forearm immobilization orthoses to allow for more functional motion.
3. T F Thinner and highly perforated material is preferable for post-surgical elbow orthoses to provide comfort and cooling.
4. T F Following a proximal radius fracture, the elbow can be immobilized in either a brace or posterior elbow orthosis.
5. T F Posterior elbow orthoses are preferred for increasing extension.
6. T F The angle of elbow immobilization is dictated by the client's comfort.
7. T F Olecranon fractures are positioned in 90 degrees of flexion.
8. T F An anterior elbow orthosis is appropriate for preventing or correcting elbow flexion contractures and for blocking elbow flexion.
9. T F The best orthosis for an extension contracture of the elbow of >30 degrees is a serial static elbow extension orthosis.
10. T F Generally, biceps tendon repairs are immobilized with the elbow in complete extension.

Review Questions

1. What are main indications for elbow immobilization orthoses?
2. What are the precautions for elbow orthotic provision?
3. When might a therapist consider serial orthotic provision with an elbow immobilization orthosis?
4. What are the purposes of immobilization orthotic provision of the elbow?
5. What are the advantages and disadvantages of a custom orthosis over a commercial orthosis for the elbow?
6. What are the indications for anterior elbow orthotic provision?
7. What are the optimal positions for molding a posterior elbow orthosis?

References

1. Blackmore S: Therapist's management of ulnar nerve compression at the elbow. In Mackin EJ, Callahan AD, Skirven TM, et al.: *Rehabilitation of the hand and upper extremity*, ed 5, St Louis, 2000, Mosby.
2. Budoff JE: Coronoid fractures, *J Hand Surg Am* 37(11):2418–2423, 2012.
3. Cabanela MF, Morrey BF: Fractures of the olecranon. In Morrey BF, editor: *The elbow and its disorders*, ed 3, Philadelphia, 2000, Saunders, pp 365–379.
4. Charalambos CP, Morrey BF: Posttraumatic elbow stiffness, *J Bone Joint Surg* 94A:1428-1437.
5. de Haan J, den Hartog D, Tuinebreijer WE, et al.: Functional treatment versus plaster for simple elbow dislocations, *BMC Musc Dis* 11:263–270, 2010.
6. Edwards SG, Cohen MS, Lattanza LL, et al.: Surgeon perceptions and outcomes regarding proximal ulna fixation: a multicenter experience, *J Should Elb Surg* 12:1637–1643, 2012.
7. Fess E, Gettle K, Philips C, et al.: Splinting for work, sports and the performing arts. In Fess E, Gettle K, Philips C, et al.: *Hand and upper extremity splinting: principles and methods*, ed 3, St Louis, 2005, Mosby, pp 470–471.
8. Flowers KR, LaStayo P: Effect of total end range time on improving passive range of motion, *J Hand Ther* 7(3):150–157, 1994.
9. Gelinas JJ, Faber KJ, Patterson SD, et al.: The effectiveness for turnbuckle splinting for elbow contractures, *J Bone Joint Surg Br* 82(1):74–78, 2000.
10. Hoisington SA, Murthy VL: Forearm fractures. In Hoppenfeld S, Murthy VL, editors: *Treatment and rehabilitation of fractures*, Philadelphia, 2000, Lippincott Williams and Williams, pp 169–190.
11. Hotchkiss R: Fractures and dislocations of the elbow. In Green DP, editor: *Rockwood and Green's fractures in adults*, ed 4, Philadelphia, 1996, Lippincott-Raven.
12. Liu HH, Wu K, Chang CH: Treatment of complex elbow injuries with a postoperative custom-made progressive stretching static elbow splint, *J Orthop Trauma* 20(6):400–404, 2006.
13. McKee RC, McKee MD: Complex fractures of the proximal ulna: the critical importance of the coronoid fragment, *Inst Course Lect* 61:227–233, 2012.
14. Morrey BF: Anatomy of the elbow joint. In Morrey BF, editor: *The elbow and its disorders*, ed 3, Philadelphia, 2000, Saunders, pp 13–42.
15. Neumann DA: The elbow and forearm complex. In Kisner C, Colby LA: *Therapeutic exercise foundations and techniques*, ed 6, Philadelphia, FA Davis.
16. Oatis CA: *Kinesiology: the mechanics and pathomechanics of human movement*, Philadelphia, 2004, Lippincott Williams and Williams.
17. Pike JM, Athwal GS, Faber KJ, et al.: Radial head fractures—an update, *J Hand Surg Am* 34(3):557–565, 2009.
18. Quach T, Jazayeri R, Sherman OH, et al.: Distal biceps tendon injuries—current treatment options, *Bull NYU Hosp Jt Dis* 68(2):103–111, 2010.
19. Rayan G: Ulnar nerve compression, *Hand Clinics* 8:325, 1992.
20. Ruch DS, Papadonikolakis A: Elbow instability and arthroscopy. In Trumble TE, Budoff JE, Cornwall R, editors: *Hand, elbow and shoulder: core knowledge in orthopedics*, St Louis, 2004, Mosby, pp 510–521.
21. Seiler 3rd JG, Parker LM, Chamberland PD, et al.: The distal biceps tendon: two potential mechanisms involved in its rupture: arterial supply and mechanical impingement, *J Shoulder Elbow Surg* 4(3):149–156, 1995.
22. Smith LK, Weiss EL, Lehmkuhl LD: *Brunnstrom's clinical kinesiology*, ed 5, Philadelphia, 1996, FA Davis.
23. Wolff AL, Hotchkiss RN: Lateral elbow instability: nonoperative, operative, and postoperative management, *J Hand Ther* 19(2):238–243, 2006.
24. Yoon A, Athwal GS, Faber KJ, et al.: Radial head fractures, *J Hand Surg Am* 37(12):2626–2634, 2012.

APPENDIX 10-1   CASE STUDIES

CASE STUDY 10-1

Read the following scenario, and use your clinical reasoning skills to answer the questions based on information in this chapter.

Laura is a 47-year-old attorney who slipped on the ice and fractured and dislocated her left elbow. She was first treated at the local emergency room, where she was casted. One week later, she was underwent open reduction internal fixation (ORIF) to the radial head, which repaired the ruptured lateral ligament of the elbow. Two days post-surgery she is referred for therapy (prior to discharge from the hospital) for a posterior elbow orthosis in 110 to 120 degrees of flexion. Laura lives alone and has two active dogs for pets.

1. Describe the appropriate orthosis for Laura. List all of the joints to include in this orthosis.
2. How should the client be positioned for fabrication of this orthosis?
3. Which bony prominences require extra protection in the orthosis? How is this accomplished?
4. What wearing schedule should be provided to Laura?

CASE STUDY 10-2

Read the following scenario, and use your clinical reasoning skills to answer the questions based on information from this chapter.

Marissa is a 42-year old office clerk who is referred for therapy with a diagnosis of ulnar neuropathy of the left hand. She reports waking up in the middle of the night with tingling sensation to the ulnar side of the forearm and hand lasting for 10 to 15 minutes. There is no atrophy of the intrinsic hand muscles of the left hand. There is significant difference in strength of grip and pinch between the two hands. Further examination reveals a positive Tinel sign to the ulnar nerve at the cubital tunnel region and positive symptoms of tingling following 30 seconds of sustained elbow flexion.

Bob is a 37-year old taxi cab driver who sustained a "terrible triad" of the right elbow from a non–work-related car accident. He underwent open reduction internal fixation (ORIF) of the distal humerus, coronoid process, and proximal radius. A hinged external fixator was applied for 11 to 12 weeks. He was referred to therapy to improve his range of motion and facilitate return to work. He came to therapy 2 weeks post-external fixator removal without an orthosis or brace. His elbow range of motion is currently 50/120. Bob performs his self-care activities independently. His main concern is being able to drive his taxi again.

1. What orthosis or brace is most appropriate for each client?
2. What wearing schedule and instructions should be provided to each client?

APPENDIX 10-2 LABORATORY EXERCISES

Laboratory Exercise 10-1 Making an Elbow Shell Pattern

1. Practice making a posterior elbow shell pattern on another person. Use the detailed instructions provided to take measurements and draw the pattern.
2. Cut out the pattern, and check for proper fit.

Laboratory Exercise 10-2 Fabricating an Elbow Orthosis

Practice fabricating an elbow immobilization orthosis on a partner. Before starting, determine the correct position for the partner's elbow. Measure the angle of elbow flexion/extension with a goniometer to ensure correct position. After fitting the orthosis and making adjustments, use Form 10-1 as a self-evaluation of the elbow immobilization orthosis, and use Grading Sheet 10-1 as a classroom grading sheet.

APPENDIX 10-3   FORM AND GRADING SHEET

FORM 10-1 Elbow immobilization orthosis

Name: _____

Date: _____

Type of elbow immobilization orthosis:

Posterior ○   Anterior ○

Elbow position: _____

After the person wears the orthosis for 30 minutes, answer the following questions. (Mark NA for non-applicable situations.)

Evaluation Areas				Comments
Design				
1. The elbow position is at the correct angle.	Yes ○	No ○	NA ○	
2. The elbow has adequate medial and lateral support (two-thirds the circumference of the elbow).	Yes ○	No ○	NA ○	
3. The orthosis supplies sufficient proximal/lateral support (1 inch proximal to axillary crease).	Yes ○	No ○	NA ○	
4. The orthosis is two-thirds the circumference of the upper arm.	Yes ○	No ○	NA ○	
5. Distally the orthosis extends to the distal palmar crease (DPC).	Yes ○	No ○	NA ○	
6. The orthosis is two-thirds the circumference of the forearm.	Yes ○	No ○	NA ○	
Function				
1. The orthosis allows full thumb and digit motion.	Yes ○	No ○	NA ○	
2. The orthosis allows full shoulder motion.	Yes ○	No ○	NA ○	
3. The orthosis provides adequate elbow support to properly secure the elbow in the orthosis and prevent elbow motion.	Yes ○	No ○	NA ○	
Straps				
1. The straps are secure.	Yes ○	No ○	NA ○	
2. The straps are adequate in length.	Yes ○	No ○	NA ○	
Comfort				
1. The orthosis' edges are smooth with rounded corners.	Yes ○	No ○	NA ○	
2. The proximal and distal ends are flared.	Yes ○	No ○	NA ○	
3. The orthosis does not cause impingements or pressure sores.	Yes ○	No ○	NA ○	
4. The orthosis does not irritate bony prominences.	Yes ○	No ○	NA ○	
Cosmetic Appearance				
1. The orthosis is free of fingerprints, dirt, and pencil and pen marks.	Yes ○	No ○	NA ○	
2. The orthotic material is not buckled.	Yes ○	No ○	NA ○	
Therapeutic Regimen				
1. The person was instructed in a wearing schedule.	Yes ○	No ○	NA ○	
2. The person was provided orthotic precautions.	Yes ○	No ○	NA ○	
3. The person demonstrates understanding of the education.	Yes ○	No ○	NA ○	
4. Client/caregiver knows how to clean the orthosis.	Yes ○	No ○	NA ○	

Discuss possible orthosis adjustments or changes you should make based on the self-evaluation. (What would you do differently next time?)

_____

_____

_____

_____

_____

_____

Discuss possible areas to improve clinical safety when fabricating the orthosis.

_____

_____

_____

_____

GRADING SHEET 10-1

Elbow Immobilization Orthosis

Name: _____

Date: _____

Type of elbow immobilization orthosis:

Posterior ○   Anterior ○

Elbow position: _____

Grade:
1 = Beyond improvement, not acceptable
2 = Requires maximal improvement
3 = Requires moderate improvement
4 = Requires minimal improvement
5 = Requires no improvement

Evaluation Areas						**Comments**
Design						
1. The elbow position is at the correct angle.	1	2	3	4	5	
2. The elbow has adequate medial and lateral support (two-thirds the circumference of the elbow).	1	2	3	4	5	
3. The orthosis supplies sufficient proximal/lateral support (1 inch proximal to axillary crease).	1	2	3	4	5	
4. The orthosis is two-thirds the circumference of the upper arm.	1	2	3	4	5	
5. Distally the orthosis extends to the distal palmar crease (DPC).	1	2	3	4	5	
6. The orthosis is two-thirds the circumference of the forearm.	1	2	3	4	5	
Function						
1. The orthosis allows full thumb and digit motion.	1	2	3	4	5	
2. The orthosis allows full shoulder motion.	1	2	3	4	5	
3. The orthosis provides adequate elbow support to properly secure the elbow in the orthosis and prevents elbow motion.	1	2	3	4	5	
Straps						
1. The straps are secure.	1	2	3	4	5	
2. The straps are adequate in length.	1	2	3	4	5	
Comfort						
1. The orthosis' edges are smooth with rounded corners.	1	2	3	4	5	
2. The proximal end is flared.	1	2	3	4	5	
3. The orthosis does not cause impingements or pressure sores.	1	2	3	4	5	
4. The orthosis does not irritate bony prominences.	1	2	3	4	5	
Cosmetic Appearance						
1. The orthosis is free of fingerprints, dirt, and pencil and pen marks.	1	2	3	4	5	
2. The orthotic material is not buckled.	1	2	3	4	5	

CHAPTER 11

Orthotics for the Fingers

Cynthia Cooper, MFA, MA, OTR/L, CHT
Lisa Deshaies, OTR/L, CHT

Key Terms
boutonnière deformity
buddy straps
central extensor tendon (CET)
collateral ligaments
extensor lag
finger sprain
flexion contracture
fusiform swelling
lateral bands
mallet finger
oblique retinacular ligament (ORL)
swan neck deformity
terminal extensor tendon
transverse retinacular ligament
volar plate (VP)

Chapter Objectives
1. Explain the functional and anatomical considerations of orthotics for the fingers.
2. Identify diagnostic indications for using finger orthoses.
3. Describe a mallet finger.
4. Describe a boutonnière deformity.
5. Describe a swan neck deformity.
6. Name three structures that provide support to the stability of the proximal interphalangeal (PIP) joint.
7. Explain the purpose of buddy straps.
8. Apply clinical reasoning to evaluate finger orthoses in terms of materials used, strapping type and placement, and fit.
9. Discuss the process of making a mallet orthosis, a gutter orthosis, and a PIP hyperextension block orthosis.

Ryland is a 23-year-old right dominant male computer programmer who jammed his right middle finger while playing softball. He developed pain and swelling of the injured distal finger, along with drooping of the distal interphalangeal (DIP) joint. His doctor diagnosed a mallet injury and sent him to occupational therapy for orthotic fabrication.

In addition to computer use, Ryland enjoys softball, golf, and bicycle riding. He expressed concern that his injury would prevent him from participating in upcoming athletic activities. He presumed that his orthotics would have to support his forearm and wrist, and he was relieved to learn that his diagnosis could be treated appropriately with a small distal finger orthotic.

Depending on the diagnosis, finger problems may require orthotics that cross the hand and wrist, or they may be treated with orthotics that are smaller. This chapter describes the smaller orthoses that are finger-based, crossing the proximal interphalangeal (PIP) and/or DIP joint, leaving the metacarpophalangeal (MCP) joint free.

Functional and Anatomical Considerations of Orthotics for the Fingers

The PIP and DIP joints are hinge joints. These joints have **collateral ligaments** on each side that provide joint stability and restraint against deviation forces. The radial collateral ligament protects against ulnar deviation forces, and the ulnar collateral ligament protects against radial deviation forces. On the palmar (or volar) surface is the **volar plate (VP)**, which is a fibrocartilaginous structure that prevents hyperextension. The **central extensor tendon (CET)** crosses the

PIP joint dorsally and is part of the PIP joint dorsal capsule. It is implicated in boutonnière deformities. The **lateral bands**, which are contributions from the intrinsic muscles, and the **transverse retinacular ligament** are additional structures that contribute to the delicate balance of the extensor mechanism at the PIP joint. They are implicated in boutonnière deformities and swan neck deformities. The **terminal extensor tendon** attaches to the distal phalanx and is implicated in **mallet finger** injuries (Figure 11-1).[6]

For any finger problem, it is always important to prioritize edema control. Treatment for edema can often be incorporated into the orthotics process. Examples of this would be the use of self-adherent compressive wrap under the orthosis or to secure the orthosis on the finger. For diagnoses that require orthotic application 24 hours per day but permit washing of the digit, it may be appropriate to fabricate one orthosis for shower use and another one for the rest of the day. In general, thinner low-temperature thermoplastic (LTT) (1/16 inch or thinner) is typically used on digits because it is less bulky yet strong enough to support or protect these relatively small body parts. On a stronger person or a person with larger hands, 3/32-inch material may be better to use than a 1/16-inch thickness. Choosing perforated versus non-perforated thermoplastic material is partly a matter of personal choice, but use caution with perforated materials because the edges may be rougher, and there can be the possibility of increased skin problems or irregular pressure, particularly if there is edema. Smaller perforations seen in microperforated materials minimize this risk.

Because finger orthoses are so small, there is an increased possibility of them being pulled off in the covers during sleep or during activity. It is often necessary to tape them in place in addition to using Velcro straps. Be careful not to apply the tape circumferentially so as not to cause a tourniquet effect. An alternative solution is to use a long Velcro strap to anchor the orthosis around the hand or wrist.

Diagnostic Indications

Commonly seen diagnoses that require finger orthoses are mallet fingers, boutonnière deformities, swan neck deformities, and finger sprains. Refer to Chapter 15 for a discussion of trigger finger. These diagnoses are discussed separately in terms of orthotic indications with consideration of wearing schedule and fabrication tips. Prefabricated orthotic options will also be addressed.

Mallet Finger

A mallet finger presents as a digit with a droop of the DIP joint (Figure 11-2). This posture often occurs as a result of axial loading with the DIP extended or else by a flexion force to the fingertip. The terminal tendon is avulsed, causing a droop of the DIP joint. A laceration to the terminal tendon may also cause this problem.[5]

With a mallet injury, the DIP joint can usually be passively extended to neutral, but the client is not able to actively extend it. This is called a *DIP extensor lag*. If the DIP joint cannot be passively extended, this is called a *DIP flexion contracture*. It is unlikely for the DIP joint to develop a **flexion contracture** early on, but this can be seen in more long-standing cases.

Orthoses for Mallet Finger

The goal of orthotics for mallet finger is to prevent DIP flexion. Some physicians prefer the DIP joint to be supported in slight hyperextension to prevent **extensor lag**, whereas others prefer a neutral DIP position. It is good to clarify this with the doctor. If hyperextension is desired, care must be taken not to excessively hyperextend because this may compromise blood flow to the area. Either way, it is important that the orthosis does not impede PIP flexion unless there are specific associated issues, such as a secondary swan neck deformity, that would justify limiting the PIP joint's mobility.

The DIP joint should be supported for approximately 6 weeks to allow the terminal tendon to heal. This terminal tendon is a very delicate structure and for this reason, the

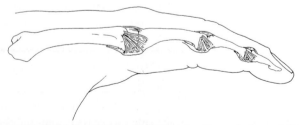

Figure 11-1 Structures that provide proximal interphalangeal (PIP) joint stability include the accessory collateral ligament (ACL), the proper collateral ligament (PCL), the dorsal capsule with the central extensor tendon (CET), and the volar plate (VP). (From Skirven TM, Callahan AD, Osterman AL, et al: *Hunter, Mackin & Callahan's rehabilitation of the hand and upper extremity,* ed 5, St Louis, 2002, Mosby.)

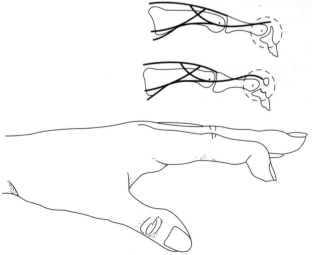

Figure 11-2 Mallet finger deformity. (From American Society for Surgery of the Hand: *The hand: examination and diagnosis,* ed 2, Edinburgh, 1983, Churchill Livingstone.)

joint should not be left unsupported or be allowed to flex for even a moment during this 6-week interval. It can be challenging to achieve this continuous DIP support, because there is also the need for skin care and air flow. Practice with the client so there is good understanding of techniques to support the DIP joint while performing skin hygiene and when applying and removing the orthosis.[2]

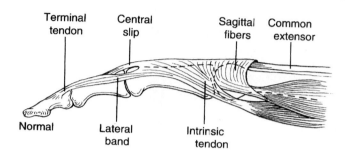

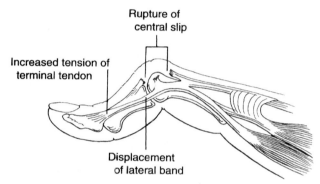

Figure 11-3 Normal anatomy and anatomy of boutonnière deformity. (From Burke SL, Higgins J, McClinton MA, et al: *Hand and upper extremity rehabilitation: a practical guide,* ed 3, St Louis, 2006, Churchill Livingstone.)

After about 6 weeks of continual support and with medical clearance, the client is weaned off the orthosis. The orthosis is usually still worn at night for several weeks. At this time it is important to watch for the development of a DIP extensor lag, and if this is noticed, to resume use of the orthotics and consult the physician.

Boutonnière Deformity

A **boutonnière deformity** is a finger that postures with PIP flexion and DIP hyperextension (Figure 11-3).[7] A boutonnière deformity can result from axial loading, tendon laceration, burns, or arthritis. The CET (also called the *central slip*) is disrupted, which leads to the imbalance of the extensor mechanism as the lateral bands displace volarly. If not treated in a timely manner, the PIP joint extensor lag may become a flexion contracture. In addition, the DIP joint may lose flexion motion due to tightness of the **oblique retinacular ligament (ORL),** also called the *ligament of Landsmeer.*

Orthotics for Boutonnière Deformity

The goal of orthotics for boutonnière deformity is to maintain PIP joint extension while keeping the MCP and DIP joints free for approximately 6 to 8 weeks. If there is a PIP flexion contracture, a prefabricated dynamic three-point extension orthosis might be used, or a static orthosis can be adjusted serially with the goal of achieving full passive PIP extension. There are various types of orthoses for boutonnière deformity, including simple volar gutter orthoses. Figure 11-4 demonstrates some common options of orthotics for the PIP joint in extension while keeping the DIP joint free. In some cases, including the DIP joint in the orthosis may be preferable because this will increase the mechanical advantage. It is usually acceptable to do this if the ORL is not tight.

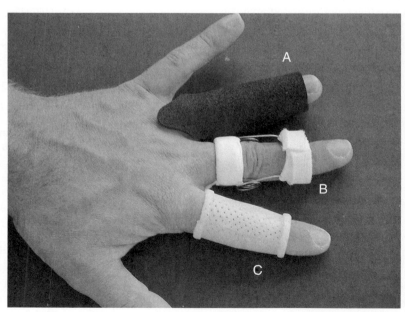

Figure 11-4 Extension orthoses. **A,** Tube. **B,** Capener. **C,** Custom. (From Burke SL, Higgins J, McClinton MA, et al: *Hand and upper extremity rehabilitation: a practical guide,* ed 3, St Louis, 2006, Churchill Livingstone.)

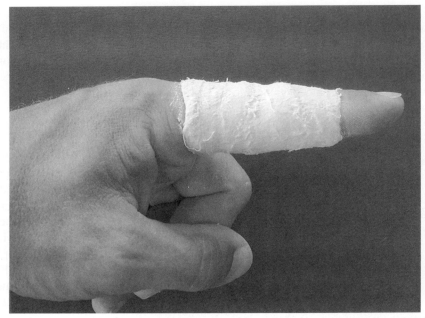

Figure 11-5 Serial cast. (From Burke SL, Higgins J, McClinton MA, et al: *Hand and upper extremity rehabilitation: a practical guide,* ed 3, St Louis, 2006, Churchill Livingstone.)

Serial casting is also an option with this diagnosis (Figure 11-5). This technique requires training and practice before being used on clients.[1] After 6 to 8 weeks of support and with medical clearance, the client is weaned off the orthosis. At this time it is important to watch for loss of PIP extension. If this is noted, adjust orthotic usage accordingly.

Swan Neck Deformity

A **swan neck deformity** is seen when the finger postures with PIP hyperextension and DIP flexion (Figure 11-6). Positionally, the swan neck deformity at the PIP and DIP is the opposite of the boutonnière deformity. It may be possible to correct the PIP and DIP joints passively, or they may be fixed in their deformity positions. There are multiple possible causes of this deformity that may occur at the level of the MCP, the PIP, or the DIP joints. As with a boutonnière deformity, the result is an imbalance of the extensor mechanism, but with a swan neck deformity the lateral bands displace dorsally. In addition to other traumatic causes, it is not uncommon for people with rheumatoid arthritis to demonstrate swan neck deformities.[3]

Orthoses for Swan Neck Deformity

The goal of orthoses for swan neck deformity is to prevent PIP hyperextension and to promote DIP extension while not restricting PIP flexion. A dorsal gutter with the PIP joint in slight flexion (about 20 degrees) can be made. If the DIP demonstrates an extensor lag, the orthosis can cross the DIP and a strap can be added to support the DIP in neutral. Less restrictive styles of orthotics are shown in Figure 11-7. These are three-point orthoses that prevent PIP hyperextension but allow PIP flexion. They can be either custom-formed or prefabricated.

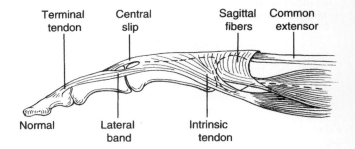

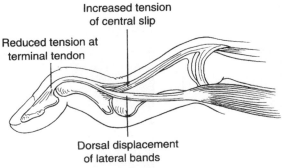

Figure 11-6 Normal finger anatomy and anatomy of swan neck deformity. (From Burke SL, Higgins J, McClinton MA, et al: *Hand and upper extremity rehabilitation: a practical guide,* ed 3, St Louis, 2006, Churchill Livingstone.)

Finger Proximal Interphalangeal Sprains

Finger sprains may be ignored by clients as trivial injuries, but they can be very painful and functionally debilitating with potential for chronic swelling and stiffness and surprisingly long recovery time. Uninjured digits are at risk of losing motion and function, which further complicates the picture.

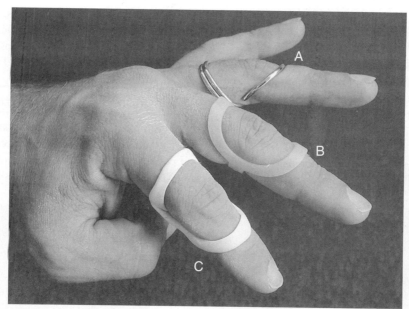

Figure 11-7 Proximal interphalangeal (PIP) hyperextension block (swan neck) orthoses. **A,** Custom-ordered silver ring orthosis. **B,** Prefabricated polypropylene Oval 8 orthosis. **C,** Custom low-temperature thermoplastic (LTT) orthosis. (From Burke SL, Higgins J, McClinton MA, et al: *Hand and upper extremity rehabilitation: a practical guide,* ed 3, St Louis, 2006, Churchill Livingstone.)

Table 11-1	Grades of Ligament Sprain Injuries	
GRADE	**DESCRIPTION**	**TREATMENT**
Mild grade I sprain	No instability with AROM or PROM; macroscopic continuity with microscopic tears. The ligament is intact but individual fibers are damaged.	Immobilize the joint in full extension if comfortable and available; otherwise immobilize in a small amount of flexion. When pain has subsided, begin AROM and protect with buddy taping or buddy strapping.
Grade II sprain	Abnormal laxity with stress; the collateral ligament is disrupted. AROM is stable but passive testing reveals instability.	Immobilize the joint in full extension for 2 to 4 weeks. The physician may recommend early ROM but avoid any lateral stress.
Grade III sprain	Complete tear of the collateral ligament along with injury to the dorsal capsule or the VP. The finger has usually dislocated with injury.	Early surgical intervention is often recommended.

AROM, Active range of motion; *PROM,* passive range of motion; *ROM,* range of motion; *VP,* volar plate.

Prompt treatment can favorably affect the client's outcome and expedite return to occupations impacted by the injury.

PIP sprains are graded in terms of severity, from grade I to III. Table 11-1 describes these grades and identifies proper treatment. PIP joint dislocations are also described in terms of the direction of joint dislocation (e.g., dorsal, lateral, or volar). PIP joint sprains are associated with **fusiform swelling,** which is fullness at the PIP that tapers proximally and distally. Edema control is critical with this diagnosis.

Orthoses for Finger Proximal Interphalangeal Sprains

The goal of orthoses for finger PIP sprains is to support the PIP joint and promote healing and stability. Orthotic options for the injured PIP joint with extension limitations are similar to those used for boutonnière deformities. If there is a PIP flexion contracture, then a dynamic or serial static PIP extension orthosis is used, or serial casting may be considered. If there has been a VP injury, then a dorsal gutter is fabricated to block about 20 to 30 degrees of PIP extension while allowing PIP flexion (Figure 11-8).

Buddy straps (Figure 11-9) are used to promote motion and support the injured digit.[4] There are many different styles to choose from. An offset buddy strap may be needed, especially for small finger injuries due to the length discrepancy between the small and ring fingers.

The physician will indicate what arc of motion is safe, according to the injury and joint stability. It is important not to apply lateral stress to the injured tissues. For example, if the index finger has an injury to the radial collateral ligament, avoid ulnar stress on it. Lateral pinch would also be problematic in this instance. Sometimes it is necessary to custom fabricate a PIP gutter that corrects lateral position as well. Figure 11-10 shows a digital orthosis that provides lateral support.

Generally speaking, PIP finger sprains are at risk for stiffness and are prone to developing flexion contractures. For this reason, a night PIP extension orthosis is often appropriate to use. But this type of injury may also present problems achieving PIP/DIP flexion as well. In this instance, orthoses can be provided along with exercises to gain flexion passive range of motion (PROM). Examples of flexion orthoses are shown in Figure 11-11. Such orthoses must be applied very gently, and tissue tolerances should be monitored carefully.

Precautions for Finger Orthotics

- Monitor skin for signs of maceration and/or pressure both on the finger affected and adjacent fingers that come into contact with the orthosis.
- Check orthotic edges and straps for signs of tightness.

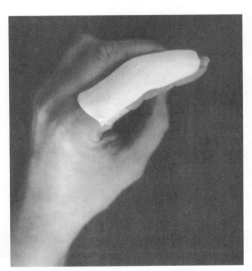

Figure 11-8 Dorsal gutter orthosis blocking about 20 to 30 degrees of proximal interphalangeal (PIP) extension. (From Fess EE, Gettle K, Philips C, et al: *Hand and upper extremity splinting: principles and methods,* ed 3, St Louis, 2005, Mosby.)

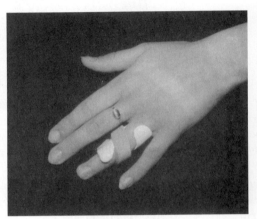

Figure 11-10 Proximal interphalangeal (PIP) extension orthosis with lateral support. (From Fess EE, Gettle K, Philips C, et al: *Hand and upper extremity splinting: principles and methods,* ed 3, St Louis, 2005, Mosby.)

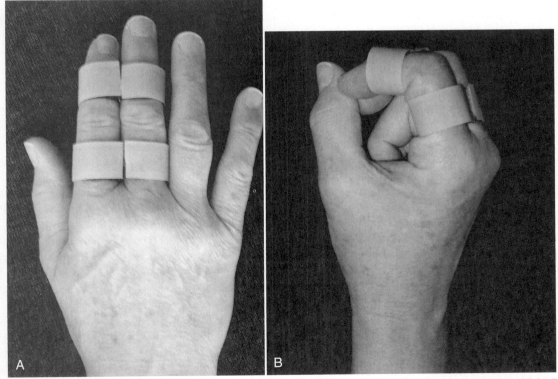

Figure 11-9 A and **B,** Examples of buddy straps for proximal interphalangeal (PIP) collateral ligament injuries. (From Burke SL, Higgins J, McClinton MA, et al: *Hand and upper extremity rehabilitation: a practical guide,* ed 3, St Louis, 2006, Churchill Livingstone.)

- Provide written instructions, and practice with clients so that they are following guidelines of orthotics care and use correctly.

Occupation Based Orthotics

Some finger orthoses may help with hand function by decreasing pain and providing stability. However, many finger orthoses can certainly interfere with daily hand use.

Understandably, clients may be tempted to remove their orthoses in order to participate in activities they enjoy. To help prevent this from happening, therapists should incorporate an occupation based approach.

Examples of Occupation Based Finger Orthoses

An elderly retired male enjoyed woodworking but was unable to use his woodworking tools comfortably due to

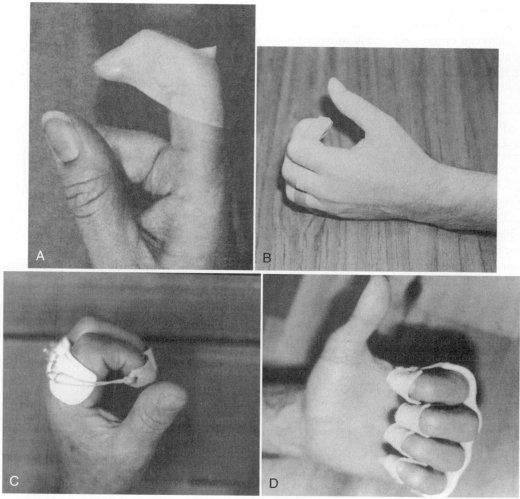

Figure 11-11 **A** to **D,** Examples of proximal interphalangeal (PIP)/distal interphalangeal (DIP) flexion orthoses. (From Fess EE, Gettle K, Philips C, et al, *Hand and upper extremity splinting: principles and methods,* ed 3, St Louis, 2005, Mosby.)

SELF-QUIZ 11-1*

Please circle either true (T) or false (F).

1. T F PIP joints are hinge joints.
2. T F A mallet finger is represented by loss of extension at the PIP joint.
3. T F An extensor lag occurs when there is loss of passive extension at the joint.
4. T F Finger sprains of the PIP joints are always trivial injuries.
5. T F Buddy straps promote motion and support an injured digit.

*See Appendix A for the answer key.

arthritis-related pain and instability of the index finger PIP joint. He expressed interest in a PIP joint protective gutter orthosis to help him use his tools. In order to determine the best position of the PIP joint orthosis, he brought his tools to therapy and demonstrated the finger position he needed. An orthosis was made that provided support during this task.

A client with a mallet injury came to clinic with maceration under the orthosis. He stated that he was wearing his orthosis in the shower and keeping the wet orthosis on his finger all day. In addition to reviewing skin care guidelines and practicing safe protected donning and doffing of the orthosis, an additional orthosis was made to use while showering. This allowed him to apply a dry orthosis after his shower. With this solution, he was able to avoid further skin maceration.

Fabrication of a Dorsal-Volar Mallet Orthoses

The dorsal-volar mallet orthosis is indicated for a mallet injury. Figure 11-12, *A,* represents a detailed pattern that can be used for any finger. Figure 11-12, *B,* shows a completed orthosis. This orthosis has some adjustability for fluctuations in edema, which can be advantageous. Nonperforated ³⁄₃₂-inch material works well for this orthosis. An alternative orthotic design is a DIP gutter orthosis. Figure 11-12, *C* represents a detailed pattern for this alternative orthosis.

1. Mark the length of the finger from the PIP joint to the tip.
2. Mark the width of the finger.
3. Cut out the pattern and round the four edges.
4. Trace the pattern on a sheet of thermoplastic material.
5. Warm the material slightly to make it easier to cut the pattern out of the thermoplastic material.
6. Heat the thermoplastic material.
7. Apply the material to the client's finger, clearing the volar PIP crease. Be gentle with the amount of hand pressure over the dorsal DIP because this is usually quite tender.
8. Maintain the DIP in extension or slight hyperextension, depending on the physician's order.
9. Allow the material to cool completely before removing the orthosis.
10. Ensure proper fit of the orthosis. The orthosis should stay in place securely with a thin ½-inch Velcro strap.
11. Trim the edges as needed.
12. Smooth all edges completely.

TECHNICAL TIPS for Proper Fit of Mallet Orthoses

1. Finger orthoses may seem easy to make because they are small. However, it may actually take extra time to fabricate them precisely. Do not be surprised if you wind up needing extra time to make and fine-tune these small orthoses.
2. Ordinary Velcro loop straps may feel bulky on small finger orthoses. Thinner strap material that is ½ inch width and less bulky can be very effective for finger orthoses.

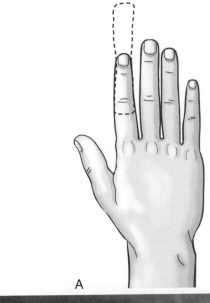

A

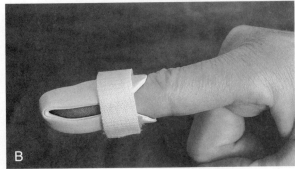

B

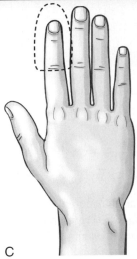

C

Figure 11-12 A, Dorsal-volar mallet orthosis pattern. **B,** Completed dorsal-volar mallet orthosis. **(C),** and DIP gutter orthosis pattern.

Prefabricated Mallet Orthoses

If there has been surgery and the client has a percutaneous pin, the orthosis must accommodate the pin. The DIP orthosis can be a volar gutter orthosis, a dorsal-volar orthosis, or a stack orthosis. A prefabricated AlumaFoam orthosis is sometimes used, but there may be inconveniences and skin issues associated with the adhesive tape that is used to secure it. Prefabricated or custom fabricated stack orthoses need to be monitored for clearance at the dorsal distal edge, because this is an area prone to tenderness and edema related to the injury (Figure 11-13).

Mallet Finger Impact on Occupation

Mallet injuries can result in awkward hand use and can also limit the freedom of flexion of uninvolved digits. It is important to teach clients to maintain active PIP motion of the involved digit and to use compensatory skills, such as relying on uninjured fingertips for sensory input.

Fabrication of a Proximal Interphalangeal Gutter Orthosis

A PIP gutter orthosis is indicated for a PIP sprain injury. Figure 11-14, *A,* represents a detailed pattern that can be used for any finger. Figure 11-14, *B,* shows a completed orthosis. Non-perforated ³⁄₃₂-inch material works well for this orthosis.

1. Mark the length of the finger from the web space to the DIP joint.
2. Mark the width of the finger, adding approximately ¼ to ½ inch on each side, depending on the size of the digit.

3. Cut out the pattern and round the four edges.
4. Trace the pattern on a sheet of thermoplastic material.
5. Warm the material slightly to make it easier to cut the pattern out of the thermoplastic material.
6. Heat the thermoplastic material.
7. Position the client's hand with the palm up to allow the material to drape.
8. Apply the material to the client's finger, clearing the MCP and DIP creases and positioning the PIP joint in the desired position. (This is typically the available passive extension.) Be gentle with the amount of hand pressure used over the PIP joint and over the sides of the joint.
9. Roll the edges of the orthosis as needed for comfort and clearance of MCP and DIP joint motions.
10. Allow the material to cool completely before removing the orthosis.
11. Ensure proper fit of the orthosis.
12. Trim the edges as needed.
13. Smooth all edges completely.

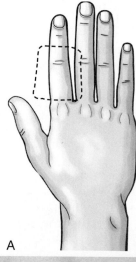

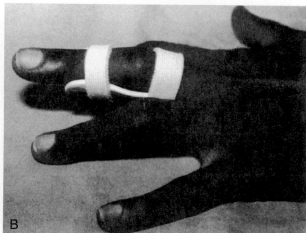

Figure 11-14 A, Proximal interphalangeal (PIP) gutter orthosis. Pattern for fabrication. **B,** and completed orthosis. (From Clark GL: *Hand rehabilitation: a practical guide,* ed 2, New York, 1998, Churchill Livingstone.)

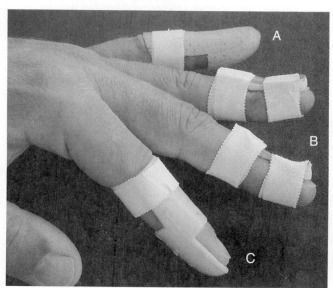

Figure 11-13 Mallet orthoses. *A,* Custom thermoplastic. *B,* AlumaFoam. *C,* Stack. (From Burke SL, Higgins J, McClinton MA, et al: *Hand and upper extremity rehabilitation: a practical guide,* ed 3, St Louis, 2006, Churchill Livingstone.)

TECHNICAL TIPS for Proper Fit of a Proximal Interphalangeal Gutter Orthosis

1. Straps should not be too tight because this can cause edema. However, straps must fit closely enough to provide a secure fit.
2. Modify the height of finger orthotic edges so that straps can have contact with the skin. If the edges are too high, the straps will not be effective.
3. If the goal is to achieve full PIP extension, consider placing a strap directly over the PIP joint but be careful to closely monitor skin tolerance.

Prefabricated Proximal Interphalangeal Orthoses

Figure 11-15 shows examples of prefabricated PIP extension orthoses. Remember that prefabricated orthoses do not always fit well or accommodate edema. Also, there can be problems with distribution of pressure, skin tolerance, and excessive joint forces.

Impact of Proximal Interphalangeal Injuries on Occupations

PIP joint injuries can limit the flexibility and function of the entire hand. Reaching into the pocket or grasping a tool may be impeded. Pain can interfere with the comfort of doing a simple but socially significant task such as a handshake. Rings may no longer fit over the injured joint. Early appropriate therapy can help restore these functions to clients.

Fabrication of a Proximal Interphalangeal Hyperextension Block (Swan Neck Orthosis)

The PIP hyperextension block orthosis is indicated for a finger with a flexible swan neck deformity. Figure 11-16, *A,* represents a detailed pattern that can be used for any finger. Figure 11-16, *B,* shows a completed orthosis. An alternate orthotic design involves wrapping a thin strip or tube of thermoplastic material in a spiral fashion (11-16, *C*).

A properly fitting orthosis effectively blocks the PIP in slight flexion when the finger is actively extended and allows unrestricted active PIP flexion. A thin (1/16 inch) non-perforated thermoplastic material (such as Orfit or Aquaplast) works well for this orthosis. It is especially important to minimize bulk if multiple fingers need

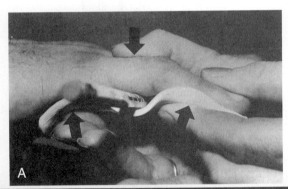

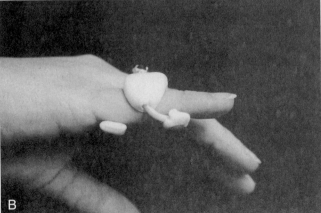

Figure 11-15 A, Prefabricated proximal interphalangeal (PIP) extension orthosis that crosses the distal interphalangeal (DIP). **B,** Prefabricated PIP extension orthosis with DIP free. (From Fess EE, Gettle K, Philips C, et al, *Hand and upper extremity splinting: principles and methods,* ed 3, St Louis, 2005, Mosby.)

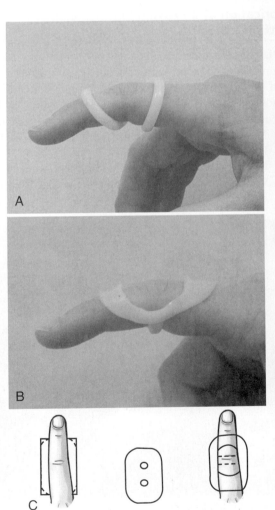

Figure 11-16 A, Spiral design proximal interphalangeal (PIP) hyperextension block orthosis. **B,** Proximal interphalangeal (PIP) hyperextension block orthosis pattern. **C,** Completed PIP hyperextention block orthosis.

orthoses on the same hand. The orthoses must not get caught on each other.

1. Mark the length of the finger from the web space to the DIP joint.
2. Mark the width of the finger, adding approximately ¼ inch on each side.
3. Cut out the pattern and round the four edges.
4. Trace the pattern on a sheet of thermoplastic material.
5. Cut the pattern out of the thermoplastic material. Cutting thin material does not require heating of the plastic first.
6. Mark location for holes, leaving an approximately ¼- to ½-inch bar of material in the center of the orthosis.
7. Punch holes.
8. Apply a light amount of lotion to the finger to enable to material to slide over the finger easily.
9. Heat the thermoplastic material.
10. Slightly stretch the holes so that they are just large enough to slide the finger through. Be careful not to overstretch because the orthosis will be too loose.
11. Slide the material over the finger, weaving the finger up through the proximal hole and down through the distal hole.
12. Center the volar thermoplastic bar directly under the PIP joint, and the dorsal distal and proximal ends of the orthosis over the middle and proximal phalanges.
13. As the orthosis is formed on the finger, keep the PIP in slight flexion (approximately 20 to 25 degrees).
14. Roll the edges of the volar thermoplastic bar as needed to allow unrestricted PIP flexion.
15. Fold the lateral sides of the orthosis volarly, and contour the material to the finger.
16. Allow the material to cool completely before removing the orthosis.
17. Ensure proper fit of the orthosis. The orthosis should be loose enough to slide over the PIP joint yet snug enough to not migrate or twist on the finger. The orthosis should allow full PIP flexion and effectively prevent the PIP from going into hyperextension.
18. Trim the edges as need.
19. Smooth all edges completely.

TECHNICAL TIPS for Proper Fit of the Hyperextension Block (Swan Neck Orthosis)

1. A common mistake is to allow the PIP joint to go into extension while fabricating the orthosis. Closely monitor the PIP position to make sure that it remains in slight flexion during the fabrication process.
2. If the PIP joint is enlarged or swollen, it may be very difficult to slide the orthosis off the finger once it is made. This can be avoided by gently sliding the orthosis back and forth over the PIP joint a few times before the thermoplastic material is fully cooled.
3. Since this orthosis is meant to enable function, make sure to minimize orthotic bulk by flattening the volar PIP bar and lateral edges as much as possible so that the edges do not impede the grasping of objects.

Prefabricated Hyperextension Block Orthoses

Swan neck orthoses are commercially available, and they offer some advantages over custom-fabricated thermoplastic orthoses. They are more durable, less bulky, and often more cosmetically pleasing to clients. Therapists use ring sizers to determine the size needed for each finger. Custom-ordered ring orthoses made of silver or gold (Figure 11-17) are attractive, unobtrusive, and flexible enough to be adjusted for fluctuations in joint swelling; however, they are more costly. Prefabricated orthoses made of polypropylene (Figure 11-18) are a less expensive alternative that offer durability and a

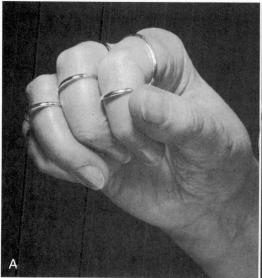
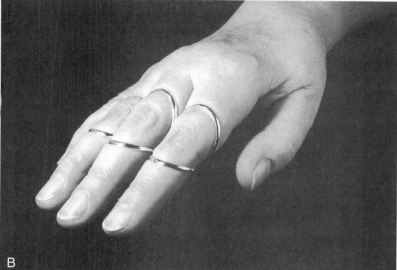

Figure 11-17 A and **B,** Custom-ordered proximal interphalangeal (PIP) hyperextension block orthoses. (From Skirven TM, Callahan AD, Osterman AL, et al: Hunter, Mackin & Callahan's rehabilitation of the hand and upper extremity, ed 5, St Louis, 2002, Mosby.)

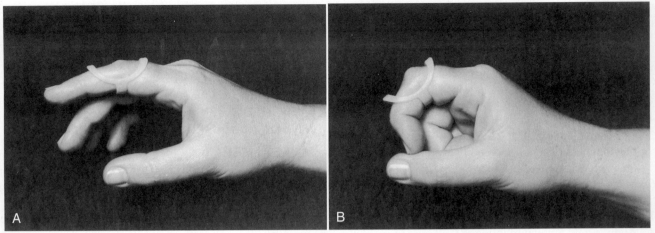

Figure 11-18 **A** and **B,** Prefabricated proximal interphalangeal (PIP) hyperextension block orthoses. (From Skirven TM, Callahan AD, Osterman AL, et al: Hunter, Mackin & Callahan's rehabilitation of the hand and upper extremity, ed 5, St Louis, 2002, Mosby.)

streamlined fit. Their fit can be slightly modified by a therapist using a heat gun, but they cannot be adjusted by clients in response to variations in joint swelling.

Impact of Swan Neck Deformities on Occupations

Swan neck deformities often cause difficulty with hand closure. PIP tendons and ligaments can catch during motion, and the long finger flexors have less mechanical advantage to initiate flexion when the PIP starts from a hyperextended position. A PIP hyperextension block should improve the client's hand function by allowing the PIP to flex more quickly and easily, enabling the ability to grasp objects.

Conclusions, Evidence Based Practice Information Chart

Table 11-2 presents one study published on PIP hyperextension block orthoses. Considering how frequently finger orthoses are used, there is a surprising lack of evidence to support their efficacy.

Despite the lack of evidence for finger orthoses, there is strong clinical support for the use of finger orthoses as a mainstay of care for many common finger problems. Finger biomechanics are very complicated. Added to this, there are multiple custom and prefabricated orthotics to select from.

These challenges can understandably obfuscate the decision-making, particularly for novice therapists. Hopefully this chapter helps therapists use sound clinical reasoning to work collaboratively with clients. Application of clinical reasoning ensures that the best orthosis is selected based on each client's clinical needs and occupational demands.

Review Questions

1. What is a mallet finger?
2. What is the posture of a finger with a boutonnière deformity?
3. What is the posture of a finger with a swan neck deformity?
4. What is fusiform swelling?
5. What structures provide joint stability and restraint against PIP deviation forces?
6. What is the difference between an extensor lag and a flexion contracture?
7. What type of finger orthosis is typically used for a swan neck deformity?
8. How is the DIP positioned when providing an orthosis for a mallet finger?
9. What position should the PIP be in when providing an orthosis for a boutonnière deformity?
10. What position should the PIP be in when providing an orthosis for a swan neck deformity?

Table 11-2 Evidence Based Practice about Silver Ring Orthoses

AUTHOR'S CITATION	DESIGN	NUMBER OF PARTICIPANTS	DESCRIPTION	RESULTS	LIMITATIONS
Zijlstra TR, Heijnsdijk, L, Rasker JJ: Silver ring splints improve dexterity in clients with rheumatoid arthritis, *Arthritis Rheum* 51: 947-951, 2004.	Prospective study	17 subjects	Clients with stable disease and finger deformities were seen by two therapists who decided by consensus which deformities a silver ring orthosis might be appropriate for. Silver ring orthosis size was measured, and temporary thermoplastic orthoses were made. Seventeen subjects received a total of 72 silver ring orthoses (64 PIP, 5 DIP, 3 thumb IP). Measurements were taken on dexterity, self-reported hand function, pain, grip and pinch strength, and clients' satisfaction at time of silver ring orthosis delivery—1 month, 3 months, and 12 months.	There was a statistically significant improvement in observed dexterity (P = 0.005 at 3 months; P = 0.026 at 12 months). There was no statistically significant change in self-reported hand function, pain, or strength. After 1 year, 48 silver ring orthoses were still regularly used by clients. Twenty-four silver ring orthoses (21 PIP, 2 DIP, 1 thumb IP) were discontinued, with main reasons cited as paresthesias and pressure on bony edges or rheumatoid nodules. Eleven of 15 clients completing a survey said they would continue to wear their silver ring orthoses.	Small sample size. Non-blinded observers. Authors cite some outcomes measures used may have lacked sensitivity to change. Decisions to treat clients with silver ring orthoses were made by therapists without input from clients' point of view.

DIP, Distal interphalangeal; *IP*, interphalangeal; *PIP*, proximal interphalangeal.

References

1. Bell-Krotoski J: Plaster serial casting for the remodeling of soft tissue, mobilization of joints, and increased tendon excursion. In Fess EE, Gettle KS, Philips CA, et al., editors: *Hand and upper extremity splinting: principles and methods*, ed 3, St Louis, 2005, Mosby, pp 599–606.
2. Cooper C: Common finger sprains and deformities. In Cooper C, editor: *Fundamentals of hand therapy: clinical reasoning and treatment guidelines for common diagnoses of the upper extremity*, ed 1, St Louis, 2007, Mosby, pp 301–319.
3. Deshaies L, Arthritis: In Pendleton HM, Schultz-Krohn W, editors: *Pedretti's occupational therapy: practice skills for physical dysfunction*, ed 7, St Louis, 2013, Mosby. pp 1103–1036.
4. Gallagher KG, Blackmore SM: Intra-articular hand fractures and joint injuries: Part II—therapist's management. In Skirven TM, Osterman AL, Fedorczyk JM, et al., editors: *Rehabilitation of the hand and upper extremity*, ed 6, Philadelphia, 2011, Mosby, pp 417–435.
5. Hofmeister EP, Mazurek MT, Shin AY, et al.: Extension block pinning for large mallet fractures, *J Hand Surg Am* 28(3):453–459, 2003.
6. Little KJ, Jacoby SM: Intra-articular hand fractures and joint injuries: Part I—surgeon's management. In Skirven TM, Osterman AL, Fedorczyk JM, et al.: *Rehabilitation of the hand and upper extremity*, ed 6. Philadelphia, 2011, Mosby, pp 402–416.
7. Rosenthal EA, Elhassan BT: The extensor tendons: evaluation and surgical management. In Skirven TM, Osterman AL, Fedorczyk JM, et al., editors: *Rehabilitation of the hand and upper extremity*, ed 6, Philadelphia, 2011, Mosby, pp 487–520.

APPENDIX 11-1   CASE STUDIES

CASE STUDY 11-1*

Read the following scenario, and use your clinical reasoning skills to answer the questions based on information in this chapter.

Ryland is a 23-year-old right dominant male who jammed his right middle finger while playing softball. He developed pain and swelling of the distal finger, along with a droop of the DIP joint. His doctor diagnosed a mallet injury and sent him to occupational therapy for orthotic fabrication.

1. What joint(s) should his finger orthosis cross? _____
    _____

2. What is the recommended orthotic wearing schedule? _____
    _____

3. List two different types of orthoses that Ryland could use. _____
    _____

4. How long is Ryland likely to need to wear his orthosis? _____
    _____

*See Appendix A for the answer key.

CASE STUDY 11-2*

Read the following scenario, and use your clinical reasoning skills to answer the questions based on information in this chapter.

Darlene is a 62-year-old left dominant female who fell and developed pain and swelling of her left ring finger PIP joint. She was diagnosed with a PIP joint injury to the radial collateral ligament and VP.

1. Should Darlene have a dorsal or volar finger orthosis? _____
   _____

2. What joint(s) should the orthosis cross, and what position should they be in? _____
   _____

3. Which fingers would be good to buddy tape or buddy strap together and why? _____
   _____

4. Darlene loved to play tennis. When she was medically cleared to play again, she experienced recurrence of swelling at the ring finger PIP joint. What might help her manage her pain and swelling so that she could play tennis again? _____
   _____
   _____

*See Appendix A for the answer key.

CASE STUDY 11-3*

Read the following scenario, and apply clinical reasoning skills to answer the questions based on information in this chapter.

Andrea is a 41-year-old right dominant law firm receptionist who has a 3-year history of rheumatoid arthritis. She was referred to occupational therapy for evaluation of orthotic needs. She presents with recent development of bilateral swan neck deformities of all fingers. She is able to actively flex her PIPs, but it is awkward and effortful to do so. She reports having difficulty with home and work tasks that involve grasping objects.

1. Do you think Andrea would benefit from PIP hyperextension block orthoses? Why or why not? _____
    _____
    _____

2. How could you and Andrea determine if orthoses will improve her hand function? _____
    _____
    _____

3. What key client factors and orthotic options would you consider in selecting the best orthoses for Andrea? _____
    _____
    _____

4. When should Andrea wear her orthoses? _____
    _____
    _____

*See Appendix A for the answer key.

APPENDIX 11-2 LABORATORY EXERCISES

Laboratory Exercise 11-1

1. The following picture shows a mallet finger gutter orthosis. What is wrong with this orthosis? _____
    _____
    _____

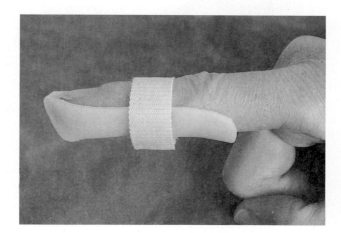

2. The following picture shows a PIP gutter orthosis. What is wrong with this orthosis? _____
    _____
    _____

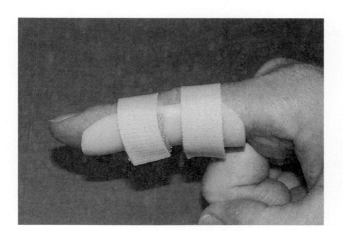

3. The following picture shows a PIP hyperextension block orthosis. What is wrong with this orthosis? _____

_____

_____

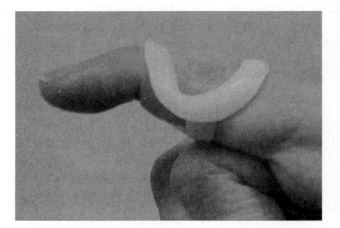

Laboratory Exercise 11-2

Practice fabricating a dorsal-volar mallet orthosis on a partner with the DIP joint in neutral. Check to be sure the PIP crease is not blocked and that full PIP AROM is available.

APPENDIX 11-3   FORM AND GRADING SHEET

FORM 11-1* Finger orthotic

Name: _____

Date: _____

After the person wears the orthosis for 30 minutes, answer the following questions. (Mark NA for non-applicable situations.)

Evaluation Areas				Comments

Design

1. The PIP position is at the correct angle.   Yes ○   No ○   NA ○
2. The DIP position is at the correct angle.   Yes ○   No ○   NA ○
3. The orthosis provides adequate support and is not constrictive.   Yes ○   No ○   NA ○
4. The orthotic length is appropriate.   Yes ○   No ○   NA ○
5. The orthotic width is appropriate.   Yes ○   No ○   NA ○
6. The orthosis is snug enough to stay in place yet loose enough to apply and remove.   Yes ○   No ○   NA ○

Function

1. The orthosis allows full MCP motion.   Yes ○   No ○   NA ○
2. The orthosis allows full PIP motion.   Yes ○   No ○   NA ○
3. The orthosis allows full DIP motion.   Yes ○   No ○   NA ○
4. The orthosis enables as much hand function as possible.   Yes ○   No ○   NA ○

Straps

1. The straps are secure, and the terminal edges are rounded.   Yes ○   No ○   NA ○

Comfort

1. The orthotic edges are smooth, rounded, contoured, and flared.   Yes ○   No ○   NA ○
2. The orthosis does not cause pain or pressure areas.   Yes ○   No ○   NA ○

Cosmetic Appearance

1. The orthosis is free of fingerprints, dirt, and pencil/pen marks.   Yes ○   No ○   NA ○
2. The thermoplastic material is free of buckles.   Yes ○   No ○   NA ○

Therapeutic Regimen

1. The client or caregiver has been instructed in a wearing schedule.   Yes ○   No ○   NA ○
2. The client or caregiver has been provided orthotic precautions.   Yes ○   No ○   NA ○
3. The client or caregiver demonstrates understanding of the orthotic program.   Yes ○   No ○   NA ○
4. The client or caregiver demonstrates proper donning and doffing of orthosis.   Yes ○   No ○   NA ○
5. The client or caregiver knows how to clean the orthosis and straps.   Yes ○   No ○   NA ○

FORM 11-1* Finger orthotic—cont'd

Discuss possible orthotic adjustments or changes you should make based on the self-evaluation. (What would you do differently next time?)

_____

_____

_____

_____

_____

_____

_____

_____

Discuss possible areas to improve with clinical safety when fabricating the orthosis.

_____

_____

_____

*See Appendix B for a perforated copy of this form.

GRADING SHEET 11-1*

Finger Orthotic

Name: _____

Date: _____

Type of finger orthosis:

Mallet finger ○   PIP gutter ○   PIP hyperextension block ○   Other _____

Grade: _____
1 = Beyond improvement, not acceptable
2 = Requires maximal improvement
3 = Requires moderate improvement
4 = Requires minimal improvement
5 = Requires no improvement

Evaluation Areas						**Comments**

Design

1. The PIP position is at the correct angle.	1	2	3	4	5
2. The DIP position is at the correct angle.	1	2	3	4	5
3. The orthosis provides adequate support and is not constrictive.	1	2	3	4	5
4. The orthotic length is appropriate.	1	2	3	4	5
5. The orthotic width is appropriate.	1	2	3	4	5
6. The orthosis is snug enough to stay in place yet loose enough to apply and remove.	1	2	3	4	5

Function

1. The orthosis allows full MCP motion.	1	2	3	4	5
2. The orthosis allows full PIP motion.	1	2	3	4	5
3. The orthosis allows full DIP motion.	1	2	3	4	5
4. The orthosis enables as much hand function as possible.	1	2	3	4	5

Straps

1. The straps are secure and the terminal edges are rounded.	1	2	3	4	5

Comfort

1. The orthotic edges are smooth, rounded, contoured, and flared.	1	2	3	4	5
2. The orthosis does not cause pain or pressure areas.	1	2	3	4	5

Cosmetic Appearance

1. The orthosis is free of fingerprints, dirt, and pencil/pen marks.	1	2	3	4	5
2. The thermoplastic material is free of buckles.	1	2	3	4	5

*See Appendix C for a perforated copy of this sheet.

CHAPTER 12

Mobilization Orthoses: Serial-Static, Dynamic, and Static-Progressive Orthoses

Sharon Flinn, PhD, OTR/L, CHT and Janet Bailey, OTR/L, CHT

Key Terms

area of force application
biopsychosocial approach
creep
dynamic orthosis
end feel
finger loops
mechanical advantage
mobilization orthosis
outrigger
serial-static orthosis
stages of tissue healing
static-progressive orthosis
torque

Chapter Objectives

1. Identify the goals of mobilization orthoses.
2. Define the types of mobilization orthoses.
3. Apply biomechanical principles to mobilization orthoses.
4. Describe common features of mobilization orthoses.
5. Review clinical considerations for mobilization orthoses.
6. Use clinical reasoning skills through a case study presentation applying the principles of mobilization orthotic provision.

Acknowledgments: A special thanks to Jean Wilwerding-Peck OTR/L, CHT for her contributions in the previous edition and to the staff at Columbus Hand Therapy for their careful review and suggestions.

It was a middle of night visit to the refrigerator for a "secret snack" that unfortunately turned into a real nightmare for David. As he reached into the refrigerator, a glass bowl fell out that cut the volar surface of his dominant right hand fingers. This happenstance resulted in a trip to the emergency room and subsequent surgery for flexor tendon repair. A few weeks later therapy was ordered to fabricate a dorsal block mobilization orthosis to allow David to perform passive flexion and active extension within the limits of the orthosis.

The primary goal of every hand orthosis is to enhance the occupational performance of a client with an upper limb impairment. As a top-down approach to intervention, a client-centered, **biopsychosocial approach** to orthotic provision is recommended as the best practice for meeting the occupation-based needs of a client.[32] In this approach, consideration of the thoughts, emotions, behaviors, and social situations of a client are of equal concern to the physical manifestations resulting from a hand injury or disease. This shifts the focus of care from a paternalistic, reductionist, biomedical model to an empowered, holistic, approach to recovery.

To further promote the quality of functional outcomes, classifications have been developed with four categories: immobilization, mobilization, restriction, and torque transmission.[2a] This chapter focuses on one type of orthosis, that of mobilization. Specifically, the goals, types, biomechanical principles, and features specific to mobilization orthoses are provided. The use of mobilization orthoses for proximal interphalangeal (PIP) flexion contractures, flexor tendon repairs, and limitations in composite finger flexion are discussed. Finally, a case study integrates the concepts of mobilization orthotic provision provided in the chapter. Given this knowledge, additional practice, and applications to various client diagnoses, the design and fabrication of mobilization orthoses will become more efficient and effective for beginning practitioners.

Goals of Mobilization Orthoses

Mobilization orthoses are selected to move or mobilize a primary or secondary joint.[1] In providing constant or adjustable tension, mobilization orthoses can achieve one of four possible goals (i.e., correction of deformities, substitute for loss of muscle function, provide controlled motion, aid in wound healing).[19] Explanations for each goal are provided. As always with any orthosis, it is important that the therapist collaborate with the referring physician on obtaining information about the client's injury, surgical intervention, and recommended treatment protocol.

Correction of Deformities

Passive range of motion limitations in a joint result from multiple factors, including trauma, prolonged immobilization, and excessive swelling that creates dense scar formations. Joint contractures contribute to muscle-tendon tightness particularly when tenodesis of the hand is absent or when excessive immobilization of secondary joints occurs. If active and passive range of motion is the same, the goal of intervention begins with decreasing the joint contracture. From there, greater active motion can be gained through mobilization orthosis provision.[13] However, if active is less than passive range of motion, or if changes in passive range of motion occur with changes in digit or wrist position, the focus of intervention attends to decreasing joint contractures and improving extrinsic and intrinsic tendon gliding.

The best results from mobilization orthotic provision are attained when the therapist initiates intervention soon after the edema and pain are managed. The best way to remodel tissue is to provide a tolerable force over time. Evidence shows a relationship between the length of time a stiff joint is held at end range and the resulting gain achieved with passive range of motion.[20] Therefore, mobilization orthotic provision is more effective when orthoses are worn over long periods of time compared to when orthoses are worn for shorter periods of time using increased levels of force. This concept of orthotics is called *low load, long duration.*

Application of external forces necessitates careful monitoring of the skin as an indication of excessive levels of pressure and/or poor distribution of forces. A general goal for a **mobilization orthosis** is to increase passive joint range of motion by 10 degrees per week.[7] Should passive range of motion not improve following 2 weeks of orthotic provision, a reevaluation of the orthosis, home program, and intervention adherence should be completed.[17] In this chapter, fabrication of a serial cast and a hand based PIP

extension orthosis are described as one approach to correct deformities.

Substitute for Loss of Muscle Function

For clients with nerve impairment, a mobilization orthosis can improve hand function.[19] The need to substitute for weak or absent muscle action occurs in conditions, such as peripheral nerve injuries, spinal cord injuries, and other debilitating neurological conditions. The need for a temporary substitution of muscle function also occurs with healing tendons in the hand. Therefore, the goals of orthotic provision are to substitute for loss of motor activity, to prevent overstretching of nonfunctional muscles, and to prevent joint deformity.

One common peripheral nerve injury is a high-level radial nerve palsy. The functional use of the hand is limited in part due to loss of muscle function for wrist and finger metacarpophalangeal (MCP) joint extension and radial abduction and extension of the thumb. An orthosis that provides passive assistance for loss of extrinsic muscle function greatly increases the functional use of the hand (see Chapter 13, Figure 13-8). Similar applications for mobilization orthoses are recommended for clients with low-level median and high-level ulnar neuropathies where the absence or weakness of intrinsic muscles to the thumb and fingers limit hand use significantly.

Another example of substitution for loss of motor function involves clients with spinal cord injuries. A client with a C7 lesion may also benefit from mobilization orthotic provision. Because of the anatomical or biomechanical effect that wrist extension has on finger flexion, a client's active wrist extension becomes the force to generate pinch through the use of a tenodesis orthosis (Figure 12-1).

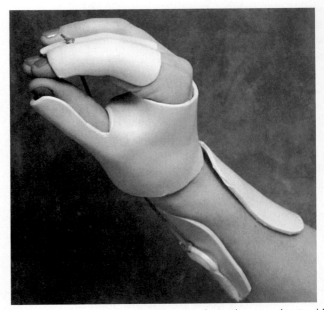

Figure 12-1 A tenodesis orthosis uses active wrist extension to aid passive finger flexion.

Clients with neurological disorders resulting from degenerative conditions (such as, Guillain-Barré, amyotrophic lateral sclerosis, and multiple sclerosis) experience muscle weakness, paralysis, and changes in sensation. Specialized mobilization orthoses may be useful in sustaining hand function, although the presence of spasticity and concerns for sensory loss might preclude candidates from this approach (see Chapter 14).

Finally, the use of mobilization orthoses is appropriate for clients with a loss in continuity of an anatomical structure as is the case with extrinsic tendon lacerations to the hand. The goals for clients following a tendon repair, especially to the flexor tendons of the hand, are threefold. First, controlled passive motion of the tendons increases the flow of nutrient-rich synovial fluids that enhance healing and prevent re-rupture of the tendon. Second, tendons that are allowed early protected mobilization have increased tensile strength compared to immobile tendons. Third, by allowing 3 to 5 mm of tendon excursion, adhesion formation between tendons and surrounding structures are minimized.[28,39] Mobilization orthoses for flexor tendon repairs assist in attaining goals by positioning the wrist and fingers in flexion to keep the repaired tendon on slack and in a protected position. A passive flexion assist from the orthosis substitutes for the loss of muscle function during the required healing period.[30] In this chapter, fabrication of a flexor tendon orthosis is described as one approach to substitute for the loss of muscle function.

Provide Controlled Motion

Mobilization orthoses are used to control motion after reconstructive surgery, such as joint arthroplasties and flexor tendon repairs. Because of altered joint mechanics in a client with rheumatoid arthritis, arthroplasties are done to reconstruct or replace joints, especially the finger MCP joints. A mobilization orthosis for this postoperative client has multiple functions. First, controlled motion and precise alignment of the repaired tissues are done while minimizing soft-tissue deformity. For example, a mobilization orthosis with an outrigger may provide forces to one finger in both extension and radial deviation. A second function of a mobilization orthosis is to maintain alignment of the MCP joints for the healing structures while allowing guarded movements of the fingers in daily activities.[19]

After flexor tendon repairs, a mobilization orthosis provides controlled motion to the healing structures in addition to substituting for loss of muscle function. Due to the protective nature of the orthosis, full finger extension is prevented and controlled extension of the fingers is allowed from the palm to a lumbrical plus position. In this chapter, fabrication of a flexor tendon orthosis is used as an example to describe one approach to control motion.

Aid in Wound Healing

The use of mobilization orthoses facilitates proper collagen alignment and scar formation that occurs in three stages of wound healing.[12] The acute stage is characterized as the inflammatory stage. In response to trauma, vasodilation brings increased numbers of leukocytes to remove damaged cells and fibroblasts to begin the healing process. The proliferative stage occurs after the initial inflammation subsides and tissues are in the early stages of healing. As the need for leukocytes decreases, the working fibroblasts begin the process of collagen formation. The chronic stage is attained when the cells are realigned and the joint response to stress is a hard end feel. Collagen continues to remodel and reorganize based on the amount of stress applied to the wound. During this stage, strength is added to the wound. Mobilization orthoses serve an important role in each stage of healing, especially following a complex trauma, surgical wound, or severe burn. In this chapter, fabrication of a composite flexion orthosis is used as an example of one approach to aid in wound healing.

Types of Mobilization Orthoses

Mobilization orthoses are divided into three types: serial-static, dynamic, and static-progressive.[42] Each type provides unique advantages for clients with limited passive range of motion and can be recommended for specific diagnostic groups of clients. A review of each orthosis type follows.

Serial-Static Orthotic Provision

The purpose of a static orthosis is to immobilize a joint. However, interpretations that the same orthosis is always static in its function are misleading.[19] From a mechanical standpoint, tissue lengthening and growth occur when it is held under constant tension that is greater than its resting tension (see Chapter 1).[3] Therefore, serial-static orthotic provision is a type of mobilization orthosis that positions a joint near its elastic limits to overcome a loss in passive range of motion.[42] A **serial-static orthosis** is easy to tolerate over long periods of time because of the low-load, end range positioning that is applied over a large surface **area of force application.** Figure 12-2 provides a schematic of the appropriate types

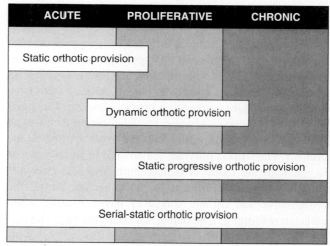

Figure 12-2 The stage of healing helps to determine the most appropriate type of orthosis.

of orthoses to use based on the three stages of healing.[12] Although a serial-static orthosis is the only orthotic type recommended across the continuum of healing, it is specifically recommended for contractures with a hard end feel[41] or when joint tightness is due to forearm muscle-tendon unit shortening.[3] In this chapter, fabrication of a serial-static orthosis is used as an example for reducing a PIP flexion contracture.

Dynamic Orthotic Provision

All dynamic orthoses are mobilization orthoses, but not all mobilization orthoses are dynamic. An orthosis is dynamic when it uses a stable static base and an elastic mobilizing component.[22] A variety of self-adjusting components can be used including rubber bands, springs, coils, Lycra, elastic thread, or monofilament line. The purpose of a **dynamic orthosis** is to apply sufficient tension that does not overpower the joint and allows the client to overcome the resistance and move in the opposite direction. In this way, active motion with a dynamic orthosis assists in lubrication of joints, flexibility of ligaments, activating muscle fibers, and maximizing tendon gliding. A dynamic orthosis is recommended primarily during the proliferative stage of healing when collagen is forming. More progress can be expected with dynamic orthotic provision in joints with less pretreatment stiffness, shorter time since surgery (<12 weeks), and in flexion rather than extension deficits.[22] For these reasons, a dynamic orthotic design may be selected over a static orthosis when active motion is preferred and when the client is developing contractures early in the treatment program. Specific applications have been recommended for commercially-available dynamic orthoses instead of custom made orthoses. These applications include (1) adhesive capsulitis of the shoulder,[21] (2) elbow extension in clients with severe burns,[37] and (3) wrist extension in clients with distal radius fractures[5] and stroke.[27] In this chapter, fabrication of a dynamic orthosis is used as an example to highlight the differences from a serial-static orthosis for reducing PIP flexion contractures.

Static-Progressive Orthotic Provision

A static-progressive orthosis includes a static orthotic base that has inelastic components to apply **torque** to a joint in order to statically position the joint as close as possible to end range.[36] Inelastic components may include Velcro tabs, progressive hinges, screws, or turnbuckles.[33,42] The position of the orthosis is adjusted by the clinician or client as the tissues lengthen in response to the stress applied by the orthosis. The tension provides the amount of force required to maintain the tissue at a maximum tolerable stretch.[36] A static-progressive orthosis is recommended during the proliferative and chronic **stages of tissue healing** when collagen is forming, remodeling, and reorganizing. The recommendations include (1) trauma to the elbow,[10] (2) limitations of forearm rotation,[31] (3) distal radius fracture and wrist injuries,[29,40] and (4) PIP joint flexion contractures.[4] In

this chapter, fabrication of a static-progressive orthosis is used as an example for increasing composite finger flexion.

Biomechanical Principles

An orthosis is an external mechanical device that requires an understanding of basic biomechanical principles.[16] In order for a mobilization orthosis to work properly, the therapist must comprehend the concept of force and how to apply it *safely* to an extremity. The goals for mobilization orthotic provision are correcting deformities, substituting for loss of muscle function, providing controlled motion, and aiding in wound healing. Knowledge of complicated mechanical calculations is not required to have a basic understanding of how to fabricate a mobilization orthosis. Several concepts for mobilization orthotic provision are presented that build on the biomechanical principles discussed in Chapter 3. They include anatomical considerations, mechanical advantage and torque, and application of force.

Anatomical Considerations

The goal of a mobilization orthosis is to restore the normal range of motion to a joint and to minimize the effects of inflammation and ensuing scar tissue. Application of an external force to healing tissues poses several clinical questions about the timing, the magnitude, and the direction of the force. During what stage in the healing process should an orthosis be used to mobilize tissue? How much force should be used? Where should the force be applied? When applying force to a contracted joint, ongoing assessment of inflammation and pain is essential before and after an orthosis is applied. Mild inflammation is acceptable, but edema should not fluctuate significantly. A mobilization orthosis applied too early after an injury can result in an increase of inflammation and a decrease in range of motion.

Soft-tissue structures respond to prolonged stress by changing or reforming. This activity is called **creep** and results from the application of prolonged force.[6] The soft tissue responds to excessive force with increased pain and a reintroduction of the inflammatory process.[17] By applying controlled stress to the tissue over a prolonged period of time, the therapist creates tension gentle enough to allow creep without tissue injury. Provided the tension remains within the tissues' elastic limits, the stress from a mobilization orthosis can positively affect the gradual realignment of collagen fibers. Important to note is this process results in stronger tensile strength of the tissue without causing microscopic tearing. The ability to alter collagen formation is greatest during the proliferative stage of wound healing but continues to a lesser degree for several months during scar maturation.[13]

Mechanical Advantage and Torque

To provide the greatest benefit from a mobilization orthosis, relevant knowledge of biomechanics is necessary.

Mechanical advantage is defined as the capacity to balance and to overcome resistance through the use of force and resistance lever arms.[34] The two lever arms represent the forces applied by the orthotic base and the dynamic portion of the orthosis. As seen in Figure 12-3, *applied force (Fa)* refers to the lever that applies force and *force resistance (Fr)* refers to the lever that applies resistance. The magnitude of the middle opposing force, *force magnitude (Fm)*, is determined by summing the opposing forces; $Fa + Fr$.[16] To calculate mechanical advantage, a ratio of the lever arm length *(la)* for the *applied force (Fa)* is divided by the lever arm length *(lr)* for the applied resistance *(Fr)*. Therefore, increasing the amount of applied force or decreasing the amount of applied resistance improves mechanical advantage.

By adjusting the length of the orthosis base or the length of an outrigger, the mechanical advantage can be altered (Figure 12-4).[33] The goal of the orthosis is to maintain a mechanical advantage of between 2:1 and 5:1, meaning that the lever arm of the applied force is between two to five times longer than the lever arm of the applied resistance.[7] An orthosis with a greater mechanical advantage will be more comfortable and durable.[16] A mobilization orthosis for MCP flexion that has a forearm and hand base will disperse pressure more effectively and provide greater mechanical advantage than a mobilization orthosis that has only a hand base, due to the longer lever arm of the applied force.

Torque is defined as the effect of force on the rotational movement of a joint.[19] The amount of torque is calculated by multiplying the applied force by the length of movement around a pivot point or axis. A relationship exists between the distance from a pivot point and the amount of force required. When achieving the same results, a force applied close to the pivot point (i.e., a short moment arm) must be greater than the force applied on a longer moment arm. This force is called *torque* because it acts on the rotational movement of a joint.

In practical terms, the force should be placed as far as possible from the mobilized joint without affecting other joints.[6a] A forearm-based dynamic wrist extension orthosis should be constructed so that its mobilizing force is on the most distal aspect of the palm, while not affecting MCP movement. An exception to placing the force as far from the mobilized joint as possible occurs with rheumatoid arthritis. If the joint is unstable, a force applied too far from the joint will result in a tilt rather than a gliding motion of the joint

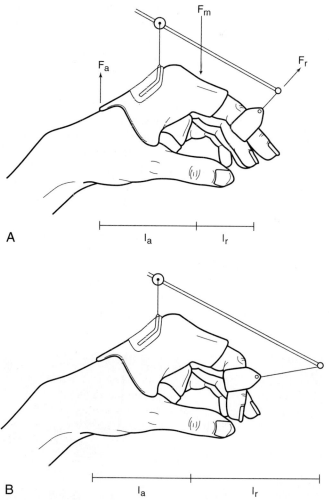

Figure 12-3 Mechanical advantage is demonstrated in two dynamic orthoses. Orthosis **A** has a better mechanical advantage than orthosis **B**.

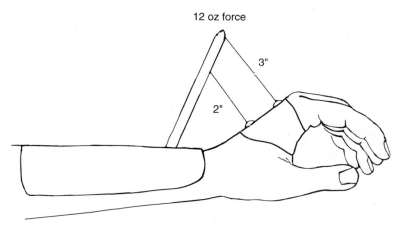

Figure 12-4 The 2-inch moment arm produces 24 inch ounces of torque. The 3-inch moment arm produces 36 inch ounces of torque.

(Figure 12-5).[23] Therefore, when fabricating an orthosis for the hand of a person with rheumatoid arthritis the force should be applied as close to the mobilizing joint as possible.

Application of Force

In dynamic orthotic provision, the direction and magnitude of the forces applied to a joint or finger are important considerations. When applying force to increase passive joint range of motion, the direction of pull must be at a 90-degree angle to the axis of the joint and perpendicular to the axis of rotation.[9] As the range of motion increases, adjustments are needed to the outrigger to maintain the 90-degree angle (Figure 12-6).[19] An extension outrigger should not pull the finger or hand toward ulnar deviation. In applying forces for finger flexion, the line of pull varies based on the number of fingers being mobilized. When one finger is mobilized, the tip of the digits should touch the palm in a small area near the thenar crease.[19] When multiple fingers are mobilized

simultaneously, the convergence point shifts to the radial middle third of the forearm (Figure 12-7).[19] Examples of these principles are depicted in Figure 12-7 and Figure 12-8.

Other important considerations include the magnitude of forces with mobilization orthotic provision. When excessive force is applied to the skin for a prolonged period, range of motion can be lost and tissue damage can occur. The amount of pressure that the skin can tolerate dictates the maximum tolerable force. As a general rule, the amount of acceptable pressure or force per unit area is 50 grams/centimeter^2.[6] This force approximates the same force as the weight of a banana resting on your palm. As the area of application where force is applied becomes larger, the force is dispersed and the pressure per unit area becomes less. A leather sling with a skin contact area on a finger of approximately 4 centimeters^2 should provide a maximum pressure of 200 grams.[19] A smaller sling with less skin contact area concentrates the pressure and is less tolerable.

Skin grafts, immature scar tissue, and fragile skin of older clients have less tolerance for sling pressure. The client's tolerance ultimately determines the amount of force. The client should report the sensation of a *gentle* stretch, not pain.[18] To avoid harm, a new orthosis should be monitored for the first 20 to 30 minutes of wear and at every treatment session thereafter. Education is critical for a client to monitor his or her orthosis for signs of pressure areas and skin breakdown, as well as how to don and doff the orthosis properly.

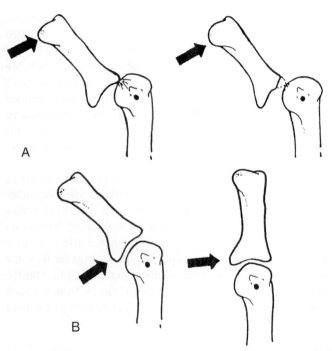

Figure 12-5 A force applied too far from an unstable joint results in "tilt" **(A)** rather than glide **(B).**

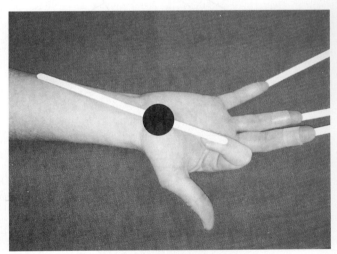

Figure 12-7 Line of pull for one digit.

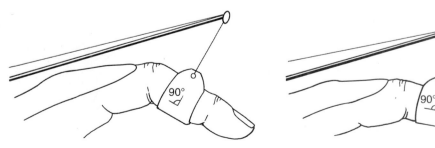

Figure 12-6 The line of tension must be maintained at 90 degrees from the long axis of the bone.

SELF-QUIZ 12-1*

Circle either true (T) or false (F).

1. T F A therapist should apply a dynamic orthosis to an extremity only when pain and inflammation are well controlled.
2. T F Creep occurs when soft tissue adapts through application of a prolonged force.
3. T F Clients who have new tissue or skin grafts have a high tolerance for pressure over those areas.
4. T F The focus of mobilization orthotic provision should be on increasing tension rather than increasing the amount of time that the orthosis is worn.
5. T F A general goal for mobilization orthotic provision is to increase passive range of motion by 10 degrees per week.
6. T F Joint end feel is an important consideration when determining whether to use static or dynamic tension.

*See Appendix A for the answer key.

Common Features of Mobilization Orthoses

The unique features of mobilization orthoses are the application of force, often done with an outrigger. The **outrigger** is a projection from the orthotic base and can be custom fabricated or a commercially available kit can be used. This is determined by the amount and position of the desired force. If the outrigger and attachment to the orthotic base is not secure, the direction of the mobilizing force may change, reducing the effectiveness of the orthosis.[11]

An outrigger can be a high or low profile (Figure 12-9). Each type has advantages and disadvantages. With a significant change in range of motion, the high-profile outrigger results in slightly less deviation from the 90-degree angle of pull than the low-profile outrigger. Clients should be seen in the clinic frequently enough so that increases in range of motion can be accommodated by regular adjustments to the outrigger, thus maintaining the 90-degree angle of pull.[2,16] It should be noted that a high-profile outrigger, on the other hand, is bulky and may decrease the client's compliance with wearing the orthosis. A low-profile outrigger requires adjustments more frequently but is more aesthetically pleasing and less cumbersome.

Outriggers are made from a variety of materials. Scraps of the thermoplastic material are rolled to form a strong tubular outrigger that can be easily adjusted and adheres well to the orthotic base. Some of the thermoplastic outriggers are made from commercially available tubes that are easily formed and provide a more uniform look.

Copper wire makes a good outrigger. A commonly used size is the ⅛-inch wire rod for its durability and ease to form with pliers or a bending jig. It takes practice to bend the wire into the desired shape. There are several different commercially available outrigger kits that add cost to the fabrication

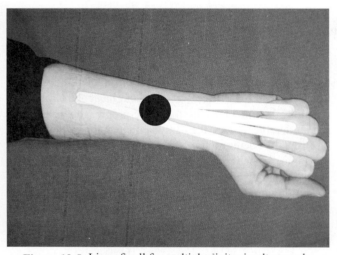

Figure 12-8 Line of pull for multiple digits simultaneously.

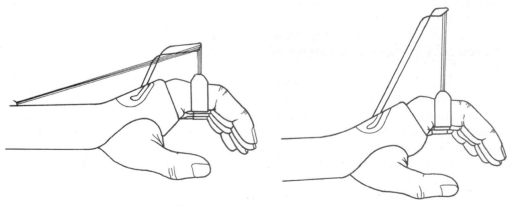

Figure 12-9 A low profile outrigger *(left)* versus a high-profile outrigger *(right)*.

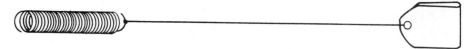

Figure 12-10 The therapist uses nonstretchable nylon string to attach finger loops to the source of tension.

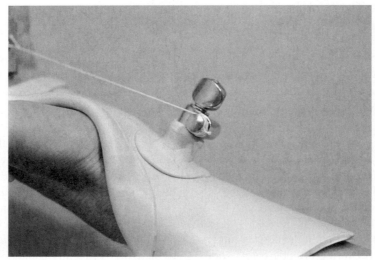

Figure 12-11 A turnbuckle can be easily adjusted to provide static tension.

of the orthosis. Extra expenses should be kept in mind, because the cost of the orthosis is determined by the price of the materials and the therapist's fabrication time.

The therapist uses various methods for applying dynamic force to a joint. **Finger loops** made from strong pliable material are usually best because of the increased conformability to the shape of the finger.[19] The therapist can supply force by using rubber bands, springs, or elastic thread. Although rubber bands are more readily available and easy to adjust, springs offer more consistent tension throughout the range. A long rubber band stretched over the maximum length of the orthosis provides more constant tension than a short rubber band.[6] Elastic thread is the easiest to apply and adjust, thereby saving time in the fabrication process. Its unique properties prevent wear even after 6 weeks of maximum stretch, making it useful for persistent finger contractures. A non-stretchable string or monofilament line is necessary to connect the finger loop to the source of the force (Figure 12-10). The choice is usually based on clinical experience and preferences, as in the end, all accomplish the same goals.

Another method of applying force is through static-progressive orthoses. Rather than providing the variable tension of a serial-static or dynamic orthosis, a **static-progressive orthosis** uses non-elastic tension to provide a constant force. An advantage of properly applied static tension is that tissue is not stretched beyond its elastic limit.[36] In place of the rubber band or spring (as used on a dynamic tension orthosis) the therapist may use a Velcro tab, turnbuckle, or commercially available static-progressive components to apply the force

(Figure 12-11). Tension is increased by gradually moving the Velcro tab more proximally on the orthotic base or adjusting the turnbuckle. The force is static rather than dynamic but is readily adjustable by the client throughout the wearing time (Figure 12-12). Because the client has control over the amount of applied tension, the static-progressive orthosis is more tolerable to wear than a dynamic tension orthosis.[36]

Critically determining whether to apply serial-static, dynamic, or static-progressive tension, the therapist must identify the **end feel** of a joint. End feel is assessed by passively moving a joint to its maximal end range. A joint with a soft or springy end feel indicates immature scar tissue. A joint with a hard end feel indicates a more mature scar tissue or long-standing contracture. An orthosis with static or dynamic tension is appropriate for a joint with a soft end feel, whereas a joint with a hard end feel responds only to static tension. Regardless of the end feel, static tension increases passive range of motion faster than dynamic tension of any joint.[35]

Another determinant in selecting the type of tension to be used with mobilization orthotic provision is the stage of tissue healing. As seen in Figure 12-2, different types of orthoses are more appropriate at various stages of healing and can assist with mobilization of hand structures.

The common features of mobilization orthoses have been described in their role to apply forces through serial-static, dynamic, and/or static-progressive types of mobilization orthoses. The following sections provide technical tips, materials and equipment, and precautions that can be used for dynamic orthotic provision.

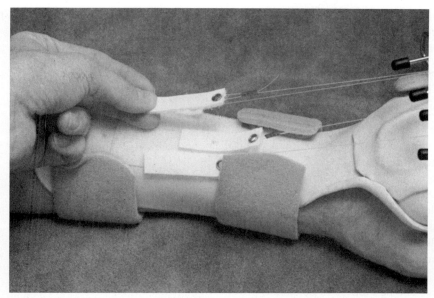

Figure 12-12 The person may adjust Velcro tabs used for static-progressive tension.

Technical Tips for Dynamic Orthotic Provision

- To apply a thermoplastic outrigger to the orthotic base, which is commonly a wrist immobilization orthosis, both surfaces need to be clean and smooth.
- Some thermoplastic materials are treated or coated to minimize the self-adherence when accidentally touched to itself. The coating can be scratched off or a bonding agent can be used to increase the self-adherence.
- After determining where the outrigger should be placed, heat both surfaces (with a heat gun or immerse in hot water), hold the surfaces together firmly while smoothing out the edges.
- Using cold spray speeds the hardening process. Alternatively, the orthosis and outrigger can be held under cold water at the sink to hasten hardening.
- To apply a wire outrigger, use a small patch of thermoplastic material. Wire conducts heat more easily than the thermoplastic material and will burn skin if touched accidentally.
- Heat the orthotic base and the thermoplastic patch, and lightly heat the end of the wire. The wire heating allows the wire outrigger to lightly "melt" into the orthotic base while the thermoplastic patch is placed over the ends of the outrigger wire and smoothed into place.
- Be careful that the wire does not deform the base or push through the thermoplastic patch.
- If the orthotic base is curved, the wire needs to be contoured to that shape before it is attached.
- The warm thermoplastic material adheres to post-operative bandages, dressings, or stockinette. Use a stockinette covering over such dressing to avoid adherence.
- If the client's skin is sensitive to the heat from the thermoplastic material, use a damp paper towel or apply the stockinette to the body part prior to applying the thermoplastic material. When the orthosis is cooled and removed, the adhering stockinette can be cut off the arm and pulled from the orthosis.
- Check the line of pull so that a 90-degree angle is present on the finger loops when axial and lateral views are observed.
- Check all joints from various angles to ensure that joints are not pulled into hyperextension, ulnar or radial deviation, or torque/rotational forces. Correct angles are particularly important when fabricating an orthosis for fractures, joint arthroplasties, or ligament repairs.

Materials and Equipment for a Dynamic Orthosis

In addition to the equipment necessary to fabricate a static orthosis, a variety of items are required to fabricate a dynamic orthosis. The following is a list of materials and equipment most commonly used, although not all items are used for every orthosis.

- Thermoplastic materials of different thicknesses with a high level of self-adhesion
- Finger loops/slings
- Nail hooks, an emery board, super glue, and super glue remover, such as acetone or fingernail polish remover
- Solvent
- Non-stretchable nylon string (e.g., outrigger line—monofilament/fishing line)
- An outrigger kit
- Wire rod (⅛ inch) with tools to bend
- Rubber bands, springs, elastic string, Velcro tabs, turnbuckles, or commercially available static-progressive components, rubber band posts
- Safety pins, paper clips, other material to make a hook or pulley, eyelets
- Pliers, wire bender, wire cutters, scissors

Fabrication of mobilization orthoses can be both challenging and fun, but very rewarding when clients' function improves due to the therapist's skills and intervention.

Precautions for a Mobilization (Dynamic) Orthosis

Specific precautions are needed when applying mobilization orthoses. The first rule of mobilization orthoses, and of all intervention, is to do no harm. Several guidelines are provided to follow this rule.[18]

- The client must be responsible enough to care for the orthosis and to follow a guided wearing schedule. A mobilization orthosis is not appropriate for a child or an adult who cannot follow instructions.
- Keep in mind normal functional anatomy and biomechanics of the upper limb.
- Apply minimal force. The amount of force should provide a low-grade stretch that is tolerable over a long period of time.[12] Signs that indicate too much force is exerted includes reddened pressure areas, cyanosis of the fingertips, and complaints of pain or numbness. A client will likely not wear an orthosis that causes discomfort.
- Keep in mind the risks of wearing an ill-fitted orthosis, such as pressure points, skin breakdown, and prolonged immobilization of noninvolved structures.
- Remember aesthetics. A client is more likely to wear an orthosis that has a finished, professional appearance. An orthosis with a low-profile outrigger may be more aesthetically pleasing than a high profile outrigger.
- Monitor and adjust the orthosis frequently for accurate fit.
- Listen to the client. The orthosis must fit well, have a tolerable amount of tension, and cause minimal interference with daily activities. Complaints by the client require reevaluation of the orthotic fit.
- Use extreme caution when applying an external force to a hand that has decreased sensation. An increased risk of skin breakdown exists if an orthosis creates an excessive amount of force in the absence of sensory feedback.
- The altered joint mechanics of a client who has rheumatoid arthritis make static orthotic provision more desirable than mobilization orthotic provision. A therapist may use mobilization orthotic provision, especially the dynamic type, on a client with rheumatoid arthritis, but only if specific indications are met. In these cases, only very gentle tension is applied as close to the joint as possible. The goal of orthotic provision is to gently stretch involved soft tissue or to provide gentle resistance to weakened muscles.[8] Caution needs to be exercised at all time to avoid adverse reactions.

Clinical Considerations for Mobilization Orthoses

Four select orthoses represent the four types of mobilization orthoses. The fabrication procedure is described for each orthosis.

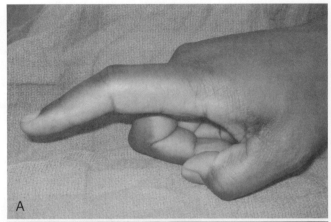

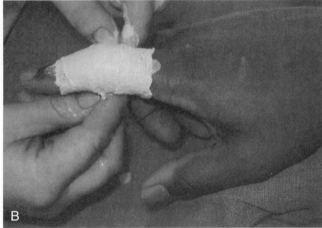

Figure 12-13 A and **B,** Demonstration of a serial cast being applied to a finger with a proximal interphalangeal (PIP) flexion contracture.

Serial-Static Casting (Orthosis) for Proximal Interphalangeal Flexion Contractures

Serial casting is an excellent way to correct PIP flexion contractures through low-load, prolonged stress. Serial casts are effective when the contracture is greater than 45 to 50 degrees or less than 20 degrees. Although a cast is worn full time, it does not interfere with function of the hand as the MCP and DIP joints remain free. The following steps are instructions for creating a serial-static orthosis (Figure 12-13, *A*).

1. Cut plaster casting tape into 1″ × 8″ lengths. A product called Specialist Extra-Fast Plaster, Green Label sets in 2 to 4 minutes.
2. Roll plaster strips into rolls.
3. Fill the small bowl with hot water. The hotter the water, the faster the plaster sets.
4. Dip one plaster roll into the hot water, squeeze the excess water from the roll, and begin wrapping the finger with no tension from the DIP crease to the MCP crease while the client extends the finger straight and the therapist applies gentle traction to the finger tip. Be careful not to pull plaster tight during rolling.
5. Smooth the plaster with wet fingers while rolling to laminate layers of plaster together (see Figure 12-13, *B*).

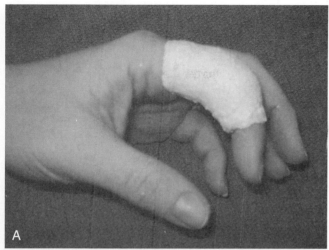

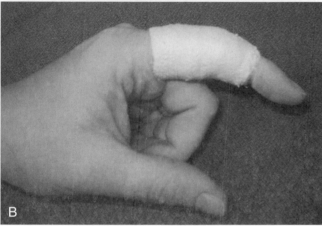

Figure 12-14 **A** and **B,** Examples of finished plaster casts for different proximal interphalangeal (PIP) flexion contractures.

6. Keep rolling plaster rolls until you have an even thickness, approximately 6 to 8 rolls.

7. Be sure to smooth the edges at the MCP and DIP joints so that the client can flex these joints.

8. Do not push down on the PIP joint to straighten finger; instead, smooth, roll, and pull along the finger to straighten the finger while the plaster is setting.

9. The plaster cast should be changed every 3 to 5 days or a maximum of 7 days if necessary.[20]

10. To remove the cast, soak the hand in warm water for approximately 5 to 10 minutes, and cut it off with small cast scissors, which are commercially available.

11. Casts are fairly durable and usually hold up during hand washing and showers, but clients may want to wrap the finger in plastic wrap (or Press-n-Seal) to maintain the integrity of the cast.

12. If the DIP joint is included because of a flexion contracture, apply ½-inch wide paper tape along the distal phalanx folding over the tip to extend approximately 1 inch from the end of the finger to give the therapist or the client the ability to hold and apply traction on the finger while rolling the plaster to the end of the finger.

13. Figure 12-14 shows completed casts in various stages of extension.

Mobilization (Dynamic) Orthotic Provision for Proximal Interphalangeal Flexion Contractures

A hand based PIP extension orthosis corrects deformities caused by muscle-tendon tightness or joint contractures. A dynamic orthosis with an outrigger is easily adjusted as the client's range of motion increases. There are several commercially available outriggers that include the components necessary to attach, assemble, and adjust as needed, for one or multiple fingers. Keep in mind that such kits increase the total cost of the orthosis. Outriggers can be fabricated "from scratch" with the common materials available in the clinic, such as thermoplastic material, outrigger wire, rubber bands, and a paperclip.

The following steps are instructions for creating a mobilization or dynamic orthosis for PIP flexion contractures. Fabricate a pattern for a dorsal based hand based orthosis, immobilizing the MCP joint of the involved finger(s) in 45 to 50 degrees of flexion. A thermoplastic material that conforms to the hand is optimal. Be sure to conform around the thumb web space and ulnar side of the hand. Avoid extending the length of the orthosis into the wrist, which may cause rubbing or irritation of the ulnar styloid. Unnecessary joints should not be hindered by the edges of the orthosis. Figure 12-15 provides a detailed pattern for the orthosis.

1. The distal edge should extend the length of the proximal phalanx but not impede PIP motion. The edges should be flared. Soft adhesive backed padding extending over the edges may be added for comfort along the dorsum of the proximal phalanx.

2. If an outrigger kit or wire outrigger is not used, the outrigger can be made from a rolled rectangular piece of thermoplastic materials or Aquaplast tubes that are approximately twice the length of the MCP and finger.

3. With the thermoplastic outrigger warm and pliable, find the center. Shape into a half square that is the width of the finger and cool. The outriggers' end should center on the middle phalanx. Using a hole punch, "cut" a half hole or notch to act as a pulley when the finger loop is attached. Immediately proximal to the metacarpal, the outrigger should bend to attach to the base of the orthosis. This angle should be approximately 45 to 50 degrees (Figure 12-16). Mark the base orthosis where the outrigger will attach with a grease marker or pencil; the marking should follow the metacarpal of the involved finger(s).

4. Remove the orthosis from the hand to attach the outrigger. To create a low profile outrigger, the outrigger should rise approximately 1 inch above the distal end of the orthosis at the proximal phalanx. Spot heat the ends of the outrigger and the base of the orthosis with a heat gun, and attach the outrigger. A bonding solvent is beneficial for a strong, permanent attachment.

5. When cool, reapply the orthosis, and add Velcro strapping; be sure to keep the orthosis from migrating distally. This can be accomplished by placing a strap around the base of the thumb and through the palm.

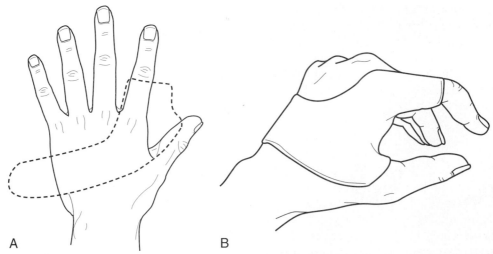

Figure 12-15 **A,** Orthotic pattern for a hand based proximal interphalangeal (PIP) extension orthosis. **B,** Orthosis formed on the hand.

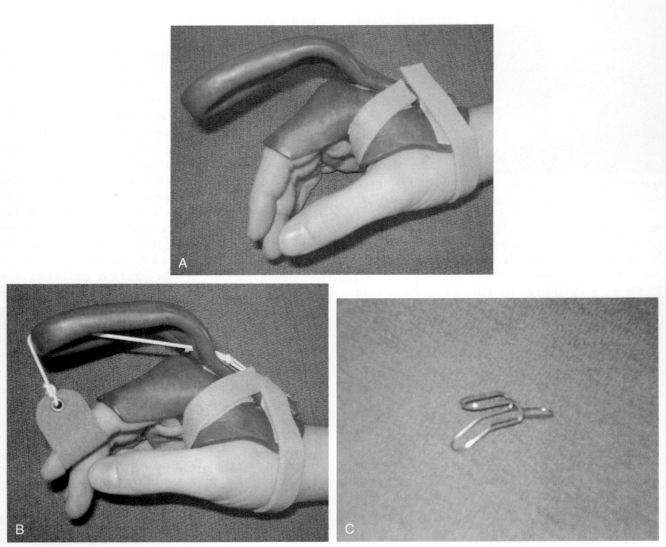

Figure 12-16 **A,** The outrigger attaches to the base and extends out over the finger. **B,** The finished orthosis, with the finger loop extending the finger, while maintaining a 90 degree angle of pull. **C,** Folding the center of the paperclip while curving the ends with needle nose pliers makes a good anchor for dynamic attachments. The loop can be threaded through the hook and then adjusted by wrapping around the hook.

6. A finger loop is made from soft leather or strapping material. Commercial finger loops are available and are comfortable. The loop should be 3 to 4 inches long and as wide as the middle phalanx. Trim the width of the finger loops if they cover the DIP and PIP flexion creases. Holes punched on both ends of the loop are threaded with monofilament line. The line is attached to a Velcro tab to create a static-progressive pull (or a rubber band or elastic thread) to create a dynamic pull (Figure 12-16, *B*).

7. If using the Velcro tab, the Velcro hook is attached to the base of the orthosis. If using the dynamic traction, use a needle nosed pliers to fold a paper clip, which makes a good hook for the attachment (Figure 12-16, *C*). The paperclip is secured with a small piece of thermoplastic material and is similar to attaching the outrigger to the base of the orthosis.

8. While the client wears the orthosis, a rubber band is threaded through the paperclip hook. The therapist pulls the finger loop over the top of the distal end of the outrigger into the notch and loop(s) around the finger. Make sure to have a 90-degree angle of pull from anterior and lateral perspectives.

9. The therapist experiments to determine the appropriate length of elastic thread or rubber band. After wearing the orthosis for 20 to 30 minutes, patients should not complain of their finger getting cold, going numb, or turning "blue." Patients should describe feeling gentle tension at the end range.

10. This orthosis is worn 20 to 30 minutes at a time, four to five times a day.

Another option for the same type of orthosis is a mobilizing PIP extension orthosis, utilizing an extender rod instead of an outrigger made out of thermoplastic material. Please refer to Evolve web site for detailed instructions on how to fabricate a mobilization orthosis for radial nerve palsy.

Dynamic Orthotic Provision for Flexor Tendon Injuries

A flexor tendon orthosis can substitute for the loss of muscle function and controlled movement while the tendon heals. A flexor tendon mobilization orthosis is one of the least complicated orthoses to fabricate because an outrigger is not required. However, it is a very demanding orthosis, because initially it must be worn 24 hours per day and removed only for therapy. Therefore, it must fit well to ensure comfort and to prevent migration. The therapist should check the physician's preference for tendon repair protocols. Although no one protocol is universally accepted,[39] the most common approaches are the Kleinert and colleagues[26] and the Duran and colleagues[15] methods. For novice therapists, it is advisable to review zones of the hand and the protocols because there are many precautions. It is strongly advisable to consult with a more experienced therapist. The following steps

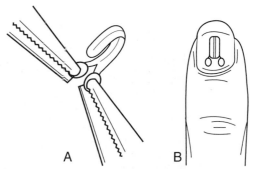

Figure 12-17 **A,** Pliers may be used to adjust the hook to fit the contour of the fingernail. **B,** The nail hook is applied to the proximal nail bed.

are instructions for creating a dynamic orthosis using modifications from both protocols.

1. To apply a nail hook to the client's proximal portion of the fingernail, use an emery board to roughen the fingernail. Apply super glue to attach the hook to the nail bed. Allow the glue to dry thoroughly before applying the force. Educate the client on the reason for the hook application. Assure the client that removal of the hook is possible. Before application of the hook to the fingernail, the hook may require an adjustment with two pairs of pliers to fit the contour of the nail (Figure 12-17, *A*). Position the hook so that the hooks point towards the nail bed. Hooks should be applied to the proximal end of the nail bed to prevent avulsion of the fingernail (see Figure 12-17, *B*). When applying the hook, do not use an excessive amount of glue. Glue that comes in a gel form may be easier to manage. Give the client extra hooks and application instructions because hooks occasionally break free from the nail bed. Alternatives to the nail hooks are adhesive Velcro loops applied to the nail or sutures placed through physician-created holes in the nail during surgery.

2. Construct the pattern for a dorsal wrist orthosis, similar to that shown in Figure 12-18 (refer to Chapter 7 for instructions). Select a thermoplastic material with the property of drapability. Remember to design the pattern to cover two-thirds the length of the forearm. The distal end of the orthosis should extend about 1 inch beyond the tips of the fingers.

3. The hand position varies according to surgeon preference. Klein[25] recommends 20 degrees wrist flexion and 40 to 50 degrees of MCP flexion. To maintain the wrist in a safe position and for ease of application, rest the forearm and hand on a foam wedge. This positions the wrist and fingers in the suggested posture (Figure 12-19, *A*). Instruct the patient not to extend the wrist to maintain the protective position. It can be helpful to have the patient use the uninvolved hand to gently prevent the wrist from extending. Since the orthosis is usually made postoperatively and the patient is wearing a bandage, cover the dressing with a stockinette sleeve (Figure 12-19, *B*) to

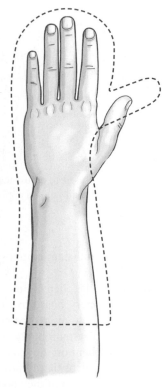

Figure 12-18 Pattern for a dorsal block orthosis that is used after a flexor tendon repair.

keep the warm thermoplastic material from sticking to the bandage (Figure 12-19, *C*). Cutting the sleeve off to remove the orthosis when cooled is easier than pulling the material off a bandage on a likely sore and swollen hand. To create a bubble to prevent pressure over the ulnar styloid, a small amount of therapy putty over the ulnar styloid makes a good temporary pad during the initial fabrication. Orthotic material with memory is helpful if needed to reform the orthosis.

4. Apply straps with hook-and-loop Velcro at the following locations: across the palmar bar, at the wrist, 3 inches proximal to the wrist, and across the proximal forearm.

5. Attach a safety pin to the strap that crosses the wrist approximately 3 inches proximal to the wrist crease. Make sure that the pulley pulls more palmarly so that the DIPs are passively flexed (Figure 12-20, *A*).

6. Apply traction using elastic thread attached to the nail hooks at the distal end and to the safety pin at the proximal end. Elastic thread is used due to its ability to stretch while maintaining a fairly constant tension. Apply the force to hold the fingers in flexion, but allow the client to achieve full active extension of the interphalangeal (IP) joints against the force of the elastic (see Figure 12-20, *B*). Full IP extension may take a few days to achieve if the client has been immobilized previously with the fingers flexed. As IP extension improves, adjust the orthosis' elastic tension

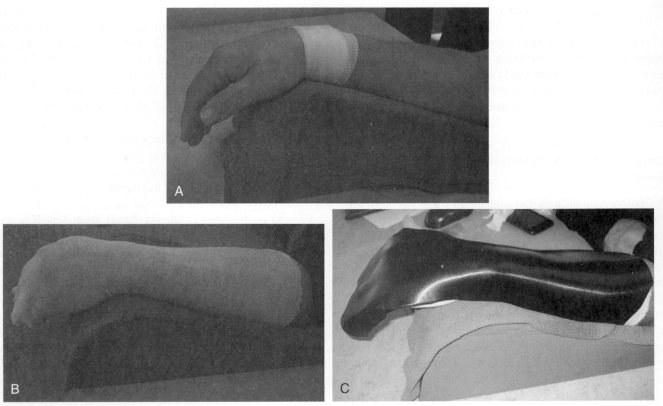

Figures 12-19 With the forearm and hand resting on the wedge, the ideal position after flexor tendon repair can be achieved with minimal discomfort to the client (A, B, C).

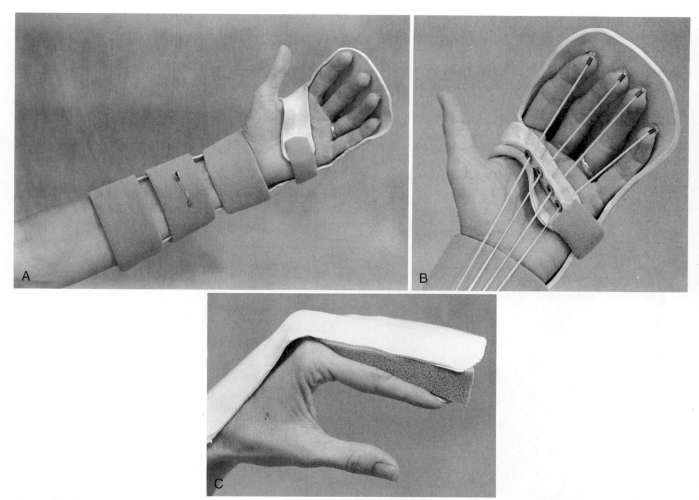

Figure 12-20 **A,** Straps are applied across the palmar bar, at the wrist, 3 inches proximal to the wrist, and at the forearm. The safety pin is fixed to the strap 3 inches proximal to the wrist crease. **B,** The person must be able to attain full IP active extension against the force of the tension. **C,** To attain full PIP extension, a wedge may be inserted.

to maintain passive finger flexion while achieving full active extension.

7. Achieving full IP extension is important because flexion contractures are common complications following flexor tendon repair.[24] If the client is unable to attain full IP extension, a wedge may be placed on the dorsum of the involved finger(s) inside the dorsal hood of the orthosis. The purpose of the wedge is to increase MCP flexion, thus decreasing flexor tension and increasing IP extension (Figure 12-20, *C*).

8. Due to the confined arrangement of tendons within the pulley system, flexor tendon injuries in zone II are highly susceptible to adhesions (Figure 12-21).[14] A palmar pulley provides greater excursion of tendons by maintaining resting position with composite flexion rather than primarily PIP flexion. The palmar bar serves to maintain the palmar arch and prevent orthotic migration. The pulley is created by firmly attaching an additional piece of thermoplastic material with eyelets for each finger. The referring physician may specify whether all digits or only the injured

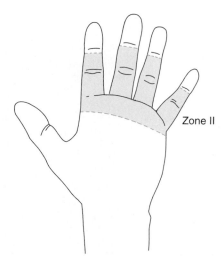

Figure 12-21 A palmar pulley may be best for tendon injuries in zone II.

digit(s) should be included (Figure 12-22). The therapist may apply a strap to the distal aspect of the fingers to maintain full IP extension. This application may reduce the loss of extension at the IP joints and is generally used for night wear or if the person is developing an IP flexion contracture. With an IP flexion contracture and with physician approval, the person may alternate between flexion traction and the extension strap during the day (Figure 12-23).

Static-Progressive Approach for Composite Finger Flexion

It is common for the fingers to become stiff after trauma to the hand or wrist. Stiffness may be due to joint pain or swelling, which prevents an ability to achieve full finger flexion.

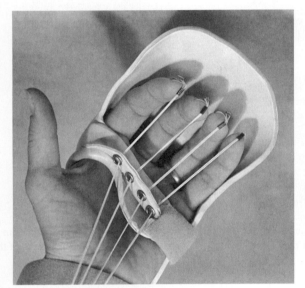

Figure 12-22 An attachment may be added to the palmar bar to increase tendon excursion in zone II injuries.

Although clients may be actively participating in a therapy program that focuses on edema control, range of motion, and tendon gliding to achieve full composite finger flexion, an orthosis that aids in wound healing or tissue remodeling through low-load prolonged stress to the joints can maximize return to function.

For the hand to function optimally, the PIP joint needs to extend and flex to the palm. Different types of grasps are important for occupational activities, such as the ability to slip the hand into a pocket, to put on a glove, grasp coins, or hold a wrench. The PIP joint can lose extension from the following:

- Crush injury
- Burn or fracture around the PIP joint
- Flexor tendon injury
- Ligament injury
- Excessive swelling of the hand following injury elsewhere
- Immobilization and disuse

There are several different ways to mobilize PIP joints to gain passive flexion with either custom fabricated or prefabricated orthoses. The following steps are instructions for creating a custom fabricated static-progressive orthosis for the hand. Static-progressive tension allows the person to maintain the tissue at a maximum tolerable stretch.[36]

1. Fabricate a volar-based wrist immobilization orthosis with the wrist in 30 to 45 degrees extension to maximize finger flexion (refer to Chapter 7 for instructions).
2. To fabricate the finger cuff, use a thinner (1/16 inch) thermoplastic material. Cut two pieces 1/2 inch to 3/4 inch wide and 1 1/2 to 2 inches long. Mold one cuff halfway around dorsum of proximal phalanx and the other cuff over distal phalanx.
3. Punch small holes using a hole punch on either side of the two cuffs. Cut a piece of monofilament line approximately 10 to 12 inches long. Tie the start of the monofilament line on one side of the distal cuff (Figure 12-24, *A*). Thread it through one side of the proximal cuff, and then

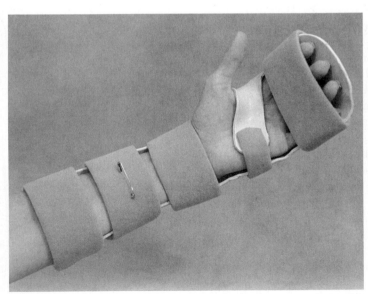

Figure 12-23 The person may use a strap to secure fingers in extension for night wear.

through the other side of the proximal cuff. Tie off on the other side of the distal cuff (Figure 12-24, *B*).

4. Find the center of the monofilament line, and slip it through the small hole at one end of a Velcro loop ½″ × 2″ to create a completed flexion cuff.

5. Repeat this for additional fingers as needed.

6. This cuff is applied to the stiff finger(s) when pulled toward the forearm. The tension should cause the finger to flex first at the DIP, then at the PIP, and finally at the MCP into the palm (composite fist).

7. Reapply the volar orthosis, and apply straps across the dorsum of the hand, at the wrist and forearm.

8. Fit the individual finger flexion cuffs, and gently pull them toward the forearm (Figure 12-25, *A*), to determine where to place the Velcro hook on the volar aspect of the wrist orthosis (Figure 12-25, *B*).

9. The cuffs should be pulled tight enough to provide gentle tension to the fingers. After each 5 minutes attempt to tighten the tension as tolerated, with the goal of wearing the orthosis 30 minutes for two times a day.

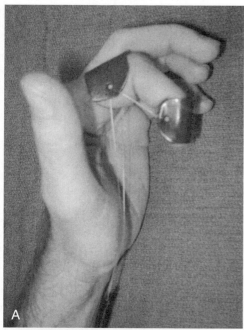

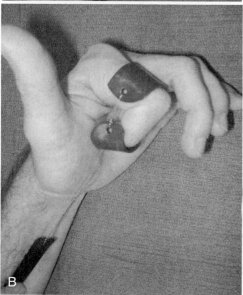

Figure 12-24 The fishing line should start from the distal cuff through both holes on the proximal cuff before ending on the other side of the distal cuff, leaving enough fishing line to loop through the Velcro tap and reaching mid way down the forearm (A, B).

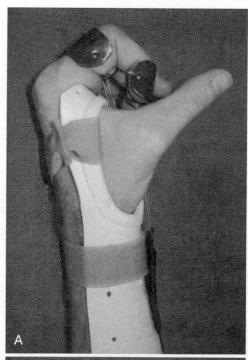

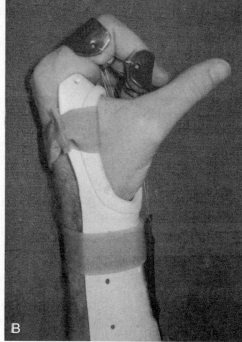

Figure 12-25 When completed, the fingers can be pulled into a composite fist position, adjusting the Velcro loop as tolerated every 5 minutes with a goal of wearing the orthosis 30 minutes at a time (A, B).

There are other options for finger cuffs, including leather, commercially available finger loops, or strapping material. Please refer to Appendix Evolve web site for another option of detailed instructions for fabrication of a composite finger flexion orthosis with static-progressive tension.

Review Questions

1. What are four possible goals of mobilization orthotic provision?
2. What criteria are used to determine whether to use static or dynamic tension?
3. What is the angle of pull between the long axis of the bone and the outrigger line that must be maintained?
4. What are the complications associated with orthotic application of too much force?
5. What is the acceptable force per unit area for sling pressure?
6. What information should the therapist gather before considering a mobilization orthosis for a client?
7. What is the difference between a high and a low profile outrigger? What are the advantages and disadvantages of each?
8. What are three methods for the application of force?
9. What are the steps for attaching a wire outrigger to the base of an orthosis?
10. What are three precautions with mobilization orthotic provision?

References

1. American Society of Hand Therapists: *Splint classification system*, Garner, NC, 1992, The American Society of Hand Therapists.
2. Austin G, Slamet M, Cameron D, et al.: A comparison of high-profile and low-profile mobilization splint designs, *J Hand Ther* 17(3):336–343, 2004.
2a. Bailey J, Cannon N, Colditz J, et al.: *Splint classification system*, Chicago, 1992, American Society of Hand Therapists.
3. Bell-Krotoski JA, Figarola JH: Biomechanics of soft-tissue growth and remodeling with plaster casting, *J Hand Ther* 8(2):131–137, 1995.
4. Benaglia PG, Sartorio F, Franchignoni F: A new thermoplastic splint for proximal interphalangeal joint flexion contractures, *J Sports Med Phys Fitness* 39(3):249–252, 1999.
5. Berner SH, Willis FB: Dynamic splinting in wrist extension following distal radius fractures, *J Orthop Surg Res* 5:53, 2010.
6. Brand PW, Hollister AM: Terminology, how joints move, mechanical resistance, and external stress: effect at the surface. In Brand PW, Hollister AM, editors: *Clinical mechanics of the hand*, St Louis, 1993, Mosby.
6a. Brand PW, Hollister A: External stress: effects at the surface. In Brand PW, Hollister AM, editors: *Clinical mechanics of the hand*, St Louis, 1993, Mosby.
7. Brand PW: The forces of dynamic splinting. Ten questions before applying a dynamic splint to the hand. In Hunter JM, Mackin EJ, Callahan AD, editors: *Rehabilitation of the hand*, ed 5, St Louis, 2002, Mosby.
8. Cailliet R: Functional anatomy and joints: injuries and disease. In Cailliet R, editor: *Hand pain and impairment*, ed 4, Philadelphia, PA, 1993, FA Davis.

9. Cannon N, Foltz R, Koepfer J, et al.: Mechanical principles. In Cannon NM, editor: *Manual of hand splinting*, New York, 1985, Churchill Livingstone.
10. Chinchalkar SJ, Pearce J, Athwal GS: Static progressive versus three-point elbow extension splinting: a mathematical analysis, *J Hand Ther* 22(1):22–37, 2009.
11. Coldiz JC: Low profile dynamic splinting of the injured hand, *Am J Occup Ther* 37(3):182–188, 1983.
12. Colditz JC: Therapist's management of the stiff hand. In Hunter JM, Schneider LH, Mackin EJ, et al, editors: *Rehabilitation of the hand*, St Louis, 1995, Mosby.
13. Colditz JC: Dynamic splinting of the stiff hand. In Hunter JM, Mackin EJ, Callahan AD, editors: *Rehabilitation of the hand*, ed 5, St Louis, 2002, Mosby.
14. Duran RJ, Coleman CR, Nappi JF, et al.: Management of flexor tendon lacerations in zone 2 using controlled passive motion post-operatively, In Hunter JM, Schnieder LH, Mackin EJ, et al.: *Rehabilitation of the hand*, St Louis, 1990, Mosby.
15. Duran R, Houser R: Controlled passive motion following flexor tendon repair in zones 2 and 3. In Curtis RM, editor: *AAOS Symposium on Tendon Surgery in the Hand*, Philadelphia, 1976, Lippincott, Williams, and Wilkins.
16. Fess EE: Splints: mechanics versus convention, *J Hand Ther* 8(2):124–130, 1995.
17. Fess EE, McCollum M: The influence of splinting on healing tissues, *J Hand Ther* 11:125–130, 1998.
18. Fess EE, Philips CA, Gettle-Harmon K, et al.: *Hand and upper extremity splinting: principles and methods*, ed 3, St Louis, 2002, Mosby.
19. Fess EE, Gettle K, Philips C, et al.: *Hand and upper extremity splinting: principles and methods*, ed 3, St Louis, 2005, Mosby.
20. Flowers K, LaStayo P: Effect of total end range time on improving passive range of motion, *J Hand Ther* 7:150–157, 1994.
21. Gaspar PD, Willis FB: Adhesive capsulitis and dynamic splinting: a controlled, cohort study, *BMC Musculoskelet Disord* 10:111, 2009.
22. Glasgow C, Tooth L, Fleming J, et al.: Dynamic splinting for the stiff hand after trauma: predictors of contracture resolution, *J Hand Ther* 24:195–206, 2011.
23. Hollister A, Giurintano D: *How joints move: clinical mechanics of the hand*, St Louis, 1993, Mosby.
24. Jebson PL, Kasdan ML: *Hand secrets*, ed 3, Philadelphia, 2006, Elsevier Mosby.
25. Klein LJ: Tendon injury. In Cooper C, editor: *Fundamentals of hand therapy: clinical reasoning and treatment guidelines for common diagnoses of the upper extremity*, St Louis, 2007, Mosby Elsevier, pp 320–347.
26. Kleinert HE, Kutz JE, Atasay E, et al.: Primary repair of flexor tendons, *Orthop Clin North Am* 4(4):865–876, 1973.
27. Lai JM, Francisco GE, Willis B: Dynamic splinting after treatment with Botulinum Toxin Type-A: a randomized controlled pilot study, *Advanced Therapy* 26(2):241–248, 2009.
28. Loth TS, Wadsworth CT: *Orthopedic review for physical therapists*, St Louis, 1998, Mosby.
29. Lucado AM, Li Z: Static progressive splinting to improve wrist stiffness after distal radius fracture: a prospective case series study, *Physiother Theory Pract* 25(4):297–309, 2009.
30. May E, Silfverskiold K, Sollerman C: Controlled mobilization after flexor tendon repair in zone II: a prospective comparison of three methods, *J Hand Surg Am* 17(5):942–952, 1992.
31. McGrath MS, Ulrich SF, Bonutti PM, et al.: Static progressive splinting for restoration of rotational motion of the forearm, *J Hand Ther* 22(1):3–8, 2009.

32. McKee PR, Rivard A: A biopsychosocial approach to orthotic intervention, *J Hand Ther* 24:155–163, 2011.

33. Morrey BF: Splinting and bracing at the elbow. In Morrey BF, editor: *The elbow and its disorders*, Philadelphia, PA, 2000, Saunders.

34. Rybski M: *Kinesiology for occupational therapy*, ed 2, Thorofare, NJ, 2012, Slack Inc.

35. Schultz-Johnson K: Splinting the wrist: mobilization and protection, *J Hand Ther* 9(2):165–177, 1996.

36. Schultz-Johnson K: Static progressive splinting, *J Hand Ther* 15(2):163–178, 2002.

37. Shanesy RR, Miller CP: Dynamic versus static splints: a prospective case for sustained stress, *J Burn Care Rehabil* 16(3 Pt 1):284–287, 1995.

38. Smith LK, Weiss EL, Lehmkuhl DL: *Brunnstrom's clinical kinesiology*, ed 5, Philadelphia, PA, 1996, FA Davis.

39. Stewart KM, van Strien G: Postoperative management of flexor tendon injuries. In Hunter JM, Schnieder LH, Mackin EJ, et al.: *Rehabilitation of the hand*, ed 5, St Louis, 2002, Mosby.

40. Sueoka SS, Detemple K: Static-progressive splinting in under 25 minutes and 25 dollars, *J Hand Ther* 24(3):280–286, 2011.

41. Recor CJ, Johnson CW: Hand therapy. In Trumble T, Rayan GM, Budoff JE, et al, editors: *Principles of hand surgery and therapy*, ed 2, Philadelphia, 2010, Saunders.

42. Trumble TE, Rayan GM, Budoff JE, et al.: *Principles of hand surgery and therapy*, ed 2, Philadelphia, PA, 2010, Saunders.

APPENDIX 12-1   CASE STUDY

CASE STUDY 12-1*

Tom is a 54-year-old mechanic who slipped on oil in his garage and broke his right dominant wrist. He had surgery for an intra-articular distal radius (Colles) fracture. His hand was severely swollen and despite early intervention by occupational therapy for edema control, tendon gliding, and range of motion, he developed stiff fingers and was unable to make a complete fist at 9 weeks post injury. He is using his hand for all activities of daily living (ADLs) and with light to moderate functional activities. He can put on a glove and slip his hand into his pocket, but he is unable to tightly grip a wrench or the steering wheel. As part of his home exercise program a mobilization orthosis is recommended to increase composite finger flexion.

1. What clinical evaluation is required before fabrication of the orthosis? Answer yes (Y) or no (N) to the following options:
   a. Evaluation of active and passive range of motion of the fingers (Y/N)
   b. Evaluation of sensibility (Y/N)
   c. ADL evaluation (Y/N)
2. What is the primary purpose of this orthosis?
   a. To increase strength in the hand
   b. To increase active extension of the fingers
   c. To increase passive flexion of the fingers
   d. Protect damaged nerves in the hand
3. What is the most desirable source of finger traction for this orthosis?
   a. Rubber band traction
   b. Spring wire
   c. Turnbuckle
   d. Elastic thread
4. How often should Tom wear the orthosis?
   a. 60 minutes, four times a day
   b. 30 minutes, two times a day
   c. 5 minutes, eight times a day
   d. 4 hours at a time

*See Appendix A for the answer key for Case Study 12-1.

FORM 12-1* Static-progressive finger flexion orthosis

After the person wears the orthosis for 30 minutes, answer the following questions. (Mark NA for non-applicable situations.)

Evaluation Areas				**Comments**
Design				
1. The orthotic trough is the proper length and width.	Yes ○	No ○	NA ○	
2. The orthotic trough supports, does not push on the arches.	Yes ○	No ○	NA ○	
3. The orthotic trough allows full motion of the finger MCP and thumb joints.	Yes ○	No ○	NA ○	
4. Adequate Velcro hooks are used on the orthotic trough to secure the number of monofilament straps.	Yes ○	No ○	NA ○	
Function				
1. The fit of the orthotic trough and straps prevents migration.	Yes ○	No ○	NA ○	
2. The monofilament allows full composite flexion when pulled.	Yes ○	No ○	NA ○	
3. Each finger cuff maintains its position on the digit with finger flexion and extension.	Yes ○	No ○	NA ○	
Straps				
1. All straps are rounded at the ends.	Yes ○	No ○	NA ○	
2. The Velcro hooks on the orthotic trough are covered to prevent snagging clothes.	Yes ○	No ○	NA ○	
3. The correct width of straps is used to increase the surface area, to diffuse pressure, and to prevent pockets of swelling.	Yes ○	No ○	NA ○	
Comfort				
1. The proximal, distal, and thenar edges of the orthotic trough are smooth and slightly flared.	Yes ○	No ○	NA ○	
2. The orthotic trough is free of impingement and pressure areas.	Yes ○	No ○	NA ○	
3. The edges of the finger cuffs are smooth.	Yes ○	No ○	NA ○	
4. The width of the finger cuffs disperses the application of forces.	Yes ○	No ○	NA ○	
5. The direction of pull for each finger cuff is accurate.	Yes ○	No ○	NA ○	
6. The tension from the finger cuffs can be adjusted to provide appropriate levels of force.	Yes ○	No ○	NA ○	
Cosmetic Appearance				
1. The orthotic trough is free of fingerprints, dirt, pencil or pen marks.	Yes ○	No ○	NA ○	
2. The orthotic trough is smooth and free of buckles or wrinkles.	Yes ○	No ○	NA ○	
Therapeutic Regimen				
1. The client is able to demonstrate correct application of the orthotic trough and to adjust finger cuffs as instructed.	Yes ○	No ○	NA ○	
2. The client is instructed in the orthotic wearing schedule.	Yes ○	No ○	NA ○	
3. The client is aware of orthotic precautions.	Yes ○	No ○	NA ○	
4. The client is knowledgeable of how to clean and care for the orthosis.	Yes ○	No ○	NA ○	

FORM 12-1* Static-progressive finger flexion orthosis—cont'd

Discuss possible adjustments or changes you would make based on the self-evaluation. (What would you do differently next time?)

_____

_____

Discuss possible areas to improve with clinical safety when fabricating the orthosis.

_____

_____

* See Appendix B for a perforated copy of this form.

GRADING SHEET 12-1*

Static-Progressive Finger Flexion Orthosis

Name: _____

Date: _____

Wrist position at rest:

Grade: _____
1 = Beyond improvement, not acceptable
2 = Requires maximal improvement
3 = Requires moderate improvement
4 = Requires minimal improvement
5 = Requires no improvement

Evaluation Areas						**Comments**
Design						
1. The orthotic trough is the proper length and width.	1	2	3	4	5	
2. The orthotic trough supports, does not push on the arches.	1	2	3	4	5	
3. The orthotic trough allows full motion of the finger MCP and thumb joints.	1	2	3	4	5	
4. Adequate Velcro hooks are used on the orthotic trough to secure the number of monofilament straps.	1	2	3	4	5	
Function						
1. The fit of the orthotic trough and straps prevents migration.	1	2	3	4	5	
2. The monofilament allows full composite flexion when pulled.	1	2	3	4	5	
3. Each finger cuff maintains its position on the digit with finger flexion and extension.	1	2	3	4	5	
Straps						
1. All straps are rounded at the ends.	1	2	3	4	5	
2. The Velcro hooks on the orthotic trough are covered to prevent snagging clothes.	1	2	3	4	5	
3. The correct width of straps is used to increase the surface area, to diffuse pressure, and to prevent pockets of swelling.	1	2	3	4	5	
Comfort						
1. The proximal, distal, and thenar edges of the orthotic trough are smooth and slightly flared.	1	2	3	4	5	
2. The orthotic trough is free of impingement and pressure areas.	1	2	3	4	5	
3. The edges of the finger cuffs are smooth.	1	2	3	4	5	
4. The width of the finger cuffs disperses the application of forces.	1	2	3	4	5	
5. The direction of pull for each finger cuff is accurate.	1	2	3	4	5	
6. The tension from the finger cuffs can be adjusted to provide appropriate levels of force.	1	2	3	4	5	
Cosmetic Appearance						
1. The orthotic trough is free of fingerprints, dirt, pencil or pen marks.	1	2	3	4	5	
2. The orthotic trough is smooth and free of buckles or wrinkles.	1	2	3	4	5	

GRADING SHEET 12-1*—cont'd

Comments:

_____

_____

_____

_____

_____

*See Appendix B for a perforated copy of this form.

CHAPTER 13

Orthotic Intervention for Nerve Injuries

Helene Lohman
Brenda M. Coppard
Mackenzie Raber

Key Terms
axonotmesis
cubital tunnel syndrome
cumulative trauma disorder (CTD)
median nerve
neurapraxia
neurotmesis
posterior interosseous nerve syndrome
pronator tunnel syndrome
radial nerve
radial tunnel syndrome
ulnar nerve
Wallerian degeneration
Wartenberg neuropathy

Chapter Objectives
1. Identify the components of a peripheral nerve.
2. Describe a peripheral nerve's response to injury and repair.
3. Describe the operative procedures used for nerve repair.
4. Explain the three purposes for orthotic intervention of nerve palsies.
5. Describe nerve injury classification.
6. Identify the locations for low and high peripheral nerve lesions.
7. Explain common causes of radial, ulnar, and median nerve lesions.
8. Review the sensory and motor distributions of the radial, median, and ulnar nerves.
9. Explain the functional effects of radial, ulnar, and median nerve lesions.
10. Identify the orthotic intervention approaches and rationale for radial, ulnar, and median nerve injuries.
11. Use clinical judgment to evaluate a problematic orthosis for a nerve lesion.
12. Use clinical judgment to evaluate a fabricated hand based ulnar nerve orthosis.
13. Apply documentation skills to a case study.
14. Summarize the importance of evidence-based practice with provision of orthoses for nerve conditions.

Your friend, Shelley, is an avid bicyclist. She bikes almost every day to work and weekly with members of several bicycling clubs. After completing a particularly rigorous event biking across the state, Shelley developed pain and a "pins and needles" feeling in the ring and little fingers of both hands. Over the next several months, she began complaining of feeling clumsy picking up objects and spreading her fingers apart to grasp items. Shelley approached you about her hand problems stating, "I believe that I might have carpal tunnel syndrome!" From listening to her symptoms and how they developed, you suspected compression of the ulnar nerve at the wrist and suggested that she go to an orthopaedic physician for a diagnosis. After her appointment, she shares with you that she did have an ulnar nerve compression at the wrist called Guyon canal syndrome, and she received an order for therapy and an orthosis.

Orthotic interventions for nerve lesions require therapists to possess a thorough knowledge of static (immobilization) and dynamic (mobilization) principles and sound critical-thinking skills. Comprehension of kinesiology, physiology, and anatomy is paramount to understanding the motor, sensory, and vasomotor implications of a nerve injury. Competence in manual muscle-testing skills is also necessary to evaluate affected muscles as nerves recover from injuries.[16] This chapter addresses peripheral nerve anatomy; nerve injury classifications; nerve repair; and types, effects, and interventions for radial, ulnar, and median nerve injuries.

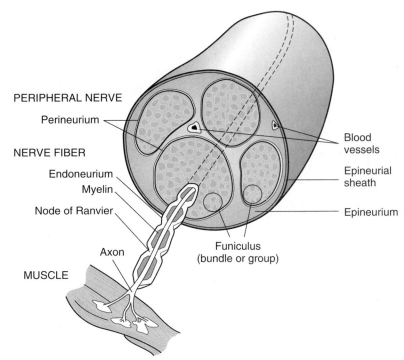

Figure 13-1 Components of a peripheral nerve: epineurium, perineurium, endoneurium, funiculi, axons, and blood vessels.

Peripheral Nerve Anatomy

A peripheral nerve consists of the epineurium, perineurium, endoneurium, funiculi, axons, and blood vessels (Figure 13-1).[34] The epineurium is made of loose collagenous connective tissue. There are external and internal types of epineurium. The external epineurium contains blood vessels. The internal epineurium protects the funiculi from pressure and allows for gliding of fascicles. The amount of epineurium varies among persons, nerve types, and along each individual nerve. The perineurium surrounds funiculi, and the endoneurium surrounds the axons. A funiculus, or fascicle, consists of a group of axons that are surrounded by endoneurium and are covered by a sheath of perineurium. An individual fascicle contains a mix of myelinated and unmyelinated fibers. The myelin sheath encapsulates the axon. Myelin is a lipoprotein, which allows for conduction of fast impulses. Each nerve contains a varied number and size of funiculi.

Nerves are at risk for injury when laceration, avulsion, stretch, crush, compression, or contusion occurs.[10] Peripheral nerves can also be attacked by viruses, bacteria, or the body's immune system.[10] Often bone, tendon, ligament, vessel, and soft-tissue injuries accompany nerve injuries.

Nerve Injury Classification

Nerve injuries are categorized by the extent of damage to the axon and sheath.[10] Nerve compression lesions often contribute to peripheral neuropathies. When a specific portion of a peripheral nerve is compressed, the peripheral axons within that nerve

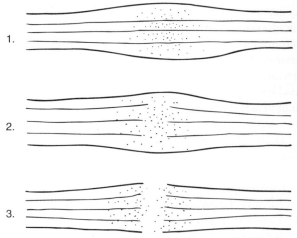

Figure 13-2 The three classifications of nerve injuries are (1) neurapraxia, (2) axonotmesis, and (3) neurotmesis.

sustain the greatest injury. Initial changes occur in the blood/nerve barrier followed by subperineural edema. This edema results in a thickening of the internal and external perineurium.[44] As the compression worsens, the motor, proprioceptive, light touch, and vibratory sensory receptor specific functions are compromised.[65] All the nerve fibers may be paralyzed after enduring severe and prolonged compression. Seddon[59] originally described three levels of nerve injury (Figure 13-2):

1. **Neurapraxia**
2. **Axonotmesis**
3. **Neurotmesis**

Later in 1968, Sunderland[66] extended the classification to five levels, which are termed as first- through fifth-degree injuries. Mackinnon and Dellon[37] describe an added sixth-degree injury.

First-Degree Injury

A first-degree injury involves the demylination of the nerve, which temporarily blocks conduction.[8,45] The prognosis for persons with neurapraxia is extremely good; recovery is usually spontaneous within 3 months.[65]

Second-Degree Injury

When a second-degree injury occurs, the axon is severed and the sheath remains intact. Specifically, **Wallerian degeneration** occurs when a nerve is completely severed or the axon and myelin sheath are damaged, and the endoneurial tube remains intact. The segment of axon and the motor and sensory end receptors distal to the lesion become ischemic and begin to degenerate 3 to 5 days after the injury.[34] The intact endoneurial tube allows for potential regrowth for the proximal part of the nerve to regenerate. With the ideal scenario, the rate of regeneration is approximately 1 inch per month. Complete recovery usually occurs if regeneration happens in a timely manner before muscle degeneration.[45]

Third-Degree Injury

A third-degree injury varies from a second-degree injury in that the "continuity of the endoneurial tube [is] destroyed from a disorganization of the internal structures of the nerve bundles"[66] and scarring is present within the tube.[24] Recovery is more complicated with possible delayed or incomplete axonal growth.[66] Because fibers are often mismatched, clients benefit from motor and sensory reeducation.[45]

Fourth-Degree Injury

With the fourth-degree of injury "the involved segment is ultimately converted into a tangled strand of connective tissue, Schwann cells, and regenerating axons which can be enlarged to form a neuroma."[66] The effects are more severe than a third-degree injury with increased neuronal degeneration, misdirected axons, less axon survival[66] and more scar tissue.[24] Complete "distal loss of function" occurs with this level of injury.[24] Surgical intervention is necessary to remove a neuroma (tumor of nerve fibers and cells).

Fifth-Degree Injury

A fifth-degree injury results in partial or complete severance of the axon and the sheath with loss of motor, sensory, and sympathetic function.[66] Without the directional guidance from an intact endoneurial tube, malaligned axon growth may lead to a complicated recovery. Microsurgery is required as the person will not restore distal functioning without surgery.[24] Occasionally, grafting is necessary if the severance gap is too large for approximation of the two nerve ends.[65]

Sixth-Degree Injury

A sixth-degree injury is a mixed injury involving a "neuroma-in-continuity."[24] This type of injury involves many of the aspects of the earlier five degrees to varying degrees.[37] Surgery needs will vary according to the specific condition, and in some cases surgery may not be required.

Nerve Repair

Peripheral nerve lesions often occur to the median, radial, and ulnar nerves. The location of the lesion determines the impairment of sudomotor, vasomotor, muscular, sensory, and functional involvement.[8] Sometimes nerves can be compressed at more than one site.[53,67] Therefore, it is important to be aware of key diagnostic procedures to determine the extent of compression.

Operative Procedures for Nerve Repair

There are four procedures used to surgically repair nerves[54]:
1. Decompression
2. Repair
3. Neurolysis
4. Grafting

Nerve decompression is the most common surgery performed on nerves. An example of surgical decompression is the transection of the transverse carpal ligament to decompress the **median nerve** or release the carpal tunnel.

Surgical nerve repairs involve microsurgical sutures to fix the epineurium. Surgical nerve repairs are classified as primary, delayed primary, or secondary.[34] A primary repair occurs within hours of the injury. A delayed primary repair occurs within 5 to 7 days after the injury. Any surgical repair performed beyond 7 days is a secondary repair.

Neurolysis is a procedure performed on a nerve that has become encapsulated in dense scar tissue. The scar tissue compresses the nerve to surrounding soft tissues and prevents it from gliding. When the client attempts to move in a way that would normally glide the nerve, the movement instead stretches the nerve, affecting circulation and chemical balance. Scars may also physically interfere with the axon regeneration.

Nerve grafting is necessary when there is a large gap in a nerve and end-to-end nerve repair is not possible. An autograft donated by a cutaneous nerve, such as the sural nerve, may fill the gap. Although the outcome from a nerve graft is somewhat unreliable, occasionally it is the only option for repair.

Purposes of Orthotic Intervention for Nerve Injuries

The three purposes for orthotic intervention of an extremity that has nerve injury are protection, prevention, and assistance with function.[3,40] If a nerve has undergone surgical repair, the physician may order application of a cast or an orthosis to place the hand, wrist, or elbow in a protective position, thus reducing the amount of tension on the repaired nerve. Avoiding tension on a repaired nerve is extremely important because outcomes of nerve repairs are directly related to the amount of tension across the repair site.[62]

Prevention of contractures is important because nerve lesions result in various degrees of muscle denervation. For example, a short opponens orthosis prevents contracture of the thumb web space after a median nerve injury.[23] Sometimes a client does not seek immediate medical attention after nerve injury resulting in contracture development that warrants orthotic intervention. For example, for a person with a claw hand deformity from an ulnar nerve injury, the therapist may fabricate a mobilizing ulnar gutter orthosis. This orthosis helps remodel the soft tissues to increase passive extension of the ring and little fingers' proximal interphalangeal (PIP) joints[10] by placing the metacarpophalangeal (MCP) joints in a flexed position. Once MCP and PIP stiffness occur, intervention focuses on regaining maximum passive range of motion (PROM). After normal PROM is regained, orthotic interventions for the muscle imbalance becomes an option.[22]

Often, function after a nerve injury can require or be enhanced by orthotic intervention. For example, a client may be better able to grasp and release objects after a radial nerve injury while wearing an elastic tension MCP and wrist extension orthosis. This orthosis assists the MCP joints to extend to open the hand for grasp and release. Without the orthosis, the wrist and MCP joints are unable to extend, and difficulty with grasp and grasp release activities results.

Upper Extremity Compression Neuropathies

Cumulative trauma disorder (CTD) is not a medical diagnosis but an etiologic label for a range of disorders.[42] The cause of CTD is not solely from engaging in work activities. Social activities, activities of daily living (ADLs), and leisure pursuits may enhance the development and exacerbation of CTD.[42] The first step in controlling the CTD comes from understanding the compressive neuropathies of the upper extremity.[68] Table 13-1 outlines the nature and intervention of compressive neuropathies that occur at the wrist, elbow, and forearm. The compressive neuropathies are discussed in more detail later in this chapter.

Locations of Nerve Lesions

The location of a nerve lesion determines the sensory and motor involvement. Lesions are referred to as low or high. Low lesions occur distal to the elbow, and high lesions occur proximal to the elbow.[5] High lesions affect more muscles and may influence a larger sensory distribution than low lesions. Therefore, knowledge of relevant anatomy is important for determining physical and functional implications of nerve injuries.

Substitutions

When a nerve lesion occurs, "there is no opposing balancing force to the intact active muscle group."[16] If a person with a nerve lesion does not receive orthotic intervention, the intact musculature overpowers the denervated muscles. Intact musculature takes over and produces movement normally generated by the denervated muscles.[13] The person learns to adapt to the imbalance through substitutions and compensation.[16,52] An example of a substitution or trick movement is the pinch that develops after a low-level median nerve injury. With the help of the adductor pollicis, the flexor pollicis longus pinches objects against the radial side of the index finger. A therapist may mistakenly think that motor return has occurred for the abductor pollicis brevis, flexor pollicis brevis, opponens pollicis, and first and second lumbricals. However, the pinch movement observed is actually a substitution.

Prognosis

Many factors affect the prognosis for recovery from nerve injury. These factors include the extent of the injury, cleanliness of the wound, method of repair, and the client's age.[10,62] Other factors that impact the recovery from nerve repair include the amount of tension on the repair, the person's general health, and whether the person smokes. Correct alignment of axons and avoidance of tension on the damaged nerve improve the prognosis. A clean wound has a better prognosis than a dirty wound.[8] Sharply severed nerves recover better than frayed nerves resulting from a crush injury or gunshot wound.[25] Nerve microsurgery "timed appropriately according to the nature and extent of the injury is essential for a favorable outcome."[10] Age is also a factor in the speed of recovery. A child's potential for regeneration is greater than an adult's.[10] Full sensory and motor return occurs often in a child but rarely in an adult.

The rate of axonal regeneration is 1 to 3 mm per day. Because nerve regeneration is slow, the therapist conducts periodic monitoring and orthotic intervention is often part of the intervention protocol. In addition, the therapist documents results of the evaluation and any changes to the orthotic intervention or exercise program.

Radial Nerve Injuries

Radial nerve palsies are very common and typically occur from midhumeral fractures or compressions.[3,15] Other causes of superficial radial nerve palsies at the wrist include pressure, edema, and trauma on the nerve from crush injuries; de Quervain tendonitis; handcuffs; and a tight or heavy wristwatch.[19] The location of the radial nerve injury determines which muscles are affected (Figure 13-3).

Three types of lesions are possible when the **radial nerve** is injured.[16] The first type of lesion involves a high level injury at the humerus resulting in wrist drop and lack

Table 13-1 Upper Extremity Compression Neuropathies

	PRESENTATION	ORTHOTIC INTERVENTION
Wrist		
Radial sensory entrapment (Wartenberg neuropathy)	Compression of the superficial radial nerve usually includes numbness, tingling, and pain of the dorsoradial aspect of the forearm, wrist, and hand. Symptoms occur during ulnar deviation of the wrist, thumb composite flexion, and forceful pronation and supination of the forearm.	Conservative intervention involves avoidance of wrist and forearm motions. Fabricate a wrist immobilization orthosis with the wrist in 20 to 30 degrees of extension. If pain occurs with thumb motion, the thumb should also be incorporated into the orthosis.
Ulnar nerve entrapment at the wrist (ulnar tunnel syndrome)	Entrapment of the ulnar nerve usually occurs in the Guyon canal. Sensory changes involve the fifth digit and ulnar side of the fourth digit. True ulnar nerve entrapment is not common.	Orthotic provision involves a dorsal hand based orthosis or a figure-eight orthosis with fourth and fifth digit in 30 to 45 degrees of flexion at the MCP joint to block MCP hyperextension. Orthosis can be dynamic (mobilization) or static. Orthosis is worn until the nerve regenerates.
Carpal tunnel syndrome (CTS)	Complaints of numbness, tingling, and paresthesias in the median nerve distribution. Persons may complain of dropping objects or cramping and aching in the wrist and hand, especially during sleep and driving. In severe cases, thenar atrophy or loss of strength of palmar abduction of the thumb are present. Positive Phalen's and Tinel signs and night pain are present.	Orthotic provision involves custom-made or prefabricated wrist orthosis with the wrist in neutral. Orthotic regimens vary, but most include nighttime wear.
Elbow and Forearm		
Radial tunnel syndrome	True radial tunnel syndrome is rare and often misdiagnosed as lateral epicondylitis. Radial tunnel syndrome presents with pain and discomfort in the extensor-supinator muscle mass in the proximal forearm. Radial tunnel syndrome has pain as the presenting symptom, not motor dysfunction.	Currently the trend is to immobilize only as much as needed to resolve the symptoms. Conservative management may involve immobilization in a volar wrist immobilization orthosis in slight extension and or Kinesio taping[51] when area is irritated to reduce tension. Another suggestion is a "yoke orthosis" for support of the middle finger MCP joint.[51]
Posterior interosseous nerve syndrome	Presentation is similar to radial tunnel syndrome. However, posterior interosseous syndrome includes weakness or paralysis of any muscles innervated by the posterior interosseous nerve and does not involve sensory loss. The ability to extend the wrist in radial deviation is present, but extension of the wrist is impaired in neutral or ulnar deviation. Loss of thumb extension and abduction and active extension of the MCP joints are also present.	It is important to provide orthotic intervention as much as possible for this condition to prevent stretch of structures innervated by the radial nerve. Various orthotic options are suggested for posterior interosseous nerve syndrome. Several options are presented in this chapter for the condition including a mobilization orthosis with the wrist in 30 to 40 degrees of extension and MCPs in neutral. Other options are to fabricate a tenodesis orthosis or a static wrist extension and dynamic MCP extension orthosis.
Cubital tunnel syndrome	Presents with localized pain to the medial side of the proximal forearm and elbow. There is numbness and tingling of the fifth digit and the medial side of the fourth digit. Advanced compression presents with hypothenar eminence atrophy. A positive Froment sign may accompany this syndrome.	Conservative intervention includes avoidance of direct pressure on the medial aspect of the elbow and on the flexor carpi ulnaris. An elbow pad may help to protect the nerve from direct pressure. During the daytime, prolonged elbow flexion should be avoided to prevent compression of the ulnar nerve and orthotic provision is usually not necessary. Orthotic provision for nighttime includes positioning the elbow in 30 to 45 degrees of flexion. If the wrist is included, it is positioned in 20 degrees of extension.

Continued

Table 13-1   Upper Extremity Compression Neuropathies—cont'd

	PRESENTATION	ORTHOTIC INTERVENTION
Pronator syndrome	Compression of the median nerve as it crosses the elbow at the origin of the pronator teres. It is associated with pain in the proximal forearm and is aggravated by resisted forearm pronation when the elbow is flexed.	One orthotic option is to place the elbow in 90 degrees flexion and forearm in neutral rotation (between supination and pronation)[64]
Anterior interosseous syndrome	Compression of the anterior interosseous branch of the median nerve is associated with pain in the proximal volar forearm followed by loss of ability to flex the IP joint of the thumb and the DIP joint of the second and third digits. There are usually no sensory complaints.	Orthotic provision may include immobilizing the elbow in 90 degrees of flexion with the forearm in neutral. Another option is to fabricate small orthoses to block index DIP and thumb IP extension or hyperextension (see Figure 13-18).

DIP, Distal interphalangeal; *IP*, interphalangeal; *MCP*, metacarpophalangeal.

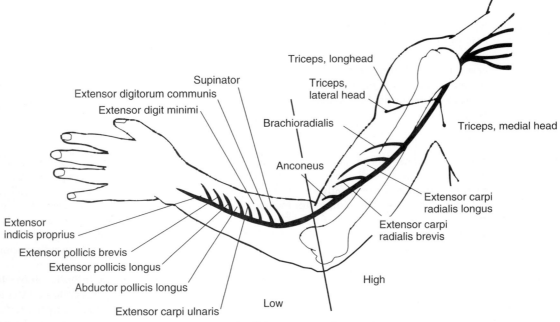

Figure 13-3 Radial nerve motor innervation.

of finger MCP extension (Figure 13-4). With this type of lesion, the triceps are rarely affected unless the injury is extremely high.

The second type of lesion involves the posterior interosseous nerve. After spiraling around the humerus and crossing the elbow, the radial nerve divides into a motor and a sensory branch.[19] The motor branch is the posterior interosseous nerve, and the sensory branch is the superficial branch of the radial nerve. Compression usually causes the posterior interosseous nerve injury, but lacerations or stab wounds can be sources of lesions to the posterior interosseous nerve. Radial tunnel syndrome and posterior interosseous nerve compression are two distinct types of compression syndromes described in the literature that occur in the same tunnel with the same nerve. As Gelberman and colleagues[26] stated, "It is difficult for the conscientious diagnostician to accept the reality that the same nerve compressed in the same anatomical site can result in two entirely different symptom complexes." Radial tunnel syndrome refers to compression of the radial nerve just distal to the elbow between the radial head and the supinator muscle,[33,62] and it is linked to repetitive forearm rotation.[14] With radial tunnel syndrome, complaints of pain are usually in the radial nerve distribution of the distal forearm[32] and the condition involves pain without muscle weakness.[18,19,26] Radial tunnel syndrome is controversial because it is complicated to diagnose a pain syndrome that does not have motor components. The condition needs to be differentiated from lateral epicondylitis, which is close to the same area.[18]

Posterior interosseous nerve compression results in rapid motor loss[26] and with no sensory loss.[19,26,35] This compression is characterized by aching on the lateral side

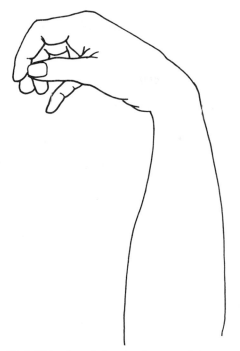

Figure 13-4 Wrist drop deformity from a radial nerve injury.

of the elbow, difficulty with MCP finger and thumb extension, and difficulty with thumb abduction. Wrist extension is intact, but the wrist tends to radially deviate due to muscle imbalance.[35]

The third type of lesion is damage to the sensory branch of the radial nerve. Compression of this superficial branch is called *Wartenberg syndrome*.[46] This lesion does not result in functional loss. However, symptoms of this nerve compression include numbness, tingling, burning, and pain over the dorsoradial surface of the hand.[63]

Functional Involvement from Radial Nerve Lesions

Table 13-2 outlines lesion locations and the muscles and motions that are affected in radial nerve lesions. After crossing the elbow and dropping below the supinator, the radial nerve divides and forms the posterior interosseous nerve.[16] Lesions and compressions of the posterior interosseous nerve at the forearm level can affect the following muscles:

- Extensor digitorum communis
- Extensor carpi ulnaris
- Abductor pollicis longus
- Extensor pollicis longus
- Extensor pollicis brevis
- Extensor indicis proprius
- Extensor digiti minimi

Loss of these muscles results in absent MCP extension of all digits, thumb radial abduction, and thumb extension. With attempts at wrist extension, strong wrist radial deviation is present. With attempts at finger extension, the MCPs flex and the PIPs extend because the extensor digitorum muscle is affected. In addition to the muscles previously

indicated, a radial nerve injury at the elbow level can affect the following muscles:

- Extensor carpi radialis longus
- Extensor carpi radialis brevis
- Supinator

In addition to the motions lost at the forearm level, an injury at the elbow level involves inability to produce radial wrist extension, MCP joint extension, thumb extension, thumb radial abduction, and weakened forearm supination.

With a high-level lesion or compression in the upper arm (i.e., axilla level), the injury affects the triceps and brachioradialis muscles. Loss of these muscles results in lost elbow extension, weak supination, absent wrist and finger extensors, and lost thumb extension and abduction.

The functional results of an axilla-level lesion include an inability to stabilize the wrist in an extended position, extend fingers and thumb, and abduct the thumb. For example, a client with a high radial nerve lesion has poor grip and coordination because of the lack of wrist extensor opposition to the flexors.[8,22] The resulting deformity is called *wrist drop* (see Figure 13-4).

Significant impairment of sensation is not present with radial nerve injuries. The superficial sensory branch of the radial nerve supplies sensation to the dorsum of the index and middle fingers and half of the ring finger to the PIP joint level (Figure 13-5). Laceration or contusion to the sensory branch of the radial nerve can be bothersome to a client. This often occurs in conjunction with de Quervain release. Sensory compromise over the dorsum of the thumb may result in hypersensitivity. An orthosis or padded device can protect the area while a desensitization program is implemented.[58]

Orthotic Intervention for Radial Nerve Injury

The client with a radial nerve injury benefits from orthotic intervention and a therapeutic program. There are several orthotic options for radial nerve injuries. Orthoses specific for diagnoses are discussed first, followed by various orthotic design options.

Orthotic Intervention for Radial Tunnel Syndrome

Currently the trend for orthotic intervention for **radial tunnel syndrome** is to immobilize only to the extent as needed to relieve symptoms. Conservative management may involve immobilization when symptomatic in a volar wrist immobilization orthosis in slight extension and/or Kinesio taping[51] to reduce tension. Another suggestion is a yoke orthosis to support the middle MCP joint (Figure 13-6).[51]

Orthotic Intervention for Posterior Interosseous Nerve Syndrome

It is important to apply orthotic intervention as much as possible for **posterior interosseous nerve syndrome** in order to prevent stretch of structures innervated by the radial nerve. Various orthotic options are suggested for posterior interosseous nerve syndrome. Examples are a mobilization orthosis

Table 13-2　Radial Nerve Lesions

AFFECTED MUSCLES	WEAK OR LOST MOTIONS
Forearm Level (Posterior Interosseous Nerve)	
Extensor digitorum communis	MCP extension of digits 2 through 5
Extensor carpi ulnaris	Wrist extension and wrist ulnar deviation
Extensor indicis proprius	Extension of the MCP of the second digit
Extensor digiti minimi	Extension of the MCP of the fifth digit
Abductor pollicis longus	Thumb abduction
Extensor pollicis longus	Thumb extension at the IP and MCP joints
Extensor pollicis brevis	MCP extension and assist CMC extension
Elbow Level	
Extensor carpi radialis longus	Radial wrist extension
Extensor carpi radialis brevis	Neutral wrist extension
Supinator	Supination
Extensor digitorum communis	MCP extension of digits 2 through 5
Extensor carpi ulnaris	Wrist extension and wrist ulnar deviation
Extensor indicis proprius	Extension of the MCP joint of the second digit
Extensor digiti minimi	Extension of the MCP joints of the fifth digit
Abductor pollicis longus	Thumb abduction
Extensor pollicis longus	Thumb extension of the MCP and IP joints
Extensor pollicis brevis	joints and assist CMC extension
Axilla Level	
Brachioradialis	Elbow flexion in neutral forearm position
Triceps	Elbow extension
Extensor carpi radialis longus	Radial wrist extension
Extensor carpi radialis brevis	Neutral wrist extension
Supinator	Supination
Extensor digitorum communis	MCP extension of digits 2 through 5
Extensor carpi ulnaris	Wrist extension and wrist ulnar deviation
Extensor indicis proprius	Extension of the MCP of the second digit
Extensor digiti minimi	Extension of the MCP of the fifth digit
Abductor pollicis longus	Thumb abduction
Extensor pollicis longus	Thumb extension at the MCP and IP joints
Extensor pollicis brevis	MCP extension and assist CMC extension

CMC, Carpometacarpal; *IP,* interphalangeal; *MCP,* metacarpophalangeal.

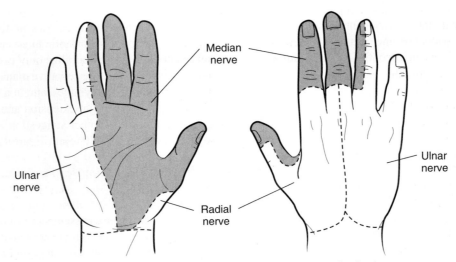

Figure 13-5　Radial, median, and ulnar nerve sensory distribution.

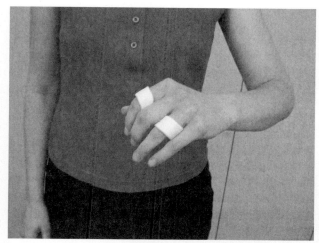

Figure 13-6 Yoke orthosis for support of the middle metacarpophalangeal (MCP) joint with radial tunnel syndrome. (From Porretto-Loehrke A, Soika E: Therapist's management of other nerve compressions about the elbow and wrist. In Skirven TM, Osterman AL, Fedorczyk JM, et al., editors: *Rehabilitation of the hand and upper extremity,* ed 6, Philadelphia, 2011, Elsevier.)

with the wrist in 30 to 40 degrees of extension and MCPs in neutral and a tenodesis orthosis that encourages wrist and finger function by facilitating wrist extension.[19]

Orthotic Intervention for Wartenberg Neuropathy
For **Wartenberg neuropathy,** a wrist immobilization orthosis is fabricated with the wrist in 20 to 30 degrees of extension. If pain occurs with thumb motion, the thumb is also incorporated into the orthosis. Refer to Chapter 8 for information on thumb orthoses.

Wrist Immobilization Orthosis
The therapist applies a wrist immobilization orthosis to place the wrist in a functional position of 30 degrees of extension.[11] When wearing a wrist immobilization orthosis, the client can usually extend the IP joints of the fingers to release an object by using the intrinsic hand muscles.[8] The therapist keeps in mind the advantages, disadvantages, and patterns of volar and dorsal wrist orthoses (see Chapter 7). A wrist immobilization orthosis is appropriate to wear on occasions when the client desires a more inconspicuous design than a mobilization orthosis. A wrist immobilization orthosis may also be more appropriate for nighttime wear than a mobilization orthosis with an outrigger. Wearing a mobilization orthosis with an outrigger at night may result in damage to the outrigger and injury to the client. Some people who have heavy demands on their hands prefer the simple wrist immobilization orthoses to the more fragile outrigger-mobilization designs. A therapist may offer both a wrist immobilization orthosis and a wrist mobilization orthosis to the person. Alternating the orthoses may maximize function. The mobilization orthosis discussed later in this chapter might be an alternative for the client to wear both day and night because it is less cumbersome.

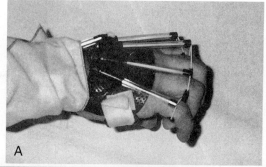

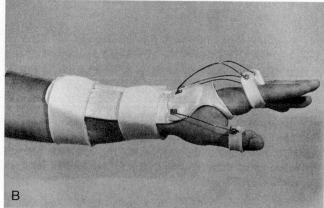

Figure 13-7 Low-profile designs with pre-purchased outrigger parts. (From Fess EE, Gettle KS, Philips CA, et al: *Hand and upper extremity splinting: principles and methods,* ed 3, St Louis, 2005, Elsevier/Mosby.)

Mobilization Extension Orthoses
Mobilization orthotic intervention for a radial nerve injury promotes functional hand usage[7] and several options exist. One option involves fabricating a dorsal wrist immobilization orthosis as the base for a mobilization extension orthosis (using elastic for the source of tension).[3] The dynamic component for this orthosis positions the MCPs in extension. Several low-profile options exist that can be made with purchased outrigger parts (Figure 13-7). The costs of utilizing purchased outrigger parts should be considered. Alternatively, the therapist can use a piece of wire or thermoplastic material to fabricate an outrigger. Refer to Chapter 12 for more information on outriggers.

A mobilization MCP extension orthosis for radial nerve injury substitutes for the absent muscle power by assisting the MCP extensors. This orthosis is worn throughout the day until the impaired musculature reaches a manual muscle testing (MMT) grade of fair (3).[10] Colditz[16] cautions that "the powerful unopposed flexors often overcome the force of the dynamic splint during finger flexion." A client who shows no clinical improvement in 3 months should return to the physician for consideration of surgical intervention.[19] Because wrist control usually returns first, the therapist modifies the orthotic design and uses a hand based mobilization orthosis after the forearm based mobilization orthosis has been worn and improvement in wrist control is demonstrated.[3,71] If only one finger is lagging in extension,

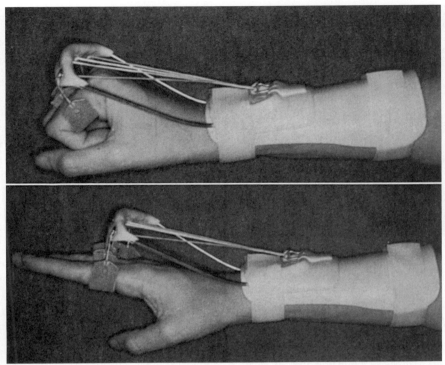

Figure 13-8 An orthosis for radial nerve injury. (From Colditz JC: Splinting the hand with a peripheral nerve injury. In Mackin EJ, Callahan AD, Skirven TM, et al., editors: *Rehabilitation of the hand and upper extremity,* ed 5, St Louis, 2002, Mosby, pp. 622-634.)

the therapist dynamically incorporates that finger into the orthosis.[71]

Another type of mobilization orthosis for radial nerve injuries is a mobilization orthosis that reestablishes the tenodesis action of the hand.[15,16,17] A tenodesis action occurs when the client flexes the wrist and the fingers extend. When the client extends the wrist, the fingers flex (Figure 13-8). The tenodesis orthosis includes a dorsal base with a low-profile outrigger that spans from the wrist to each proximal phalanx. This orthosis is sometimes called a *dynamic tenodesis suspension orthosis.*[29] Finger loops are worn on each proximal phalanx and a nylon cord attached from the finger loops is stretched to a point on the dorsal base.

The tenodesis orthosis has many advantages. First, the design allows the palmar surface of the hand to be relatively free for sensory input and normal grasp.[16] The wrist is not immobilized and only moves with the natural tenodesis effect, while the thumb can move independently.[15] In addition, the hand arches are maintained.[16] The components of the tenodesis orthosis "follow the contours of the hand and take up less space."[41] As wrist extension returns, the client continues to wear the orthosis because it does not immobilize the wrist and it enhances the strength of the wrist extensors for functional tasks.[16] Therefore a hand based orthosis is not required. The low-profile design enhances the performance of functional tasks.

There are some disadvantages with the tenodesis orthosis. Because finger MCP flexion and extension mobilize as a group, independent finger motion is not achieved. An additional orthotic component can be added if the thumb is to be included in the orthosis. Because the orthotic design supports the weight of the hand through the finger cuffs, wearing the orthosis can be fatiguing.[40] The tenodesis orthotic design is usually not sturdy enough for people with high load demands on their hands.[58]

Fabrication of a Mobilization Orthosis for Radial Nerve Palsy

A unique mobilization orthosis for radial nerve palsy is a static wrist extension and dynamic MCP extension orthosis, which was originally designed by Mark Walsh and Sue Blackmore with adaptations by the Philadelphia Hand Center Therapy Department. Besides radial nerve palsy, this orthosis may be used with other conditions which require immobilization, such as post cerebrovascular accidents (CVAs).[69] The instructions are based on an adaptation for making the orthosis with moleskin loops. The original design by Walsh and Blackmore is fabricated slightly differently. Walsh's design includes slits approximately ¼ inch wide and 1 inch long between each of the fingers, leaving enough material distally to heat the area whereby a 3/32-inch wire is pushed into the material. The wire creates a bar to support the elastic between each finger. The elastic is woven through this part of the orthosis (Figure 13-9).

Steps for fabricating a mobilization orthosis for radial nerve palsy can be found in the following procedure.

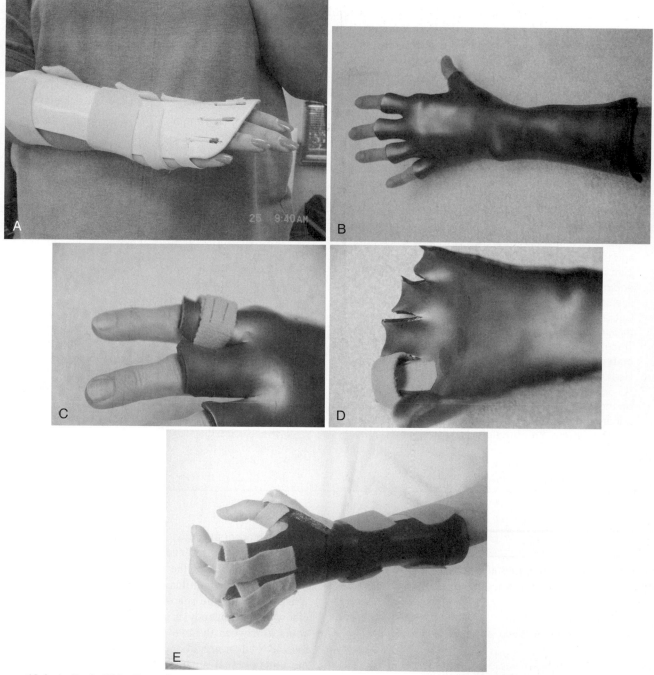

Figure 13-9 **A,** Static Wrist Extension and MCP Mobilization Extension Orthosis for Radial Nerve Palsy originally designed by Mark Walsh and Sue Blackmore. **B, C,** and **D,** Adapted Static Wrist Extension and MCP Mobilization Extension Orthosis using moleskin and elastic finger loops.

PROCEDURE | **for Mobilization Orthosis for Radial Nerve Palsy**

1. Position the person's hand palm-side up on a piece of paper. The wrist should be as neutral as possible with respect to radial and ulnar deviation. The fingers are abducted and the thumb is radially abducted.
2. Trace the hand and forearm. With the person's hand still on the paper, mark X's corresponding to (Figure 13-10):
   - Each web space between the fingers

- PIP joints (both ulnar and radial sides) of all four fingers
- IP joints (both ulnar and radial sides) of the thumb
- Two-thirds the length of the forearm
- ¼ to ½ inch lateral and parallel from the side of the little finger PIP joint on the ulnar side of the hand
- ¼ to ½ inch lateral and parallel from the ulnar side of the thumb IP joint

Continued

PROCEDURE   **for Mobilization Orthosis for Radial Nerve Palsy—cont'd**

3. Draw the pattern (see Figure 13-10). Start with the PIP joint of the index finger radial side, and draw a straight line across the joint to the ulnar side. Draw a straight line down from the ulnar side of the PIP joint to the marking at the web space between the index and middle fingers. Continue the same process of drawing lines across the PIP joints and connecting them to a line down to the marking at the base of the web space for all digits. Connect the line from the little finger to the marking ¼ to ½ inch outside of the PIP joint, and continue the line down the side of the forearm curving it to adjust to the forearm muscle bulk. End the line at the two-thirds marking. Connect the line that is ¼ to ½ inch parallel to the index finger to the middle of the thumb IP joint curving it to follow the "C" shape of the index and thumb. From the middle of the thumb. cross the IP joint and curve the line down the side of the forearm ending it at the two-thirds marking. Connect the two lines at the two-thirds marking.

4. Cut out the pattern making certain to completely cut through web space marks.

5. Trace the pattern onto the sheet of thermoplastic material.

6. Heat the thermoplastic material.

7. An option is to place padding on the dorsal MCPs and on the ulnar styloid during orthotic formation and later adhere the padding to the orthosis.

8. Cut the pattern out of the thermoplastic material. Wait until later to cut out the markings between the web spaces so that they do not adhere together. Another approach is to cut the area between the web space as

a "V" shape to prevent the thermoplastic material from sticking together.

9. Position the person's upper extremity on a table with the elbow resting on a pad (folded towel or foam wedge) and the forearm in a pronation. Place the wrist and hand in the following position:
   - Wrist: Approximately 10 to 20 degrees extension
   - Index through small MCPs: Neutral
   - Thumb: Functional position of palmar abduction

10. Reheat the thermoplastic material, and cut out the markings between the web spaces.

11. Mold the warmed thermoplastic material over the dorsum of the wrist and hand, making sure to conform the orthosis around the proximal phalanx of each finger and thumb. Push out the material at the area of the ulnar styloid or use Theraputty over the styloid.

12. Make any adjustment for proper fit, and position the orthosis on the person.

13. Once the orthosis is formed, cut a piece of ½-inch to ¾-inch elastic to comfortably fit over and around each proximal phalanx within the orthosis. Allow the elastic material to overlap ½ inch to ¾ inch. After the size of loop is determined, using a small stapler place two staples in the elastic to secure each loop.

14. Remove the orthosis; be careful that the elastic pieces stay in the proper place for each finger.

15. With strips of moleskin that are approximately ¾ inch × 4 inches, secure loops in place for each finger and thumb.

16. Apply straps to the wrist and forearm. When placing the orthosis on the person, position the staples on the dorsal side of the orthosis.

Ulnar Nerve Injuries

Ulnar compression syndromes are the second most common upper extremity compression neuropathies.[52] An ulnar nerve

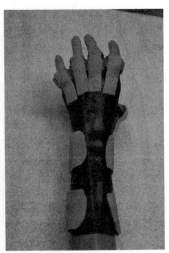

Figure 13-10 Pattern for dorsal base of Static Wrist Extension and MCP Mobilization Extension Orthosis.

lesion can occur in conjunction with a median nerve lesion.[20] Lesions to the **ulnar nerve** often result from a fracture of the medial epicondyle of the humerus, a fracture of the olecranon process of the ulna, or a laceration or ganglia at the wrist. Typically, the site of ulnar nerve compression at the elbow is the epicondylar groove, or where the ulnar nerve courses between the two heads of the flexor carpi ulnaris muscle.[52] Ulnar nerve compressions at the wrist level within the Guyon canal are less common.[52] Wrist-level injuries usually result from compression because of the superficial nature of ulnar nerve within the Guyon canal (Table 13-1).[52]

McGowan[39] developed a grading system for ulnar nerve conditions: grade I manifesting with paresthesias and clumsiness; grade II exhibiting interosseous weakness and some muscle wasting; and grade III involving paralysis of the ulnar intrinsic muscles. Ulnar nerve injuries at the elbow are classified as acute, subacute, or chronic.[52] Acute injuries result from trauma. Subacute injuries develop over time and involve continual elbow compression, such as a factory worker whose elbow is continuously positioned on a table while doing work. Both acute and subacute injuries respond to conservative interventions, such as reducing elbow flexion during tasks and/or orthotic intervention.

Chronic conditions require surgery, especially if daily living tasks are severely impacted.[52] Clinically, a person with an ulnar nerve compression at the elbow (**cubital tunnel syndrome**) complains of discomfort on the medial side of the arm and numbness and tingling in digits 4 and 5.[31] Prolonged flexion and force from occupations or sports such as baseball and tennis are common causes of ulnar nerve compression and irritation.[23]

Regardless of the cause or location, if a deformity results from an ulnar lesion it is called a *claw hand*. Anatomically, this deformity occurs because the MCP joints of the ring and little fingers are positioned in hyperextension. The fourth and fifth digits are incapable of fully extending the PIP and distal interphalangeal (DIP) joints because of the unopposed action of the extensor digitorum communis and the extensor digiti minimi (Figure 13-11). This position occurs because the lumbricals and the intrinsic muscles responsible for interphalangeal (IF) extension are paralyzed.[8]

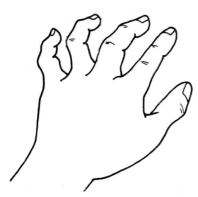

Figure 13-11 A claw hand deformity caused by an ulnar nerve injury.

Functional Implications of Ulnar Nerve Injuries

In the early stages of an ulnar nerve injury, a person may have difficulty performing ADLs and may experience hand fatigue. Muscle weakness is not usually evident until after the condition progresses.[52] Table 13-3 identifies the muscles that the ulnar nerve innervates in a low-level or wrist lesion and a high-level lesion that occurs at or above the elbow. If an ulnar nerve lesion occurs just distal to the elbow, the extrinsic muscles of the hand are lost because they are innervated distal to the elbow. At the wrist level, compression of the ulnar nerve in the distal part of the ulnar tunnel results in different functional effects based on the zone location of the nerve.[28,52]

Generally, the functional result from a high- or low-level ulnar nerve lesion is loss of pinch and power grip strength.[10,22] The client is unable to grasp an object fully because of the denervation of the finger abductors, atrophy of the hypothenar eminence, inability to oppose the little finger to the thumb, and ineffective pinch with the thumb.[8,56] The loss of the first dorsal interosseous and the adductor pollicis leads to unstable pinching of the thumb and index finger.[8] Loss of lateral finger movements and diminished sensory feedback can affect functional occupational activities, such as typing on a computer[56] and other daily tasks. With a high lesion, the loss of the flexor digitorum profundus of the ring and small fingers further compromises hand

Table 13-3 Ulnar Nerve Lesions	
AFFECTED MUSCLES	**WEAK AND LOST MOTIONS**
Low Level (Wrist Level)	
Abductor digiti minimi	MCP abduction of the fifth digit
Flexor digiti minimi	MCP flexion of the fifth digit and opposition
Opponens digiti minimi	Opposition of the fifth digit
Lumbricals to the fourth and fifth digits	MCP finger flexion and IP extension to the fourth and fifth digits
Dorsal interossei	MCP abduction of the digits
Palmar interossei	MCP adduction of the digits
Flexor pollicis brevis (deep head)	MCP and CMC flexion of the thumb and opposition
Adductor pollicis	Adduction of the CMC joint and MCP flexion
High Level (At or above the Elbow Level)	
Flexor carpi ulnaris	Wrist flexion and ulnar deviation
Flexor digitorum profundus of the fourth and fifth digits	Flexion of the DIP and PIP joints joint of the fourth and fifth digits
Abductor digiti minimi	MCP abduction of the fifth digit
Flexor digiti minimi	MCP flexion of the fifth digit and opposition
Opponens digiti minimi	Opposition of the fifth digit
Lumbricals to the fourth and fifth digits	MCP flexion and IP extension to the fourth and fifth digits
Dorsal interossei	MCP abduction of the digits
Palmar interossei	MCP adduction of the digits
Flexor pollicis brevis (deep head)	MCP and CMC flexion of the thumb and opposition
Adductor pollicis	Adduction of the CMC joint and MCP flexion

CMC, Carpometacarpal; *DIP,* distal interphalangeal; *IP,* interphalangeal; *MCP,* metacarpophalangeal.

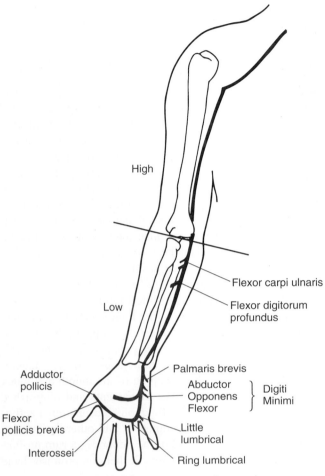

High

Low

Flexor carpi ulnaris

Flexor digitorum profundus

Adductor pollicis

Palmaris brevis

Abductor
Opponens   } Digiti
Flexor   } Minimi

Flexor pollicis brevis

Little lumbrical

Interossei

Ring lumbrical

Figure 13-12 Ulnar nerve motor innervation.

grasp.[10] In addition, the client presents with weakened wrist ulnar deviation.

Another characteristic of ulnar nerve injuries is a posture called *Froment sign,* which functionally results in flexion of the thumb IP joint during pinching activities.[9] Froment sign is apparent because the adductor pollicis, the deep head of the flexor pollicis brevis, and first dorsal interosseous muscle are not working. Because of these losses, performance of the fine dexterity tasks of daily living is remarkably affected.

The sensory distribution of the ulnar nerve typically innervates the little finger and the ulnar half of the ring finger on the volar and dorsal surfaces of the hand (see Figure 13-5). Clients who have ulnar nerve compression can experience numbness, tingling, and paresthesia in this nerve distribution. When designing an orthosis for ulnar nerve lesions, the therapist monitors the areas of decreased sensation for pressure sores and skin irritation. Figure 13-12 illustrates the muscles an ulnar nerve lesion affects.

Orthotic Interventions for Ulnar Nerve Injury

Interventions for ulnar nerve compression or injury at the elbow and wrist levels require modification of activities that contribute to the development of the problem.

Orthotic Intervention for Ulnar Nerve Compression at the Elbow

A common intervention for compression at the cubital tunnel is an elbow orthosis with the elbow flexed 30 to 45 degrees.[1,30] If the wrist is included, it is positioned in neutral to 20 degrees of extension. Incorporating the wrist into the orthotic design decreases the effects from flexor carpi ulnaris contraction.[52]

The elbow orthosis helps prevent repetitive or prolonged elbow flexion, especially beyond 60 to 90 degrees. Prolonged elbow flexion can stress the ulnar nerve via traction[30,60] and increase pressure in the cubital tunnel.[38] This flexed position commonly occurs during sleep or with computer usage.[9,60] For sporadic or mild symptoms, the elbow orthosis may be worn during the night for approximately 3 weeks.[6] If demonstrating dysthesia, decreased sensibility, and continuous symptoms, the client may wear the elbow orthosis all the time.[6,11,52] However, it is generally recommended that instead of daytime elbow orthosis wear, the patient is educated to avoid flexing the elbow and or resting the elbow on a surface during activities.

Many therapists recommend a soft orthosis for comfort. Several soft elbow orthoses allow some movement but limit flexion to less than 45 degrees. When fabricating a rigid elbow orthosis, the therapist chooses a thermoplastic material with the following properties (see Chapter 3 for additional information):

- Rigidity so that the material is strong enough to support the weight of the elbow
- Self-bonding to help with formulation of the crease at the elbow
- Conformability and drapability to mold the material over the bony olecranon process

When fabricating the orthosis, the therapist may utilize an assistant to help stabilize the arm or use an elastic wrap bandage. A tuck in the thermoplastic material is close to the elbow joint, as shown in Figure 13-13, *A*. Care must be taken that strapping does not provide pressure over the medial elbow area, where the nerve crosses.[52] Another fabrication option is an anterior approach as shown in Figure 13-13, *B*. Thermoplastic material with conformability and drapability works well for this anterior-based orthosis.

Hand Based Orthotic Intervention for Ulnar Nerve Injury

The orthosis for an ulnar nerve lesion (Figure 13-14) positions the ring and little fingers in 30 to 45 degrees of MCP flexion[10,12] as a strong counterforce to prevent a claw hand deformity.[10] This position (30 to 45 degrees of MCP flexion) prevents attenuation of the denervated intrinsic muscles and the MCP volar plates of the ring and little fingers[16] and corrects the claw hand deformity of MCP hyperextension and PIP flexion. With the MCPs blocked in flexion, the power of the extensor digitorum communis is transferred to the IP joints and allows them to extend in the absence of the

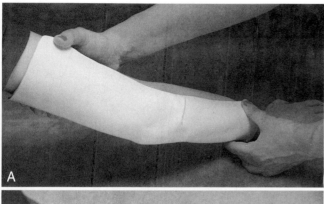

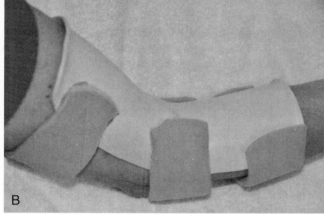

Figure 13-13 A, The arm and elbow position during molding of an elbow orthosis. **B,** An anterior based elbow orthosis.

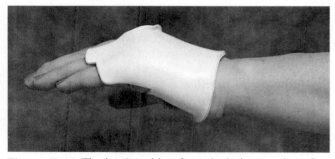

Figure 13-14 The hand position for orthotic intervention of an ulnar nerve injury in a static orthosis.

intrinsic muscles. Ultimately, the orthosis facilitates functional grasp.[10]

A client usually wears an immobilization orthosis continuously with removal only for hygiene and exercise. Some therapists recommend day time usage only.[50] Colditz[16] suggests the fabrication of a less bulky orthosis to keep from impeding the palmar sensation and function of the hand. One such orthosis is the figure-eight orthotic designed by Kiyoshi Yasaki and developed at the Hand Rehabilitation Center in Philadelphia, Pennsylvania (Figure 13-15).[10] The instructions in the following procedure include one method to fabricate a figure-eight hand based orthosis for an ulnar nerve injury.

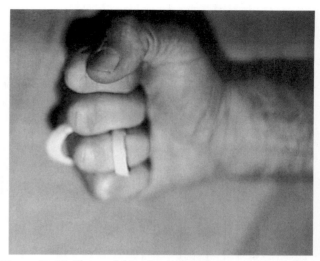

Figure 13-15 Figure-eight orthosis for ulnar nerve injury. (From Little KJ, Jacoby SM: Intra-articular hand fractures and joint injuries: part 1—surgeon's management. In Skirven TM, Osterman AL, Fedorczyk JM, et al., editors: *Rehabilitation of the hand and upper extremity,* ed 6, St Louis, 2011, Mosby, p. 406.)

PROCEDURE	for Fabrication of an Orthosis for Ulnar Nerve Injury

1. Cut a ½-inch strip of thermoplastic material approximately 12 to 14 inches long (Figure 13-16).
2. Heat the strip of thermoplastic material.
3. Position the arm with the elbow resting on a towel on a table and the hand in an upright position. Position the ring and small fingers in 30 to 45 degrees of MCP flexion. (IPs are in extension.)
4. Determine the midpoint of the strip, and place it midway between the ring and little fingers on the dorsal side of the fingers at the level of the MCP joints over the proximal phalanx.
5. Wrap one end of the strip around the ulnar side of the little finger to the volar surface and one end of the strip around the radial side of the ring finger to the volar (palmar) surface.
6. On the volar surface, cross straps (proximal to the MCP joints) over each other at the level of the metacarpals circling the ring and little finger.
7. Bring the straps back around to the dorsal surface proximal to the heads of the MCP joints. Overlap the straps approximately 1 inch, and adhere the pieces together.
8. Roll any areas that could interfere with function, such as rolling the area on the volar surface distal to the second and third digits and around the thenar crease.

Mobilization Orthoses for Ulnar Nerve Injuries

With a mobilizing (dynamic) orthosis, the therapist places the hand in the same position with the fourth and fifth digits in 30 to 45 degrees of MCP flexion. The therapist uses a mobilization orthotic design that includes finger loops attached to the ring and little fingers' proximal phalanges (Figure 13-17). The rubber band is connected to a soft wrist

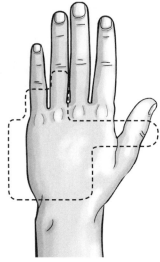

Figure 13-16 A hand based pattern for an ulnar nerve orthosis.

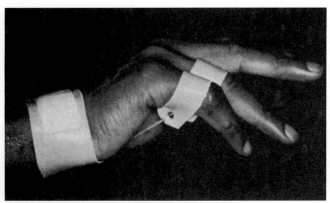

Figure 13-17 An extension mobilization orthosis for an ulnar nerve injury. (From Colditz JC: Splinting the hand with a peripheral nerve injury. In Mackin EJ, Callahan AD, Skirven TM, et al., editors: *Rehabilitation of the hand and upper extremity,* ed 5, St Louis, 2002, Mosby, pp. 622-634.)

cuff and uses traction to pull the two fingers into MCP flexion. The client wears the orthosis throughout the day with removal for hygiene and exercise. Physicians usually prescribe this type of orthosis when there is a need for a strong force to prevent hyperextension contractures at the MCP joints. To supplement this orthosis, a positioning (immobilization) nighttime orthosis may be necessary.

Another mobilization option for orthotic intervention of the ulnar nerve lesion is a spring-wire-and-foam orthosis, which is available commercially or can be custom made. Persons appreciate the low-profile design of the spring-wire-and-foam orthosis, and adherence tends to be high.[58]

Median Nerve Lesions

Traumatic median nerve lesions result from humeral fractures, elbow dislocations, distal radius fractures, dislocations of the lunate into the carpal canal, and lacerations of the

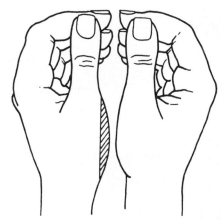

Figure 13-18 The classic median nerve deformity called an *ape* (or *simian*) *hand.* Note the thenar muscle atrophy of the left hand.

volar wrist.[10] The classic deformity associated with median nerve damage is called an *ape* (or *simian*) *hand* because the thenar eminence appears flattened due to denervation. A loss of thumb opposition occurs (Figure 13-18). The thumb is positioned in extension and adduction next to the index finger because of the unopposed action of the extensor pollicis longus and the adductor pollicis.[8] The thumb web space may contract, and the fingers may show trophic changes. In addition, a slight claw deformity of the index and middle fingers may occur because of the loss of lumbrical innervation.[56]

Functional Involvement from a Median Nerve Injury

The median nerve innervates the muscles depicted in Figure 13-19 (Table 13-4) in a low-level or wrist lesion and a high-level lesion involving the elbow or neck area. The impact on function from a median nerve lesion results in clumsiness with pinch and a decrease in power hand grip.[8] With lack of sensation in the fingers, skilled functions are difficult to perform with the hand. Power grip is affected because the thumb is no longer a stabilizing force due to the loss of the abductor pollicis brevis, flexor pollicis brevis, and opponens pollicis. Weakness in the lumbricals of the index and middle fingers further affects skilled movements of the hand.[7] The sensory areas innervated by the median nerve are used for identifying objects, temperature, and texture.[3]

Higher lesions can weaken or impair forearm pronation, wrist flexion, thumb IP flexion, and flexion of the proximal and distal IP joints of the index and middle fingers. Compression syndromes that occur from higher median nerve injuries are pronator syndrome and anterior interosseous syndrome. Pronator syndrome often results from strong and repetitive pronation and supination motions with the most common compression site between the two heads of the pronator teres.[46] Anterior interosseous syndrome is rare and is characterized by a vague discomfort in the proximal forearm. It usually involves compression of the deep head of the pronator teres. Clinically, the person presents with an inability to

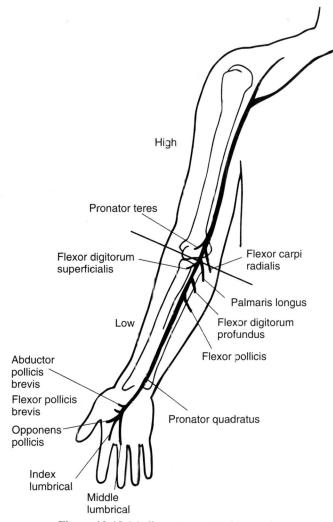

Figure 13-19 Median nerve motor innervation.

Labels on figure:
High
Pronator teres
Flexor digitorum superficialis
Flexor carpi radialis
Palmaris longus
Low
Flexor digitorum profundus
Flexor pollicis
Abductor pollicis brevis
Flexor pollicis brevis
Opponens pollicis
Pronator quadratus
Index lumbrical
Middle lumbrical

make an O with the thumb and index finger because usually there are no sensory losses with this condition.[46]

Thoracic outlet syndrome is sometimes initially considered an ulnar nerve injury or a high-level median nerve injury because it can initially resemble such nerve compressions.[43] Because median nerve injuries occur throughout the extremity, it is possible that a person be mistakenly thought to have one type of median nerve injury when he or she actually has another. Therefore, the astute therapist carefully considers the symptoms present for each person. For example, a person may have pronator syndrome instead of carpal tunnel syndrome (CTS) if[46,53,54]:

- Pain is experienced with resisted pronation and passive supination activities
- A positive Tinel sign at the proximal forearm is present
- Tenderness of the pronator muscle is evident
- "Numbness in the thenar eminence in the distribution of the palmar cutaneous branch of the median nerve" is present[53]
- Nocturnal symptoms are absent
- Muscle fatigue is present

- Thenar atrophy is absent
- Phalen's test is negative

CTS is a likely diagnosis for persons who have complaints of night pain, symptoms with repetitive wrist movements (especially flexion), weakness in thumb opposition and abduction, a positive Phalen's test, and a positive Tinel sign at the wrist.[52] If a person is referred with a diagnosis of CTS and actually has symptoms of pronator syndrome, the therapist calls the referring physician and discusses examination findings.

Frequently in persons with these syndromes, surgical procedures are required to decompress the nerve.[7] On occasion, a physician may request an orthosis for conservative management of mild cases. For example, for a mild case of **pronator tunnel syndrome** the physician may prescribe an elbow orthosis to position the forearm in neutral between pronation and supination and the elbow in flexion (Table 13-5).[9] This elbow position takes tension off the nerve, and the forearm position prevents compression via pronator contraction or stretch.

The median nerve's classic course and sensory distribution include the volar surface of the thumb, index, middle, and radial half of the ring fingers and the dorsal surface of the distal phalanxes of the thumb, index, middle, and radial half of the ring finger (see Figure 13-5). Clients who have median nerve compression can experience numbness, tingling, and paresthesia in this nerve distribution. Because the area of sensory distribution is large, the therapist monitors and educates clients or caregivers about the associated risks and prevention of skin injury or breakdown.

Orthotic Interventions for Median Nerve Injuries

Understanding the functional effects of the muscular loss resulting from a median nerve injury or compression syndrome is important because it influences the therapist's orthotic provision. With a median nerve lesion, if the therapist is able to maintain good passive mobility of the joints, extensive orthotic intervention may be unnecessary and occasional night orthotic intervention may be sufficient.[22]

Orthotic Intervention for Pronator Syndrome

Clients with pronator syndrome should avoid resisted pronation and passive supination.[54] Other than changing activities that contribute to pronator syndrome, the person may benefit from orthotic intervention. One orthosis option is to place the elbow in 90 degrees flexion and forearm in neutral rotation.[64]

Orthotic Intervention for Anterior Interosseous Nerve Compression

Besides the suggestion to avoid elbow extension and extreme forearm pronation and supination, orthotic intervention options are recommended for anterior interosseous nerve compressions. One option is to immobilize the elbow in

Table 13-4   Median Nerve Lesions

AFFECTED MUSCLES	WEAK AND LOST MOTIONS
Low Level (Wrist Level)	
Abductor pollicis brevis	Abduction of the CMC and MCP joints of the thumb, weak extension of the IP joint, and opposition
Flexor pollicis brevis (superficial head)	Flexion of the MCP and CMC joints and opposition
Opponens pollicis	Thumb opposition
First and second lumbricals	IP extension and MCP flexion of the second and third digits
High Level (Elbow or Neck Level)	
Flexor pollicis longus	IP thumb flexion and weakness with flexion of the MCP and CMC joints
Lateral half of the flexor digitorum profundus to the second and third digits	DIP and PIP flexion of the second and third digits
Pronator quadratus	Forearm pronation
Pronator teres	Forearm pronation and elbow flexion
Flexor carpi radialis	Flexion and radial deviation of the wrist
Palmaris longus	Wrist flexion
Flexor digitorum superficialis	Flexion of the PIP joints second through fifth digits and weak flexion of the MCP joints and wrist flexion
Abductor pollicis brevis	Abduction of the CMC and MCP joints of the thumb, weak extension of the IP joint, and opposition
Flexor pollicis brevis (superficial head)	Flexion of the MCP and CMC joints and opposition
Opponens pollicis	Thumb opposition
First and second lumbricals	IP extension and MCP flexion of the second and third digits

CMC, Carpometacarpal; *DIP,* distal interphalangeal; *IP,* interphalangeal; *MCP,* metacarpophalangeal; *PIP,* proximal interphalangeal.

Table 13-5   Orthotic Interventions for Peripheral Nerve Lesions

ORTHOSIS	POSITION
Radial	
Wrist immobilization orthosis	Wrist in 30 to 40 degrees of extension
Mobilization dorsal-based MCP extension orthosis	Wrist in 30 to 40 degrees of extension; MCPs in dynamic extension
Tenodesis orthosis (described by Colditz) (Other options for radial nerve orthotic provision are listed within the chapter)	Dorsal base using the tenodesis effect with MCPs in dynamic extension
Ulnar	
Elbow orthosis	Elbow in 30 to 45 degrees of flexion
Hand based immobilization anticlaw orthosis	MCPs of fourth and fifth digits in 30 to 45 degrees of MCP flexion
Median	
Dorsal- or volar-based wrist orthosis	Wrist in neutral
Ulnar gutter wrist orthosis	Wrist in neutral
Thumb web spacer orthosis or C bar orthosis	Thumb in 40 to 45 degrees of palmar abduction

MCP, metacarpophalangeal.

90 degrees flexion and the forearm in neutral. As discussed, impairments to the anterior interosseous nerve results in difficulty making an O with the thumb and index finger flexed. To compensate for this deficit, the therapist fabricates a small thermoplastic orthosis to block thumb IP and index DIP extension (Figure 13-20).[16]

Orthotic Intervention for Carpal Tunnel Syndrome

The most common type of median nerve compression is CTS. Compression at the wrist occurs because of a discrepancy in the volume of the rigid carpal canal and its contents, consisting of the median nerve and flexor tendons. Some conditions (such as, diabetes, pregnancy, Dupuytren disease,

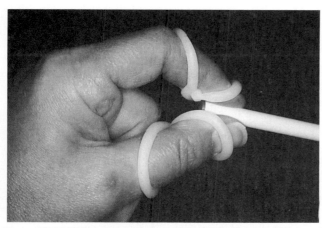

Figure 13-20 To encourage fingertip to thumb prehension, these small orthoses help someone with anterior interosseus nerve palsy. (From Colditz JC: Splinting the hand with a peripheral nerve injury. In Mackin EJ, Callahan AD, Skirven TM, et al., editors: *Rehabilitation of the hand and upper extremity,* ed 5, St Louis, 2002, Mosby, pp. 622-634.)

and carpometacarpal [CMC] arthritis) are associated with CTS. Home, leisure, and occupational activities involving repetitive or sustained wrist flexion, extension, and ulnar deviation; forearm supination; forceful gripping; and pinching all contribute to the development and exacerbation of CTS. Vibration, cold temperatures, and constriction over the wrist can also be contributing factors.[4,21,49,57,70] When manifestations of CTS are primarily sensory and occur from overuse or occupational causes, orthotic intervention of the wrist often reduces pain and symptoms.[7]

Often, other therapeutic interventions need to accompany the orthotic intervention program for CTS. Other interventions include ergonomic adaptations for home, leisure, and work environments; education on prevention; activity modifications; range of motion program with emphasis on tendon gliding exercises; and edema control techniques.[55] See Chapter 7 for an overview of efficacy studies on carpal tunnel intervention.

Usually, any orthosis for CTS positions the wrist as close to neutral as possible.[47] This neutral position maximizes available carpal tunnel space, minimizes median nerve compression, and facilitates pain relief.[36,43] A wrist immobilization orthosis is commonly worn at night and sometimes during home, leisure, or work activities that involve repetitive stressful wrist movements.[48] As discussed in Chapter 7, the wearing schedule can vary. Minimally, nighttime wear is required[48] to prevent extreme wrist postures that often occur during sleep.[55] Immobilization orthotic intervention with CTS has shown to improve long-term nerve conduction outcomes when consistently worn every night.[61] The wearing schedule is carefully monitored to prevent weakening of the muscles as a result of inactivity.[43] The orthosis may exacerbate symptoms if the person fights against the orthosis.[58]

Volar Wrist Immobilization Orthosis

Some clients and therapists prefer volar wrist orthoses, which provide adequate support to the wrist. A volar wrist orthosis

with a gel sheet or elastomer putty insert may be beneficial to control scar formation after carpal tunnel release surgery. A disadvantage of the volar wrist orthotic design for CTS is that the orthosis may interfere with palmar sensation.[7] Positioning the wrist in the orthosis is important. A poorly-designed wrist orthosis may compress the carpal tunnel area of the wrist. Some people may benefit from a volar wrist orthosis because it also immobilizes the MCP joints (see Chapter 7).

Dorsal or Ulnar Gutter Wrist Immobilization Orthoses

Other orthotic intervention approaches for CTS include fabrication of dorsal, ulnar gutter, or circumferential wrist orthosis. An advantage of the dorsal wrist orthosis is that there is no thermoplastic material directly over the carpal tunnel, thus avoiding compression. However, a disadvantage of the dorsal wrist orthosis is that it may not provide as much support and distribute pressure as well as the volar wrist orthosis. Some therapists fabricate the dorsal orthosis with a larger palmar area to increase support. An ulnar gutter wrist orthosis positions the wrist in neutral and is less likely to compress the carpal tunnel. A circumferential wrist orthosis provides a high degree of wrist immobilization (see Chapter 7).

Some clients may be more comfortable with soft prefabricated wrist orthoses that are appropriately sized based upon manufacturer recommendations. The therapist must check the orthosis on the person to ensure a correct fit for function and preservation of hand structures based on clinical reasoning.[2]

Orthotic Intervention for Median Nerve Injuries with Thumb Involvement

For a client who has a median nerve injury involving the thumb, which occurs in the later stages of CTS, the therapist addresses loss of thumb opposition for functional grasp and pinch. The orthosis positions the thumb in opposition and palmar abduction, which assists the thumb for tip prehension. A C bar between the thumb and the index finger helps maintain the thumb web space. The thumb web space is a common site for muscular shortening of the adductor pollicis after median nerve damage. The orthotic design is usually static. A person with a median nerve injury with thumb involvement may benefit from a hand based thumb spica orthosis (see Chapter 8).

For a low-level median nerve injury, the therapist may fabricate a thumb web spacer orthosis (Figure 13-21). The web spacer orthosis allows free wrist mobility.[7] If the therapist fabricates a mobilization thumb orthosis, a static thumb spica orthosis may be incorporated into the orthotic intervention program for nighttime wear.

Orthotic Intervention for Combined Median and Ulnar Nerve Injuries

Sometimes with extensive injuries, both median and ulnar nerves are involved. In that case, orthotic intervention to

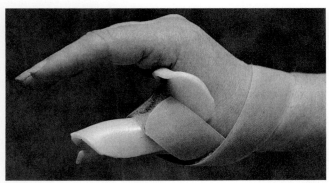

Figure 13-21 A thumb web spacer orthosis for median nerve injury.

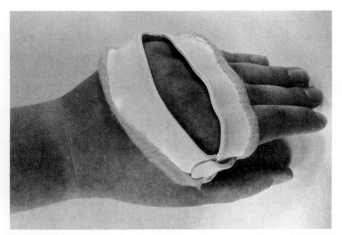

Figure 13-22 This orthosis inhibits metacarpophalangeal (MCP) extension with a combined median and ulnar nerve. (From Fess EE, Gettle KS, Philips CA, et al: *Hand and upper extremity splinting: principles and methods,* ed 3, St Louis, 2005, Elsevier Mosby.)

prevent further deformities entails designs that are similar to a singular nerve injury but with all digits included. The thumb may be included if it is affected (Figure 13-22).

Summary

Orthotic intervention for nerve injuries involves a comprehensive knowledge of the muscular, sensory, and functional implications for each client. There are various orthotic interventions for nerve injuries (Table 13-6). However, the therapist must note that these are general guidelines and physicians and experienced therapists may have other protocols for positioning and orthotic intervention.

Patient Safety Tips and Precautions Box

- Be aware of natural reactions to a nerve injury, including skin changes, muscle imbalance with possible deformity and joint contracture, and circulatory changes such as cold skin.
- Avoid heavy lifting or resistance, as well as forceful or repetitive motions.
- Pay attention to potential pressure areas from the orthosis.
- Pay attention to cleaning the orthosis and wound care management.
- Do not neglect nail care despite orthotic intervention.
- Be aware of protecting versus overprotection. Overprotection of injury while wearing the orthosis may cause decreased motion and put the client at further risk for contractures or deformity.
- Be aware of substitution motions, which are a normal reaction after a nerve injury to protect and decrease pain. These unnatural movements may cause further harm to a recovering nerve and put the client at risk for muscle imbalance.

Review Questions

1. Which factors are important in the prognosis of a peripheral nerve lesion?
2. What are the common deformities resulting from radial, ulnar, and median nerve lesions?
3. What are the functional implications of radial, ulnar, and median nerve lesions?
4. What are the orthotic intervention options for radial nerve injuries? In which position should the therapist place the hand?
5. What is the proper type, position, and thermoplastic material needed for fabrication of an orthosis for ulnar nerve compression at the elbow?
6. What is the proper orthotic position for a claw hand deformity? Why is this a good position?
7. What are the advantages and disadvantages of the different approaches to wrist orthotic intervention for CTS?
8. What is the appropriate position in which to place a hand with a median nerve lesion that includes thumb symptoms?

Table 13-6   Evidence Based Practice about Orthotic Provision for Radial and Ulnar Nerve Deficits

AUTHOR'S CITATION	DESIGN	NUMBER OF PARTICIPANTS	DESCRIPTION	RESULTS	LIMITATIONS
Svernlov B, Larsson M, Rehn K, et al: Conservative treatment of the cubital tunnel syndrome, *J Hand Surg European Volume 2*: 201-207, 2009.	Randomized control trial with three groups	70 participants (39 women and 31 men)	"The purpose of this randomized study was to evaluate the efficacy of treatment with a brace or nerve gliding exercises in patients with mild or moderate ulnar neuropathy at the elbow" (p. 201). Three groups of subjects received basic information on ulnar nerve anatomy, explanation of body mechanics, and how to avoid provocation of symptoms. Group A used a prefabricated Neoprene elbow brace at night for 3 months. Group B was instructed to perform nerve gliding exercises with therapist supervision and direction for 3 months. Group C, the control group, was only given the previously stated written information.	Six participants showed no improvements and demanded surgery; however the remaining 89.5% showed subjective and objective improvement. Activity impairment as measured by the COPM improved in all groups at a 6 month follow up, however there were no significant differences between the groups. Grip strength showed no statistical improvement or differences between groups. All groups shared an improvement in daytime pain with a visual analogue scale, yet there was no statistical difference between groups.	Because of the consistent improvement in all three groups regardless of level of education or intervention provided, it is impossible to say whether the improvement was due to the variables of the study or due to spontaneous recovery of the ulnar nerve. Small sample size and attrition for follow-up visits also limit the study results. Adherence to home exercise programs within the study were only monitored for one group (group B) by participant attendance to a nerve gliding group once during the study duration, but this does not ensure that the nerve gliding home program (or using orthotic intervention in group A) was followed as directed.
Apfel E, Sigafoos G: Comparison of range-of-motion constraints provided by splints used in the treatment of cubital tunnel syndrome: a pilot study, *J Hand Ther* 19:384-392, 2006.	Multiple-subject experimental design	Three cadaver arms were used of varying sizes to include small, small/medium, and medium	"The purpose of this article is to assess the range-of-motion constraints of 5 nighttime elbow orthoses commonly used in the treatment of cubital tunnel syndrome" (p. 384). Researchers hypothesized that all five orthoses would have the same restriction on elbow range of motion.	The AliiMed Cubital Tunnel Syndrome Support orthosis allowed the most elbow flexion. The Hely & Weber orthosis allowed the least amount of flexion and was the only orthosis to limit extension. The Pil-O-Splint Elbow Splint with stay and the Folded Towel all restricted flexion less than the criteria of 90 degrees.	The fact that subjects were cadaver arms instead of human participants is the largest limitation. Use of cadaver arms makes it impossible for this study to account for tissue differences in the arm of a living person, orthosis comfort and functional use, and actual alleviation of symptoms for cubital tunnel syndrome. Sizes and genders for the cadaver arms were also dependent only on availability. Small sample size is another limitation. Only a limited number of orthoses (five) were tested as well, limiting the study results.

Continued

Table 13-6 Evidence Based Practice about Orthotic Provision for Radial and Ulnar Nerve Deficits—cont'd

AUTHOR'S CITATION	DESIGN	NUMBER OF PARTICIPANTS	DESCRIPTION	RESULTS	LIMITATIONS
Hannah SD, Hudak PL: Splinting and radial nerve palsy: a single-subject experiment, *J Hand Ther* 14:195-201, 2001.	Single-subject experimental design	Single-subject (1 study participant)	The aim of this study was to compare the client's response to four interventions: no orthosis (baseline), static collar wrist cock-up orthosis, dynamic tenodesis orthosis, and dorsal wrist cock-up with dynamic finger extension orthosis. The participant wore each orthosis for 3 weeks, documenting time worn and activities performed.	Following the three 3-week trials, the study participant was allowed to choose whichever orthosis she felt was the most beneficial for another 3-week trial. She chose both the static volar wrist cock-up orthosis and the dynamic finger extension orthosis. Using the DAH, the TEMPA, and the COPM, the dynamic finger extension orthosis showed the most improvement in perceived disability, functional abilities, and satisfaction with performance. Despite lack of improvement with the volar cock-up orthosis, the participant chose it because she found it supportive, easy to put on, and less conspicuous than others.	Researchers were not blind to the interventions (types of orthoses). No re-administration of the TEMPA was completed at the end of each 3-week interval. The two dynamic orthoses had an added thumb component to assist in grasp and release of objects, which may have exaggerated findings of the functional differences among orthoses. Alternative research methods are needed to further understand the effects of using an orthosis for radial nerve palsy and other nerve conditions. Another limitation is that both the tenodesis suspension orthosis and dorsal wrist dynamic finger extension orthosis had components that encouraged thumb abduction for grasp and release. This may have magnified the functional differences between the dynamic orthoses and the volar wrist cock-up orthosis.
Hong CZ, Long HA, Kanakamedala V, et al: Splinting and local steroid injection for the treatment of ulnar neuropathy and the elbow: clinical and electrophysiological evaluation, *Arch Phys Med Rehabil* 77(6):573-576, 1996.	Randomized control trial	10 participants (12 nerves)	The aim of this study was to compare the effects of using an orthosis at the elbow to the effects of using an orthosis combined with steroid intervention for ulnar neuropathy. The study participants were randomized with Group A receiving a steroid injection and an orthosis and Group B, using the orthosis alone. Orthosis wearing was monitored, and participants were disqualified if they did not meet the required time. Motor nerve conduction was measured by patient report and also myoelectrically to detect returns in ulnar nerve function. Participants were tested at 1 month and 6 months.	The study demonstrated that orthosis application offered a significant decrease in symptoms and increase in conduction velocity for both groups at 1 and 6 months. The addition of a steroid injection did not appear to create a significant difference in reducing symptoms of study participants. Based on this study, it seems as though using an orthosis is an adequate intervention for ulnar neuropathy at the elbow because the addition of a steroid injection did not appear to offer additional benefits.	One limitation of this study was the lack of population diversity. The participants in this study were gathered from a local VA facility and were all males with an average age of 59.1 years. Authors of the study cite this as a possible reason for poor response to local steroid injection.

COPM, Canadian Occupational Performance Measure; *DAH,* ***; *TEMPA,* ***; *VA,* US Department of Veterans Affairs.

SELF-QUIZ 13-1*

In regard to the following questions, circle either true (T) or false (F).

1. T F With neurapraxia, the prognosis is extremely good because recovery is usually spontaneous.
2. T F Functionally, a client diagnosed with a radial nerve injury has a poor grip.
3. T F The main purpose of orthotic intervention for a nerve injury is to immobilize the extremity.
4. T F The claw hand deformity occurs only with a low-level ulnar nerve injury.
5. T F The therapist should position an elbow orthosis in 90 degrees of flexion for a client who has an ulnar nerve compression at the elbow level.
6. T F For an ulnar nerve orthosis, the therapist should position the ring and little fingers in approximately 30 to 45 degrees of MCP flexion.
7. T F The proper orthosis for a radial nerve injury is a wrist immobilization or dynamic wrist and MCP extension orthosis.
8. T F The therapist should immobilize radial, ulnar, and median nerve injuries only in static orthoses.
9. T F Froment sign is an identifying posture of a median nerve injury.
10. T F Functionally, a client diagnosed with an ulnar nerve injury has loss of pinch strength and power grip.
11. T F The therapist may use a thumb web spacer orthosis for a median nerve injury.
12. T F Low-level nerve injuries occur only distal to the wrist.

*See Appendix A for the answer key.

SELF-QUIZ 13-2*

Match the following nerve conditions with the appropriate upper extremity positions required for conservative orthotic intervention.

1. Ulnar tunnel syndrome
2. Pronator syndrome
3. Anterior interosseous syndrome
4. Radial tunnel syndrome
5. Posterior interosseous nerve syndrome
6. Cubital tunnel syndrome
7. Wartenberg neuropathy
8. Carpal tunnel syndrome (CTS)

a. 90 degrees elbow flexion and neutral forearm and or a small orthoses to block index DIP and thumb IP extension or hyperextension
b. 30 to 45 degrees MCP flexion of the fourth and fifth digits
c. 20 to 30 degrees wrist extension
d. 30 to 40 degrees wrist extension and neutral MCP extension
e. 30 to 45 degrees elbow flexion
f. 90 degrees elbow flexion and neutral forearm
g. Slight wrist extension
h. Neutral wrist

*See Appendix A for the answer key.

References

1. Aiello B: Ulnar nerve compression in cubital tunnel. In Clark GL, Shaw EF, Aiello WB, et al, editors: *Hand rehabilitation: a practical guide*, New York, 1993, Churchill Livingstone.
2. Apfel E, Sigafoos GT: Comparison of range-of-motion constraints provided by splints used in the treatment of cubital tunnel syndrome: a pilot study, *J Hand Ther* 19(4):384–392, 2006.
3. Arsham NZ: Nerve injury. In Ziegler EM, editor: *Current concepts in orthotics: a diagnosis-related approach to splinting*, Germantown, WI, 1984, Rolyan Medical Products.
4. Barnhart S, Demers PA, Miller M, et al.: Carpal tunnel syndrome among ski manufacturing workers, *Scand J Work Environ Health* 17(1):46–52, 1991.
5. Barr NR, Swan D: *The hand: principles and techniques of splintmaking*, Boston, 1988, Butterworth Publishers.
6. Blackmore SM: Therapist's management of ulnar nerve neuropathy at the elbow. In Mackin EJ, Callahan AD, Skirven TM, et al, editors: *Rehabilitation of the hand*, ed 5, St Louis, 2002, Mosby, pp 679–689.
7. Borucki S, Schmidt J: Peripheral neuropathies. In Aisen ML, editor: *Orthotics in neurologic rehabilitation*, New York, 1992, Demos Publications.
8. Boscheinen-Morrin J, Davey V, Conolly WB: Peripheral nerve injuries (including tendon transfers). In Boscheinen-Morrin J, Davey V, Conolly WB, editors: *The hand: fundamentals of therapy*, Boston, 1987, Butterworth Publishers.
9. Cailliet R: *Hand pain and impairment*, ed 4, Philadelphia, 1994, FA Davis.
10. Callahan A: Nerve injuries. In Malick MH, Kasch MC, editors: *Manual on management of specific hand problems*, Pittsburgh, 1984, American Rehabilitation Educational Network.

11. Cannon NM, editor: *Diagnosis and treatment manual for physicians and therapists*, ed 3, Indianapolis, 1991, The Hand Rehabilitation Center of Indiana.

12. Cannon NM, Foltz RW, Koepfer JM, et al.: *Manual of hand splinting*, New York, 1985, Churchill Livingstone.

13. Clarkson HM, Gilewich GB: *Musculoskeletal assessment: joint range of motion and manual muscle strength*, Baltimore, 1989, Williams & Wilkins.

14. Cohen MS, Garfin SR: Nerve compression syndromes: finding the cause of upper-extremity symptoms, *Consultant* 37:241–254, 1997.

15. Colditz JC: Splinting for radial nerve palsy, *J Hand Ther* 1:18–23, 1987.

16. Colditz JC: Splinting the hand with a peripheral nerve injury. In Mackin EJ, Callahan AD, Skirven TM, et al.: *Rehabilitation of the hand*, ed 5, St Louis, 2002, Mosby, pp 622–634.

17. Crochetiere WJ, Goldstein SA, Granger GV, et al.: The Granger orthosis for radial nerve palsy, *Orthotics and Prosthetics* 29(4):27–31, 1975.

18. Dang AC, Roder CM: Unusual compression neuropathies of the forearm, part I: radial nerve, *J Hand Surg* 34(10):1906–1914, 2009.

19. Eaton CJ, Lister GD: Radial nerve compression, *Hand Clinics* 8(2):345–357, 1992.

20. Enna CD: *Peripheral denervation of the hand*, New York, 1988, Alan R. Liss.

21. Feldman RG, Travers PH, Chirico-Post J, et al.: Risk assessment in electronic assembly workers: carpal tunnel syndrome, *J Hand Surg Am* 12(5):849–855, 1987.

22. Fess EE: Rehabilitation of the patient with peripheral nerve injury, *Hand Clinics* 2(1):207–215, 1986.

23. Fess EE, Gettle KS, Philips CA, et al.: *Hand splinting principles and methods*, ed 3, St Louis, 2005, Elsevier Mosby.

24. Fox IK, Mackinnon SE: Adult peripheral nerve disorders: nerve entrapment, repair, transfer, and brachial plexus disorders, *Plast Reconstr Surg* 127(5):105e–118e, 2011.

25. Frykman GK: The quest for better recovery from peripheral nerve injury: current status of nerve regeneration research, *J Hand Ther* 6(2):83–88, 1993.

26. Gelberman RH, Eaton R, Urbanisk JR: Peripheral nerve compression, *J Bone Joint Surg Am* 75:1854–1878, 1993.

27. Greene DP, Roberts SL: *Kinesiology movement in the context of activity*, St Louis, 1999, Mosby.

28. Gross MS, Gelberman RH: The anatomy of the distal ulnar tunnel, *Clin Orthop Relat Res* 196:238–247, 1985.

29. Hannah SD, Hudak PL: Splinting and radial nerve palsy: a single-subject experiment, *J Hand Ther* 14(3):195–201, 2001.

30. Harper BD: The drop-out splint: an alternative to the conservative management of ulnar nerve entrapment at the elbow, *J Hand Ther* 3:199–210, 1990.

31. Hong CZ, Long HA, Kanakamedala V, et al.: Splinting and local steroid injection for the treatment of ulnar neuropathy at the elbow: clinical and electrophysiological evaluation, *Arch Phys Med Rehabil* 77(6):573–576, 1996.

32. Hornbach Culp: Radial tunnel syndrome. In Mackin EJ, Callahan AD, Skirven TM, et al.: *Rehabilitation of the hand*, ed 5, St Louis, 2002, Mosby.

33. Izzi J, Dennison D, Noerdlinger M, et al.: Nerve injuries of the elbow, wrist, and hand in athletes, *Clin Sports Med* 20(1):203–217, 2001.

34. Jebson PJL, Gaul JS: Peripheral nerve injury. In Jebson PJL, Kasdan ML, editors: *Hand secrets*, Philadelphia, 1998, Hanley & Belfus.

35. Kleinert MJ, Mehta S: Radial nerve entrapment, *Orthop Clin North Am* 27(2):305–315, 1996.

36. Kruger VL, Kraft GH, Deitz JC, et al.: Carpal tunnel syndrome: objective measures and splint use, *Arch Phys Med Rehabil* 72(7):517–520, 1991.

37. Mackinnon SE, Dellon AL: *Surgery of the peripheral nerve*, New York, 1988, Thieme Medical Publishers, Inc.

38. MacNicol MF: Mechanics of the ulnar nerve at the elbow, *J Bone Joint Surg Br* 62(53):518, 1980.

39. McGowan AJ: The results of transposition of the ulnar nerve for traumatic ulnar neuritis, *J Bone Joint Surg Br* 23:293–301, 1950.

40. McKee P, Nguyen C: Customized dynamic splinting: orthoses that promote optimal function and recovery after radial nerve injury: a case report, *J Hand Ther* 20:73–88, 2007.

41. McKee P, Nguyen C: Low-profile dorsal dynamic wrist-finger-thumb-assistive-extension orthosis for high radial nerve injury-fabrication instructions, *J Hand Ther* 20:70–72, 2007.

42. Melhorn JM: Cumulative trauma disorders and repetitive strain injuries: the future, *Clin Orthop Relat Res* 351:107–126, 1998.

43. Messer RS, Bankers RM: Evaluating and treating common upper extremity nerve compression and tendonitis syndromes …without becoming cumulatively traumatized, *Nurse Pract Forum* 6(3):152–166, 1995.

44. Novak CB, Mackinnon SE: Nerve injury in repetitive motion disorders, *Clin Orthop Relat Res* 351:10–20, 1998.

45. Novak CB, Mackinnon SE: Evaluation of nerve injury and nerve compression in the upper quadrant, *J Hand Ther* 18:230–240, 2005.

46. Nuber GW, Assenmacher J, Bowen MK: Neurovascular problems in the forearm, wrist, and hand, *Clin Sports Med* 17(3):585–610, 1998.

47. Nuckols T, Harber P, Sandin K, et al.: Quality measures for the diagnosis and non-operative management of carpal tunnel syndrome in occupational settings, *J Occup Rehabil* 21(1):100–119, 2011.

48. Ono S, Chapham PJ, Chung KC: Optimal management of carpal tunnel syndrome, *Int J Gen Med* 3:235–261, 2010.

49. Ostorio AM, Ames RG, Jones J, et al.: Carpal tunnel syndrome among grocery store workers, *Am J Int Med* 25:229–245, 1994.

50. Peck J: Personal communication, March 2013.

51. Porretto-Loehrke A, Soika E: Therapist's management of other nerve compressions about the elbow and wrist. In Skirven TM, Osterman AL, Fedorczyk JM, et al, editors: *Rehabilitation of the hand and upper extremity*, ed 6, Philadelphia, PA, 2011, Mosby.

52. Possner MA: Compressive neuropathies of the ulnar nerve at the elbow and wrist, *Instr Course Lect* 49:305–317, 2000.

53. Rehak DC: Pronator syndrome, *Clin Sports Med* 20(3):531–540, 2001.

54. Saidoff DC, McDonough AL: *Critical pathways in therapeutic intervention: upper extremities*, St Louis, 1997, Mosby.

55. Sailer SM: The role of splinting and rehabilitation, *Hand Clinics* 12(2):223–240, 1996.

56. Salter MI: *Hand injuries: a therapeutic approach*, Edinburgh, London, 1987, Churchill Livingstone.

57. Schottland JR, Kirschberg GJ, Fillingim R, et al.: Median nerve latencies in poultry processing workers: an approach to resolving the role of industrial "cumulative trauma" in the development of carpal tunnel syndrome, *J Occup Med* 33(5):627–631, 1991.

58. Schultz-Johnson K: Personal communication, October 1999.
59. Seddon HJ: Three types of nerve injury, *J Neurol* 66:237–288, 1943.
60. Seror P: Treatment of ulnar nerve palsy at the elbow with a night splint, *J Bone Joint Surg Br* 75(2):322–327, 1993.
61. Sevim S, Dogu O, Camdeviren H, et al.: Long-term effectiveness of steroid injections and splinting in mild and moderate carpal tunnel syndrome, *Neurol Sci* 25(2):48–52, 2004.
62. Skirven TM, Callahan AD: Therapist's management of peripheral-nerve injuries. In Mackin EJ, Callahan AD, Skirven TM, et al, editors: *Rehabilitation of the hand*, ed 5, St Louis, 2002, Mosby, pp 599–621.
63. Skirven T, Osterman AL: Clinical examination of the wrist. In Mackin EJ, Callahan AD, Skirven TM, et al.: *Rehabilitation of the hand*, ed 5, St Louis, 2002, Mosby, pp 1099–1116.
64. Slutsky DJ: New advances in nerve repair. In Skirven TM, Osterman AL, Fedorczyk JM, et al.: *Rehabilitation of the hand and upper extremity*, ed 6, Philadelphia, 2011, Elsevier Mosby, pp 611–618.
65. Spinner M: Nerve lesions in continuity. In Hunter JM, Schneider LH, Mackin EJ, et al.: *Rehabilitation of the hand*, ed 3, St Louis, 1990, Mosby, pp 523–529.
66. Sunderland S: The peripheral nerve trunk in relation to injury: a classification of nerve injury. In Sunderland S, editor: *Nerves and nerve injuries*, Baltimore, 1968, Williams & Wilkins, pp 127–137.
67. Upton AR, McComas AJ: The double crush in nerve entrapment syndromes, *Lancet* 2:359–362, 1973.
68. Vender MI, Truppa KL, Ruder JR, et al.: Upper extremity compressive neuropathies, *Physical Medicine and Rehabilitation: State of the Art Reviews* 12(2):243–262, 1998.
69. Walsh M: Personal communication, June 2012.
70. Wieslander G, Norback D, Gothe C, et al.: Carpal tunnel syndrome (CTS) and exposure to vibration, repetitive wrist movements and heavy manual work: a case-referent study, *Br J Ind Med* 46(1): 43–47, 1989.
71. Ziegler EM: *Current concepts in orthotics: a diagnosis-related approach to splinting*, Germantown, WI, 1984, Rolyan Medical Products.

APPENDIX 13-1   CASE STUDIES

CASE STUDY 13-1*

Read the following scenario, and answer the questions based on information in this chapter.

Sally is a 52-year-old woman who is employed at a bank. She primarily works on the computer and sleeps with her elbow bent. Over time Sally develops compression of the ulnar nerve at the elbow, which is manifested by interosseous weakness, a positive Froment sign, complaints of discomfort on the medial side of the arm, and continuous numbness and tingling in digits 4 and 5.

1. Functionally, what might Sally have difficulty doing?
2. What is the correct orthosis for her condition?
3. What are the correct positions for her joints in the orthosis?
4. After being fitted with a custom thermoplastic orthosis, Sally complains that she does not like the hard feel of the material. What would you do?
5. What is your suggested wearing schedule?
6. What other lifestyle adjustments would be suggested?

*See Appendix A for the answer key.

CASE STUDY 13-2*

Read the following scenario, and answer the questions based on information in this chapter. Indicate all answers that are correct.

Diana sustained a fall breaking the middle third of her right humeral shaft. Diana later reflected that it was a classic beautiful summer evening when the fall happened. She had been taking a leisurely walk with her fiancé, and when walking across a bridge, she turned around to admire the view. In the dark she did not see a pole sticking out of the middle of the bridge. This led to a fall on the hard surface of the bridge. In the emergency room the physician identified not only a fracture of the right humeral shaft, which needed to be set, but a complete transaction of the radial nerve. After surgery you (the therapist working with her) have been ordered to provide therapy for Diana and an orthosis for her radial nerve condition.

1. Which of the following motion difficulties would you expect to see with Diana?
   a. Difficulty with abduction of the carpometacarpal (CMC) joint of the thumb, weakness with thumb opposition and with IP extension, and weakness with metacarpophalangeal (MCP) flexion of the second and third digits.
   b. Difficulty with MCP extension, wrist extension, thumb abduction and extension as well as weakness with elbow flexion/extension, wrist extension, and deviation.
   c. Difficulty with wrist flexion and adduction, flexion of the distal interphalangeal (DIP) of the fourth and fifth digit, MCP flexion of the fifth digit and opposition, and abduction and adduction at the MCP joints. Difficulty also with some thumb motions, especially with thumb adduction.
   d. Diana will not have motion difficulties and will only experience sensory difficulties.
2. What type of orthosis might you consider providing?
   a. Volar wrist orthosis
   b. Dynamic tenodesis suspension orthosis
   c. Thumb immobilization orthosis
   d. Elbow extension orthosis
3. What is the functional advantage of this orthosis?
   a. The design allows the dorsal surface of the hand to be relatively free
   b. The wrist and thumb can move
   c. The fingers are not immobilized
   d. The hand is completely free to move
4. What would be your suggested wearing schedule?
   a. Only during painful activities
   b. All the time with removal for hygiene
5. What could be another orthosis option for Diane?
   a. Mobilization orthosis in wrist and MCP joint extension
   b. Thumb immobilization orthosis
   c. Static orthosis with fourth and fifth digits in 30 degrees of flexion
   d. Thumb web spacer orthosis

*See Appendix A for the answer key.

APPENDIX 13-2   LABORATORY EXERCISES

Laboratory Exercise 13-1* MCP Extension Hand Based Orthosis

Read the following scenario, and answer the questions based on information from the chapter.

Maria is a 36-year-old right-handed woman who presents with left forearm level posterior interosseous nerve syndrome. The physician referred Maria to a therapist for orthotic fabrication and a home exercise program. The therapist wrote the following SOAP note:

   S: *"I really want to get better fast."*

   O: *Pt. presented with posterior interosseous nerve syndrome. Manual muscle testing (MMT) scores for the extensor digitorum communis, extensor digiti minimi, extensor indicis, abductor pollicis longus, and extensor carpi ulnaris were all 0 (zero). Pt. reports no pain in the left upper extremity (LUE). A left dorsal forearm based MCP mobilization extension orthosis was fabricated and fitted. Pt. was instructed how to don and doff the orthosis and how to grasp and release objects. Pt. was also instructed verbally and given written information on the wearing schedule, orthotic care, and precautions. Pt. was given a home exercise program to be completed five times daily.*

   A: *Pt. was receptive to the orthosis and home exercise program. Pt. was able to independently grasp objects while wearing the orthosis. Anticipate compliance with wearing schedule and home exercise program.*

   P: *Will monitor needs for modifications of the orthosis and home exercise program.*

   Several appointments later, the client regained muscle strength with an MMT score of fair (3) wrist extensors. Fabricated a left dynamic MCP extension hand based orthosis. The therapist encouraged the patient to continue with activities of daily living (ADLs) and the home exercise program and initiated gentle strengthening activities. The orthotic-wearing schedule and home exercise program were modified. The client was instructed to complete the program five times daily. The client had no complaints and was able to independently grasp light objects while wearing the orthosis.

   Write the next progress note.

*See Appendix A for the answer key.

Laboratory Exercise 13-2 Anticlaw Orthosis

On a partner, practice fabricating a hand based orthosis in the anticlaw position for a client who has an ulnar nerve lesion. Refer to options provided in the chapter (figure-eight orthosis, hand based static orthosis, or hand based mobilization orthosis). Before starting, determine the position to place the person's hand. Remember to position the MCP joints of the ring and little fingers in approximately 30 to 45 degrees of flexion. After fitting the orthosis and making all adjustments, use Form 13-1. This check-off sheet is a self-evaluation of the orthosis. Use Grading Sheet 13-1 as a classroom grading sheet.

FORM 13-1* Anticlaw orthosis

Name: _____

Date: _____

Answer the following questions after the orthosis has been worn for 30 minutes. (Mark NA for non-applicable situations.)

Evaluation Areas				**Comments**

Design
1. The orthosis prevents hyperextension of the MCP joints of the ring and little fingers.   Yes ○   No ○   NA ○

Function
1. The orthosis allows full wrist motions.   Yes ○   No ○   NA ○
2. The orthosis allows full function of the middle and index fingers.   Yes ○   No ○   NA ○

Straps (if used)
1. The straps avoid body prominences.   Yes ○   No ○   NA ○
2. The straps are secure and rounded.   Yes ○   No ○   NA ○

Comfort
1. The edges are smooth with rounded corners.   Yes ○   No ○   NA ○
2. The proximal end is flared (if appropriate).   Yes ○   No ○   NA ○
3. Impingements or pressure areas are not present.   Yes ○   No ○   NA ○
4. Orthosis pressure is well distributed over the proximal phalanx of the ring and little fingers.   Yes ○   No ○   NA ○

Cosmetic Appearance
1. The orthosis is free of fingerprints, dirt, and pencil or pen marks.   Yes ○   No ○   NA ○
2. The orthosis is smooth and free of buckles.   Yes ○   No ○   NA ○

Therapeutic Regiment
1. The person has been instructed in a wearing schedule.   Yes ○   No ○   NA ○
2. The person has been provided with orthosis precautions.   Yes ○   No ○   NA ○
3. The person demonstrates understanding of the education.   Yes ○   No ○   NA ○
4. Client/caregiver knows how to clean the orthosis.   Yes ○   No ○   NA ○

Discuss possible adjustments or changes you would make based on the self-evaluation.

_____

_____

_____

Discuss possible areas to improve with clinical safety when fabricating the orthosis.

_____

_____

_____

*See Appendix B for a perforated copy of this form.

GRADING SHEET 13-1*

Anticlaw orthosis

Name: _____

Date: _____

Grade: _____

1 = Beyond improvement, not acceptable
2 = Requires maximal improvement
3 = Requires moderate improvement
4 = Requires minimal improvement
5 = Requires no improvement

Evaluation Areas						**Comments**
Design						
1. The orthosis prevents hyperextension of the MCP joints of the ring and little fingers.	1	2	3	4	5	
Function						
1. The orthosis allows full wrist motions.	1	2	3	4	5	
2. The orthosis allows full function of the middle and index fingers.	1	2	3	4	5	
Straps (if used)						
1. The straps avoid body prominences.	1	2	3	4	5	
2. The straps are secure and rounded.	1	2	3	4	5	
Comfort						
1. The edges are smooth with rounded corners.	1	2	3	4	5	
2. The proximal end is flared (if appropriate).	1	2	3	4	5	
3. Impingements or pressure areas are not present.	1	2	3	4	5	
4. The pressure is well distributed over the proximal phalanx of the ring and little fingers.	1	2	3	4	5	
Cosmetic Appearance						
1. The orthosis is free of fingerprints, dirt, and pencil or pen marks.	1	2	3	4	5	
2. The orthosis is not buckled.	1	2	3	4	5	

CHAPTER 14

Orthotic Provision to Manage Spasticity

Salvador Bondoc

Key Terms

biomechanical
composite extension
contracture
minimalist design
Neoprene
neurophysiologic
orthosis
plaster bandage
serial casting
spasticity
stretch reflex
submaximum range
task-oriented approach

Chapter Objectives

1. Define *spasticity*.
2. Compare the strengths and weaknesses of dorsal and volar forearm platforms.
3. Discuss orthotic design based on a neurophysiologic rationale.
4. Discuss orthotic design based on a biomechanical rationale.
5. Differentiate between the elastic and contractile properties of muscle, and describe their implications on using an orthosis.
6. Describe the difference between submaximum and maximum ranges as they relate to spasticity using an orthosis.
7. Describe the properties of alternative materials to thermoplastics and plaster and fiberglass casts used for neurologic orthoses.
8. Successfully fabricate and clinically evaluate the proper fit of a dorsal forearm-volar hand immobilization orthosis.
9. Use clinical judgment to correctly analyze two case studies.

Spasticity is defined as a velocity-dependent increase in muscle tone due to hyperactive **stretch reflex**.[3,38] The defining feature of velocity-dependence is highlighted when clinicians assess spastic tone by the degree and extent of resistance to passive stretch. Some scholars have expanded on the definition of **spasticity** to highlight other manifestations of impaired motor control including the loss of normal reciprocal inhibition and abnormal co-activation of agonist and antagonist muscles during active movement.[8,34,40] This definition has important implications toward therapy management using a problem-solving and evidence-based approach.

The onset of spasticity is associated with upper motor neuron lesions (UMNLs) seen in many common central nervous system (CNS) conditions, such as cerebrovascular accident, cerebral palsy, traumatic brain injury, spinal cord injury, and multiple sclerosis. During the acute stages following the onset of the lesion, spasticity affects motion by restricting active and passive movement in the direction of the agonist (e.g., spasticity in the flexors limits agonistic extension). From acute to chronic stages, the loss of upper motor neuron (cortical) inhibition on the reflex arc[63] continues to perpetuate the spasticity, which further exacerbates the loss of motion. Movement restriction brought on by spastic or hypertonic muscles lead to **contracture** formation or tissue shortening in the immobile muscles. Muscles atrophy, sarcomeres are lost, and muscle fibers undergo fibrotic changes.[15,47,55] This state of shortening of spastic muscle further increases the muscle's sensitivity to stretch[27] and, therefore, greater resistance to agonist movement and more subsequent loss of motion. In addition to the muscle shortening, contractures may also develop to the soft tissues that surround the joints where the spastic muscles cross, causing joint stiffness, and in severe cases, joint ossification or arthrodesis. Unabated spasticity may cause pain and muscle spasms with either passive or active movement further leading to immobility. Thus, with the onset of spasticity, a negative cycle of neurological and biomechanical pathophysiologic processes ensues. Early intervention and ongoing management is key to abating the impairment process.

Given the complexity of spasticity, effective management requires a multi-disciplinary effort. Medical management is conducted primarily through the use of pharmacologic agents. These agents vary in their pharmacokinetics and therapeutic effects, including a generalized reduction in the excitability of the spinal reflex arc (via oral or intrathecal medications) or by localized functional denervation of muscles (via nerve block or neurotoxin injections).[24] Medical management must be complemented by rehabilitative intervention with major considerations to the pathophysiologic processes associated with spasticity and their functional consequences.

Rehabilitative intervention for spasticity should be multi-pronged with the goals of maintaining biomechanics, preventing further musculoskeletal and neuromuscular impairments and pain, regaining motor control, and relearning functional limb use. To achieve these goals, the use of multiple modalities including orthotics, is necessary. (A discussion of other modalities or therapeutic procedures goes beyond the scope of this chapter). Furthermore, the development of an intervention plan should be individualized. Specific to the use of orthoses to manage spasticity, there is no one-size-fits-all approach. The therapist's challenge is to use clinical reasoning to problem-solve the issues brought on by spasticity and minimize their negative impact on function and activity. It must be stressed that the use of orthotic devices is only part and parcel of a comprehensive intervention plan for persons with neurologic conditions with UMNL manifestations.

In terms of research-based evidence, studies present conflicting recommendations making the practice of orthotic provision to manage spasticity controversial. Systematic reviews such as those by Hellweg and Johannes,[28] Autti-Ramo, Suoranta, Anttila, and colleagues,[2] and Mortenson and Eng[44] favor the use of orthoses to manage spasticity, while systematic reviews by Lannin and Herbert[36] and Katalinic, Harvey, and Herbert[32] provide counter-evidence for the use of orthoses as modality for spasticity management. Furthermore, a comprehensive review of theory and evidence indicate that "static splinting has not been able to demonstrably reduce either spasticity or contracture and since it was shown to do neither, a subsequent effect on activity was also not detected."[37] This statement should however not be construed as a call to abandon the practice of orthotic provision altogether. To reiterate, orthoses should not be regarded as the sole modality to manage spasticity but rather an important component of a multi-dimensional and multi-disciplinary approach. An in-depth understanding of the pathophysiologic process of spasticity, knowledge of current evidence to manage spasticity, and sound clinical judgment are keys to a successful orthotic intervention program.

Orthotic Designs for the Neurologically Impaired Hand

Applying orthotics to the neurologically impaired upper extremity is a widespread and long-held practice in physical rehabilitation. However, there remains a lack of consensus among practitioners and researchers on which approach is best. Two surveys of practitioners, conducted 30 years apart, illustrate this lack of consensus in terms of when orthotics is indicated and which design and theoretical rationale is preferred.[1,46] Scholars have criticized the continued use of orthoses for persons with neurologic impairment in the clinic for its lack of "effect in reducing spasticity... or in preventing contracture."[37] Katalinic, Harvey, and Herbert[32] further concluded that stretch (as often accomplished through orthotic provision for the hand) "does not produce clinically important changes in joint mobility, pain, spasticity or activity limitation."[32] Although these evidence-based statements may be bothersome to adherents of clinical traditions, they should not be construed as a call to abandon orthotic provision altogether. Instead, clinicians should undergo deep critical reflection on how orthoses should be used in practice. It should be noted that results of systematic reviews and meta-analyses are aggregates of select information to answer a broad clinical question. Nuances of original studies are lost. In an attempt to generate homogeneity, many smaller studies including "n = 1" or single case designs and case series studies are routinely excluded from systematic reviews, even though they are considered acceptable alternatives to large randomized experiments. Given that clients are unique not only in their clinical manifestations but also in how they respond to rehabilitative interventions, it may be argued that managing spasticity is an "n = 1" practice. Evidence-based reasoning requires that clinicians not only critically appraise the evidence but also to reflect on the individual client's needs and how they match with the evidence.

Client-centered practice indicates that the client's needs and concerns are the main consideration. To that end, therapists need to consider the individualization of the intervention plan based on the client's presentation. Not all clients with neurological impairment present with the same muscle tone, not all clients with spasticity benefit from the same orthotic type and prescription, and not all clients require an **orthosis.** In the same manner, clinical rationale for orthotic provision varies including inhibition of tone, management or prevention of contractures, or active facilitation of neuromotor recovery. It stands to reason that depending on the goal or indications of the orthosis and the clinical presentation of the client, clinicians vary in their designs and prescriptions for use. Ways in which designs vary may be categorized on the basis of theoretical orientation, biomechanics, and overall practical considerations. However, key to a successful management is constant monitoring of the client's response and ongoing problem-solving with the client to attain therapeutic goals.

Design Based on Theory

There are two prevailing theoretical orientations that inform the use of orthoses for spasticity: neurophysiologic and biomechanical. From a **neurophysiologic** perspective, orthoses may be used to influence muscle tone by either inhibition or facilitation. From a **biomechanical** perspective, orthoses may be used to provide stretch to muscles to minimize the onset of contractures brought on by spasticity. The biomechanical orientation is discussed in later sections.

In general, design incorporating the neurophysiologic perspective varies according to: (1) location of the hand-wrist-forearm platform and (2) the configuration of the hand component (including the position of the digits). Rehabilitation science literature contains proponents for volar platforms[6,48,65] and dorsal platforms.[9,11,31,56] Dorsal platform adherents argue that cutaneous stimulation of the volar surface of the hand and forearm triggers greater spasticity.[14,29,41] Volar platform adherents argue that sustained pressure on flexor tendon insertions result in muscle relaxation.[19,57] Both assertions have yet to be proven through well-designed empirical methods because other authors see no greater advantage for one platform design over the other.[36,43,53] Both volar- and dorsal-based forearm platforms may be custom-fabricated (refer to Chapter 12) or prefabricated, which can be accessed through vendors and catalogs. Figure 14-1 is an example of a prefabricated orthosis.

In terms of the configuration of the hand component, one design approach based on neurophysiologic theory relies on the positioning of the thumb and fingers. As with the platform location, the positioning of the digits in either flexion over a rigid cylinder[19,20,52] or extension and abduction using

a "finger spreader"[4,13,65] is purported to reduce spasticity. Earlier designs did not incorporate a forearm platform to provide support to the wrist and take advantage of biomechanical leverage to maintain the position of the orthosis on the hand. Over the years, commercial providers of orthoses and expert clinicians (through textbooks) have incorporated the forearm platform as an important design feature (Figure 14-2). Examples of the cone configuration are the Rolyan Deluxe Spasticity Hand Splint and the Comfy Adjustable Cone Hand Orthosis. An example of the finger spreader configuration is the Rolyan Deluxe Spasticity Hand

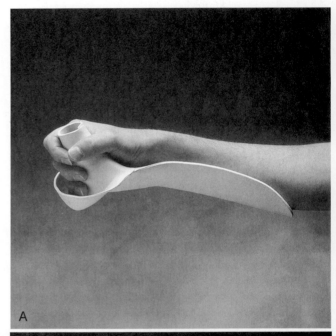

A

Figure 14-1 Prefabricated resting hand orthosis. (Courtesy of North Coast Medical, Gilroy, CA.)

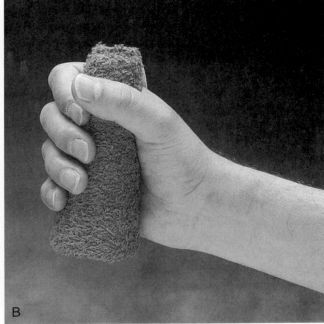

B

Figure 14-2 A, Prefabricated cone orthosis with forearm trough. **B,** Prefabricated cone orthosis without forearm trough.

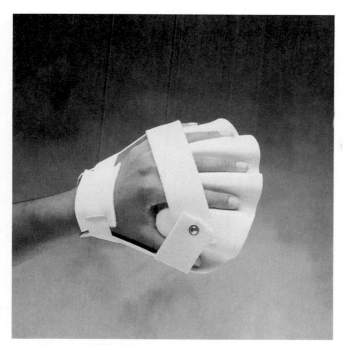

Figure 14-3 Prefabricated finger spreader/ball orthosis.

Splint (Figure 14-3). Adding a forearm component not only improves the leverage of the orthosis but also prevents the spastic long flexors from acting on the wrist.

There are two types of cylindrical orthotic designs for the hand component found in the literature: cone orthoses and dowel orthoses. Cone orthoses are constructed of rigid thermoplastic material with the smaller end placed radially and the larger end placed ulnarly to provide maximum palmar contact. The optimal contact is designed to provide deep tendon pressure on the wrist and finger flexor insertions at the base of the palm. Farber[19] observed that the total contact from the hard cone provides maintained pressure over the flexor surface of the palm, thus assisting in the desensitization of hypersensitive skin. MacKinnon and colleagues[39] adapted the standard hard cone to a solid wood dowel that asserts pressure on the palmar aspect of the metacarpal heads and exposes a larger surface area of the palm for sensory input compared to a cone. Although the shape of the hand may appear similar, the authors' rationale could not be any more different from each other. Pressure on tendon insertion created by the cone orthosis was intended to inhibit spasticity,[20] whereas the pressure applied on the palmar surface around the metacarpal head region by the hard dowel was purported to provide facilitation of the deep hand intrinsics.[18,39] The efficacy of these orthotic designs has yet to be evaluated through studies with a larger sample and more rigorous methods.

In contrast to keeping the fingers in a flexed position, there are proponents of orthoses that require maintaining finger and thumb abduction and extension. Largely based on neurodevelopmental treatment,[4,13] the position of digital extension and abduction is considered a reflex-inhibiting pattern (RIP) that inhibits flexor spasticity of the hand.

From Bobath's original foam block design that spreads the fingers apart, clinicians developed versions with more rigid and custom molded thermoplastic materials that also incorporates the wrist and forearm.[16,35] The abducted thumb component is key to the RIP effect (relaxation of spasticity) and for proper fit and comfort.[16] The elements of RIP pattern described earlier are to be contrasted with that of Pizzi, Carlucci, Falsini, and colleagues[49] where the RIP pattern for the hand is described as the "...wrist in 30 degrees of extension, normal transverse arch, thumb in abduction and opposition with the pads of the 4 fingers, and metacarpal and proximal interphalangeal joints in 45 degrees of flexion."[49]

Design Based on Biomechanics

Orthoses may be designed to address the biomechanical properties of muscles. Muscles are made of contractile and elastic components.[21] The contractile components are comprised of the myofilaments that respond to neural excitation. These myofilaments are serially arranged into myofibrils, which are bundled to form muscle fibers. The elastic components of a muscle are part of connective tissue, along with collagen, that wraps around and runs in parallel with the muscle fibers and muscles tissues. The maintenance of the number of the contractile myofilament units, or sarcomeres, and the size of the muscle are use-dependent. Therefore, lack of use or disuse leads to muscle atrophy via reduction in the size or number of sarcomeres especially when the muscle is in a shortened state.[25] Muscle disuse in persons with CNS conditions is brought on by lack of motor control, muscle weakness, decreased movement or immobilization, and spasticity. Confounding the loss of muscle mass is the onset of contractures, which causes a decrease in range of motion.

Contractures or shortening of soft tissues may occur to the joint capsule that is immobilized and to the connective tissue surrounding the inactive or disused contractile muscle tissues. The onset of contractures is time-dependent; that is, with prolonged immobility or lack of use, there is loss of elasticity to the soft tissues, which makes for increased resistance to passive or active stretch. In spastic muscles, the presence of contractures may accentuate the stretch reflex sensitivity[27,42] further, causing the muscles to shorten at rest and become more resistant to movement in the antagonist direction. The stretch reflex can be triggered at any point of the range of motion arc, thus limiting free range of motion. This phenomenon makes clinical measurement of spasticity challenging because it may be masked by the presence of contractures.

Given the biomechanical properties of muscles, an intervention program for spasticity incorporates promoting muscle activity to address disuse atrophy and maintaining the elasticity of tissues through stretch to address the onset of contractures. Stretch for the hand, wrist and/or elbow may be best achieved through prolonged orthotic use or casting. Orthoses may be preferred if the intervention plan requires active use since they are removable. Casts are preferred if prolonged and sustained stretch is needed especially when the spasticity is severe and the soft tissue contractures significantly limit range of motion. For the lower extremity, full weight bearing may suffice to maintain the requisite stretch.[63]

Controversies exist regarding the amount of time needed to sustain the stretch to maintain soft tissue length. In a meta-analysis conducted by Katalinic, Harvey, and Herbert,[32] there is a wide variation in the frequency and duration in the application of stretch to address contractures in persons with neurologic conditions. The pooled outcomes neither favor the control nor the intervention (stretch). Study results varied in relationship to the immediate, short-term, and long-term effects of the intervention. In spite of the variations in intervention protocol and outcomes, the authors concluded the following: "regular stretch does not produce clinically important changes in joint mobility, pain, spasticity or activity limitation in people with neurological conditions."[32] It must be noted that studies included in the meta-analysis are exclusively randomized control or controlled clinical trials. Thus studies that do not have a control or comparison group were excluded.

Adding to the confusion is the debate on how much stretch is applied. Lannin and Ada[37] criticized the use of submaximal orthotic positioning (5 to 10 degrees below maximum passive range) citing the "functional" position described in textbooks is not supported by evidence and contradictory to findings about the benefits of maximal stretch. Many authors recommended positioning the spastic muscles in optimal stretch to achieve an inhibitory effect.[20,27,56,61] On the other hand, some authors recommended orthotic positioning with the wrist and hand in extension but with substantial consideration to the point when the stretch reflex is triggered.[42,48,53,60] Scherling and Johnson[54] suggested that wrist extension of 10 to 15 degrees and metacarpophalangeal (MCP) joint extension of −45 degrees offers a good starting position that is less likely to trigger the stretch reflex while gradually introducing passive stretch to the spastic muscles.

Given the dynamic nature of spasticity, the optimal position may not be the same for all clients. Even with the same client, spasticity can fluctuate at any given time. Anecdotal reports from clients indicate that the time of day, type of activity, fatigue/energy levels, emotional status and weather may influence tone. In consideration of this issue, therapists should adopt a concept of spasticity management as a 24-hour/day regimen. With regards to the use of orthoses, there are alternatives that are flexible or conformable to the fluctuations in a client's tone. Examples of softer, more dynamic materials found to be effective in managing the spastic arm and hand include Lycra[17,26] and **Neoprene.**[10,59] Neoprene-based thumb orthoses such as the TheraKool Breathable Neoprene Thumb Spica and the Benik Pediatric Neoprene Glove are commercially available (Figure 14-4). Another design that combines both flexible and rigid components is the SaeboStretch (Saebo Inc., Charlotte, NC) where

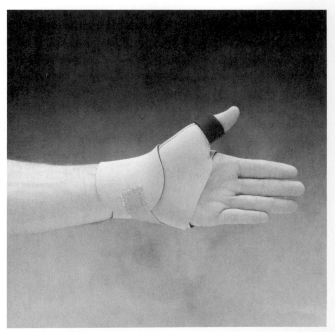

Figure 14-4 Prefabricated Neoprene thumb orthosis.

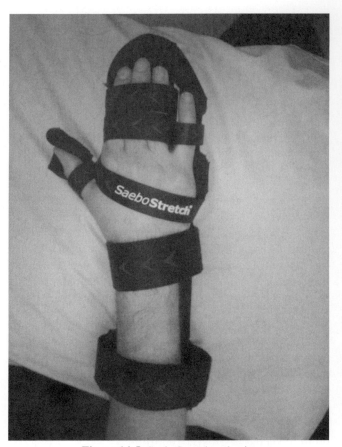

Figure 14-5 SaeboStretch orthosis.

the forearm volar platform is made of thin rigid metal and the flexible metal-based volar hand component is interchangeable (Figure 14-5). The metal components are padded adequately with Neoprene-based material, and the straps vary in widths according to the body part and are made of rigid silicone material. While case reports have been described,[5] the orthosis requires further examination through rigorous empirical studies.

With various conflicting evidence to draw from, the best recommendation is always to be judicious in the interpretation of the studies and consider the client's unique clinical presentation. Since a client's neuromuscular presentation varies, a successful intervention plan is one that is consistently monitored and adjusted as needed in response to the client's changing status.

Managing the Neurologically-Impaired Hand using a Problem-Solving Approach

When a client sustains an UMNL, a clinical syndrome consisting of impaired reflex function (hyperreflexia), muscle weakness, and impaired motor control is expected. As described earlier, spasticity, though associated with UMNL, may not be clinically manifested. In a longitudinal study of clients with stroke conducted by Wissel and colleagues,[64] nearly 25% developed spasticity in the first 2 weeks of onset. Some of the clients with initial spastic manifestation, have a decrease in spasticity to levels that are not clinically detectible, whereas others have a worsening condition especially if early intervention is not provided. There are clients who develop spasticity at a much later time; yet, still many will not develop any spasticity. With or without spasticity, the focus of intervention is on regaining active function and preventing secondary impairments (i.e., disuse, atrophy, and contractures).

Many clients who develop spasticity are preceded with a flaccid/hypotonic and a reflexive/hyporeflexive presentation. When muscles are flaccid, the hand rests in a dependent position, such as a "wrist drop" with an "ape hand" posture. The dropped wrist position is due to lack of extensor muscle control while the ape hand position of hyperextended MCP joints with partial interphalangeal flexion is due to the passive tension of the extensor digitorum caused by the flexed wrist. To preserve the normal length-tension balance between the flexors and the extensors of the wrist and hand, an orthosis that positions the wrist in slight extension and the digits in **composite extension** is recommended. (Note: Composite means that the entire kinematic chain of a digit involving MCP, proximal interphalangeal (PIP), and distal interphalangeal joints are positioned as a unit). The resting position of the hand places the digits in partial flexion (due to passive tension of the elastic components of the flexors). This position keeps the joints in extension, which provides gentle, static stretch to the flexors to preserve the length of the muscle fibers. A volar forearm hand immobilization orthosis is appropriate as a resting and positioning device especially when muscle tone is considered flaccid. With a greater than neutral extension of the wrist, the orthosis may facilitate edema reduction to the hand.

In clients with acute UMNL, there is propensity for flexor contractures. Early anticipation of the contracture and subsequent preventive orthotics in extension is good practice.

Over time, the elastic properties of the muscle adapts to the position of static stretch. Depending on the extent to which the extensors of the digits needed to approximate the requisite aperture size for the hand during pre-grasp and release, the orthosis can be adjusted to increase the stretch on the flexors. For example, to actively grasp a water bottle, the wrist is stabilized in slight extension and the fingers and the thumb must compositely extend to an aperture slightly greater than the diameter of the bottle. Therefore, the clinician must assess whether the client can be passively stretched pain-free in composite wrist, hand, and elbow extension that approximates the desired hand-wrist position during reach-to-grasp. The therapist trains the client to tolerate this position through an orthosis. The elbow is included in the assessment of composite extension since the wrist and finger flexors are attached proximal to and can influence kinematics at the elbow joint. However, orthotic provision including the elbow is not necessary. Positioning the elbow in extension and encouraging motion in elbow extension assists with providing stretch to proximal and distal attachments of the hand and wrist flexors.

Using a **minimalist design**,[62] a dorsal forearm based orthosis with a volar hand immobilization component and dorsal thumb extension is recommended to achieve passive stretch to the flexors. Unlike an entirely volar forearm and hand configuration, this "crowbar" design offers better leverage by pulling the "dropping" hand rather than pushing it into extension. As the client's hand evolves with spasticity, the orthosis is adjusted with increased wrist extension while maintaining the digits extended to provide constant stretch to the finger and thumb flexors. Even with significant muscle stiffness, the orthotic design is mechanically more advantageous in dispersing pressure over a large surface area unlike in volar designs where significant flexor spasticity pulls the wrist and the MCP joints into greater flexion and away from orthosis contact. This design creates a three-point friction and concentrated pressure areas. The following are instructions on how to fabricate a dorsal forearm volar hand immobilization orthosis with a dorsal thumb extension component (Figure 14-6).

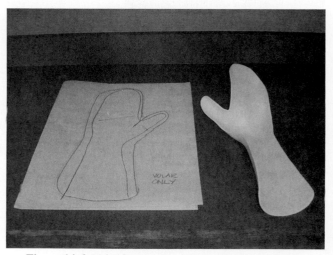

Figure 14-6 Volar forearm hand immobilization orthosis.

Dorsal Forearm Volar Hand Immobilization Orthosis Construction

Material

The ideal thermoplastic material for this orthosis has moderate drape and resistance to stretch, moderate to excellent rigidity and memory, and low flexibility. The recommended dimensions are non-perforated to 1% perforated (for rigidity) and ³⁄₃₂″ to ⅛″ thickness depending on the severity of tone. Rolyan Ezeform, Kay-Splint III Basic, TailorSplint, and PolyFlex II meet these criteria.

Pattern Making

1. Place the hand and wrist in a neutral position over a tracing paper (Figure 14-7). If the client has significant spasticity, the therapist may trace the less involved hand and then invert the pattern on the thermoplastic material prior to cutting.
   a. Trace the forearm (Figure 14-8) and hand (Figure 14-9), and mark the following anatomical locations: posterior one-third of the forearm, radial and ulnar styloids and the middle of the second and fifth proximal phalanges.
   b. Exclude the thumb by not terminating at the first web space distally and at the base of the first metacarpal proximally. Connect the two thumb points to create a straight edge.

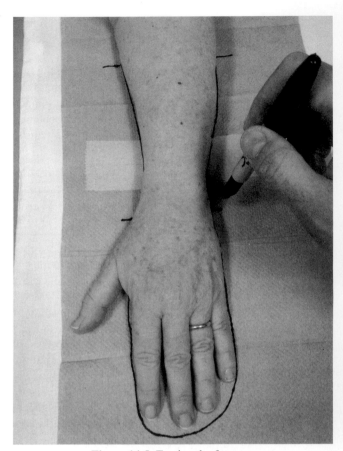

Figure 14-8 Tracing the forearm.

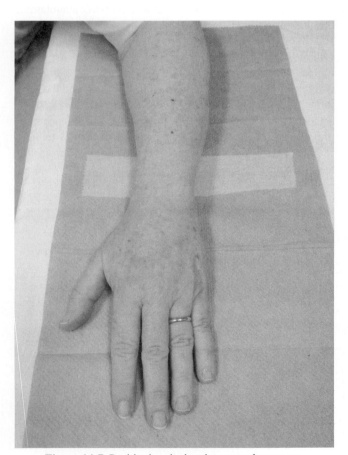

Figure 14-7 Positioning the hand to trace the pattern.

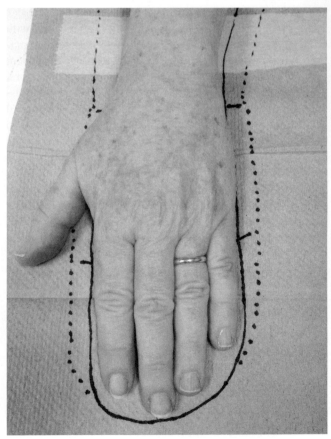

Figure 14-9 Tracing the hand.

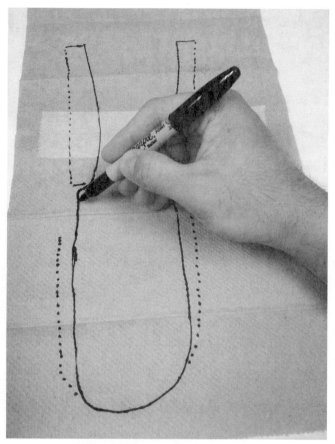

Figure 14-10 Completing the pattern.

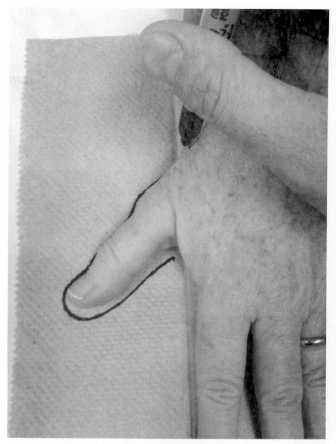

Figure 14-11 Tracing the thumb.

c. Draw an arc that connects the phalangeal points. Cut a slit along this arc (Figure 14-10).

d. Trace the thumb on a separate piece of paper (Figure 14-11). For the thumb, create ¼-inch margins on the medial and lateral sides and a 1-inch margin proximally.

2. Mark ¾-inch margins on the radial and ulnar side of the forearm, and ½-inch margins on the radial and ulnar side of the wrist shown in Figure 14-12. Complete the pattern by drawing trim lines along the margins. The distal and proximal ends may not require additional margin because most thermoplastic materials appropriate for this type of orthosis tend to elongate when heated and draped on the body. The position of wrist extension may also create excess thermoplastic material during fabrication.

3. Transfer the hand-forearm and thumb patterns on the thermoplastic material. Mark the phalangeal arc using the slit on the pattern (refer to Step 1c).

a. Using a box cutter, cut the thermoplastic material in a rectangular configuration that contains the pattern, prior to trimming the pattern to shape.

b. Punch holes at the ends of the phalangeal arc using a leather puncher (Figure 14-13).

c. Heat the material slightly, and trim the thermoplastic material by the pattern. Cut a slit along the phalangeal arc as shown in Figure 14-14. Do not heat the material to its maximum heating point to maintain its optimal integrity prior to molding.

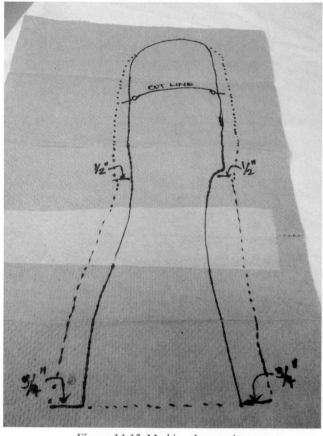

Figure 14-12 Marking the margins.

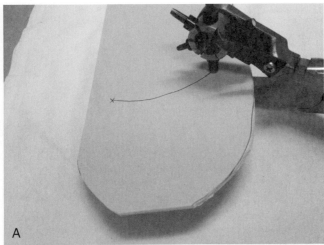

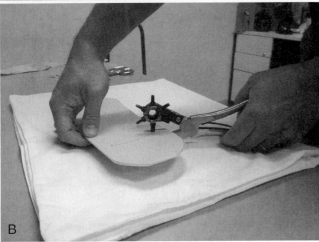

Figure 14-13 A and **B,** Punching holes for the phalangeal arc.

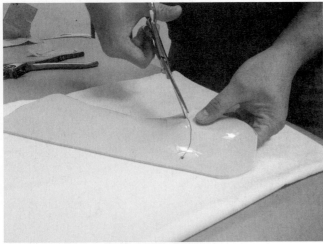

Figure 14-14 Trimming the thermoplastic for the thumb piece.

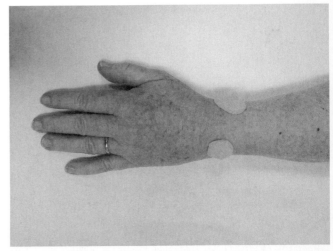

Figure 14-15 Padding bony prominences.

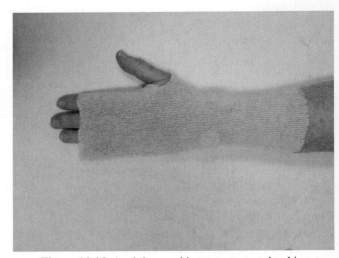

Figure 14-16 Applying stockinette to protect the skin.

Fabrication

4. Prior to molding, establish the optimal wrist position by performing the following:
    a. Place the forearm on a table surface with the elbow flexed at 80 to 90 degrees, the wrist flexed, and the hand resting freely over the edge of the table.
    b. Stabilize the forearm against the elbow, and support the hand by the distal palm and fingers while maintaining the fingers in composite extension.
    c. Slowly extend the wrist passively to minimize the stretch reflex response (spastic tone). Feel for a palpable stretch until the PIP and distal interphalangeal joints begin to passively or reflexively flex. Use this as a reference angle for optimal wrist extension. A goniometric measurement may be useful to have an estimate of the optimal position. Note however that this angle may change during fabrication, because some clients will respond to the heat and/or pressure of the thermoplastic material with either relaxation or excitation of spasticity. Ideally, the greater the composite wrist and finger extension is, the more the stretch can be optimized.
5. Apply foam padding to the ulnar head and radial styloid (Figure 14-15).
6. Apply a stockinette cover to the hand and forearm (Figure 14-16).
7. Heat the thermoplastic material to the recommended time and optimum temperature per the manufacturer's instructions.

8. Begin the molding process by inserting the fingers through the phalangeal slit so that the fingers are supported to the proximal phalanx. Drape the rest of the material over the dorsum of the hand and the dorsal wrist and forearm (Figure 14-17).

9. Stabilize the hand by maintaining the digits in extension. Fold the ulnar and radial margins dorsally from the digits to the wrist (Figure 14-18).

10. While the material remains warm, contour the dorsal platform on the wrist and forearm to maintain the wrist and fingers in optimal composite extension (Figure 14-19).

11. Heat the lateral and medial folds, and seal them against the body of the orthosis (Figure 14-20).

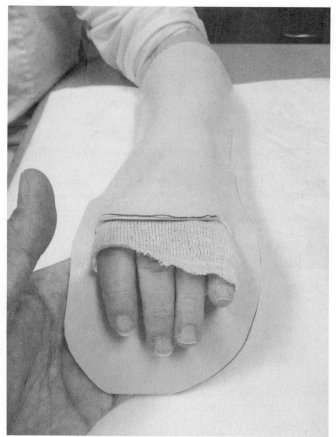

Figure 14-17 Draping the thermoplastic.

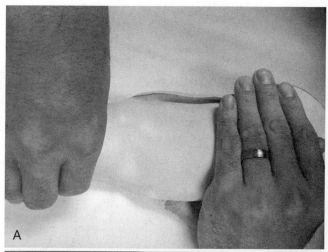

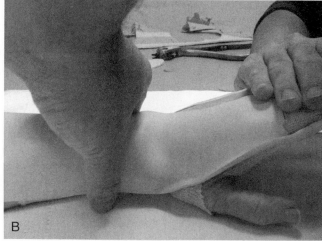

Figure 14-19 **A** and **B,** Molding the wrist and forearm.

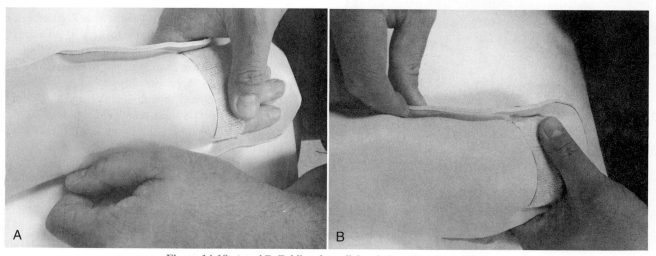

Figure 14-18 **A** and **B,** Folding the radial and ulnar sides for stability.

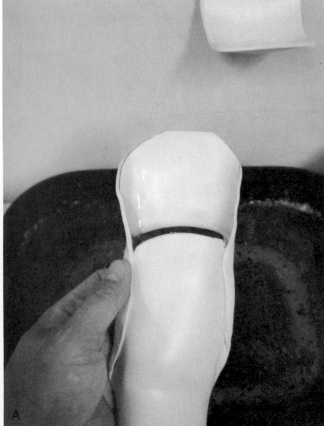

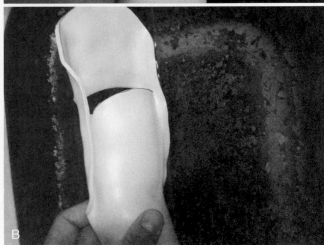

Figure 14-20 A and **B,** Finishing and reinforcing the radial and ulnar folds.

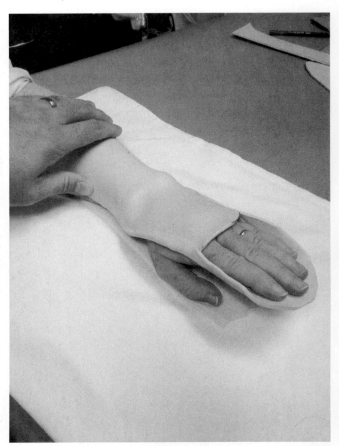

Figure 14-21 Smoothing the edges of the orthosis.

12. Smooth the edges, and fit the orthosis to the client (Figure 14-21).
13. Apply a 1½″ to 2″ rough adhesive-backed Velcro on the proximal forearm aspect of the dorsal platform. Secure the orthosis on the client using a 2″ wide Neoprene strap (Figure 14-22).
14. Apply thin foam padding on the corresponding contours created by the ulnar head and radial styloid pads (Figure 14-23).

15. Reapply the orthosis on the client, and check for comfort (Figure 14-24). Ensure that the edges of the hand opening do not touch or cause pressure on the metacarpal heads.
16. Heat the thumb component, and drape thermoplastic material on the dorsal aspect of the thumb while the orthosis is on (Figure 14-25, *A*). Maintain the thumb in optimal extension and abduction (see Figure 14-25, *B*). Take caution when positioning the thumb by observing its color. Too much pressure or stretch causes the thumb to blanch and/or turn dark red to bluish purple.
17. Spot heat the proximal end of the thumb platform, and smooth it against the orthosis to keep it adhered. For materials that have coating that prevents bonding, sand or scrape the surface coating or apply an adhesive agent prior to finishing (Figure 14-26).
18. Apply adhesive-back rough-side Velcro to the dorsal aspect of the hand and the thumb (Figure 14-27).
19. Secure the hand and the thumb with a 1½″ and 1″ wide Neoprene strap, respectively (Figure 14-28).
20. Optional step: The purpose of the hand strap is to prevent the hand (palm) and wrist to lag volarly and the fingers from migrating proximally. This strap maintains the MCP joints in neutral. In rare occasions during the course of wear, the MCP joints may become hyperextended and the PIP joints flexed due to unexpected increase in long

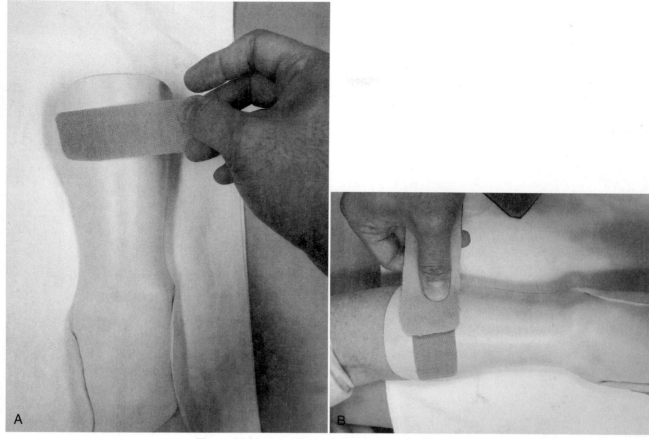

Figure 14-22 **A** and **B,** Applying straps to the forearm.

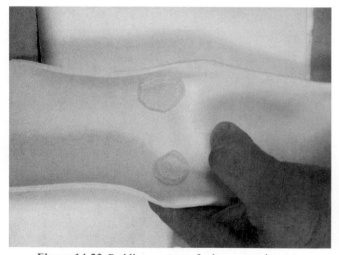

Figure 14-23 Padding contours for bony prominences.

flexor tone. To prevent this "buckling" of the fingers, an extra strap over the proximal phalanx may be applied. The strap should not go over the PIP joint so as not to cause PIP hyperextension.

Orthotic Provision and Task-Oriented Intervention

At the earliest sign of volitional control of a mass movement pattern, the orthotic program is complemented with intensive task-oriented practice with or without therapeutic modalities that facilitate active control of the extensors to gain in

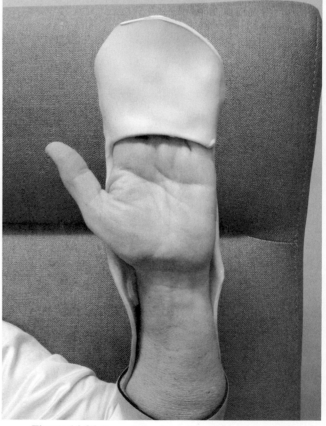

Figure 14-24 Reapplying the splint to assess comfort.

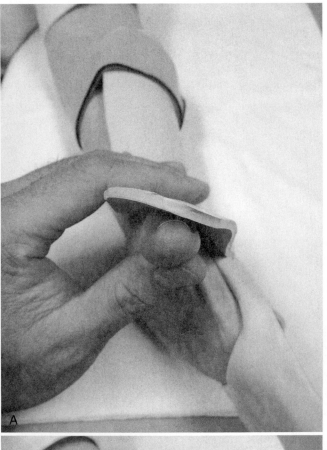

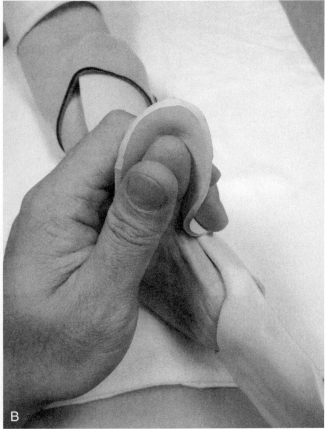

Figure 14-25 **A** and **B,** Molding the thumb component.

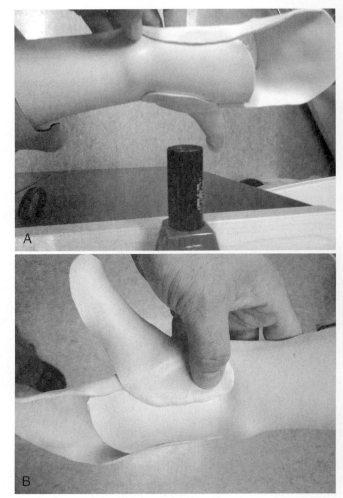

Figure 14-26 **A** and **B,** Spot-heating and bonding the thumb component to the rest of the orthosis.

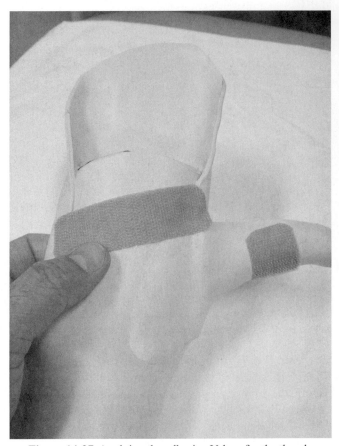

Figure 14-27 Applying the adhesive Velcro for the thumb.

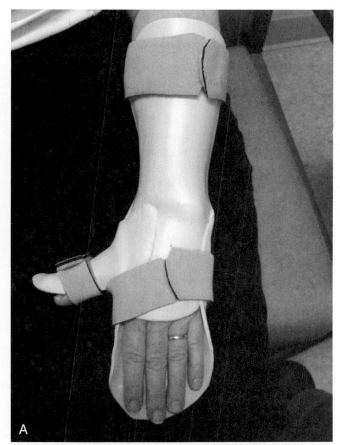

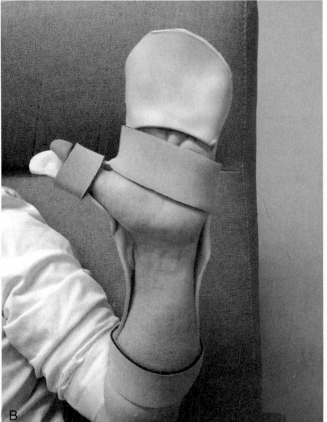

Figure 14-28 A and **B,** Reapplying/applying the straps for the forearm and thumb.

passive motion which translates into daily functioning. The practice of positioning the hand and wrist to maintain the required alignment for arm and hand use in various daily living activities is deemed an effective method to prepare a client for intensive task training.[58]

The need to constantly monitor the success of the orthotic program in relation to the client goals cannot be over emphasized. As suggested in the study conducted by Wissel and colleagues,[64] many clients may not develop spasticity; and of those who do, a few have diminished to full resolution of spasticity over time. Therefore, orthoses to manage the secondary effects of spasticity may outlast their usefulness. However, clients with diminished motor control, especially in hand opening for pre-grasp and release and in achieving precision grip (e.g., picking up a pen or finger food), regardless of the presence and severity of spasticity, may require a different orthosis. This orthosis constrains select joints or positions for certain digits to enable more active and functional use of the hand. For example, a client with a cortical thumb or thumb-in-hand resting posture (i.e., the thumb is flexed and adducted into the palm), a short opponens, or C-bar orthosis may accomplish two purposes:

1. The orthosis preserves the soft tissue integrity of the structures around the thumb including the first web space.
2. The orthosis positions the thumb in opposition and palmar abduction to facilitate precision or cylindrical grip during task practice (Figure 14-29).

An alternative orthosis is a Neoprene- or Lycra-based thumb extension design.[10,17,59]

As discussed in the beginning of the chapter, there are two predominant theoretical orientations that guide the use of orthotic provision for the neurologically impaired hand—neurophysiologic and biomechanical. With neurorehabilitation shifting toward more contemporary models of task-oriented and repetitive task training, therapists consider **task-oriented approaches** when it comes to the use of orthoses. Another example of an orthosis that promotes intensive active practice of the hand is the SaeboFlex (Saebo Inc., Charlotte, NC). The SaeboFlex orthosis is a dynamic forearm-based orthosis that positions the wrist in slight extension and the digits in composite extension through spring-loaded traction (Figure 14-30). A client wearing the orthosis is trained to actively flex the fingers in limited excursion by grasping large diameter balls against the resistance of the spring-loaded mechanisms followed by active relaxation of the finger flexors (Figure 14-31). As demonstrated in a number of studies,[7,22,30] the device when used in intensive repetitive task-training facilitates gains in hand and arm function for persons with strokes.

Serial Casting to Manage Spasticity

In clients with significant joint and muscle stiffness due to severe spasticity and prolonged immobilization, **serial casting** presents an evidence-based solution that translates into

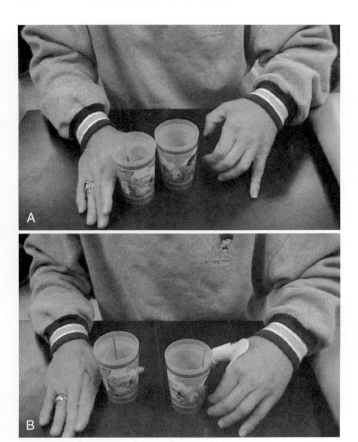

Figure 14-29 A, Client with thumb extensor weakness unable to grasp a cup. **B,** Client with thumb short opponens orthosis more able to grasp a cup.

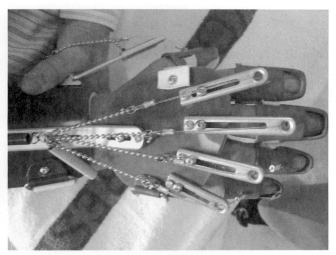

Figure 14-30 SaeboFlex dynamic orthosis.

increases in active and passive range of motion.[45,50,51,60] In addition to providing sustained passive stretch, the circumferential nature of the cast creates a warming effect on the soft tissue for increased relaxation.[33] While effective, serial casting is known for various complications, such as pressure sores, pain, and swelling.[50] Therefore, it is highly recommended that a therapist who is a novice in casting,

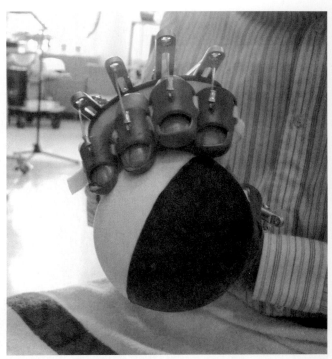

Figure 14-31 Using the SaeboFlex to assist with hand extension after grasping ball.

receive on-the-job or post-professional training and appropriate supervision from an experienced practitioner before attempting the procedure.

Circumferential casting techniques involve specialized fabrication skills and orthopedic casting materials. Solid serial casting is designed to increase range of motion and decrease contractures caused by spasticity through a series of periodic cast changes. Typically, the affected joint is casted in submaximal range (5 to 10 degrees below maximum passive range). Cast change schedules range from every other day for recent contractures to every 5 to 7 days for chronic contractures. Blood circulation, edema, skin condition, sensation, and range of motion are closely monitored during the casting process. The serial progression of the cast is discontinued when range of motion gains are no longer noted between a couple of cast changes. When no range of motion gains are noted, a final cast with bivalve configuration is applied daily to maintain range of motion.[23]

Therapists use plaster or synthetic resin materials such as fiberglass or stretch bandage with polyurethane resin for casting. Plaster is a cost-effective choice if the practitioner desires to gradually increase passive range of motion by using a series of static orthoses in brief intervals. A **plaster bandage** is easy to handle, and it conforms/drapes easily to body parts. However, the disadvantages of using plaster casts include: porousness (non-water resistant), difficulty with maintenance, potential for allergic reactions, and heaviness compared to lighter weight alternatives. Fiberglass and bandage orthopedic resin materials are more costly and require specialized training. These are lighter in weight, more durable, and ideal for long-term use. A review of studies[45,50] on serial casting reveals preference for synthetic materials for reasons not clearly specified. Both materials require six to eight layers of thickness for adequate strength. They harden in 3 to 8 minutes (depending on water temperature). A special type of synthetic material made of bandage impregnated with polyurethane resin (Delta Cast Conformable, Depuy Orthopedics, Warsaw, IN) is layered to focus the rigidity on certain regions thereby decreasing the need for multiple layers. Both plaster and synthetic bandages emit heat as a byproduct in the curing process.

Materials, Tools, and Equipment

Specialized casting tools include the following:
- Electric cast saw
- Hand cast spreader
- Bandage scissors
  Casting program materials include the following:
- Plaster or fiberglass casting tape (2″, 3″, 4″, 5″)
- Nylon or cotton stockinette (2″, 3″, 4″, 5″)
- Rubber gloves (specialized casting gloves for fiberglass)
- Plastic water bucket
- Drop sheet to protect client
- Cast padding

Plaster Casting Procedures[23]

1. Measure and record joint range of motion.
2. The client should be sitting or lying comfortably and should be draped with sheets or towels to protect clothing and skin. Explain the procedure to the client clearly and reassure as needed. Some clients with brain injuries may be agitated during the casting procedure. In such cases, the therapist must discuss the use of sedative agents with the referring physician to accomplish the task.
3. Tubular stockinette is placed over the extremity to be casted, extending it at either end 4 to 6 inches beyond where the cast ends.
4. Determine the targeted position of the extremity. Direct another person (therapist or aide) how and where to hold the extremity.
5. Strips of stick-on foam can be placed on either side of an area that may be susceptible to skin breakdown.
6. Apply cast padding in a taut fashion around the extremity, ending after three or four layers are applied. Extra padding or felt may be added if needed over bony prominences. Padding is applied 1 to 2 inches above the end of the stockinette.
7. Dip the plaster roll five to six times in warm water. Squeeze excess moisture from the roll.
8. Apply plaster to the extremity in a spiral fashion, moving proximally to distally.
9. Direct the person assisting to stretch the joint minimally as the plaster is being applied. The casting assistant should not apply direct pressure to the plaster as it is setting (breakdown or ischemia inside the cast can occur from this loading point effect). Rather, the

assistant should stretch the joint above and below the cast or apply pressure with the entire surface of the hand to evenly distribute pressure.
10. Apply four to five layers of plaster. Smooth the plaster surface in a circular fashion as the plaster sets. Pay special attention to smoothing proximal and distal edges to prevent skin breakdown.
11. Before applying the last layer, turn back the ends of stockinette onto the cast. This gives a smooth finished surface to cast edges. Apply the last layer of plaster below this edge.
12. Instruct the casting assistant to maintain stretch on the joint until the plaster has set (3 to 8 minutes).
13. The plaster completely dries in 24 hours. Weight bearing on the casted extremity should be avoided until then.
14. Clean any dripped plaster from the client's skin, elevate the extremity comfortably, and check both ends of the cast for tightness. Check the client's circulation regularly. Some authors[12] recommend a post-casting management program of bivalve casting in order to maintain increased range of motion and tone reduction.

Fiberglass Casting Procedures[23]

1. Plastic gloves must be worn by anyone touching the fiberglass material during fabrication. Initially and throughout the procedure, the plastic gloves are coated with petroleum jelly or lotion. Fiberglass adheres to the skin or unlubricated gloves and is difficult to remove. Prepare the limb with padding and stockinette. Practice with the casting assistant to position the joint correctly.
2. Submerge the fiberglass roll in cool water, and gently squeeze it six to eight times. Remove the roll from the water, and apply it dripping wet to the extremity to facilitate handling of the material.
3. Fiberglass roll packages should be opened one at a time and applied within minutes. Fiberglass hardens and does not bond to itself when left exposed to air.
4. Fiberglass must overlap itself by half a tape width.
5. Blot the exterior of the cast with an open palm in a circular fashion after all layers are applied. This facilitates maximum bonding of all layers. Rubbing in a longitudinal fashion disrupts the fiberglass bond.
6. If one layer of the cast is allowed to cure (harden), subsequent layers will not bond well. All three to four layers are applied in efficient succession.
7. During the first 2 minutes after immersion, the fiberglass is molded while the extremity is maintained in the desired position. The extremity is held stationary during the last few minutes of the 5- to 7-minute setting time.
8. The cast is completely set in 7 to 10 minutes. Thereafter, the cast may be removed using a cast saw. Cast saws should be operated only by those individuals with training and experience.

The fiberglass cast can be made into a working bivalve in the following manner[23]:

1. Using the cast saw, cut the cast into anterior and posterior sections. Remove the cast with the cast spreader.
2. Remove the padding and stockinette from the extremity with the cast scissors and discard.
3. Inspect both fiberglass shells for protrusions and rough edges. Trim the edges of each shell and file smooth.
4. For soiled cast padding, use cotton padding to reline the shells, taking care to rip padding edges off to provide a smooth inner surface with no ripples. Reline with the same amount of padding used to fabricate the original cast. Extend the padding over all edges and sides of the shells.
5. Fold the padding over the edges of the shells, and secure with adhesive tape.
6. Cut a length of the stockinette approximately 4 to 6 inches longer than the length of the shell. Line each shell with stockinette. Secure both ends with adhesive tape.
7. Fashion straps using wide webbing and buckles. These straps can be taped or sewn onto stockinette covering the shell. Bivalves can also be secured with Ace wraps.
8. Carefully wean the client into the bivalve, modifying and adjusting as needed.

Review Questions

1. How do the biochemical and neurophysiological approaches to hand orthotic provision differ?
2. Why would an orthosis that positions in submaximal range be less beneficial and potentially harmful to a client with evolving muscle tone?
3. What are the strengths and weaknesses of orthotic dorsal versus volar forearm platforms?
4. What is an appropriate rationale for orthotic design based on a biomechanical rationale?
5. What is the difference between the elastic and contractile properties of muscles, and what are the implications for orthotic provision?
6. What are the material options for casting?
7. What are two major characteristics for each of the materials below?
   - Plaster bandage
   - Fiberglass bandage
   - Neoprene or Lycra

References

1. Adrienne C, Manigandan C: Inpatient occupational therapists hand-splinting practice for clients with stroke: a cross-sectional survey from Ireland, *J Neurosci Rural Pract* 2(2):141–149, 2011.
2. Autti-Ramo I, Suoranta J, Anttila H, et al.: Effectiveness of upper and lower limb casting and orthoses in children with cerebral palsy: an overview of review articles, *Am J Phys Med Rehabil* 85:89–103, 2006.
3. Basmajian J, Burke M, Burnett G, et al.: *Illustrated Stedman's medical dictionary*, ed 24, London, 1982, Williams & Wilkins.
4. Bobath B: *Adult hemiplegia: evaluation and treatment*, London, 1987, William Heinemann, Medical Books.
5. Bondoc S: *Management of the neurologic upper extremity with focus on the hand: an evidence base approach and practical solutions*, Chicago, IL, 2012, A Seminar presented at the Rehabilitation Institute of Chicago in November.
6. Brennan J: Response to stretch of hypertonic muscle groups in hemiplegia, *Br Med J* 1:1504–1507, 1959.
7. Butler AJ, Blanton S, Rowe VT, et al.: Attempting to improve function and quality of life using the FTM protocol: a case report, *J Neurol Phys Ther* 30(3):148–156, 2006.
8. Burridge JH, McLellan DL: Relation between abnormal patterns of muscle activation and response to common peroneal nerve stimulation in hemiplegia, *J of Neur*, (69)353–361.
9. Carmick J: Case report: use of neuromuscular electrical stimulation and a dorsal wrist splint to improve the hand function of a child with spastic hemiparesis, *Physical Therapy* 77(6):661–671, 1997.
10. Casey CA, Kratz EJ: Soft splinting with neoprene: the thumb abduction supinator splint, *Am J Occup Ther* 42(6):395–398, 1988.
11. Charait S: A comparison of volar and dorsal splinting of the hemiplegic hand, *Am J Occup Ther* 22:319–321, 1968.
12. Copley J, Watson-Will A, Dent K: Upper limb casting for clients with cerebral palsy: a clinical report, *Aust Occup Ther J* 43:39–50, 1996.
13. Davies P: *Steps to follow: a guide to the treatment of hemiplegia*, New York, 1985, Springer-Verlag.
14. Dayhoff N: Re-thinking stroke soft or hard devices to position hands, *Am J Nurs* 75(7):1142–1144, 1975.
15. Dietz V, Ketelsen UP, Berger W, et al.: Motor unit involvement in spastic paresis. Relationship between leg muscle activation and histochemistry, *J of Neurol Sci* (75)86–103.
16. Doubilet L, Polkow L: Theory and design of a finger abduction splint for the spastic hand, *Am J Occup Ther* 32:320–322, 1977.
17. Elliott CM, Reid SL, Alderson JA, et al.: Lycra arm orthoses in conjunction with goal-directed training can improve movement in children with cerebral palsy, *NeuroRehabilitation* 28(1):47–54, 2011.
18. Exner C, Bonder B: Comparative effects of three hand splints on bilateral hand use, grasp, and arm-hand posture in hemiplegic children: a pilot study, *Occup Ther J Res* 3:75–92, 1983.
19. Farber SD: *Neurorehabilitation: a multidisciplinary approach*, Toronto, 1982, WB Saunders.
20. Farber SD, Huss AJ: *Sensorimotor evaluation and treatment procedures for allied health personnel*, Indianapolis, 1974, Indiana University Foundation.
21. Farmer SE, James M: Contractures in orthopaedic and neurological conditions: a review of causes and treatment, *Disabil Rehabil* 23(13):549–558, 2001.
22. Farrell JF, Hoffman HB, Snyder JL, et al.: Orthotic aided training of the paretic upper limb in chronic stroke: results of a phase 1 trial, *Neurorehabilitation* 22:99–103, 2007.
23. Feldman PA: Upper extremity casting and splinting. In Glenn MD, Whyte J, editors: *The practical management of spasticity in children and adults*, Malvern, PA, 1990, Lea & Febiger.
24. Gelber DA, Jozefcyk PB: Therapeutics in the management of spasticity, *Neurorehabil Neural Repair* 13:5–14, 1999.
25. Goldspink G, Williams P: Muscle fibre and connective tissue changes associated with use and disuse. In Ada L, Canning C, editors: *Key issues in neurological physiotherapy*, Oxford, 1990, Butterworth Heinmann.

26. Gracies JM, Marosszeky JE, Renton R, et al.: Short-term effects of dynamic lycra splints on upper limb in hemiplegic patients, *Arch Phys Med Rehabil* 81(12):1547–1555, 2000.

27. Gracies JM: Pathophysiology of impairment in patients with spasticity and use of stretch as a treatment of spastic hypertonia, *Phys Med Rehabil Clin N Am* 12:747–768, 2001.

28. Hellweg S, Johannes S: Physiotherapy after traumatic brain injury: a systematic review of the literature, *Brain Inj* 22:365–373, 2008.

29. Jamison S, Dayhoff N: A hard hand-positioning device to decrease wrist and finger hypertonicity: a sensorimotor approach for the client with non-progressive brain damage, *Nursing Research* 29:285–289, 1980.

30. Jeon HS, Woo YK, Yi CH, et al.: Effect of intensive training with a spring-assisted hand orthosis on movement smoothness in upper extremity following stroke: a pilot clinical trial, *Top Stroke Rehabil* 19(4):320–328, 2012.

31. Kaplan N: Effect of splinting on reflex inhibition and sensorimotor stimulation in treatment of spasticity, *Arch Phys Med Rehabil* 43:565–569, 1962.

32. Katalinic OM, Harvey LA, Herbert RD: Effectiveness of stretch for the treatment and prevention of contractures in people with neurological conditions: a systematic review, *Phys Ther* 91(1):11–24, 2011.

33. King T: Plaster splinting as a means of reducing elbow flexor spasticity: a case study, *Am J Occup Ther* 36:671–673, 1982.

34. Knutson E, Martensen A: Posture and gait in Parkinsonian patients. In Bles, Brandt, editors: *Disorders of posture and gait*, Amsterdam, 1986, Elsevier.

35. Langlois S, Pederson L, MacKinnon JR: The effects of splinting on the spastic hemiplegic hand: report of a feasibility study, *Canadian J Occup Ther* 58(1):17–25, 1991.

36. Lannin NA, Herbert RD: Is hand splinting effective for adults following stroke? A systematic review and methodological critique of published research, *Clinical Rehabilitation* 17:807–816, 2003.

37. Lannin N, Ada L: Neurorehabilitation splinting: theory and principles of clinical use, *NeuroRehabilitation* 28:21–28, 2011.

38. Little JW, Massagli TL: Spasticity and associated abnormalities of muscle tone. In DeLisa JA, Gans BM, editors: *Rehabilitation medicine: principles and practice*, ed 3, Philadelphia, 1998, Lippincott-Raven, pp 997–999.

39. MacKinnon J, Sanderson E, Buchanan D: The MacKinnon splint: a functional hand splint, *Canadian J Occup Ther* 42:157–158, 1975.

40. Mayer NH: Spasticity and the stretch reflex, *Muscle and Nerve* 6(suppl 6):51–513, 1997.

41. Mathiowet V, Bolding D, et al.: Immediate effects of positioning devices on the normal and spastic hand measured by electromyography, *AJOT* (37)247–254, 1983.

42. McPherson J, Becker A, Franszczak N: Dynamic splint to reduce the passive component of hypertonicity, *Arch Phys Med Rehabil* 66:249–252, 1985.

43. McPherson J, Kreimer D, Aalderks M, et al.: A comparison of dorsal and volar resting hand splints in the reduction of hypertonus, *Am J Occup Ther* 36(10):664–670, 1982.

44. Mortenson PA, Eng JJ: The use of casts in the management of joint mobility and hypertonia following brain injury in adults: a systematic review, *Phys Ther* 83:648–658, 2003.

45. Moseley AM, Hassett LM, Leung J, et al.: Serial casting versus positioning for the treatment of elbow contractures in adults with traumatic brain injury: a randomized controlled trial, *Clin Rehabil* 22:406–417, 2008.

46. Neuhaus B, Ascher E, Coullon B, et al.: A survey of rationales for and against hand splinting in hemiplegia, *Am J Occup Ther* 35:83–90, 1981.

47. O'Dwyer NJ, Ada L, et al.: Spasticity and muscle contracture following stroke, *Brain* (Pt 5)1737–1749, 1996.

48. Peterson LT: *Neurological considerations in splinting spastic extremities*, Menomonee Fall, WI, 1980, Rolyan Orthotics Lab.

49. Pizzi A, Carlucci G, Falsini C, et al.: Application of a volar static splint in poststroke spasticity of the upper limb, *Arch Phys Med Rehabil* 86:1855–1859, 2005.

50. Pohl M, Mehrholz J, Ruckriem S: The influence of illness duration and level of consciousness on the treatment effect and complication rate of serial casting in patients with severe cerebral spasticity, *Clin Rehabil* 17(4):373–379, 2003.

51. Pohl M, Ruckriem S, Mehrholz J, et al.: Effectiveness of serial casting in patients with severe cerebral spasticity: a comparison study, *Arch Phys Med Rehabil* 83(6):784–790, 2002.

52. Rood M: Neurophysiological reactions as a basis for physical therapy, *Phys Ther Rev* 34(9):444–449, 1954.

53. Rose V, Shah S: A comparative study on the immediate effects of hand orthoses on reduction of hypertonus, *Australian Occup Ther J* 34(2):59–64, 1987.

54. Scherling E, Johnson H: A tone-reducing wrist-hand orthosis, *Am J Occup Ther* 43(9):609–611, 1989.

55. Sinkjaer T, Taft E, Larsen K, Andreassen S, Hansen H: Non-reflex and reflex mediated ankle joint stiffness in multiple sclerosis patients with spasticity, *Muscle Nerve* 16:69–79, 1993.

56. Snook JH: Spasticity reduction splint, *Am J Occup Ther* 33:648–651, 1979.

57. Stockmeyer SA: An interpretation of the approach of Rood to the treatment of neuromuscular dysfunction, *Am J Phys Med* 46(1):900–961, 1967.

58. Taub E, Uswatte G, Bowman MH, et al.: Constraint-induced movement therapy combined with conventional neurorehabilitation techniques in chronic stroke patients with plegic hands: a case series, *Arch Phys Med Rehabil* 94(1):86–94, 2013.

59. Ten Berge SR, Boonstra AM, Dijkstra PU, et al.: A systematic evaluation of the effect of thumb opponens splints on hand function in children with unilateral spastic cerebral palsy, *Clin Rehabilitation* 26(4):362–371, 2012.

60. Tona JL, Schneck CM: The efficacy of upper extremity inhibitive casting: a single subject pilot study, *Am J Occup Ther* 47(10):901–910, 1993.

61. Ushiba J, Masakado Y, Komune Y, et al.: Changes of reflex size in upper limbs using wrist splint in hemiplegic patients, *Electromyogr Clin Neurophysiol* 44(3):175–182, 2004.

62. Van Lede P: Minimalistic splint design: A rationale told in a personal style, *Journal of Hand Therapy* 15(2):192–201, 2002.

63. Watanabe T: The role of therapy in spasticity management, *Am J Phys Rehab* 83(suppl):45–49, 2004.

64. Wissel J, Schelosky LD, Faiss JH, Mueller J: Early development of spasticity following stroke: A prospective, Observational trail, *J Neurology* 257(7):1067–1072, 2010, . http://dx.doi.org/10.1007/s00415-010-5463-1.

65. Zislis JM: Splinting of hand in a spastic hemiplegic patient, *Arch Phys Med Rehabil* 45:41–43, 1964.

APPENDIX 14-1   CASE STUDY

CASE STUDY 14-1

Read the following scenario, and answer the questions based on information in this chapter.

Bertha is a 78-year-old client who is a resident of a long-term care facility, and she experienced an ischemic cerebrovascular accident (CVA) 2 months ago. She was admitted to the hospital for 12 days and returned to the facility for short-term rehabilitation. Prior to the CVA, Bertha was independent in dressing and toileting, ambulatory using a walker, and able to participate in recreational activities. After a 2-week period of flaccidity, wrist and finger flexion spasticity emerged. Outside of the therapy schedule, the hand rests in wrist flexion most of the day. The dorsum of the hand is significantly edematous causing the fingers to assume the position of deformity with the metacarpophalangeal (MCP) joints in slight hyperextension and the interphalangeal (IP) joints partially flexed. Pain-free range of motion is limited to 10 degrees of wrist extension. Composite finger extension can only be accomplished pain-free with the wrist in 5 degrees of extension. No active wrist motion is present, but reflexive digit flexion is emerging. From a position of maximum wrist flexion, the stretch reflex is elicited at −15 degrees of wrist extension until slightly past neutral. The family is concerned about Bertha's hand becoming deformed. The nursing plan of care has been to position the hand elevated on a pillow resting on Bertha's lap. The palm and the web spaces are moist, and a faint odor is detected along with slightly macerated skin. Additionally, the thumb is tightly flexed across the palm, thus causing skin irritation to the thumb web space.

1. Which of the following orthotic designs is most appropriate for Bertha? Explain your rationale.
   a. A dorsal-based forearm platform with a volar hand component that positions the wrist and fingers in tolerable composite extension
   b. A volar finger spreader that positions the wrist and fingers statically in maximum extension
   c. A volar-based forearm platform and hard cone that positions the wrist in submaximal extension and fingers in partial flexion
   d. A volar forearm-based hand immobilization orthosis that stretches and positions the wrist and the fingers in composite extension
   e. A plaster cast that places the wrist in maximum extension and the fingers in a current resting position
2. The nursing staff reports that the orthosis is not applied regularly because Bertha's edema worsens with wear. Meanwhile, Bertha's hand at rest continues to be in the position of deformity of MCP joint hyperextension and PIP and DIP joint flexion. How would you modify the intervention approach?
   Four weeks have passed, and Bertha's hand and arm function as well as occupational performance are being assessed. Bertha has been wearing the orthosis consistently for several hours daily. The edema has reduced significantly, the joints remain passively mobile but the spasticity is causing more muscle tightness. Bertha is also getting more active mass grasp and partial release of 20 degrees of composite finger extension with effort—adequate to grasp and release a dish towel. There is evidence that the wrist stabilizers that are activating as grip on an object can be sustained for a few seconds duration before the hand fatigues. The thumb rests in an adducted and flexed position and is not able to engage in gross grasp tasks. The first web space and the thumb flexors are tight, but they can be passively positioned in extension and palmar abduction.
3. Which of the following orthotic designs should be considered for Bertha at this time? Explain your answer.
   a. A finger spreader that positions the thumb in radial abduction and does not incorporate the wrist
   b. A hard cone that positions the thumb in opposition and does not incorporate the wrist
   c. A short (hand based) opponens orthosis positioning the thumb in abduction with partial extension/opposition
   d. An orally inflatable orthosis that positions the wrist, fingers, and thumb in extension
   e. A Neoprene thumb abduction and extension orthosis that extends to the forearm radially
4. What specific suggestions would you offer the health care team and the family to encourage increased functional hand skills while Bertha is wearing the orthosis?

*See Appendix A for the answer key.

APPENDIX 14-2   **LABORATORY EXERCISE**

Laboratory Exercise 14-1

1. Practice fabricating a dorsal forearm based with volar hand immobilization orthosis on a partner. Use a goniometer and an acrylic cone to position the hand and wrist correctly.
2. After fitting the cone, use Form 14-1. This is a check-off sheet for self-evaluation of the hard-cone wrist and hand orthosis. Use Grading Sheet 14-1 as a classroom grading sheet.

APPENDIX 14-3 FORM AND GRADING SHEET

FORM 14-1* Dorsal forearm based with volar hand immobilization orthosis

Name: _____

Date: _____

Answer the following questions after the orthosis has been worn for 30 minutes.
(Mark NA for non-applicable situations.)

Evaluation Areas				Comments

Design

1. The wrist position is at the correct angle. — Yes ○ No ○ NA ○
2. The digits are in composite extension. — Yes ○ No ○ NA ○
3. The thumb is positioned in palmar abduction and extension. — Yes ○ No ○ NA ○
4. The hand platform extends slightly beyond the fingers. — Yes ○ No ○ NA ○
5. The orthosis is two-thirds the length of the forearm. — Yes ○ No ○ NA ○
6. The orthosis is half the width of the forearm. — Yes ○ No ○ NA ○

Function

1. The wrist is positioned in the target range. — Yes ○ No ○ NA ○
2. The fingers are positioned to provide gentle stretch to the flexors. — Yes ○ No ○ NA ○
3. The thumb position preserves the first web space. — Yes ○ No ○ NA ○

Straps

1. The straps avoid bony prominences. — Yes ○ No ○ NA ○
2. The straps are secure and rounded. — Yes ○ No ○ NA ○

Comfort

1. The edges are smooth with rounded corners. — Yes ○ No ○ NA ○
2. The proximal end is flared. — Yes ○ No ○ NA ○
3. Impingements or pressure areas are not present. (The ulnar styloid is relieved.) — Yes ○ No ○ NA ○

Cosmetic Appearance

1. The orthosis is free of fingerprints, dirt, or ink marks. — Yes ○ No ○ NA ○
2. The orthotic material is not buckled. — Yes ○ No ○ NA ○

Therapeutic Regimen

1. The person/caregiver has been instructed in a wearing schedule. — Yes ○ No ○ NA ○
2. The person/caregiver has been provided with orthotic precautions. — Yes ○ No ○ NA ○
3. The person/caregiver demonstrates understanding of the education. — Yes ○ No ○ NA ○
4. Person/caregiver knows how to clean the orthosis. — Yes ○ No ○ NA ○

Discuss adjustments or changes you would make based on the self-evaluation.

_____

_____

_____

GRADING SHEET 14-1*

Dorsal Forearm Based with Volar Hand Immobilization Orthosis

Name: _____

Date: _____

Grade: _____

1 = Beyond improvement, not acceptable
2 = Requires maximal improvement
3 = Requires moderate improvement
4 = Requires minimal improvement
5 = Requires no improvement

Evaluation Areas						**Comments**
Design						
1. The wrist position is at the correct angle.	1	2	3	4	5	
2. The digits are in composite extension.	1	2	3	4	5	
3. The thumb is positioned in palmar abduction and extension.	1	2	3	4	5	
4. The hand platform extends slightly beyond the fingers.	1	2	3	4	5	
5. The orthosis is two-thirds the length of the forearm.	1	2	3	4	5	
6. The orthosis is half the width of the forearm.	1	2	3	4	5	
Function						
1. The wrist is positioned in the target range.	1	2	3	4	5	
2. The fingers are positioned to provide gentle stretch to the flexors.	1	2	3	4	5	
3. The thumb position preserves the first web space.	1	2	3	4	5	
Straps						
1. The straps avoid bony prominences.	1	2	3	4	5	
2. The straps are secure and rounded.	1	2	3	4	5	
Comfort						
1. The edges are smooth with rounded corners.	1	2	3	4	5	
2. The proximal end is flared.	1	2	3	4	5	
3. Impingements or pressure areas are not present. (The ulnar styloid is relieved.)	1	2	3	4	5	
Cosmetic Appearance						
1. The orthosis is free of fingerprints, dirt, or ink marks.	1	2	3	4	5	
2. The orthotic material is not buckled.	1	2	3	4	5	
Therapeutic Regimen						
1. The person/caregiver has been instructed in a wearing schedule.	1	2	3	4	5	
2. The person/caregiver has been provided with orthotic precautions.	1	2	3	4	5	
3. The person/caregiver demonstrates understanding of the education.	1	2	3	4	5	
4. Person/caregiver knows how to clean the orthosis.	1	2	3	4	5	

CHAPTER 15

Orthotic Intervention for Older Adults

Marlene A. Riley
Helene Lohman

Key Terms

ecchymosis
integumentary system
prefabricated
soft orthosis
working memory

Chapter Objectives

1. Describe special considerations for orthotic intervention with older adults in different environments.
2. Identify the complexity of age-related changes, medical conditions, and medication side effects that may impact orthotic provision.
3. Recognize how an older adult's performance in occupations and activities may influence orthotic use and design based on the Occupational Therapy Practice Framework.[2,36]
4. Select appropriate prefabricated orthoses.
5. Select appropriate materials to fabricate custom orthoses.
6. Describe factors that influence methods of instruction about safe use and care of an orthosis for an older adult and/or caregiver.

Anthony is a 75-year-old male who plays basketball at the senior center. He does not consider himself to be "old" and would not think of going to a senior center except that his friend invited him to join the indoor basketball team. He plays three times per week despite pain in his thumbs. The senior center director routinely invites health care professionals to provide free screenings. A hand therapist was requested to offer a screening due to the director's observation that a number of older adults complained of hand problems during participation in activities. Anthony attended the screening and asked if there was anything he could wear to help his thumbs. He said he had "his father's hands"

and was interested in learning about braces that may help decrease his pain. The therapist recommended bilateral prefabricated thumb carpometacarpal (CMC) MetaGrip orthoses because they would be appropriate for someone who is active and requires a durable orthoses (Figure 15-1).

Lucille is a 78-year-old widow who lives alone. She just completed 5 months of chemotherapy for colon cancer and complains of weakness, numbness, and cold intolerance in her hands. Her history is significant for flexor tenosynovitis in her dominant hand ring finger. She is pleased that her cancer seems to be in remission. She feels very despondent that she is not able to drive or prepare meals due to the difficulty that she is experiencing with her hands. Her son accompanies Lucille to an outpatient physical rehabilitation setting. Part of the therapy intervention for Lucille includes an orthosis to restrict metacarpophalangeal (MCP) flexion for trigger finger.[15] There are a variety of trigger finger designs to choose from including a lightweight custom fabricated thermoplastic type (Figure 15 -2, A), a silver ring that resembles jewelry (see Figure 15-2, B), a soft prefabricated Neoprene orthosis (see Figure 15-2, C) and a prefabricated high temperature thermoplastic orthosis (see Figure 15-2, D). Considerations for this decision include the availability of materials, payment source, and client input. In addition to the trigger finger orthosis, Lucille may benefit from wearing a lightweight Atlas nitrile-coated garden glove to reduce cold intolerance and assist with gripping objects (Figure 15-3).

Anthony and Lucille are both older adults who benefit from orthoses to improve their ability to participate in daily activities. Although close in age, their stories illustrate the broad range of knowledge and skills necessary when making decisions about orthotic provision for older adults. Anthony is an active, independent older adult whose primary goal is to decrease hand pain. Lucille has a complicated medical history and requires on-going therapy to address her decline in function.

Late adulthood spans from age 65 until the end of life.[5] According to the Department of Health and Human Services Administration on Aging, almost one in every eight, or 12.9%, of the population is an older American.[12] By 2030 the older adult population is projected to represent 19.3% of the total population.[12] Only 4.1% of the 65 and older population in 2009 lived in institutional settings, such as nursing homes. However, the percentage increases dramatically with age to 14.3% for persons 85 and older. The 85 and older population was projected to increase by 36% from 4.2 million in 2000 to 5.7 million in 2010. A new projection suggested that the 85 and older population will increase by 15% to 6.6 million in 2020.[12] The growth of the older adult population is a significant reason that the Bureau of Labor Statistic's employment projections rise by 26% for occupational therapists and 30% for physical therapists, between 2008 and 2018.[9]

Over 25% of community-resident Medicare beneficiaries older than 65 in 2007 had some limitation in function that prevented them from being fully independent in performing

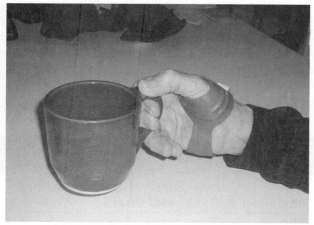

Figure 15-1 Thumb Carpometacarpal Push Metagrip Orthosis designed in consultation with Judy Colditz, Hand Lab.

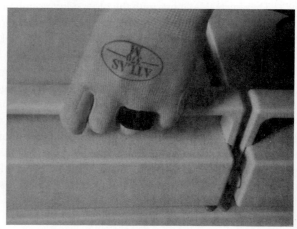

Figure 15-3 370 Atlas Lightweight nitrile-coated garden glove to reduce cold intolerance and assist with gripping objects worn under or over an orthosis.

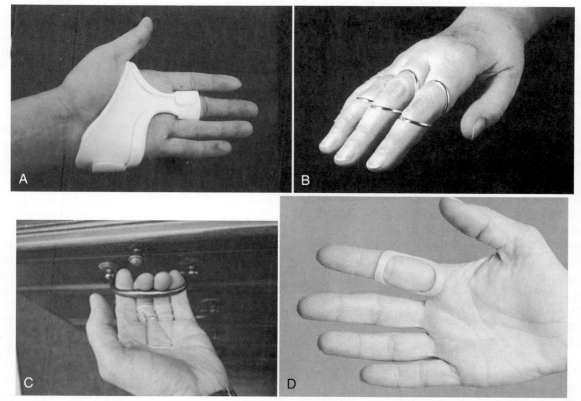

Figure 15-2 **A,** Thermoplastic orthosis to restrict metacarpophalangeal (MCP) flexion for trigger finger. **B,** Siris Silver Ring Trigger Finger for chronic recurring flexor tenosynovitis. **C,** Neoprene TFSTrigger Finger Solution. **D,** Oval-8 for trigger finger. (**B,** Courtesy of Silver Ring Company. **D,** Courtesy of 3-Point Products, Stevensville, Maryland.)

one or more activities of daily living (ADLs). An additional 14.6% reported difficulties with instrumental activities of daily living (IADLs).[12] Musculoskeletal dysfunction is one of the major causes of disability in older adults resulting in decreased mobility and fine motor control.[30] The development of hand problems in older adults significantly impacts global physical functioning.[35] According to McKee and Rivard,[21] an orthosis that includes the needs of the client in the design process improves the ability to function by "relieving pain, providing protection and joint stabilization."[21] Therapists who work with the older adult population need to have a strong foundation of interventions, including orthotic provision to improve functional abilities in ADLs and IADLs.

Fundamental principles of clinical examination, design, and fabrication of orthoses do not change as people age. Therapists do, however, need to be aware of special considerations necessary to accommodate the unique needs of older adults. When designing an orthosis for an older adult, the therapist considers the special needs of the individual, the goals of the orthosis, and the orthotic materials available. Clinical reasoning to determine the most effective orthosis for an older adult should consider:

- Age-related changes in body functions
- Medical history, including current medications
- Least restrictive designs impacting mobility
- Choice of lightweight but supportive materials
- Choice of materials for skin integrity maintenance
- Simple designs for donning and doffing
- Awareness of payer source and cost effectiveness (e.g., prefabricated vs. custom)
- The environment

Treatment Settings and Orthotic Designs

The older adult's environment is an important consideration for clinical decision making. Therapists provide interventions to older adults in multiple settings. Table 15-1 presents specific considerations and goals specific to different settings. The older adult's living situation (e.g., living at home, apartment, long-term care setting, assisted living center, and so on) is important when the therapist determines the most appropriate orthosis. For example, an 80-year-old woman with osteoarthritis (OA) who performs her self-care and requires the use of her hands throughout the day may benefit from a thumb carpometacarpal (CMC) immobilization orthosis to improve her daily function. In contrast, a long-term care resident with multiple cerebrovascular accidents (CVAs) may require an orthosis to maintain sufficient range of motion (ROM) for dressing and bathing. Hand ROM is necessary to prevent skin maceration in the palm caused by sustained full-finger flexion. A prefabricated resting orthosis that is easily adjusted, such as the Comfy Hand-Wrist-Finger Orthosis (Figure 15-4, *A*) or a custom thermoplastic cone-shaped orthosis (see Figure 15-4, *B*) can prevent secondary contractures. Therapists who treat older adults during the

acute stage of an illness must be aware of risk factors to prevent secondary complications, such as loss of passive range of motion (PROM), edema, and skin breakdown.

Age-Related Changes and Medical Conditions Impacting Orthotic Intervention

In addition to typical age-related changes, older adults' body systems are vulnerable to chronic medical conditions. For instance, someone referred for a hand orthosis following a CVA may have other conditions more prevalent with aging, such as diabetes and OA. In addition to obtaining a thorough medical history to determine the appropriate goals of an orthosis, the therapist needs to be familiar with how different medical conditions concurrently affect hand function.

Table 15-2 provides a summary of age-related changes and health conditions that affect the design and approach to

Table 15-1 Considerations for Orthotic Design in Different Settings	
TREATMENT SETTING	**SPECIAL CONSIDERATIONS AND GOALS**
Short term: Acute hospital/ICU Sub-acute/SNF Comprehensive inpatient rehabilitation	• Goals are to prevent secondary complications, such as loss of ROM and compromised skin integrity, while monitoring recovery • Positioning orthoses, such as a resting hand orthosis and neutral ankle/foot orthosis • Forward information related to the orthosis to the discharge setting
Long term: Assisted living Long term care Geropsychiatry	• Choose materials that are safe for clients who may have cognitive impairments or restricted mobility • Train staff members to monitor skin integrity when orthoses are used long-term (e.g., after discharge from skilled rehabilitation)
Community-based: Home health Outpatient Wellness center	• Provide pictures and written instructions for use and care of orthoses and phone contact information in case questions arise • Orthoses are typically used to enable functional participation in ADLs and IADLs; orthoses must be versatile and durable

ADL, Activity of daily living; *IADL*, instrumental activity of daily living; *ICU*, intensive care unit; *ROM*, range of motion; *SNF*, skilled nuring facility.

orthotic intervention. The following client factors[2] are based on selected classifications from the World Health Organization's (WHO's) International Classification of Functioning, Disability and Health (ICF)[36] as they relate to considerations for orthotic intervention.

Mental Functions

Therapists assess cognitive status to determine the older adult's ability to understand the orthosis' purpose, wearing schedule, and precautions. **Working memory** impairment may prevent the older adult from recalling the orthosis' storage location or application procedure. Sometimes a therapist can ascertain memory problems by noting how an older adult follows directions during orthotic fabrication. If memory is a problem, the therapist establishes a routine schedule for wear and care, fabricates a simple design, and labels the orthosis for easy application.

If the older adult has significant cognitive impairments, the therapist educates the caregiver(s) about the orthosis'

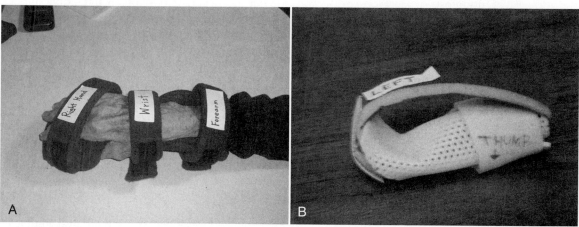

Figure 15-4 A, Comfy Hand-Wrist-Finger Orthosis is an example of an adjustable prefabricated orthosis. **B,** A custom lightweight cone-shaped orthosis assists with keeping fingers out of the palm.

Table 15-2 Summary of Age-Related Changes and Medical Conditions Impacting Orthotic Interventions

BODY FUNCTIONS	TYPICAL AGE-RELATED CHANGES AND ASSOCIATED CONDITIONS	COMMON ORTHOSES AND GENERAL HINTS
Mental function: Cognition	Memory impairment Dementia	Assess individual's ability to understand the orthosis' purpose, schedule, and precautions. Establish routine schedule. Develop habit of keeping orthosis in same location when not in use. Provide thorough training to caregivers.
Sensory functions: Vision Hearing Touch Pain Temperature and pressure	Acuity loss (presbyopia) Cataracts Glaucoma Diabetic retinopathy Age-related macular degeneration (ARMD) Hearing loss (presbycusis) Diminished sensibility Joint pain Decreased ability to regulate body temperature to diffuse heat Hypersensitivity to cold	Written instructions should be simple. Use large font and provide high contrast. Use contrasting colors for orthosis and straps. Use tactile labels to mark reference points on orthosis. Use compensatory techniques, such as visual scanning. Use guidelines for talking to the hearing impaired (see Box 15-2). Share guidelines with family and caregivers. Perform visual skin checks; if vision is also impaired, instruct a caregiver how to do it. Consider if a soft orthosis or padding is an appropriate alternative to a rigid orthosis. Use neutral or resting positions for pain relief. Use an adjustable orthosis or adjustable straps to modify according to comfort level. Use an orthosis that can be easily removed. Use a stockinette on the extremity. Choose lightweight multi-perforated materials. Provide a textured glove to wear under or over the orthosis.

Continued

Table 15-2   Summary of Age-Related Changes and Medical Conditions Impacting Orthotic Interventions—cont'd

BODY FUNCTIONS	TYPICAL AGE-RELATED CHANGES AND ASSOCIATED CONDITIONS	COMMON ORTHOSES AND GENERAL HINTS
Neuromusculoskeletal and movement-related functions: Neurological Skeletal	Cerbrovascular accident (CVA) Peripheral neuropathies • Chemotherapy • Carpal tunnel • Cubital tunnel Parkinson disease Idiopathic essential tremors Ostoporosis • Wrist fractures (Colles) Osteoarthritis (OA) • Heberden (DIPs) and Bouchard (PIPs) nodes • Thumb trapeziometacarpal involvement Loss of mobility	Use inhibition techniques to assist with application of anti-spasticity orthoses (refer to Chapter 14). Use resting hand and foot drop orthoses for flaccid extremities. Assess both sensory and motor function. Use a wrist orthosis in neutral. Position the elbow joint in 30 to 45 degrees of flexion. Provide elbow padding. Provide instruction on positioning and ergonomics (refer to Chapter 13). Use orthotic material to fabricate a base to hold assistive devices. Choose a thermoplastic material with memory and moderate resistance to stretch if serial adjustments are indicated. Choose a prefabricated tubular design with D-rings for ease of application if fracture is healed. Immobilize PIPs/DIPs to rest joints. Use lightweight thermoplastic material. Ensure orthosis is easily donned and doffed. Use a hand-based thumb CMC custom or prefabricated design Keep the orthosis within reach or easy walking distance. Maintain a consistent storage location. Keep the orthosis simple for easy application and removal. Permanently attach one end of each strap to the orthosis. Use D-ring straps.
Cardiovascular and hematologial functions	Peripheral vascular disease (PVD)	Use inhibition techniques to assist with application of anti-spasticity orthoses (refer to Chapter 14). Use resting hand and foot-drop orthoses for flaccid extremities. Consider a foot-drop orthotic design to float the heels and avoid pressure. Use volar knee extension orthosis for below knee amputations. Choose a thermoplastic material with maximum resistance to stretch. Monitor skin carefully due to loss of sensation.
Digestive, metabolic and endocrine functions	Diabetes • Peripheral neuropathies • Trigger finger • De Quervain disease • Dupuytren disease	Assess sensory and motor function. Educate to perform visual inspections. Use closed cell padding to prevent pressure. Keep fingertips and toes visible. Restrict MCP flexion. Immobilize thumb/wrist. Hand based (no thumb) resting orthosis.
Genitourinary functions	End-stage renal disease (ESRD) Bladder conditions	In the presence of forearm AV fistulas, straps must be loose and easily adjusted to avoid constriction with fluctuations in edema. Orthoses may be contraindicated for insensate hands. For incontinence or frequent nocturnal urination, provide instructions on quick and safe removal of orthoses.
Skin functions	Fragile skin: • Corticosteroid adverse effect • Skin tears • Delayed wound healing	Use stockinette or arm sleeves. Use gel orthotic pads or pressure relief padding. Use lightweight thermoplastic materials or soft prefabricated orthoses. Inspect skin frequently. Modify wearing schedule to prevent skin maceration.

AV, Arteriovenous; *CMC,* carpometacarpal; *DIP,* distal interphalangeal; *MCP,* metacarpophalangeal; *PIP,* proximal interphalangeal.

purpose, wearing schedule, care, correct application, and precautions. Individuals with later-stage dementias often posture in flexed positions and thus the caregiver(s) may require recommendations to maintain skin integrity. If there are cognitive impairments, or if a caregiver is involved, the risks versus the benefits of an orthosis must be carefully weighed against alternative positioning, such as the use of pillows or dense foam wedges. In addition, the therapist may consider using D-ring straps for a person with dementia who is constantly trying to remove the orthosis. Refer to Box 15-1 for a summary of general hints for orthotic instructions.

Sensory Functions

Vision

Older adults are particularly vulnerable to conditions that affect the visual system. Cataracts, glaucoma, age-related macular degeneration, and diabetic neuropathy are the primary conditions of visual impairment in older adults. According to the National Eye Institute,[23] more than two-thirds of people with visual impairment are older than 65 years of age. Decreased vision plays a role in non-adherence of orthotic wear. For example, some older adults may be unable to apply their orthoses because of poor figure/ground discrimination. Older adults may have difficulty seeing how the straps attach and may be unable to visually inspect their skin. Using color thermoplastic material and contrasting color straps may assist the older adult who has poor visual discrimination. Bright colors may prevent the orthosis from being easily lost or mistakenly sent to the laundry.

When receiving orthotic instructions by demonstration, older adults who have correctable vision should wear their glasses. The therapist asks older adults to demonstrate proper orthotic application and removal. Simple, large-print instructions are best for this population. A high contrast of ink and paper is helpful. The use of direct lighting and magnification devices help with reading instructions and with performing skin inspections.

For older adults who have macular degeneration (i.e., distorted or loss of central vision), cataracts or poor visual acuity, the therapist encourages the use of compensatory techniques during application and removal of the orthosis and during skin inspections. Compensatory techniques include eye scanning, head turning, and use of tactile labels to mark reference points on orthoses (Figure 15-5).

Auditory System

According to the American Federation for Aging Research, approximately 30% of older adults between 65 and 74 years of age and 50% of adults age 75 or older have hearing loss.[1] Hearing impairment influences verbal explanations and statements. Sometimes hearing problems can be detected during the initial interview or during orthotic fabrication. Therapists should not rely solely on printed information to relay instructions, because some older adults may be unable to read or have visual impairments that make reading difficult or impossible. The therapist needs to use more tactile cues when positioning the person for orthotic intervention. When talking to a person who is hearing impaired, the therapist should use the guidelines outlined in Box 15-2.

Touch

Somatosensory function of two-point discrimination declines with age.[32] Because the decline is gradual over the life cycle, older adults may not be aware of their diminished sensibility. Vision is the primary sense used to compensate for decreased tactile sensation. When both vision and touch sensory functions decline, the older adult is at greater risk for compromised skin integrity.

Tactile sensation may become impaired secondary to poor positioning of older adults with limited mobility. Decreased sensation may contribute to compression neuropathies of the

---

Box 15-1   General Hints for Orthotic Instructions

- Keep the orthotic design simple for easy donning and doffing. Observe the client's/caregiver's ability to don and doff the orthosis.
- Label the orthosis with individual's name, right or left extremity, hand or foot, and additional landmarks to identify how to properly position the orthosis.
- Provide written and oral instructions that include application, wearing schedule, and precautions for discharge.
- Identify a consistent location to store the orthosis within easy reach.
- Keep straps attached to the orthosis.
- Provide a picture of the orthosis on the extremity. Observe privacy regulations, and avoid public posting of information related to client's care.
- A dark colored orthosis provides better contrast with light colored bed linens.

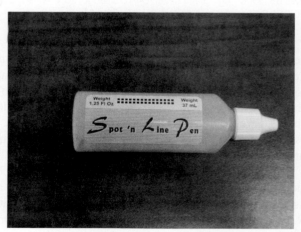

Figure 15-5 Tactile label markers, such as the Spot n' Line Pen, can be used to mark reference points on an orthosis for an older adult with impaired vision.

Box 15-2   Guidelines for Talking to the Hearing Impaired

- Seat or position the hearing-impaired person to see the face of the person speaking.
- Whenever possible, face the person with impaired hearing on the same level during verbal communication.
- Before talking, gain the older adult's attention by using touch, gesture, and eye contact.
- Use visual aids when possible. Take a photograph or draw a diagram that shows correct orthotic application.
- Use demonstration as part of the instructions.
- Keep hands away from face while talking.
- If the person misses statements, rephrase the statements rather than repeat the same words.
- Reduce background noises during verbal communication. When possible, work with the person one-on-one in a quiet room.
- Do not shout because doing so distorts voices. Talk in a normal voice but at close range.
- Avoid chewing gum during verbal communication, because this makes speech more difficult to understand.
- Be aware that people hear better if they are vertical rather than horizontal. If a person is standing or sitting, sound waves are directed into the ears. If a person is lying on a bed, sound waves are dispersed over the head.
- Recognize that persons with hearing impairments may not hear as well if they are tired or ill.
- If hearing is better in one ear, direct speech toward that ear. Never shout directly into the ear.
- Ask client to repeat the instructions back to you.

Data from Lewis SC: *Older adult care in occupational therapy,* Thorofare, NJ, 1989, Slack; Barlowe E, Siegal DL, Edwards F, et al: Vision, hearing, and other sensory loss associated with aging. In Doress PB, Siegal DL, editors: *Ourselves, growing older,* New York, 1987, Simon & Schuster, pp. 365-379; Hills GA: The changing realm of the senses. In Lewis BB, editor: *Aging: the health care challenge,* ed 4, Philadelphia, 2002, FA Davis.

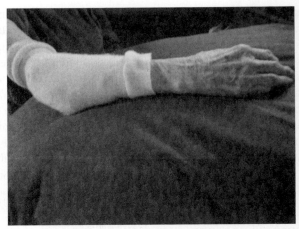

Figure 15-6 Heelbo padded soft elbow sleeve protector to decrease pressure on the ulnar nerve.

Pain

Perception of pain is variable among individuals regardless of age. A visual analog scale and careful history, including assessment of location and particular activities that increase or decrease pain, are part of the initial assessment. It is important to assist the client to find a balance between resting joints in the orthosis and actively using the hand.

Neuromusculoskeletal and Movement-Related Functions

Skeletal System

Several neurologic and orthopedic problems are more common in older adults.[19] The skeletal system is most affected by aging. Osteoporosis and OA are common diagnoses that often require orthotic intervention. The National Osteoporosis Foundation reports that the loss of bone density accelerates after menopause.[24] Thus, fractures are common in older adults. Some older adults may sustain multiple fractures, commonly resulting from a fall (e.g., hip and distal radius fracture). Therapists may encounter such patients in a variety of settings (inpatient or outpatient) depending on the severity and healing progression.

The distal radius is especially vulnerable to fractures. A common fracture of the distal radius, Colles fracture, often occurs after falling on an outstretched arm.[25] Sustaining a Colles fracture can be associated with functional declines in physical performance in hand strength and walking speed.[25] A volar wrist orthosis is generally indicated after removal of an arm cast or external fixator for immobilization (see Chapter 7). As the fracture heals, the goal may change to one of mobilization, which can be achieved by serial adjustments to a thermoplastic orthosis to improve wrist extension. When treating a Colles fracture or any upper extremity condition, it is important to determine if there are other etiologies causing upper extremity impairments. For example, a thorough assessment of a client referred with a wrist injury may reveal pre-existing sensory loss in the dermatome distribution of C6-C7 due to compression of cervical nerve roots

median or ulnar nerves. Cubital tunnel syndrome, a compression of the ulnar nerve at the elbow level, may result from constant pressure on flexed elbows while sitting in a wheelchair or from prolonged bed confinement. A padded elbow sleeve (Figure 15-6) or a padded elbow orthosis to restrict elbow flexion greater than 30 to 45 degrees prevents further pressure on the nerve.[28]

Compression of the median nerve at the wrist may be due to prolonged wrist flexion posturing or secondary to an associated medical condition, such as rheumatoid arthritis (RA) or diabetes. A prefabricated wrist orthosis in neutral with D-ring straps is easier to don and can be used to prevent nerve compression (Figure 15-7; see Chapter 13 for further discussion of these conditions).

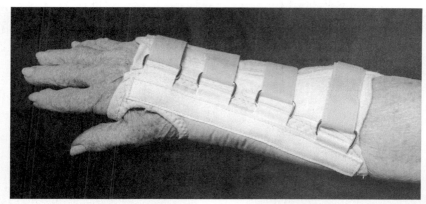

Figure 15-7 This D-ring orthosis has a circumferential design that holds the orthosis in place during application.

caused by OA. The sensory loss might otherwise have only been associated with the wrist fracture. In older adults who have multiple medical conditions, the source of decreased sensorimotor function in the hand requires careful medical evaluation.

In addition to OA of the cervical spine, hand joints are frequently affected. The initial onset OA typically occurs between the ages of 40 and 50.[26] Primary OA results from idiopathic or known causes. Secondary OA results from congenital joint abnormalities, genetics, infections, and metabolic or endocrine disorders.[26] Most older adults have evidence of some cartilage damage.[6] Hand OA is characterized by enlarged distal interphalangeal (DIP) joints (Heberden nodes) and enlarged proximal interphalangeal (PIP) joints (Bouchard nodes).[26] The nodes typically cause more discomfort in the index finger because of the demands placed on the joints during pinch activities. An immobilization orthosis for the DIP joint is a conservative measure to decrease pain (Figure 15-8). Surgical fusion may be warranted for more advanced cases.

OA of the thumb at the CMC joint is another common reason for an orthotic referral. Initial conservative management usually requires a hand-based thumb immobilization orthosis (see Chapter 8). Individuals with this condition benefit from education on joint protection techniques to break the pain cycle. As discussed in Chapter 8, there are different approaches to orthotic intervention for arthritic hands. One of the most prevalent approaches is to fabricate a removable hand based orthosis to immobilize only the CMC joint.[16]

Chronic flexion of the thumb MCP joint, or an adduction contracture leads to a hyperextended interphalangeal (IP) joint. The hyperextended joint can be conservatively treated with a figure-eight orthosis to improve stability and function of the thumb (Figure 15-9).

Neurological System

Central nervous system (CNS) disorders are some of the most common causes of disability in older adults.[3] Progression of cardiovascular disorders may lead to CVAs resulting in abnormal tone on one side of the body. When making

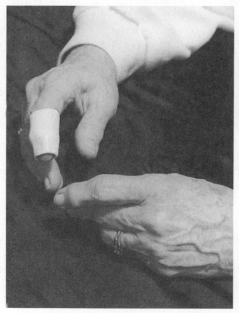

Figure 15-8 Enlarged distal interphalangeal (DIP) joints from osteoarthritis (OA) may become painful and benefit from immobilization to decrease pain.

an orthosis for an older adult with abnormal tone, it may be important to consider principles involved with orthotic design related to a coexisting condition, such as OA of the thumb CMC joint. Orthokinetic properties of materials should be cautiously selected because they may affect tone (see Chapter 14).

Some neurological conditions cause tremors, which are particularly problematic for older adults. Tremors may be associated with Parkinson disease, idiopathic essential tremors, or tremors secondary to medication side effects. Orthoses may be used as a base to hold assistive devices to improve self-care function in the presence of tremors. An adaptation may be made to an orthosis that is required for a coexisting diagnosis. Thermoplastic material may be used to fabricate a base to hold self-care utensils, such as a spoon, or to stabilize a pen to write (Figure 15-10).

Peripheral neuropathies may be due to adverse effects of chemotherapy.[17] Persons over age 65 account for 60% of

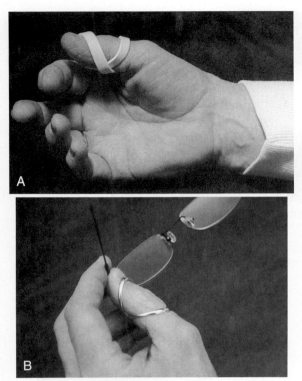

Figure 15-9 A, A tri-point figure-eight design stabilizes the thumb interphalangeal (IP) joint to prevent hyperextension during pinch. **B,** Siris Swan Neck on the IP joint of the thumb to prevent hyperextension. (**B,** Courtesy of Silver Ring Company.)

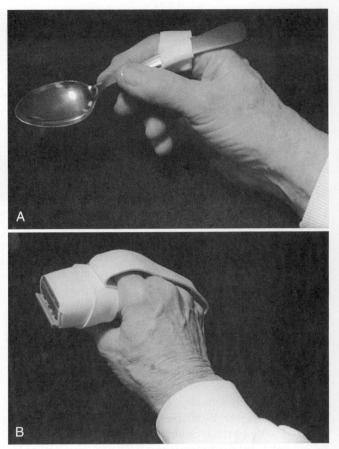

Figure 15-10 A, Example of a hand based orthosis used as a base for an activity of daily living (ADL) device. **B,** Example of how thermoplastic material is used to adapt an ADL device.

newly diagnosed cancer cases.[4] Protocols for orthotic intervention of the particular nerve involved are used. Careful monitoring of skin must be routinely completed due to loss of sensation.

Cardiovascular and Hematologic Functions

Many older adults have cardiovascular disease, which may be the primary or secondary reason for referral. Older adults with cardiovascular disease may have limited energy. The therapist educates the older adult to store the orthosis in close proximity in order to conserve energy.

Peripheral vascular disease is a common accompanying condition for those who have cardiovascular disease. When fitting someone with a lower extremity orthosis, precautions for peripheral vascular disease are observed. The temperature of the thermoplastic material is carefully checked, and a double layer of stockinette should be considered instead of applying warm material directly to the skin. Older adults who have less ability to dissipate heat are vulnerable to burn or torn skin. Older adults with decreased cognition and thin skin, they may not be aware of the potential for burns. Poor circulation results in delayed wound healing after skin breakdown. Foot drop orthoses should float on the heel to avoid pressure. A volar knee extension orthosis may be indicated to prevent flexion contractures following a below knee amputation (BKA).

Digestive, Metabolic, and Endocrine Functions

Digestive System
Dehydration, alcohol abuse, chronic disease, or poor diet in older adults may cause nutritional deficiencies.[26] Sensory testing is carefully completed with individuals who have digestive disorders and nutritional deficiencies because they may also present with impaired nerve function. Poor wound healing may be the result of a poor nutritional status. The condition of the skin and nails is observed to determine appropriate materials and orthotic care. Review of lab values give therapists insight into nutritional status.

Endocrine System
Diabetes mellitus (DM), a disorder of the endocrine system, is a common condition reported by the Centers for Disease Control and Prevention,[10] which affects up to 17% of older adults. Individuals with long-standing DM have an increased incidence of other conditions that must be considered before an orthosis is made.

A careful sensory evaluation determines whether there are peripheral neuropathies in the hands or feet.[20] In the presence of diminished sensation, pressure caused by an orthosis may not be perceived by the older adult and may lead to skin breakdown. Straps must never cause constriction, especially if there is associated peripheral vascular disease. These considerations are particularly important when someone, regardless of age, with diabetes is referred for a foot-drop orthosis, a knee extension orthosis after a BKA, or a finger flexion contracture secondary to a CVA.

Individuals with DM are at greater risk of associated conditions[11] that may require orthotic intervention for the upper extremity, such as carpal tunnel syndrome, trigger finger stenosing tenosynovitis, and Dupuytren disease (tenosynovitis).[15] When stenosing tenosynovitis occurs at the first dorsal extensor compartment on the radial aspect of the wrist, it is referred to as *de Quervain disease* (tenosynovitis). Conservative management includes a thumb spica orthosis (Figure 15-11) (refer to Chapter 8).

A flexion contracture of the palmar fascia may resemble Dupuytren disease and is another example of a soft-tissue condition associated with DM.[11] Idiopathic Dupuytren disease is most common in men age 45 and older.[26] These individuals have limited extension of their fingers or thumbs with nodules at the palmar base of the involved digits. An orthosis is not effective in preventing contractures because the contracted tissue of Dupuytren disease does not respond to low-load prolonged stress. Therefore, surgical intervention is necessary if the contracture is limiting function.[16] Orthotic intervention with a hand immobilization orthosis to regain extension of the digits[14] is appropriate only after a surgical release of the fascia (see Chapter 9).

Genitourinary Functions

Kidneys are part of the urinary system and have an endocrine function. When treating individuals with end-stage renal disease (ESRD), it is important to identify the subcutaneous arteriovenous (AV) fistula. AVs are typically located on the forearm and used for vascular access for hemodialysis. As a result of the radial artery anastomoses with the cephalic vein, vascularity distal to the AV is compromised[26] and can result in edema and peripheral neuropathies that

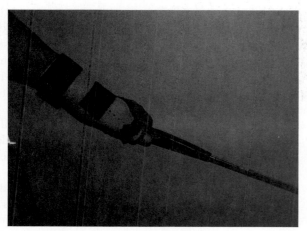

Figure 15-11 An example of a prefabricated orthosis for de Quervain disease is the Liberty Wrist and Thumb Spica.

affect sensorimotor hand function. Orthoses should be used selectively because any source of pressure could cause skin breakdown in an insensate hand with compromised vascularity.

Older adults often go the bathroom during the night for a variety of reasons. The presence of co-morbidities, medication usage, and a variety of factors more prevalent in older persons influences the sleep-wake cycle.[8] If an older adult needs to wear an orthosis during sleep periods, the history includes urinary function and a review of possible sleep-related disorders. With orthotic wear during sleep, it is especially important that the orthosis is easily donned and doffed for bathroom hygiene.

Skin Functions

Aging of the **integumentary system** includes thinning of the epidermis and dermis.[30] Older adults with little subcutaneous fat are more susceptible to pressure sores. Fragile older adults are more likely to have skin tears. A **soft orthosis,** padding to line the orthosis or a protective skin sleeve should be considered.

Medications and Side Effects

Many older adults take medications that cause side effects[31] that may affect orthotic provision. A list of medications should be included in the history before an orthotic decision is made. Corticosteroids are commonly prescribed for chronic conditions, such as RA and chronic obstructive pulmonary disease (COPD). Long-term steroid use can lead to **ecchymosis** (bruising), osteoporosis, and thin skin that is vulnerable to skin tears. Long-term steroid use can also lead to delayed wound healing. Anticoagulants, such as heparin, are prescribed for collagen vascular disorders. Side effects of anticoagulants include increased risk of ecchymosis and edema from minor soft-tissue trauma.

Antihistamines for respiratory conditions and psychotropic medications for mental conditions can cause tremors. When designing orthoses for older adults who take these medications, the additional risks of fragile skin, osteoporosis, bruising, edema, or tremors are factored into the orthotic design. In older adults, sleep medications may affect orthotic wear. For example, the person may not notice problems if the orthosis becomes uncomfortable during the night, thus increasing the possibility of skin breakdown. In addition, the older adult may be noncompliant with the wearing schedule and wear the orthosis too long.[18]

Purposes of Orthoses for Older Adults

With the plethora of conditions that may affect older adults, the purpose of orthotic intervention may include, but are not limited to, the following:
* Prevent ROM loss
* Reduce pain

- Improve occupational performance
- Manage contractures
- Decrease edema
- Protect skin integrity
- Substitute for loss of sensorimotor function

Range of Motion

The design of an orthosis should always allow full ROM of non-involved joints. Serial mobilization orthotic intervention is generally the preferred method to improve ROM for an older adult. An orthosis that is serially adjusted to improve ROM is easier to manage because the therapist has better control over the amount of force applied. For example, a volar wrist extension immobilization orthosis after a distal radius fracture may require several progressive adjustments to improve wrist extension (see Chapter 7).[22]

Pain Reduction

With acute and chronic conditions, one goal of orthotic intervention is to reduce pain by providing support and rest to the involved joints. In addition to the design of the orthosis to rest specific joints, the wearing schedule should provide the appropriate balance between rest and activity. The hand based thumb immobilization orthosis worn for CMC OA is an example of an orthosis removed periodically for ROM and reapplied during activities that otherwise cause pain and stress to the joint.

Improvement of Occupational Performance

An orthosis may improve or maintain an older adult's function. When possible, it is preferable to adapt the environment rather than restrict ROM in an orthosis. For example, rather than wearing a wrist orthosis for use during shaving, the therapist makes adaptations from thermoplastic material on an electric razor to allow an older adult to remain independent (see Figure 15-10, *B*). If adapting the environment is not effective, then an orthosis may be indicated.

Contracture Management

Loss of mobility and neurologic conditions place an older adult at increased risk of developing contractures.[27] Changes in the older adult's connective tissue and cartilage increase the risk for contractures, especially during inactivity.[27] Appropriate goals may be to prevent further contracture, decrease pain, or enable better skin care. Therapists determine whether or not to provide an orthosis by weighing the risks of additional complications that may arise from orthotic wear, such as contributing to skin breakdown.

If the orthosis is applied while PROM is still within normal limits, it may be possible to prevent a contracture. If the loss of PROM is recent, orthotic intervention may improve ROM and correct the contracture. An example is a foot-drop orthosis to gradually position the ankle at 90 degrees after loss of active ankle dorsiflexion. Therapists commonly use hand immobilization orthoses to prevent further deformity when there is a loss of active hand or wrist ROM.

Edema Management

With loss of active range of motion (AROM) combined with diminished circulation, edema can lead to secondary shortening of soft tissue. It is important to prevent edema through techniques such as elevation and AROM. The edematous hand is positioned in an orthosis to counteract adaptive tissue shortening and residual contractures. The position of deformity caused by edema in the hand results in thumb adduction, MCP extension, and IP flexion.[33] To prevent deformity, the wrist is positioned in an intrinsic plus position. The intrinsic plus position consists of approximately 20 to 30 degrees of wrist extension, the thumb in palmar abduction to level of comfort, and the fingers in MCP flexion with the PIP and DIP joints in extension (see Chapter 9). Adjunctive techniques may be necessary to treat edema unless AROM returns. Wearing a pressure garment, such as an Isotoner glove, concurrently with the orthosis may help control edema. If the non-involved side of an older adult also appears edematous, a systemic cause, such as congestive heart failure (CHF), may be present.

Protection of Skin Integrity

The combination of impaired cardiovascular function and changes associated with aging, such as diminished sensation and thinning of the dermis and epidermis, creates the risk for loss of skin integrity. The heel is the most vulnerable area for skin breakdown in the lower extremity. Use of a foam positioning orthosis or foot-drop orthosis with the heel elevated from the orthotic surface may prevent pressure sores from developing. Older adults who hold their hands in a fisted position or continually flex their elbows, knees, and hips create an environment conducive to skin breakdown.

The accumulation of perspiration within the skin folds allows bacteria to grow.[29] This constant posturing and the resulting bacteria growth may cause joint contractures, skin maceration, and possible infection. A thermoplastic orthosis, a hand roll, or a palm protector positions the involved joints in submaximum extension, allowing adequate hygiene of the hand. To accomplish any of these goals, the therapists use the following guidelines:

- An orthosis should not impede function unnecessarily. For example, the orthosis should not prevent an older adult from safely grasping an ambulation device or interfere with wheelchair propulsion.
- An orthosis should not exacerbate a pre-existing condition. For example, an older adult who demonstrates a flexor-synergy pattern may wear a functional position orthosis at night for pain and contracture management. The older adult may also have CMC OA in the thumb.

Although there are many approaches to positioning for CMC OA, one approach is the use a functional position orthosis that places the thumb MCP and IP joints in extension and the CMC joint in 45 degrees of abduction, midway between radial and palmar abduction. This thumb position differs from that of a functional positioning orthosis, which places the thumb in palmar abduction and opposition to the pads of the index and middle fingers.

- An orthosis should not limit the use of uninvolved joints.

Substitution for Loss of Sensorimotor Function

When there is a nerve compression severe enough to cause loss of motor function, an orthosis may substitute for the lost function. In the case of median nerve compression, an orthosis often positions the thumb in opposition to the index finger. If the ulnar nerve is affected, the fourth and fifth MCP joints are blocked in slight flexion to prevent a claw deformity with MCP hyperextension and IP flexion of the fourth and fifth digits. See Chapter 13 for more information on orthotic intervention for nerve conditions.[15] In the case of damage to the peroneal nerve, an ankle-foot orthosis can substitute for loss of ankle dorsiflexion (see Chapter 17).

Orthotic Intervention Process for an Older Adult

Assessment

During initial assessment, the therapist completes a comprehensive rehabilitative evaluation to determine whether orthotic intervention is indicated. All components of a therapy evaluation are essential for determining effective intervention strategies. (See Chapter 5 for a discussion of a hand examination). The therapist pays special attention to the cognitive, sensory, physical, and ADL status of the older adult to determine the usefulness of orthotic intervention as part of the plan of care. The results of the evaluation are used to develop a list of problems to be addressed. Typical goals include those listed in the section "Purposes of Orthotics for Older Adults." The therapist documents functional goals of the orthosis. Additional problems associated with aging (such as, decreased vision, cognition, and hearing) are considered when providing orthotic instructions to the older adult or caregiver.

During the initial assessment, the therapist notes any current use of adaptive devices and techniques. For example, an older adult may already have an orthosis for a chronic condition, such as de Quervain disease. The therapist evaluates the orthosis for its functional purpose, proper fit, and wearing schedule.

Observation during the assessment is vital to determine the purpose and orthotic design. It is important to observe and assess movement of the extremities in relation to the trunk. For example, an older adult who has hemiplegia with a spastic upper extremity may wear a hand orthosis resting on the chest and causing pressure.

Material Selection, Instruction, and Follow-Up Care

The choice of thermoplastic material, straps, and padding varies and is based on the older adult's needs.

Material Selection

Depending on client considerations and the goal(s) of the orthosis, the optimal material may be rigid, lightweight, multi-perforated, less rigid thermoplastic material, or soft fabrics and foams. Selection of a low-temperature thermoplastic material is determined by the following:

- Extent to which an older adult's joint can assume and maintain a gravity-assisted position
- Size of the orthosis
- Performance requirements of the orthosis
- The padding requirements
- Weight of the material
- Therapist's skill level
- Environment

If the older adult is physically and cognitively able to hold the limb in the desired position, the therapist uses a material with high drapability and conformability to ensure an intimate fit. The therapist positions the older adult's extremity to ensure that gravity assists in the draping of the material over the extremity. Material with a high degree of conformability allows for a precise fit, thus increasing comfort and decreasing the risk of migration and friction over bony prominences.

Some older adults cannot assume positions that allow gravity to assist during molding. Older adults may be anxious and respond to the stretch applied during orthotic intervention by exhibiting increased tone. In such situations, or during the fabrication of large orthoses, materials with resistance to stretch are helpful. A material that lightly sticks to the stockinette placed on the older adult facilitates antigravity orthotic intervention (see Chapter 3). Pre-shaping techniques are helpful when fabricating an orthosis for an older adult with diminished cognition or abnormal tone.

Thinner thermoplastic materials (e.g., $\frac{3}{32}$ inch, $\frac{1}{16}$ inch) are less rigid. The therapist selects the thinnest material that can perform effectively. Minimizing the weight of an orthosis increases comfort and enhances adherence. Strength increases with more contouring to the underlying body part. Older adults usually appreciate lightweight orthoses, because they are more comfortable.

Strapping Material

Wide, soft, foam-like strapping material distributes pressure over more surface area than thin, firm straps. The softer strapping accommodates slight fluctuations of edema. Fragile skin tolerates soft straps well. Neoprene or Velfoam materials are good choices for straps, and they can be easily cut to the desired width. They can also be fringed to decrease pressure against skin. In order to prolong the durability of soft strapping material, it is beneficial to sew standard Velcro loop over the area where the Velcro hook attaches. For older adults who have fragile skin, the therapist designs the V-loop strap to completely cover the hook portion on the orthosis' surface. This prevents skin abrasion or the catching the orthosis on clothing and blankets. The use of pre-sewn, self-adhesive straps reduces the chance of losing straps.

There are advantages and disadvantages of using D-ring straps. An advantage is that D-ring straps provide mechanical leverage to effectively tighten the strap. Using D-ring strapping is advantageous for an older adult with dementia and does not understand the orthosis' purpose. Similarly D-ring straps are useful for clients who experience difficulty spontaneously removing the orthosis. A disadvantage of using D-ring straps is that an older adult who has diminished dexterity may have difficulty threading the strap through the D-ring. However, if the ends of the straps are doubled over or looped, the strap will not de-thread through the D-ring.

Padding Selection

The two basic types of padding are open-cell foam (absorbent) and closed-cell foam (non-absorbent). Open-cell padding absorbs moisture, is more difficult to keep clean, and can become a breeding ground for bacteria. Padding should be bonded with the thermoplastic material before molding to ensure a proper fit to accommodate the thickness of the padding. A composite thermoplastic material (i.e., with attached padding) can be placed in a resealable plastic bag before being immersed in heated water to keep it dry during fabrication (Figure 15-12, *A*). Some padding, such as Plastazote (see Figure 15-12, *B*), is available in a variety of thicknesses. The thinner widths can be used to pad an orthosis, and the thicker widths can be used to fabricate an entire soft orthosis. Other materials, such as gel pads, can be used if more pressure relief is needed.

Padding may be required on the outside of an orthosis. The therapist provides cushioning to the outside of an orthosis if the involved extremity rests against another body part. For example, an older adult who has hemiplegia and a flexed upper extremity may rest the orthosis against the rib cage, or a right ankle orthosis may press against the left leg when the older adult is side lying.

Choosing the correct strapping, padding, and thermoplastic materials are important. Clinical judgment and the ability to make adaptations is beneficial for these clients, because they are most prone to contractures and pressure sores with illness.[7] Orthoses should fit well, achieve their goal(s), and be acceptable to the older adults and the caregivers.

Technical Tips

Therapists acquire technical skills through practice. With orthotic provision to older adults, one or more of the following technical tips may be helpful:

* Choose a material that has a slightly longer working time. For example, when fabricating a hand immobilization orthosis (see Chapter 9), partially pre-shape the hand portion of the resting pan before applying it to the older adult. Complete the pre-shaping on a hand of similar size.
* During the molding process, use Theraband or an elastic bandage to temporarily secure the forearm trough. This activity allows attention focused on the contouring of the hand and wrist parts of the orthosis.
* Pre-pad bony prominences using circular pieces of adhesive-backed foam or gel padding. Mold the orthosis over padding. Then place the foam or gel pad inside the orthosis to ensure intimate congruous contact.
* Apply a stockinette to the extremity, and ask the adult to wear the orthosis concurrently to maintain skin hygiene and prevent pressure areas. Loss of skin elasticity and adipose tissue make older persons prone to skin breakdown.

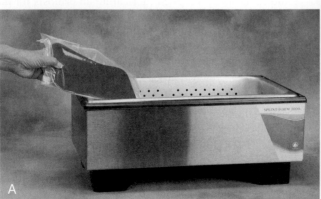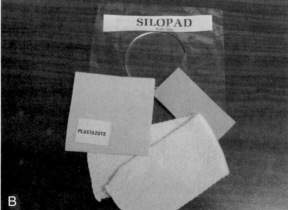

Figure 15-12 A, A composite thermoplastic material put in a re-sealable plastic bag before placement in heated water keeps the padding dry. **B,** Padding, such as Plastazote, a gel Silopad pad and/or stockinette may be indicated if skin integrity is a concern. (**A,** Courtesy of North Coast Medical.)

- Use uncoated and self-bonding material for orthoses if darts or tucks are necessary. Therapists often use this type of design for ankle, knee, and elbow orthoses.
- Use a coated material for thumb immobilization orthoses. Often the thumb IP joint is enlarged or deformed, thus making application and removal of a closed circumferential orthosis difficult or impossible. Use of a coated material allows circumferential wrapping around the proximal phalanx of the thumb. After hardening, the overlap on the proximal phalanx pops open to allow an easier removal of the thumb. If self-bonding materials are preferred, use a wet paper towel between the overlapping surfaces to prevent bonding.
- For serial repositioning, select a material that has a high resistance to stretch and memory.
- For a painful or deformed extremity, use the opposite extremity and reverse it to make the pattern.
- To ease the fabrication process when working among multiple settings, create orthotic boxes or travel kits containing all necessary supplies.[34]

Older Adult and Caregiver Instructions and Follow-Through

Clear client and caregiver instructions and consistent follow-through are important for successful orthotic intervention. Many factors influence adherence to an orthotic wearing schedule. The person responsible for the orthotic wearing schedule and care is the older adult or caregiver(s). See Box 15-3 for information on adherence issues.

Instructions to Caregivers
Older adults unable to care for themselves need caregiver assistance. Caregivers are often family members or staff members from an agency or facility. When fitting an orthosis to an older adult, the therapist provides thorough instructions to the caregiver. Instructions include information regarding the (1) orthosis' purpose, (2) wearing schedule, (3) orthotic care, and (4) precautions or safety factors. The therapist informs caregivers about who and when to contact if a problem occurs. For example, for a client who has fluctuating edema, tone, and PROM, the caregiver is instructed on how to adjust the straps of the orthosis.

The therapist gives oral and written instructions to the caregiver and demonstrates any procedure the caregiver is to perform. The therapist asks the caregiver to demonstrate the application of the orthosis, corrects mistakes, and asks the caregiver to repeat the demonstration until it is mastered.

The therapist labels parts of the orthosis for easier application (e.g., right/left, thumb/wrist/forearm). When possible, use photographs of proper orthotic position, offer a written wearing schedule, discuss a list of precautions and safety factors, and consistently update an orthotic maintenance sheet.

Therapists include instructions in the chart to ensure staff follow-through. The therapist speaks with the immediate caregivers to determine a realistic orthotic regimen. All staff

members involved with an older adult's care must receive instructions about the wearing schedule, precautions, and safety factors, particularly for those adults who wear orthoses for a portion of the day or evening. The wearing schedule may require modification to match the staff schedule.

When appropriate, the therapist instructs caregivers about the use of inhibition techniques to facilitate proper orthotic application. The therapist also teaches the older adult and caregivers about the importance of intermittent PROM and active-assisted ROM to the immobilized joints when appropriate.[13]

Skin Care
Maintenance of skin integrity is important for older adults who need long-term orthotic intervention. The orthosis must be clean for application. A good cleaning method involves the use of isopropyl alcohol. Chlorine is appropriate for removal of stains. Neither an autoclave, nor a washing machine is appropriate to clean an orthosis. After removal of the orthosis, thoroughly wash and dry the hand. To manage

---

Box 15-3 Factors that Influence Adherence to Orthotic Care and Wear Schedule

Older Adult Who is Responsible
- Explain the purpose and goals of the orthosis to the older adult and caregiver.
- Provide simple written and oral instructions.
- Use positive reinforcement for correct follow-through.
- Listen to the adult's complaints, and make adjustments as necessary.
- Use repetition with instructions as needed.
- Consider using analogies for instructions (e.g., "This is just like cleaning your dentures.")
- Ensure older adults wear their glasses, dentures, and hearing aids.
- Label the orthosis for easy application when necessary.
- Ask if the older adult has any questions about the orthotic wearing schedule and care instructions.

Caregiver (Family and/or Staff) Responsible
- Provide simple written and oral directions.
- Explain the purpose of the orthosis.
- Demonstrate proper orthotic application and removal.
- Encourage the caregiver to demonstrate the correct procedure several times.
- Use pictures to demonstrate correct application.
- In an institutional setting, ensure that the orthotic-wearing schedule and hand hygiene are part of the older adult's care plan.
- Educate the caregiver about precautions and safety. Provide contact information to report problems if they arise.
- Label the orthosis for easy application.
- Ask if the caregiver has any questions about the orthotic wearing schedule and care instructions.

moisture, have the older adult wear a stockinette under the orthosis or use powder.

Wearing Schedule

To determine the wearing schedule, the therapist considers the goals of the orthosis. The goals determine whether a daytime, nighttime, or an intermittent wearing schedule is the most beneficial. For example, an intermittent wearing schedule helps the palm or skin to dry and prevents potential skin maceration. A nighttime wearing schedule is most appropriate if the older adult uses the extremity for functional assistance during the day.

SELF-QUIZ 15-1*

In regard to the following questions, circle either true (T) or false (F).

1. T F Observing the older adult's skin condition is important when the therapist is making orthotic intervention decisions.
2. T F The therapist should apply closed-cell foam after the formation of the orthosis.
3. T F To ensure intimate contour, the therapist should use a material with high drapability for an older adult who has spasticity.
4. T F The therapist should use wide straps on an orthosis for an older adult who has fragile skin.
5. T F A functional position orthosis is always appropriate to position the arthritic hand.
6. T F Older adults are more prone to joint contractures than younger persons who have similar diagnoses.
7. T F After orthotic completion for an older adult in a long-term care facility, there is little follow-up needed by the therapist.
8. T F A younger person is more prone to skin breakdown than an older adult.
9. T F Orthotic materials may be used to adapt ADL devices.
10. T F Medication use does not affect orthotic design.
11. T F It is always important to initially evaluate the entire upper extremity for an older adult with any injury.
12. T F People with diabetes are at greater risk of associated conditions that may require orthotic intervention.
13. T F Poor positioning of older adults with limited mobility may contribute to neuropathies of the median and ulnar nerves.
14. T F When fitting an orthosis on an older adult with cardiovascular disease, the therapist should consider precautions for peripheral vascular disease.

*See Appendix A for the answer key.

SELF-QUIZ 15-2*

Critical-Thinking Case Scenarios

1. You are fabricating a volar hand immobilization orthosis for an older adult who is unable to actively supinate the forearm. You choose a material that has high drapability and moldability. Is this the best choice? Why?
2. You are treating an 86-year-old woman one year after a CVA. Since that time she has held her left hand in a fisted position. Gentle passive extension is painful. The palm is macerated from perspiration. She does not have active motion in the left hand and does not use the hand for functional assistance during ADLs. Which type(s) of positioning device(s) would be appropriate?
3. An older adult who has RA complains of pain in the wrists and metacarpal phalangeal joints. The therapist provides hand immobilization orthoses to rest all of the joints of the wrist and hands at night. What problems can you anticipate with this orthotic provision?
4. You fabricate a functional position hand immobilization orthosis for an older adult who has spasticity and hemiplegia and is in a flexor-synergy pattern. The older adult wears the orthosis at night for pain relief and contracture management. When the older adult is in bed, the orthosis is positioned against the rib cage. What can you do to relieve the pressure?
5. You fabricated a hand immobilization orthosis for an older adult with hemiplegia and CHF. You are concerned about the fluctuating edema noted in the hemiplegic hand. How would you modify the orthosis and straps?

*See Appendix A for the answer key.

Review Questions

1. What are the accommodations that a therapist can make for each of the following problems: edema, ecchymosis, fragile skin, contracture, diminished cognition, sensory loss, and motivation?

2. What are four possible goals of orthotic intervention with older adults?

3. Why are older adults prone to develop contractures?

4. What are five medical conditions more prevalent in older adults? What are the implications for orthotic intervention?

5. What are three common medication side effects that older adults typically experience? How might the side effects impact orthotic intervention?

6. How do instructions and selection of orthotic materials vary with an individual living independently in the community versus an individual in an inpatient setting?

7. What are three specific orthotic adaptations for older adults who have impaired cognition, sensory function, and poor adherence?

References

1. American Federation for Aging Research (AFAR). 2011. Hearing. Retrieved from http://www.afar.org/infoaging/healthy-aging/hearing/hearing-resources/.

2. American Occupational Therapy Association: *Occupational therapy practice framework: domain and process*, ed 3, *Am J Occup Ther*, 68(Suppl):S1–S48, 2014.

3. Bello-Haas VD: Neuromusculoskeletal and movement function. In Bonder BR, Bello-Haas VD, editors: *Functional performance in older adults*, ed 3, Philadelphia, 2009, FA Davis, pp 130–176.

4. Berger NA, Savvides P, Koroukian SM, et al.: Cancer in the elderly, *Trans Am Clin Climatol Assoc* 117:147–156, 2006.

5. Berk L: *Development through the lifespan*, ed 5, Boston, 2010, Allyn & Bacon.

6. Bland JH, Melvin JL, Hasson S: Osteoarthritis. In Melvin JL, Ferrell KM, editors: *Rheumatologic rehabilitation series: adult rheumatic diseases*, Bethesda, MD, 2000, AOTA.

7. Bliss MR, Bennett GJ: Pressure sores. In Tallis RC, Fillit HM, editors: *Brocklehurst's textbook of geriatric medicine and gerontology*, ed 6, London, 2003, Churchill Livingstone, pp 1347–1366.

8. Bloom HG, Imran A, Alessi CA, et al.: Evidence-based recommendations for the assessment and management of sleep disorders in older persons, *J Am Geriatr Soc* 57(5):761–789, 2009.

9. Bureau of Labor Statistics: *Occupational outlook handbook*. (website) http://www.bls.gov/oco/. Accessed March 3, 2014.

10. Centers for Disease Control and Prevention: Distribution of age at diagnosis of diabetes among adult incident cases aged 18-79 years, United States, 2011. *Diabetes public health resource*: (website) http://www.cdc.gov/diabetes/statistics/age/fig1.htm. Accessed March 3, 2014.

11. Cagliero E, Apruzzese W, Perlmutter GS, et al.: Musculoskeletal disorders of the hand and shoulder in clients with diabetes mellitus, *Am J Med* 112(6):487–490, 2002.

12. Department of Health and Human Services: Profile of older Americans. *Administration on aging*: (website) http://www.aoa.gov/AoARoot/Aging_Statistics/Profile/index.aspx. Accessed March 3, 2014.

13. Dittmer DK, MacAurthur-Turner DE, Jones IC: Orthotics in stroke, *Physical Medicine and Rehabilitation State of the Art Review* 7(1):171, 1993.

14. Evans RB: Therapeutic management of Dupuytren's contracture. In Skirven TM, Osterman AL, Fedorczyk J, et al, editors: *Rehabilitation of the hand and upper extremity*, ed 6, St Louis, 2011, Mosby, pp 281–288.

15. Fess EE, Gettle K, Philips CA, et al.: *Hand and upper extremity: principles and methods*, ed 3, St Louis, 2005, Elsevier/Mosby.

16. Hurst L: Dupuytren's disease: surgical management. In Skirven TM, Osterman AL, Fedorczyk J, et al.: *Rehabilitation of the hand and upper extremity*, ed 6, St Louis, 2011, Mosby, pp 266–280.

17. Kautio AL, Haanpaa M, Kautiainen H, et al.: Burden of chemotherapy-induced neuropathy—a cross-sectional study, *Support Care Cancer* 19(12):1991–1996, 2011.

18. Knauf JJ: Drugs commonly encountered in hand therapy. In Weiss S, Falkenstein N, editors: *Hand rehabilitation: a quick reference guide and review*, ed 2, St Louis, 2005, Elsevier, pp 441–446.

19. Lewis CB, Bottomley JM: *Geriatric rehabilitation: a clinical approach*, ed 3, Upper Saddle River, NJ, 2008, Pearson Education, Inc.

20. Liu W, Lipsitz LA, Montero-Odasso M, et al.: Noise-enhanced vibrotactile sensitivity in older adults, patients with stroke, and patients with diabetic neuropathy, *Arch Phys Med Rehabil* 83(2):171–176, 2002.

21. McKee P, Rivard A: Orthoses as enablers of occupation: client-centered splinting for better outcomes, *Canadian J Occup Ther* 71(5):306–314, 2004.

22. Michlovitz S, Festa L: Therapist's management of distal radius fractures In Skirven TM, Osterman AL, Fedorczyk J, et al, editors: *Rehabilitation of the hand and upper extremity*, ed 6, St Louis, 2011, Mosby, pp 949–962.

23. National Eye Institute: National plan for eye and vision research: Low vision and blindness rehabilitation. *NIH* (website): http://nei.nih.gov/strategicplanning/np_low.asp. Accessed March 3, 2014.

24. National Osteoporosis Foundation: Are you at risk? (website): http://nof.org/articles/2.

25. Nordell E, Jarnlo G, Thorngren K: Decrease in physical function after fall-related distal forearm fracture in elderly women, *Advances in Physiotherapy* 5(4):146–154, 2003.

26. Porter RS, Kaplan JL, editors: *The Merck manual for health care professionals* (website): http://www.merckmanuals.com/professional/geriatrics.html. Accessed March 3, 2014.

27. Portnoi V, Ramzel P: Contractures. In Mezey MD, editor: *The encyclopedia of older adult care: the comprehensive resource on geriatric and social care*, New York, 2001, Springer, pp 161–163.

28. Porretto-Loehrke A, Soika E: Therapist's management of other nerve compressions about the elbow and wrist. In Skirven TM, Osterman AL, Fedorczyk J, et al, editors: *Rehabilitation of the hand and upper extremity*, ed 6, St Louis, 2011, Mosby, pp 695–709.

29. Redford JB: Orthotics and orthotic devices: general principles, *Physical Medicine and Rehabilitation: State of the Art Reviews* 14(3):381–394, 2000.

30. Sandmire DA: The physiology and pathology of aging. In Robnett RH, Chop WC, editors: *Gerontology for the health care professional*, ed 2, Boston, 2010, Jones & Bartlett, pp 53–113.

31. Skidmore-Roth L: *Mosby's nursing drug reference*, ed 25, St Louis, 2012, Mosby.

32. Stevens JC, Patterson MQ: Dimensions of spatial acuity in the touch sense: changes over the lifespan, *Somatosens Mot Res* 12(1):29–47, 1995.

33. Strickland JW: Biologic basis for hand and upper extremity splinting. In Fess EE, Gettle K, Philips CA, et al.: *Hand and upper extremity: principles and methods*, ed 3, St Louis, 2005, Elsevier/Mosby, pp 87–103.

34. Swedberg L: Splinting the difficult hand, *WFOT-Bulletin* 35: 15–20, 1997.

35. Thomas E, Croft PR, Dziedzic KS: Hand problems in community-dwelling older adults: onset and effect on global physical function over a 3-year period, *Rheumatology* 48:183–187, 2009.

36. World Health Organization: *International classification of functioning, disability, and health (ICF)*, Geneva, Switzerland, 2001, World Health Organization. Note: This chapter includes content from previous contributors—Serena M. Berger, MA, OTR; Maureen T. Cavanaugh, MS, OTR; and Brenda M. Coppard, PhD, OTR/L, FAOTA.

APPENDIX 15-1   CASE STUDIES

CASE STUDY 15-1*

Ruby is a 90-year-old right-hand-dominant female who lives in an assisted living center. She was referred to occupational therapy to be evaluated and treated for an orthosis and activity of daily living (ADL) interventions. She is 2 years status post a trigger finger release of the right middle finger and has right thumb carpometacarpal (CMC) osteoarthritis (OA). Ruby no longer experiences triggering of the middle finger. However, she does have some loss of active metacarpophalangeal (MCP) extension. Ruby reports enjoying crocheting, but she finds that she has progressively crocheted less due to pain in her thumb. Upon observation of self-care performance, due to loss of active MCP extension of the middle finger, Ruby is noted to use only index-to-thumb opposition for activities that require pinch.

1. The therapist needs to consider which of the following in order to determine the most appropriate orthosis?
    a. Post-operative trigger finger protocols
    b. Biomechanical principles of pinch with occupational therapy
    c. Materials for custom orthotic designs
    d. Prefabricated orthoses for trigger finger
2. The orthotic design should incorporate a combination of which of the following? Circle all that apply.
    a. Thumb CMC immobilization
    b. Thumb CMC mobilization
    c. Middle finger extension assist
    d. Middle finger MCP flexion block
3. Goals for the orthosis should include which of the following? Circle all that apply.
    a. Thumb mobilization
    b. Improved occupational performance
    c. Pain reduction
    d. Substitute for loss of motor function
4. In order to promote occupational performance, which of the following is least significant?
    a. Self-care function
    b. Leisure interest
    c. Location and degree of pain
    d. Age

*See Appendix A for the answer key.

CASE STUDY 15-2*

Edward is a 74-year-old male who lives with his wife on a farm in a rural setting. He was recently discharged from an inpatient rehabilitation facility to his home. Edward receives home care services that include physical therapy, occupational therapy, and nursing. His referring diagnosis is left CVA with right hemiplegia. Medical history is significant for congestive heart failure (CHF), and chronic obstructive pulmonary disorder. Edward's chief complaints are limited endurance and decreased use of his right upper extremity.

   Upon evaluation, Edward presents with bilateral upper extremity tremors, good return of function at the shoulder and elbow, minimal active wrist extension, finger and right hand (dorsum) edema, and enlarged distal interphalangeal (DIP) finger joints. Although he is referred for orthotic intervention at this time, he was not fitted with an orthosis during his inpatient stay, because he was showing signs of motor return and was receiving daily treatment to prevent loss of motion.

1. Goals for the orthosis should include which of the following? Circle all that apply.
   a. Prevent loss of range of motion (ROM)
   b. Substitute for loss of sensorimotor function
   c. Decrease pain
   d. Decrease edema
2. What orthosis do you recommend?
   a. Wrist immobilization orthosis with D-ring straps
   b. Thumb immobilization orthosis
   c. Soft Neoprene prefabricated orthosis
   d. Prefabricated Comfy Wrist/Hand/Finger Orthosis or similar adjustable prefabricated orthosis
3. What type of straps would you choose?
   a. Long, soft, wide straps
   b. Thin loop straps
   c. D-ring straps cut to the exact size
   d. Wide hook straps
4. What wearing schedule would you suggest?
   a. Wear orthosis at all times
   b. Remove orthosis only for hygiene
   c. Wear orthosis only during the day
   d. Wear orthosis at night and periodically during the day to encourage motion
5. What is the most likely cause of the enlarged DIP joints?
   a. Rheumatoid arthritis (RA)
   b. Osteoporosis
   c. OA
   d. Peripheral vascular disease

*See Appendix A for the answer key.

APPENDIX 15-2   LABORATORY EXERCISE

Laboratory Exercise 15-1*

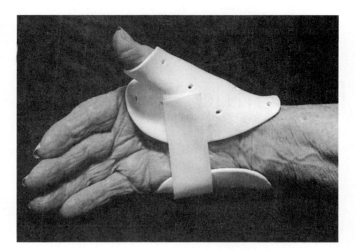

1. What problems are identified in the orthosis made for someone with thumb carpometacarpal (CMC) osteoarthritis (OA)?

_____
_____
_____

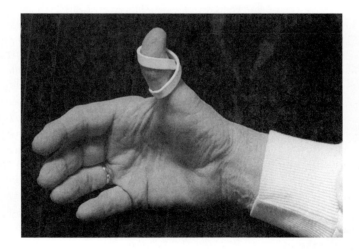

2. How would the orthosis shown in the figure be modified for someone with hyperextension of the thumb interplangeal (IP) joint?

_____
_____
_____

*See Appendix A for the answer key.

CHAPTER 16

Orthoses for the Pediatric Population

Deborah A. Schwartz
Ann McKie
Linda Gabriel

Key Terms
arthrogryposis
brachial plexus palsy
camptodactyly
cerebral palsy (CP)
clinodactyly
congenital hand anomalies
congenital trigger finger
constriction band syndrome
Erb palsy
hypoplasia
radial clubhand
spasticity
syndactyly
tone

Chapter Objectives
1. Identify common diagnoses affecting the pediatric upper extremity.
2. Examine the impact of upper extremity orthoses on child development.
3. Describe common surgical procedures for select diagnoses and the postsurgical orthoses.
4. Describe orthoses fabricated specifically for the pediatric upper extremity.
5. Identify when thermoplastic versus soft orthotics are appropriate.
6. Describe challenges of orthotic fabrication for the pediatric population.
7. Describe wearing schedules and precautions for pediatric orthoses.
8. Discuss the importance and role of family members and other caregivers in orthotic intervention for children.
9. Assess and critique correct orthotic fitting.
10. Identify safety issues of orthotic intervention for children.
11. Identify resources for the purchase of prefabricated pediatric soft orthoses.
12. Examine current evidence for pediatric orthotic intervention.
13. Apply knowledge of pediatric orthotic intervention to a case study.

Li Ann is a 6-year-old female with left-sided hemiplegia secondary to an in utero stroke. She has full passive elbow motion, but she is limited in passive forearm and wrist motion due to posturing in wrist flexion and pronation. Full active motion is limited at the elbow, forearm, and wrist. Li Ann has trouble grasping toys with her left hand because increased tone causes her wrist to flex as she reaches. Her fingers on her left hand curl into a fist, and she holds her thumb in adduction. However, passive motion of all digits is full. Note that with her wrist held in extension, Li Ann's volitional grasp and release improves (Figure 16-1).

The therapist considers the following questions: In what ways might orthoses assist Li Ann's function or prevent loss of function? Which orthoses are appropriate interventions for Li Ann? What other interventions might enhance Li Ann's volitional grasp and release, and how might orthoses be required with concurrent interventions?

This chapter is an introduction to the most common conditions that affect the pediatric population and may require upper extremity orthotic intervention. A short description of each diagnosis is offered only as an overview. It is beyond the scope of this chapter to describe every pediatric hand condition. More detailed information is found in the cited references and in texts and journals. Orthotic fabrication is a therapeutic intervention utilized for children with orthopedic conditions and/or with developmental disabilities. Surgical

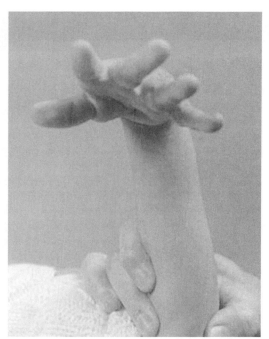

Figure 16-1 Child with cerebral palsy (CP). (Courtesy of Orfit Industries.)

interventions for congenital hand anomalies are described with the postsurgical orthoses commonly required. General orthotic fabrication principles discussed in previous chapters apply to the pediatric population, but there are differences inherent in fabrication. This chapter addresses proper selection of orthotic materials, orthotic design, steps of orthotic fabrication, and tips for working with children and their caregivers. Typical orthoses fabricated for the pediatric population include elbow, forearm rotation, resting hand, wrist, and thumb orthoses. Children may benefit from commercially available orthoses. The measurements for and recommendations of a variety commercial orthoses are described. The purpose of this chapter is to guide the novice therapist in applying knowledge of orthotic fabrication to the special needs of children with injuries, congenital hand anomalies, and/or developmental disabilities.

Purpose of Orthoses for Pediatrics

The intents of pediatric orthoses are protective, preventive, or enhancement to the child's upper extremity function and skill development. Similar to orthotic provision for adults, pediatric orthoses may address issues at single or multiple joints. Orthoses may be applied in a variety of locations (e.g., shoulder to the distal interphalangeal [DIP] joints).

The different orthoses presented in this chapter are one small part of a comprehensive intervention program. A comprehensive intervention plan is developed beginning with an assessment of the child and incorporating all elements of the Occupational Therapy Practice Framework.[3] Using the Practice Framework as a guide ensures that the delivery of occupational therapy services is client-centered and focused on occupations of importance to the child, the role within the family, and the performance of play and learning, especially within the contexts of home and school environments. One quick method to apply the Practice Framework is to incorporate the following areas during evaluation:

* Areas of occupation: Make clinical observations of the child participating in activities. Does the use of an orthosis limit or improve function? What skill(s) does the child need to develop that might be enhanced with an orthosis?
* Client factors: Assess the child's muscle tone, range of motion (ROM), strength, and contractures. Will an orthosis improve or prevent further loss of any of these components?
* Performance skills: Evaluate the child's ability to reach, grasp, bear weight on the affected limb(s), and stabilize and manipulate objects. What are the child's sensory status, visual capabilities, and cognitive level? Will the use of an orthosis affect such systems?
* Context: Note the child's home and school environments. How does the use of an orthosis affect performance in these settings?

Goals

The goals of orthotic intervention for children are similar to those for adults. Goals may include:
* Support the upper extremity
* Protect during healing
* Position for improved function
* Assist weaker muscle groups to improve function
* Facilitate or maintain tissue length and joint alignment
* Prevent deformity

However, orthotic fabrication for children involves more than simply making smaller sized orthoses.

Previous chapters discussed mechanical principles and orthotic fabrication techniques that apply to children. Orthotic fabrication for a child is different from orthotic fabrication for an adult in several key areas, including the following:

1. Different proportions between the palm and length of fingers in the growing hand versus the adult hand exist.[18]
2. Children are constantly growing and therefore require more frequent orthotic adjustments and/or new orthoses to accommodate for growth.
3. In many cases, the parents or teachers are responsible for applying and removing the orthosis. They must understand the importance of the orthosis, wear and care schedule, and precautions.
4. Foundational movement patterns are set during the first 2 to 3 years of life. Interventions with orthoses assist the child to develop more typical movement patterns.

Development

Working with children requires a thorough understanding of normal and abnormal child development, knowledge of the specific pediatric conditions, and current evidence-based intervention practices, including orthoses. The parent or caregiver must be included in the orthotic process from the beginning to ensure adherence to the intervention plan.

Normal Hand Development

Understanding normal hand development is required prior to orthotic fabrication. The upper extremity begins as a small outgrowth of tissue on the lateral body wall of the fetus, beginning on day 26 of gestation, even before growth of the lower extremity.[20] This small area contains all of the necessary information to form the limb. Development of the upper extremity proceeds proximally to distally. By the 31st day, the area of the hand is present. Fingers are evident by days 36 to 41. Bone, joint, muscle, and vascular development follows. Formation of the upper extremity is completed by the eighth week of fetal development.[20]

Abnormal Hand Development

Abnormal hand development may be affected by intrinsic factors (e.g., chromosomal abnormalities or mutant genes), extrinsic (i.e., environmental) factors, or a combination of the two. These factors contribute to the arrest of development of the forming limb or to the destruction of structures already formed.

Fine Motor Skill Development

A detailed description of hand and fine motor skill development is beyond the scope of this chapter. However, the therapist fabricating an orthosis considers the infant or child's current level of fine motor skills and thinks about how the orthotic intervention impacts future hand skill development. Through sensory exploration and play, children learn about their environments. Wearing an orthosis interferes to some degree with the ability to explore and play. The therapist provides appropriate scheduling of orthotic wear to ensure ample opportunities for play and development of grasp and release patterns. Table 16-1 is a guide of the development of gross and fine motor skills during the first year. Children develop these skills in a predictable manner. Proper orthotic selection takes this progression into account.

Atypical Upper Extremity Motor Development

Atypical upper extremity development occurs when the infant or child develops patterns of movement that compensate for weakness, spasticity, contractures, deformity, tightness, and/or sensory abnormalities. For example, if a child has an adducted thumb, grasp may result in using the ulnar fingers. Ulnar deviation and wrist flexion are reinforced with this pattern, whereas radial musculature may be overstretched and weakened through non-use. This topic is discussed later in this chapter in the "Cerebral Palsy" section.

Table 16-1	Gross and Fine Motor Skill Development
APPROXIMATE AGE	**GROSS AND FINE MOTOR SKILL**
Birth to 2 months	Physiological flexion
2 months	Grasp reflex
3 months	Hands together in supine
4 months	Objects held in midline, bears weight on forearm
5 months	Two handed approach to objects, extended arm weight-bearing, displays some supination of forearm
6 months	Weight shifts on extended arms in prone, sits with straight back, elbows fully extend
7 months	Purposeful release, may pull to stand
8 months	Creeps on hands and knees
9 months	Reaches with active supination
10 months	Pokes with index finger
12 months	One hand stabilizes while one hand manipulates
15 months	Develops release with precision

Adapted from Hogan L, Uditsky T: *Pediatric splinting: selection, fabrication, and clinical application of upper extremity splints*, San Antonio, TX, 1998, Therapy Skill Builders.

Common Pediatric Upper Extremity Conditions

Children born with **congenital hand anomalies** require special consideration and a team approach. Intervention involves family members, therapists, surgeons, and teachers. The most common congenital anomalies include:

1. Common congenital hand anomalies
   a. Radial deficiency/radial clubhand
   b. Hypoplastic thumb
   c. **Congenital trigger finger**
   d. Syndactyly
   e. Camptodactyly
   f. Clinodactyly
2. Brachial plexus palsy
3. Arthrogryposis
4. Juvenile idiopathic arthritis
5. Cerebral palsy

Common Congenital Hand Anomalies

Radial Deficiency/Radial Clubhand

Radial deficiencies refer to all congenital hand anomalies with failure of formation along the radial border of the upper extremity.[24] This includes deficient or absent thenar muscles; shortened, unstable, or absent thumb; and shortened or absent radius, commonly referred to as **radial clubhand** (Figure 16-2). Radial deficiency conditions may occur in isolation, but commonly occur to some degree in

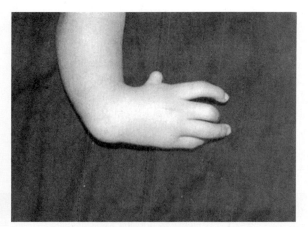

Figure 16-2 Radial clubhand. (Courtesy of Orfit Industries.)

association with each other and in the presence of other syndromes.

Orthotic intervention is typically initiated immediately after birth. A program of passive stretching along with orthoses is introduced.[5] The orthosis is molded on the radial border of the forearm and places the hand in a central position relative to the forearm. The orthosis is worn fulltime until the baby begins to use the hands. Padding or lining the orthosis with moleskin or Neoprene is important due to the increased prominence of the ulnar styloid. Full arm casting may be utilized to correct the positioning of the hand, wrist, and elbow.[23] As the child grows and when orthoses can no longer maintain the correction, surgical intervention may be necessary to enhance function. Banskota and colleagues[5] recommend surgery for the wrist prior to 2 years of age because children quickly acquire adaptive functional skills. A delayed surgery may interfere with normal hand skill development.

For children with radial deficiencies, common immobilization orthoses include radial gutter type wrist orthoses (Figure 16-3) (refer to Chapter 7), forearm orthoses (refer to Chapter 7), resting hand orthoses (refer to Chapter 9), and elbow orthoses (refer to Chapter 10). Serial static and static progressive mobilization orthoses stabilize and position the wrist. These orthoses (and passive motion) align the wrist in a more neutral position and maximize function. Children benefit from nighttime resting hand orthoses once full passive motion is achieved. Resting hand orthoses maintain digital alignment and prevent flexion contractures of the digits. A wrist support often improves functional grasp of the digits. Orthoses are fabricated to protect the upper extremity after surgery. With growth, children may require multiple surgeries and need frequent orthotic adjustments.

A number of challenges exist when fabricating an orthosis for a child with radial deficiency. These include:
- Lack of a thumb to hook the thermoplastic material around during fabrication and wear.
- Tendency of the orthosis to migrate proximally and/or distally.
- Frequent serial adjustments of the orthosis are necessary with gains in passive range of motion (PROM).

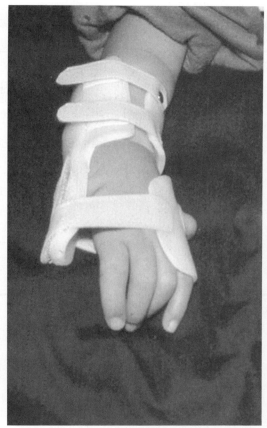

Figure 16-3 Radial clubhand with orthosis.

- Wrist orthosis should allow full digital motion.
- Children may develop a scissoring pattern of prehension with the index and middle digits for function when the thumb is absent.
- Elbow may need to be included in the orthosis for leverage and mechanical length.

Hypoplastic Thumb

Hypoplasia of the thumb refers to a spectrum of thumb disorders ranging from mild underdevelopment of the thumb anatomy to complete absence of the thumb (Table 16-2).[24]

Children with congenital thumb aplasia (total absence of the thumb) or hypoplasia (Figure 16-4) are severely impaired functionally.[20] They lack an active thumb, which plays a key component in hand function. Surgical procedures vary from tendon transfers to enhance thumb function (for mild cases of thumb hypoplasia) to pollicization (creating a thumb from the index finger when the thumb is absent).

Box 16-1 lists the indications for thumb hypoplasia orthotic intervention. Thumb orthoses (Figure 16-5) for children with thumb hypoplasia include the carpometacarpal (CMC), metacarpal (MP) and interphalangeal (IP) joints as needed. Such orthoses maintain an adequate first web space, hold the thumb in a functional position, and correct or prevent deformity. The appropriate thickness of thermoplastic material is based on the size of the child's hand. For small children and infants, even ⅟₁₆-inch thick thermoplastic material may be too heavy.

Table 16-2   Hypoplasia/Aplasia of the Thumb

TYPE	FINDINGS	TREATMENT
I	Minor generalized hypoplasia	Augmentation
II	Absence of intrinsic thenar muscles	Opponensplasty
	First web space narrowing	First web release
	UCL insufficiency	UCL reconstruction
III	Similar findings as type II plus:	A: Reconstruction
	Extrinsic muscle and tendon abnormalities	B: Pollicization
	Skeletal deficiency	
	A: Stable carpometacarpal (CMC) joint	
	B: Unstable CMC joint	
IV	Pouce flottant or floating thumb	Pollicization
V	Absence	Pollicization

UCL, Ulnar collateral ligament.

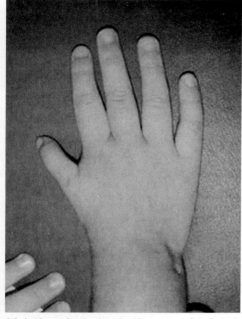

Figure 16-4 Hypoplastic thumb. (Courtesy of Orfit Industries.)

A commercially available soft thumb orthosis, a ribbon, or a thin Neoprene strap in the web space may work best.

Congenital Trigger Finger

There is some controversy as to whether pediatric trigger finger is an acquired deformity or a congenital anomaly. In either case, orthotic intervention and stretching exercises can be successful. The evidence for the protocol includes full-time hyperextension orthotic intervention for 6 to 12 weeks followed by nighttime wear. Shiozawa and colleagues[28] recommended an immobilization orthosis at the first physician evaluation. These authors found that wearing an orthosis significantly reduced the need for further surgical intervention. Surgical release of the A-1

Box 16-1   Indications for Orthotic Fabrication for Thumb Hypoplasia

Preoperatively
Orthoses to preserve and/or increase the first web space

Postoperatively
Orthoses to protect the tendon transfers during healing
Orthoses to protect pollicization of the index finger (in its new position)

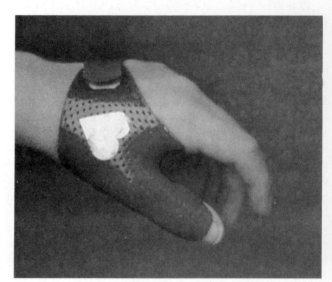

Figure 16-5 Thumb orthosis. (Courtesy of Orfit Industries.)

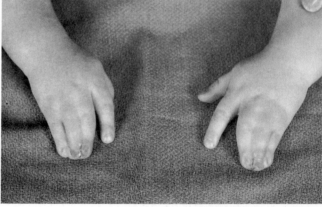

Figure 16-6 Syndactyly. (From Burke SL, Higgins J, McClinton MA, et al: *Hand and upper extremity rehabilitation: a practical guide,* ed 3, St Louis, 2006, Elsevier Churchill Livingstone.)

pulley may occur when there is no resolution after 1 year of conservative management.[32]

Syndactyly

Syndactyly (Figure 16-6) refers to the webbing of fingers. Syndactyly is classified as complete (full length of the fingers) or incomplete. Syndactyly may involve the skin only (simple syndactyly), or it may involve fusion of the bones (complex syndactyly).[31] Syndactyly is treated by surgical release for functional and cosmetic improvement. Surgery is typically performed before patterns of prehension are established.

For postsurgical syndactyly release, a web spacer or finger separator is formed from silicone or elastomer putty to maintain pressure on the surgically corrected interdigital web space. Highly conforming thermoplastic material is utilized. Web creep or the repeated fusion of the skin between the released digits may reoccur and is a significant complication that may require an additional surgical release.[23] The type of orthoses used in the treatment of syndactyly include a resting hand orthosis with finger separators made from pellets of thermoplastic material or elastomer. Another option is a finger orthosis in extension.

Several challenges arise when providing an orthosis after syndactyly release. These include protecting the skin graft; keeping the orthosis on the involved hand; maintaining the interdigital web space; keeping the fingers straight; and achievement of a smooth, non-hypertrophic scar. Often, these issues are alleviated by providing an orthosis that incorporates the entire hand, covered by a sock puppet (Figure 16-7).

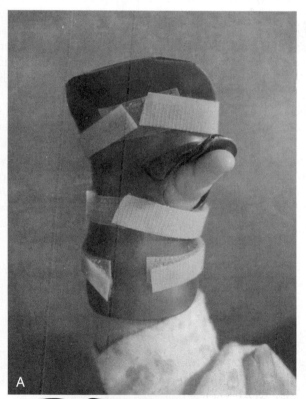

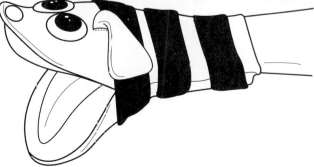

Figure 16-7 Resting hand for infant. (Courtesy of Orfit Industries.)

Camptodactyly

Camptodactyly is a non-traumatic, flexion contracture of the proximal interphalangeal (PIP) joint that typically affects the little finger.[32] There are three basic types of camptodactyly:

- Type I appears in infancy and is present in both males and females. Type I affects the little fingers on both hands and may involve the ring and long fingers.
- Type II presents in adolescence and is more common among females. Type II worsens during growth spurts.
- Type III is a more severe form of camptodactyly and may involve multiple digits of both hands. Type III is associated with additional congenital anomalies.

Intervention for camptodactyly typically involves either mobilization or immobilization orthoses and stretching regimens, especially during growth spurts. Surgery may be a treatment option. There is some evidence for the success of continuous orthotic wear to correct simple camptodactyly in young children.[20] Types of orthoses for camptodactyly are PIP extension orthoses, including immobilization, mobilization, and/or static progressive orthoses.

Orthoses are typically worn full-time at night until skeletal maturity is reached. Serial casting and/or static progressive orthoses may be more effective for rigid deformities. Younger children may require a forearm based orthosis to prevent removal.

Challenges providing orthoses for camptodactyly include difficulty keeping orthoses on the child's little finger only. Frequent orthotic adjustments are required during periods of growth. The best results occur when orthotic intervention is initiated early.

Clinodactyly

Clinodactyly refers to radioulnar deviation of the finger. Minor angulation, especially of the little finger, is so common that it is considered a normal variant. Pathologic clinodactyly is usually described as greater than 10 or 15 degrees. Clinodactyly is usually present bilaterally and is caused by an abnormally shaped middle phalanx. Orthotic and surgical intervention might not be necessary when there is no functional impairment.[32]

Brachial Plexus Palsy at Birth

Brachial plexus palsy is an injury that occurs at birth. The typical posture of a child with brachial plexus palsy includes a shoulder that is adducted and internally rotated, an extended elbow, a pronated forearm, and a flexed wrist and digits. The thumb may be flexed in the palm. Most babies born with brachial plexus palsy recover spontaneously within the first 2 months. Those babies who do not recover by 3 months have permanent impairments of ROM, decreased strength, and a smaller upper extremity.[1] Typically, the injury affects the C5 and C6 roots of the brachial plexus (**Erb palsy**). The palsy can affect C7 root or even C8 and T1 (global brachial plexus palsy). Initial intervention is PROM to all joints.

Further intervention depends on the severity of the paralysis. Children may have limitations in ROM at every joint and may develop contractures of the elbow, forearm, and wrist. Orthoses (Figure 16-8) are used for positioning, preventing deformities, and enhancing function.

Early intervention is the key to maximizing development of motor patterns. If an infant shows signs of muscle weakness or limited active range of movement, soft elastic orthoses are recommended. Signs of contracture development at the elbow, forearm, wrist, thumb, or digits indicate the need for immobilization or static progressive orthoses.

Orthotic intervention for brachial plexus palsy includes immobilization orthoses (e.g., elbow positioning, wrist extension, forearm supination, thumb positioning, and nighttime resting orthoses). Static progressive and/or mobilization orthoses may be used to lengthen tight structures and release joint contractures. Soft elastic orthoses that supinate the forearm and promote thumb opposition are used to improve functional skills. Challenges in fabricating orthoses for brachial plexus palsy include providing constant orthotic adjustments as the child grows. Adjustments ensure that the orthosis does not interfere with function.

Surgical Options for Brachial Plexus Palsy

There are multiple surgical procedures for children who do not spontaneously recover full upper extremity motion. Early surgery may include neurolysis, nerve grafts, or nerve transfers. Other surgeries typically occur between ages 2 to 10. Surgery may include tendon transfers, free muscle transfers, arthrodesis, osteotomies, and others. Postoperative care requires protective orthoses, depending on the specific surgical procedure.[1,27]

Arthrogryposis/Arthrogryposis Multiplex Congenita

Classic **arthrogryposis** or arthrogryposis multiplex congenita (Figure 16-9) typically involves all four extremities. A pronounced lack of muscle mass and flexion creases are apparent. Joints have decreased ROM with an inelastic end range. Typical posturing includes internally rotated and adducted shoulders, extended elbows, pronated forearms, flexed and ulnarly deviated wrists, partially flexed fingers, and adducted thumbs.[32] Interventions address increasing or maintaining joint ROM, with the ultimate goal of independence in activities of daily living (ADLs). Often, bimanual patterns of upper extremity function are utilized, due to lack of muscle strength. Elbow, forearm, and wrist contractures may benefit from orthotic intervention and stretching programs. Children who lack passive elbow flexion are particularly compromised with an inability to self-feed. When

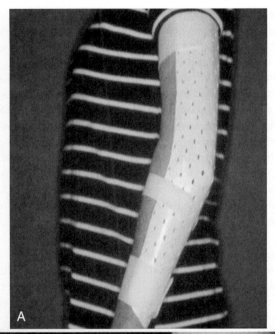

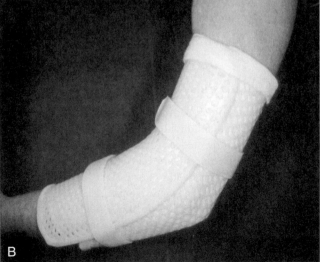

Figure 16-8 Elbow orthoses for positioning. (Courtesy of Orfit Industries.)

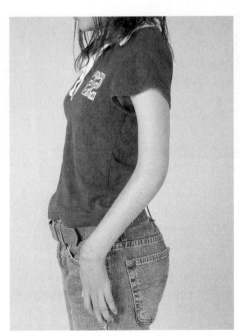

Figure 16-9 Child with arthrogryposis.

passive elbow flexion is present, children can utilize mobilization elbow flexion orthoses or other strategies (e.g., table top propping or trunk swaying) to assist in self-feeding (refer to Chapter 10).

Multiple surgical procedures may be considered for children with arthrogryposis including tendon transfers, posterior elbow capsulotomy, wrist arthrodesis or carpectomy, and thumb procedures. Orthotic intervention prior to surgery to increase passive joint ROM or stretch tight contractures may be necessary. Postsurgical protective and positioning orthoses are often provided.

The purpose determines which type of orthotic intervention is appropriate for children with arthrogryposis. Soft elastic and/or thermoplastic immobilization orthoses for elbow, forearm, wrist, fingers, and thumb may be used to maintain or increase ROM. Orthotic intervention may improve the span of reach, quality and strength of grasp, and weight-bearing. The orthoses protect the joint post-surgery.

The challenges of fabricating orthoses for children with arthrogryposis include providing orthoses that allow maximal function while trying to preserve joint positioning. These children often require multiple surgeries and orthotic adjustments. Serial static and static progressive orthoses are fabricated for maximal passive stretching of tight joints and contractures. Bilateral use of immobilization orthoses may severely impair function; therefore, consider wearing schedules carefully. Resting hand orthoses worn at night may be used to preserve and maintain joint motion and positioning.

Juvenile Idiopathic Arthritis

The term *juvenile idiopathic arthritis (JIA)* is the newer term for what used to be called *juvenile rheumatoid arthritis*. JIA encompasses different subsets of the disease.[7] Common to all subsets is the onset prior to age 17 and episodes lasting at least 6 weeks.[21] The disease is more prominent in females than males. JIA is a chronic, potentially lifelong disease causing joint inflammation. Goals of orthotic intervention are to preserve normal joint function and to prevent deformity and disability. Orthotic intervention should accompany joint protection techniques. Immobilizing orthoses are offered during periods of increased joint pain and inflammation to support and position joints. Mobilization orthoses are offered to enhance function in weak joints. Studies of adults with rheumatoid arthritis showed that patients using functional wrist orthoses reported decreased pain and improved function with orthotic use.[12]

Types of orthoses fabricated for children with JIA may include immobilization orthoses for the elbow, forearm, wrist (dorsal or volar based) fingers and thumb. These orthoses:

* Protect the joints during flare-ups
* Prevent further deformity
* Support weak and inflamed joints
* Improve function of grasp and reach

Cerebral Palsy

Cerebral palsy (CP) (Figure 16-10) is a lifelong disorder of sensory-motor development that originates from insult to the developing brain. CP is characterized by impaired ability to move and maintain posture and balance. Eighty-five percent of CP etiology is congenital, originating in utero or at the time of labor and delivery. The remaining 15% is acquired during early childhood from injury, poisoning, illness, and other causes.[10] CP ranges from mild to severe and can affect development of movement in one or all of the limbs, including the head and trunk. **Spasticity,** fluctuating muscle **tone,** muscle weakness, and/or reflex-dominated movement patterns are the hallmarks of impaired movement quality. These symptoms relate to where the initial brain damage occurred.[19] Co-occurring conditions (such as, seizures, cognitive deficits, attention deficits and visual, auditory and other sensory disorders) are frequent and affect motor development.

Atypical Motor Development

A deep understanding of the development of movement is essential when providing intervention for CP and is beyond the chapter's scope. Key to appropriate and timely intervention is the notion that, "Compensatory movement patterns develop and often become more extreme as the child ages because new functional sensorimotor patterns often are built on inefficient or inadequate foundations."[10]

At birth, spastic CP of the upper extremities usually presents as weakness with a prolonged period of fisting. Atypical and immature patterns of weight-bearing, limited active movement, and weakness contribute to both excessive and diminished ROM in infants. For example, by 5 months typically developing infants push up into forearm prop. As infants tip from side to side, weight is transferred to the ulnar forearm and functionality moves from the ulnar to the

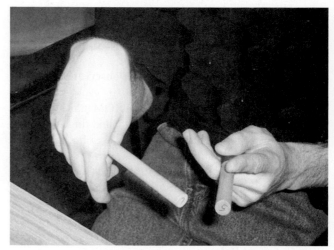

Figure 16-10 Older child with cerebral palsy (CP). (From Burke SL, Higgins J, McClinton MA, et al: *Hand and upper extremity rehabilitation: a practical guide,* ed 3, St Louis, 2006, Elsevier Churchill Livingstone.)

radial side of the hand.[2] In a child with CP, if forearm prop is delayed (due to trunk and arm weakness), persistence of grasp typical of a 4 month old is seen (i.e., adducted thumb and grasp attempts with the ulnar fingers only).[9] Infants with CP may attempt to grasp using atypical and immature patterns. Such patterns fail to serve as building blocks for more refined grasp development.[14] Likewise, limited experience in upper extremity weight bearing, unequal muscle strength between agonist and antagonist muscles leads to an inability to fully elongate shoulder flexors and elbow extensors. Inexperience in forearm prop leads to locking in pronation for stability and non- or limited development of supination.[9] Full elongation of the wrist and finger flexors is present in typically developing children when they prop on extended arms, creep, and engage the thumb in grasp. With CP, children's inexperience with these milestones leads to underdeveloped range in wrist and finger extensors. Problems at the wrist are compounded if the child is allowed to creep while bearing weight on the dorsum of the hand. This destructive movement pattern overstretches and further weakens the already weak wrist extensors. Intervention of these movement patterns when first emerging improves the course of the child's motor development.

When evaluating for potential orthotic intervention for a child with CP, view the whole child and observe movement patterns during a typical day within the context of overall development. Therapists should:

- Observe the infant during supine, prone, and sitting positions for patterns of mobility, weight-bearing, reach, and grasp.
- Watch toddlers play and note patterns of weight-bearing, reach, and grasp, but also transitional patterns of movement (i.e., sitting to creeping or lying to standing). These observations give a clear understanding whether the orthosis being considered will facilitate or inhibit function.
- Observe preschoolers and older children during play, school-related tasks and self-care activities. If children are able to verbalize, ask them what they can do with their arms and hands. Note what types of activities they struggle to perform.

Specific upper extremity function observations should include:

- Any limitations or hypermobility in ROM at the shoulder, elbow, forearm rotators, wrist, thumb and fingers
- Components of movement that appear to be diminished or absent during reach and weight-bearing
- How the hand is incorporated into activities (e.g., hand used to stabilize a toy, hand neglect, sensation, volitional control of hand/digits, bilateral use, type of grasp pattern, etc.)

Orthotic Intervention for Children with Cerebral Palsy

Individuals with CP usually benefit from orthoses throughout their lives. Orthoses address issues of weakness and spasticity (Figure 16-11), muscle fiber and connective tissue

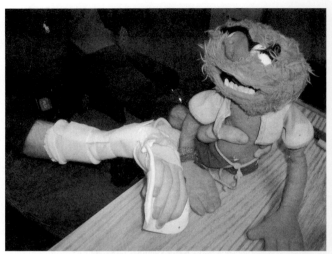

Figure 16-11 Anti-spasticity orthosis. (Courtesy of Orfit Industries.)

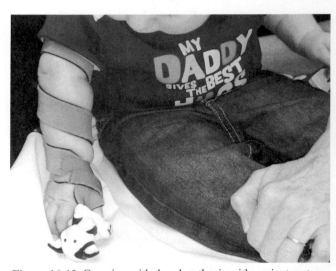

Figure 16-12 Grasping with thumb orthosis with supinator strap.

shortening, and maladaptive compensatory movement patterns. Orthoses address poorly aligned or subluxed joints, and hygiene and skin integrity. All of these concerns are addressed through a comprehensive program of stretching, muscle strengthening, anti-spasticity medications, dynamic garments, and orthoses. Constraint induced movement therapy, botulinum toxin type A (Botox), and electrical stimulation are emergent therapies used in conjunction with orthoses. Surgical interventions are used when less invasive techniques are inadequate. Orthoses are often an important component of presurgical and postsurgical intervention.

Types of Orthoses Used for Children with Cerebral Palsy

The intent of orthotic intervention determines the appropriate orthosis for children with CP. Orthoses may be fabricated for different purposes. Orthoses assist children to develop more typical movement patterns (Figure 16-12). Elastic soft orthoses augment movement in weaker muscle groups.[8,25]

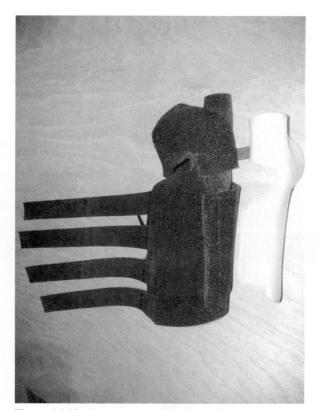

Figure 16-13 Neoprene wrist hand orthosis with ulnar stay.

These orthoses are made of Lycra, Neoprene, or similar elastic material and are worn during active play. Soft orthoses include shoulder-based rotation straps, flexible elbow extension orthoses (to assist with weight-bearing and reach), forearm rotation straps, Neoprene thumb orthoses, and Neoprene wrist-hand orthoses.

Other orthoses block abnormal, nonproductive movement patterns, such as excessive wrist flexion, ulnar deviation, or thumb adduction. Rigid or semi-rigid stays may be added to soft elastic orthoses. Examples of these orthoses include Neoprene thumb orthosis with web stay, Neoprene wrist-hand orthosis with wrist stay and ulnar hand trough (Figure 16-13), and Neoprene elbow band with an extension stay along the flexor surface of the elbow.

Functional thermoplastic orthoses block unwanted motion while allowing function. Examples include a dorsal wrist immobilization orthosis and a thumb abduction orthosis. These orthoses optimally position joints for function.

Orthoses reduce contractures, maintain ROM, and protect skin integrity. Orthoses that completely immobilize the joint and restrict function are best worn when the child is resting or napping. Immobilization orthoses include resting hand, elbow extension, thermoplastic thumb, and cone orthoses.

Orthoses assist in increasing ROM over time. Serial static and static progressive orthoses are fabricated for a stiff elbow, wrist, fingers, or thumb and may be used in combination with other interventions (refer to Chapter 12).

Postsurgical orthoses immobilize and protect joints, muscles, and soft tissues. Physicians typically determine the specifications for the orthosis and wearing schedule.

Finally, custom orthoses assist with specific skills to increase the child's functional repertoire, such as a pointer orthosis (Figure 16-14). The bases for such custom orthoses are common orthotic patterns, such as a wrist immobilization orthosis that has a component added for the assist of function.

The challenges of orthotic fabrication for children with CP include the need to make adjustments as the child grows and develops. Implementing weight-bearing orthoses in a timely manner may be a difficult task. Therapists must be aware of the child's tone and how it affects function. Muscle tone may increase when a child is fearful, ill, cold, irritable, or when experiencing a growth spurt. In a small hand, the weight and bulkiness of the orthotic material may present a barrier to movement. Therefore, the therapist needs to use thin thermoplastic materials ($\frac{1}{16}$ inch to $\frac{1}{12}$ inch) or soft orthoses during function for the very young. In children with CP, the wrist and long finger flexor muscles dominate over the extensor muscles. Over time, the muscles may shorten in length if not positioned in a resting hand orthosis (see Figure 16-12).

Because ulnar muscles dominate over radial muscles, wrist extension orthoses are designed to block excessive ulnar deviation. Due to the strength of the proximal muscles, there is a higher probability over time for hyperextension and subluxation at the thumb MCP joint.

When fabricating orthoses for children, it is always crucial that the parent and/or caregiver understand the reasons for the orthosis and be able to follow through with the wearing schedule. The child may need multiple orthoses. The therapist plans an appropriate wearing schedule to prioritize and accommodate the child's needs. For example, many children with CP need soft orthoses during the day to assist with function. But because soft orthoses do not maintain stretch on the wrist and long finger extensors, children also need resting hand orthoses at night to maintain ROM in the extensors

Hints for Orthotic Fabrication for Children with Increased Tone

Fabricating an orthosis on a child who has increased tone is challenging. With experience, therapists gain insight into methods that optimize the process. The following are hints for the novice therapist who is fabricating an orthosis for a child with increased tone:

- Choose a quiet location and minimize other activity.
- Be conscious of lighting and room temperature.
- Invite parents/caregivers to assist if they can calmly help.
- Position the child in a comfortable position so that muscle tone is as close to normal as possible.
- Speak calmly and slowly, and handle the child's extremity gently.
- For a calming effect, use soft music, sing, or read a story.

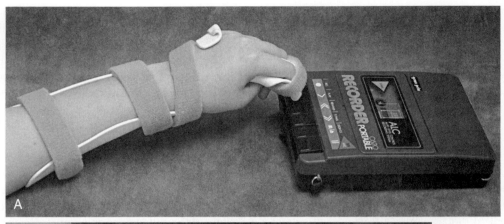

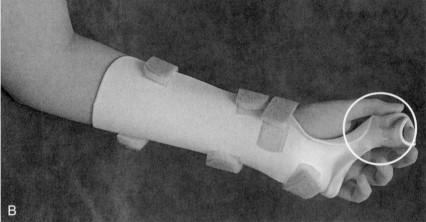

Figure 16-14 Orthosis with pointer.

- Do not use toys to distract the child because they can cause overexcitement resulting in a crossover affect and increase tone.
- Prevent any sudden quick movements.

Cerebral Palsy and Botox Injections

Recent studies examined the benefits of a combined intervention strategy incorporating injections of Botox with orthotic fabrication for treatment of spastic muscles in the upper and lower extremities. This Botox injection causes a temporary weakening of the spastic muscles. One study demonstrated significant results following injections and the use of static nighttime upper extremity orthoses for children with spasticity.[22] Botox injections cause muscle relaxation, reductions in spasticity, and increased joint ROM. These results led to improved functional skills and fine motor function.

Cerebral Palsy and Surgery

Surgical procedures considered for children with CP include arthrodesis, contracture and joint release, tendon transfers, and muscle lengthening procedures. Postoperative care requires a variety of protective orthoses depending on the specific surgical procedure.

General Principals for Orthotic Fabrication

After a thorough initial evaluation and interview with the child and parents or caregivers, the key to successful orthotic fabrication is prioritizing the needs of the child.

- Create a list of the abilities and deficits.
- Prioritize the needs in accordance to age and ability to perform.
- Incorporate the family's stated outcomes and the child's stated outcomes.
- Fabricate an orthosis that first addresses one or two primary needs.
- Fabricate other orthoses to meet additional needs, and schedule alternate wear among the various orthoses.
- Reassess the fit of each orthosis and need for it frequently!

Consider the goal(s) for the orthosis (Box 16-2). Positioning orthoses mobilize joints, reduce contractures, provide stability, rest the extremity, and provide proper joint alignment. Functional orthoses enable continuation or improvement of existing function and can substitute for weak or absent muscles. Improvement or prevention of hygiene problems is assisted with orthotic intervention. Protective orthoses keep the child safe or prevent undesired behaviors.[18]

Box 16-2   Goals of Pediatric Orthoses

Orthoses for Positioning	Orthoses for Function	Orthoses for Hygiene	Orthoses for Protection
Mobilize joints, reduce contractures Provide stability Rest the extremity Provide proper alignment	Enable existing function to continue Improve existing function Substitute for weak or absent muscles Augment benefits of therapy	Improve or prevent a hygiene problem	Keep the child safe Prevent undesired behaviors

---

Always use a problem-based approach for orthotic intervention. Although a diagnosis helps predict probable outcomes with a given orthotic intervention, applying critical analysis allows for creative interventions.

Approaches to Pediatric Orthotic Fabrication

Several approaches are used for pediatric orthotic fabrication:
- To encourage motivation and acceptance of the orthosis, engage the child in design and color selections.
- Monitor the orthosis frequently due to growth. Consider not only the physical growth, but also psychomotor and mental growth.
- Children have unique hands that require custom designs and individualized intervention plans.
- It is essential that family/caregivers are invested.

Safety Tips and Precautions

When working with children, be mindful of safety. Consider the location of tools, equipment, and the positioning of the child. The following safety guidelines are important:
- Place sharp tools and scissors out of reach.
- Do not leave scissors or other equipment unattended on the counter or table.
- When using hot water for orthotic fabrication, avoid splashing. Always cover the hydrocollator or fry pan when in use.
- Children's skin may be sensitive to heat and may react to thermoplastic materials. Allow the material to cool adequately before placing on the skin.
- Sharp edges on the orthosis' corners can scratch or cut skin. Smooth sharp edges and round corners on the orthosis and strapping materials. Securely attach straps and other small pieces to the orthosis so that they cannot be pulled off and swallowed.
- Verify that the thermoplastic material does not contain toxic ingredients.
- Use latex-free Neoprene.

Steps for Orthotic Fabrication

Once the goals are established, the orthotic fabrication process is initiated. The child and environment are prepared. The therapist designs the orthosis, selects the orthotic material, and makes the pattern. All three aspects are considered together. The orthotic design takes into account the child's unique hand shape and size, its purpose, intended wearing schedule, and the most effective material.

Prepare the Child

Position the child so that the effects of abnormal tone and postural reflexes on the arm and hand are at a minimum. This position depends on the assessment results of the child and may differ from how the child is typically positioned. It is important to provide external stability through equipment or handling for children who have not acquired internal stability of proximal joints. This stability may involve a seating system or other adaptive equipment. For the infant or young child, it may be possible for the parent to hold the child and provide external stability with the therapist's instructions.

It is important to reduce the child's fearfulness and maximize adherence. If the therapist does not already have a relationship with the child, spend time to allow the child to warm up. Even if the child knows the therapist, a brief time is provided to allow the child to acclimate to the equipment and setup for orthotic intervention. The therapist has toys, music, books, stickers, or other materials to establish a reciprocal interaction with the child before starting the fabrication process. With an infant, the therapist talks in a soothing voice and touches the child in a playful manner before fabrication. With an older child, the therapist shows the child what to expect by first fabricating an "orthosis" on a doll or stuffed animal or by making "thermoplastic jewelry," or other play objects.

When appropriate, the child is given the opportunity to touch and feel the material while it is warm and soft and again after it becomes cool and hard. The child's response to tactile stimuli is noted, and if signs of tactile defensiveness occur, the therapist follows sensory processing guidelines for improving sensory system modulation. If colored thermoplastic material is available, the child is encouraged to select a color. For some children, decorating the orthosis with stickers or leather stamps encourages acceptance.

Giving children a role to play in the fabrication process may increase adherence. The child's role may include keeping time by counting, holding the end of the Ace wrap, or any other task the therapist invents to keep the child involved. However, if associated reactions are present, it is best for the child to be involved without exerting effort because this may increase tone. Although preparing the child takes a few extra minutes at the beginning of a session, it can save hours of frustration in having to reschedule or remake an orthosis because of lack of adherence.

Prepare the Environment

Thoughtful preparation is especially important for orthotic intervention of children because of short attention spans. In addition to having orthotic and play materials close at hand, it is recommended that the therapist plan to have a second pair of adult hands to help with the fabrication.[4] This additional person might be a parent, teacher, paraprofessional, or another therapist. Extra help is especially important if the child has increased tone, is not able to follow verbal instructions, or is likely to be uncooperative. The therapist clearly explains the helper's role so that efforts assist the process and not hinder it. This usually involves maintaining the child's overall position, calming or entertaining the child, holding the arm just proximal to the joint being positioned, or stabilizing the material once in place and while it is cooling.

Design

Orthoses can be fabricated on the volar, dorsal, ulnar, radial borders, or circumferentially. Circumferential orthoses do not tend to migrate distally, especially when fabricated from a highly conforming material. Circumferential orthoses, which cover both the dorsal and volar surfaces, are more comfortable to take on and off than clamshell orthoses. Circumferential designs are strong and supportive. The number of joints included in the orthoses is considered. Although it is not usually recommended to include uninvolved joints in the typical adult orthosis, when working with the pediatric population, uninvolved joints might be included to maintain the position and keep the orthosis in place. When creating a soft elastic orthosis, the elastic quality of the orthosis must cross the joint and pull in the same direction as the muscles do if intended to assist the weaker muscles.

Selection of Orthotic Materials

Pediatric orthoses are made of many different types of materials, depending on the purpose of the orthosis and the age and needs of the child. Thermoplastic materials are commonly used for the fabrication of static orthoses, or those that require restricting motion at certain joints. Soft orthoses are commonly made of materials such as Neoprene. Soft orthoses may not totally immobilize a joint, but they provide support and allow greater freedom of movement. Children with athetosis or involuntary flailing movements should be protected from possible harm from the orthosis by selection of a soft material or by covering a thermoplastic material with a mitt or sock.

When working with Neoprene, take thickness into account. Although 3.0 mm is commonly used, consider 1.5 mm thickness because it is less bulky in a small hand. Check the stretch because the elastic quality is more prominent in one direction. It is possible to find Neoprene with one side smooth nylon and the other a Velcro-receptive material. Such material eliminates the need to sew on Velcro loop where it is intended to adhere.

With Neoprene be alert to the possibility of skin irritation or rash. According to Stern and colleagues[29] "skin contact with Neoprene poses two dermatological risks: allergic contact dermatitis (ACD) and miliaria rubra (i.e., prickly heat)." Although Neoprene hypersensitivity is rare, the authors recommend that therapists screen patients for a history of dermatologic reactions; instruct clients to discontinue use and inform the therapist if a rash, itching, or skin eruptions occur. Cases of adverse skin reactions are reported to the manufacturer of the Neoprene material. The authors recommend that therapists limit their own exposure to Neoprene and Neoprene glue because exposure to thiourea compounds may contribute to allergic reactions.

Thermoplastic materials range in conformability, thickness, stretch, and rigidity. For an orthosis designed to stretch a tight web space, utilize a highly conforming material. Otherwise the skin may breakdown from the high resistance and unyielding shape. Generally, thermoplastic materials with a high plastic content have more conformability—whereas materials with high rubber content have less stretch but are less likely to be indented with fingerprints during fabrication. When making an orthosis that counteracts the forces of spasticity, it is especially important to select a thermoplastic material that resists stretch (i.e., one with high rubber content), because it is necessary to apply considerable pressure to obtain the desired position of the wrist, thumb, and fingers.[4] For children with spasticity or larger limbs, a ⅛-inch thick thermoplastic material might be the best selection. Smaller hands require thinner thermoplastic materials of 1/12 inch and 1/16 inch.

Some products combine the properties of plastic and rubber. Usually rubberlike (or combination) thermoplastic material is necessary when one is working against spasticity, even though it is less rigid than the plastic type. If necessary, a reinforcement component is added to the orthosis. Selecting a material with a high degree of memory is helpful when one is working with a child whose movements may be unpredictable and require the therapist to start over (sometimes more than once!). These plastics are elastic-like and self-adhere easily. Self-adherence can be problematic. One way to reduce the stickiness of the thermoplastic material is adding a tablespoon of liquid soap or shampoo to the hot water.[18] Ultimately with all these suggestions for thermoplastic materials, the therapist's experience and preferences affect the choice. (See Chapter 3 for a review of orthotic material.)

Pattern Making

Pattern making for a pediatric orthosis may be challenging, and intervention approaches are based on the child's developmental level. Older children can be encouraged to participate in the process by having them trace their own hands on the paper. Infants and toddlers might best be approached while napping or feeding. Younger children can be enticed to play a game where their hands are placed on the table.

Making a photocopy of the child's hand may be helpful. A pattern drawn on a larger-sized hand can be reduced by a photocopier to obtain the correct size.[18]

Using flexible material (such as, paper towels or aluminium foil) to create the pattern allows the therapist to easily check the pattern on the child. Sometimes, it is not possible to make an accurate pattern. Children with abnormal tone may be unable to lay their hands on a table surface for an accurate tracing. In this case, the pattern must be held under the extremity in whatever position is least stressful. The therapist may consider using an uninvolved contralateral side to start a pattern, given that there is some symmetry of anatomy. Another approach is for the therapist to best estimate the design and sizing. It may be helpful to plan on extending the thermoplastic material beyond that of the finished product to give leverage to help hold joints in position. The extra thermoplastic material is cut away when the essential part of the orthosis is finished and hardened.[16] For patterns that tear, masking tape is used for repairs or to reinforce contours.

Heating the Thermoplastic Material

The therapist heats the water to the temperature range recommended by the manufacturer. After cutting out the orthosis, it may be necessary to reheat the plastic to obtain the desired degree of pliability before the molding process. Before placing the plastic on a child's extremity, the therapist dries off the hot water and makes sure the plastic is not too hot. Check the material's temperature by placing it against one's face or anterior portion of the forearm. Checking the material's temperature is especially important when spot heating with a heat gun because this method tends to result in higher surface temperatures.

Some children may be hypersensitive to temperature and react negatively, even though the temperature does not feel hot to the therapist. Because many children cannot communicate that the plastic feels too hot, the therapist watches the child's facial expressions and listens for vocalizations that indicate discomfort. The child's arm and hand can be moistened with cold water prior to molding. Another option is placing a wet piece of paper towel over the extremity, or waiting longer for the plastic to cool. Some therapists use a stockinette to protect the extremity. However, care must be taken that it does not wrinkle under the plastic during fabrication.

Hastening the Process

Time is of the essence when one is working with a moving target, a rebellious little one, or a difficult-to-position extremity. Rubber-based plastics, which are necessary to resist stretch, are somewhat slower to harden. Once the plastic is in place on the extremity, an ice pack can be rubbed on the orthosis to hasten the setting process. A rubber glove filled with ice chips can easily serve the purpose. After being partially hardened, the orthosis is carefully removed and put into a pan of ice water or placed under a faucet of cold running water. A Thera-Band roll cooled in a freezer helps form the orthosis, which accelerates the cooling process.

A spray coolant may be used, but only with great care to spray after the orthosis is off the child. The spray is directed away from the child. The use of coolant spray is avoided with children who are unable to keep their heads turned away from the direction of the spray and those who have frequent respiratory problems.

An Ace wrap is useful to hold an orthosis in place while the therapist works on other portions of the orthosis—although this maintains heat and may increase setting time. The therapist should not apply the wrap or Thera-Band too tightly and should flare the edges of the forearm trough away from the skin after formation of the orthosis.

Padding

Padding, or some form of pressure relief, may be necessary over bony areas to prevent skin problems. Padding does not compensate for pressure resulting from a poorly-made orthosis. Padding takes up space, a factor the therapist considers before formation. Otherwise, the amount of pressure against the skin may increase. A variety of paddings exist, including closed- and open-cell foam and gel products. Pressure-relief padding with a gel insert is useful in protecting bony areas for children with little subcutaneous fat.

To ensure proper fit, the therapist lays the padding on the child's extremity before molding the plastic or places it on the thermoplastic material before molding the orthosis. When molding with padding, the stretch of the thermoplastic material and the contourability may be compromised. Therefore, the therapist adds padding only if necessary. In addition, padding becomes soiled and needs to be replaced. For more information on padding, see Chapter 3.

Another way to create pressure relief around a bony prominence without using padding is to cover the prominence with a small amount of firm therapy putty before forming the orthosis. The putty creates a built-in bubble and is removed from the orthosis after cooling.[18] Thin forms of padding are used to create friction and reduce migration or shifting of orthoses, or for covering edges. Microfoam tape is useful for this purpose, especially on small orthoses.

Strapping

Many creative strapping solutions exist to keep orthoses on children (Figure 16-15).

The therapist considers strength, durability, elasticity, and texture when the strap is against the skin. Strapping with sharp edges is avoided with younger children and those with sensitive skin. The wider the strap, the more force is dispersed if the entire strap width is in full contact with the skin. Strap material may need to be cut narrower, especially around the wrist and fingers, to be proportionate to the size of the child's hand.

D-ring straps are often used to increase the likelihood of nonremoval. Fasteners that require a two-handed release prevent easy removal. Swivel snaps, rings, and/or metal C-rings from hardware stores can be incorporated into strapping mechanisms.

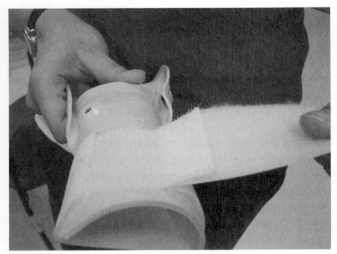

Figure 16-15 Extra Velcro strap for closure. (Courtesy of Orfit Industries.)

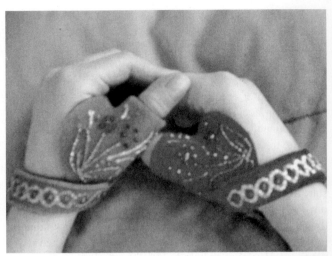

Figure 16-16 Buttons on dorsum of orthosis. (Courtesy of Orfit Industries.)

Straps can be secured at each end with Velcro hook, which is attached to the orthosis. Velcro hook allows straps to be easily replaced when they become soiled, which is important if the child drools or mouths the orthosis. However, loose straps easily become lost and many times are not placed on the orthosis at the correct angle or location. An alternative is to secure the strap at one end with a rivet or strong contact adhesive. Another option is to create an extra attachment with Velcro hook that allows the child to open the orthosis. When soiled, straps are removed and a new strap is attached. See Chapter 3 for more detailed information about attaching straps.

Increasing the likelihood that the child will not remove straps or the orthosis requires knowledge of child development and creativity. For infants and toddlers, consider the use of an Ace or Coban wrap to secure the orthosis. Children at certain ages (2- and 3-year-olds) are in the developmental stage of asserting their autonomy and may resist the parent's choice of clothing, food, or orthotic application. In this case, using principles of behavior analysis (such as, shaping or rewarding successive approximations, finding times during the day when the child is most likely to be compliant, and contingent use of praise and attention) are helpful. Actively involving the child in choosing colors and decorations may increase the child's willingness to wear the orthosis (Figure 16-16). Strap critter patterns are provided by Armstrong,[4] along with suggestions for using decorative ribbon, fabric paints, or shoelace charms. Armstrong suggests describing the orthosis as something cool to wear and providing the child with language to explain to peers, such as, "This is my shield or my princess glove."

If positive methods to prevent orthotic removal do not work, therapists use creativity to keep the little "Houdinis" in their orthoses, especially young children who do not understand cause and effect. Some child-proof methods include using shoelaces, buttons (Figure 16-17), buckles, or socks/stockinette/puppets. Lacing is done by punching holes along the lateral edges of the orthosis and lacing with wide decorative shoelaces. The therapist places padding under the laces and against the

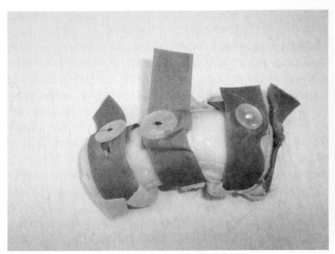

Figure 16-17 Decorated Neoprene orthoses.

skin. To secure the laces, the therapist uses a "bow biter" (a plastic device available in children's shoe departments) to hold the laces in place.[11] Depending on the function of the orthosis, a sock puppet worn over the orthosis may be used as camouflage (see Figure 16-7). Care must be taken not to provide any attachment that the child could bite off and swallow.

Providing Instruction for Orthotic Application

Those responsible for applying the child's orthosis (i.e., teachers, nursing staff, or parents) should be part of the assessment process and provide input on the orthotic design and agree with the need for the orthosis. They must understand the orthosis' purpose, rationale, precautions, and risks of incorrect usage. The correct application of the orthosis may not be obvious to those unfamiliar with orthotic intervention.

The more complex the orthosis, the more detailed and explicit the instructions are. This is especially true when there are multiple care providers. The therapist provides written instructions along with a phone number and/or email address to contact for questions or concerns. A demonstration of the steps involved in donning the orthosis are provided, followed by an opportunity for the caretaker to practice applying the orthosis under supervision. A photograph of the child with the orthosis in the correct position is often an effective teaching tool if it does not conflict with policies regarding confidentiality.

Correct placement of straps is facilitated by writing a number or placing a small design on the strap end and a corresponding number or design on the orthosis. The therapist does everything possible to take the guesswork out of putting on the orthosis. Instruct caregivers to inspect the skin every time the orthosis is removed to assess for signs of excessive pressure.

Wearing Schedules

Wearing schedules vary according to the purpose of the orthosis, the child's tolerance, musculoskeletal status, occupations, and daily routines. Orthoses may be worn for long or short intervals during the day, at night, during functional activities, or a combination. It is necessary to gradually increase the wearing time initially to build up the child's tolerance for the orthosis and to make any modifications that become apparent with use.

When the purpose of the orthosis is to increase functional use, wearing the orthosis should occur during times when the child is engaged in occupations. If the purpose is tone reduction, the orthosis is worn prior to activities or occupations. When the purpose of the orthosis is to prevent a contracture, the orthosis is worn when the child is not engaged in occupations. Finally, if the orthosis is used to treat an existing contracture, it is necessary to wear it for prolonged periods of time.

The total time spent wearing the orthosis during a 24-hour period appears to be more important than whether it is worn continuously or intermittently.[18] The length of time an orthosis can be worn is affected by how much force is applied to achieve the desired position, which causes stress on the joints, muscles, and skin. Ultimately, wearing schedule decisions are based on developing and maintaining clinical competence, clinical reasoning, and collaborating with the child and/or family members or care providers.

The wearing schedule only works if the orthosis is placed on the child during the recommended times. Incorporating the orthotic schedule into the child's regular routine may increase adherence, because it becomes less of a special chore for the parent, teacher, caregiver, or nursing staff. The therapist documents the agreed-upon wearing schedule and provides written copies to parents, caregivers, teachers, nurses, and child care providers. As the child's developmental or ROM status changes, the therapist evaluates the wearing schedule and possibly the orthotic design to make modifications.

Precautions

The skin is inspected frequently during the initial wearing phase. A distinct red area or generalized redness that does not disappear within 15 to 20 minutes after removal indicates excessive pressure and the need for revision.[17,18] During periods of monitoring, the therapist should be aware of any problems associated with joint compression, pressure on nerves, compromised circulation, and dermatologic reactions. Children's growth spurts often come without obvious signals and during those times, therapists and caregivers should be extra vigilant.

Evaluation of the Orthosis

A plan is made to reassess the orthosis on a regular basis to ensure proper fit and function. When possible, the therapist has the child don the orthosis 1 hour before the reassessment. This allows observation of how the orthosis is donned and whether the orthosis migrates. A poorly-fitting orthosis can do more harm than good.

Special Pediatric Orthoses

Resting Hand Orthosis

The purpose of a resting hand orthosis is to prevent a contracture or deformity, to prevent an existing deformity from becoming worse, or to gradually improve or reduce a deformity (deformity-reduction orthosis). Children who are at the greatest risk of developing a contracture are those with moderately to severely increased tone or those with severely decreased tone who have no active movement. For children with severely increased muscle tone and tightly fisted hands, an additional purpose may be maintenance of skin hygiene.

Features

The components of a resting hand orthosis for a child are the same as those described in Chapter 9, except for the shape of the thumb trough and C bar. Components include a forearm trough, a pan for the fingers, a thumb trough, and a C bar. If spasticity is present in the thenar muscles, the thumb is positioned in partial radial abduction to elongate the opponens muscle. Sustained stretch of tight thenar muscles may inhibit tone in the hand.[25]

For children with moderately to severely increased tone, the ideal position of the wrist, fingers, and thumb may not be possible. Because its purpose is to prevent or reduce joint deformity, the orthosis provides as much elongation of the tight muscles as possible without causing excessive stress. The child should be able to tolerate wearing the orthosis for several hours to obtain the maximum benefit.

If the orthosis places the hand into the maximum range of passive motion, the forces generated may compromise circulation, cause skin breakdown, elicit pain, or reduce the length of time the child tolerates wearing the orthosis. Therefore, the orthosis places the wrist joint in submaximal range,[15,17] which is a position especially important at the wrist to allow for finger extension. Low-load prolonged stretch provided by casts or orthoses is the best conservative way of increasing PROM.[13] When flexor spasticity is severe, using a serial static orthosis may be necessary.[13,15]

The therapist determines the best orthotic position by handling the child's extremity and feeling the amount of passive resistance. After achieving the desired position manually, the therapist notes the angles of the joints involved and where pressure is applied to obtain this position. Handling the joints and feeling the resistance from muscles determines the most therapeutic position and the location of force application during orthotic fabrication and strap application.

Process to Fabricate a Resting Hand Orthosis

Thermoplastic Material Selection
When making an orthosis that counteracts the forces of spasticity, the therapist selects a low-temperature thermoplastic material that resists stretch. A considerable amount of pressure is applied on the material to obtain the desired position of the wrist, thumb, and fingers. This pressure can indent and inadvertently stretch materials that have conformability. Usually a thermoplastic material containing a high rubber content has the desired working characteristics (see the Steps for Orthotic Fabrication section).

Pattern
The pattern includes the measurements and markings of landmarks (see Chapter 9). Because the thumb position is different from the traditional resting hand orthosis, the thumb trough and C bar are shaped differently. After the pattern is drawn and cut out, it is fitted to the child for further modifications. While making the pattern and molding the orthosis, position the child to minimize the effects of abnormal tone and postural reflexes on the body and the extremities.

Padding
Before forming the orthosis, the therapist considers the need for padding to allow the additional space necessary. Because padding places some restrictions on forming the orthosis and keeping it clean, it should not be used unless the assessment shows risk for skin problems. Creating bubbled-out areas over bony areas may be sufficient to avoid skin problems.

Forming the Orthosis
Before placing the plastic on the child's extremity, the therapist pre-stretches the edge of the orthosis that forms the C bar. The therapist then places the soft plastic on the web space of the thumb. If available, an assistant stands beside the child and secures the forearm trough. The therapist forms the orthosis into the palmar arches and around the wrist and thumb. To obtain the desired contour and fit, the therapist needs to be aggressive when molding into the palm and around the thenar eminence—especially if working against spasticity.

The therapist forms the orthosis so that the bulk of pressure positioning the thumb is directed below the thumb metacarpophalangeal (MCP) joint and distributed along the thenar eminence. This formation is necessary to avoid hyperextension and possibly dislocation of the thumb MCP joint.[15] The thumb trough cradles the thumb and extends about ½ inch beyond the end of the thumb. The IP joint of the thumb is slightly flexed, and the C bar fits snugly into the web space and contours against the radial side of the index finger.

Forearm Trough
After completing the wrist, palm, and thumb portion, the therapist completes the forearm trough. (See Chapter 9 for guidelines on securing the forearm in the trough and avoiding pressure points.) If the edges of the trough are too high, the straps bridge (i.e., the straps are raised from the skin's surface and do not follow the contour of the forearm, thus losing contact to the skin surface). To keep the forearm securely in place, the straps have maximum surface contact. If not secure, the forearm may rotate in the trough or the orthosis may shift distally, and the position of the wrist, fingers, and thumb are compromised.

Pan
Finally, the therapist forms the finger pan to position the fingers. The pan may require reheating because controlling all joints at the same time is difficult. (See Chapter 9 for the correct width and height of the pan.) In addition, the distal portion of the pan extends about ½ inch beyond the fingertips to allow for growth and for safety purposes. When forming the curve of the pan, contours into the proximal and distal transverse arches.

Straps
The correct placement of straps is as important as correct formation of the orthosis, especially when the orthosis is positioning joints against increased muscle tone. The straps and orthosis work together to create the necessary leverage and distribute pressure. If the forearm, palm, fingers, and thumb do not stay in the correct position, the benefit of the orthosis is greatly reduced. The optimum location and angle of each strap is determined in relation to the forces being applied by abnormal muscle tone.

The forearm trough requires two straps for an older child. However, for a smaller child or an infant, one wide strap across the forearm may be sufficient. Stability is provided at the proximal and distal areas of the forearm. If considerable wrist flexion is present, two straps are necessary to provide three points of pressure to secure the wrist.

One strap extends directly across the wrist distal to the ulnar styloid, and a second strap is angled from the thumb web space across the dorsum of the hand and secured proximal to the MCP joints on the ulnar side. Otherwise, one strap across the dorsum of the hand may be sufficient. If there is considerable finger flexion, straps may be needed across each of the three phalanges. Finally, the therapist adds a strap between the MP and IP joints of the thumb. When making a small orthosis for a young child, cut the straps narrower.

Adaptations
The resting hand orthosis provides a basic form for positioning the child in good alignment and serves as an inhibitor of hypertonicity. However, often the therapist deviates from the basic form to truly meet the needs of the child. One way the

orthosis is adapted is the addition of finger separators (also described in Chapter 9) to abduct the fingers and assist in tone reduction. Separators are created by bubbling the material between digits or attaching a roll of thermoplastic material between the digits. Finger separators are also fabricated from thermoplastic pellets or elastomer.

Pellets are softened in hot water and kneaded together to the shape and size required. The pellets have 100% memory and are attached in the same way as any other thermoplastic material. Because of the puttylike consistency, pellets work well for individualized finger separators—such as for children who have arthrogryposis and different deformities in each finger.[18]

Elastomer is a silicone-based putty that is used in pediatric orthoses for thumb positioning or finger spacers. Pellets and elastomers are available from many product catalogs. The putty types of elastomers "with a gel catalyst or the 50/50 mix are probably the easiest to work with because they can be mixed in the hand and varied in stiffness by adding more or less catalyst."[4] Another option for modelling is Permagum, a silicone rubber dental-impression material.[6] Elastomers and pellets may also be used to maintain the palmer arches or as a base for a small hand orthosis.[16]

The therapist may choose to use a dorsal-based resting orthosis[4,30] as an alternative to the palmar-based orthosis already described. This design is illustrated in Chapter 9. The dorsal-based orthosis avoids sensory input to the forearm flexors, although it is somewhat more difficult to fabricate. For a child with very tight wrist flexors, donning the dorsal-based resting orthosis is easier than the palmar-based orthosis. The child's fingers are placed into the finger slot (with the fingers sufficiently positioned through the slot to support the MCP joints), pressure is placed across the wrist flexors, and slowly the forearm trough can be levered down onto the dorsum of the forearm. Armstrong[4] is a good source of information on fabricating this orthosis.

Infants with congenital finger contractures often need resting hand orthoses. However, when all digits are not affected, the orthosis is altered to free nonaffected digits to engage in movement and sensory experiences. Resting hand orthoses may be made with alternative materials, especially for infants. The therapist selects a semirigid pliable material for neonatal orthoses, because it is less likely to cause abrasions. Bell and Graham[6] describe the use of Permagum, a silicone rubber dental impression material for neonatal orthoses. Several layers of adhesive cloth tape may also be an effective semirigid support.

Precautions

For orthotic provision against increased muscle tone, the therapist considers biomechanical principles of force distribution. The therapist monitors for any undesired lateral forces on the fingers or wrist that may result in poor anatomic alignment, dislocation, or deformity. The therapist is aware of any circulation compromise or pressure on nerves. The therapist's observations elicit important information from the child, parent, or caregiver—especially when assessing very young children or those with communication dysfunction.

Follow the same precautions for this orthosis as with any other orthosis. (See Chapter 6 for guidance in determining problems with skin, bone, or muscles.) For a child who has increased tone, the therapist shortens the initial wearing time to 15- to 20-minute intervals on the first day. The therapist carefully inspects the skin. A distinct red area or generalized redness on the skin that does not disappear within 15 to 20 minutes after orthotic removal indicates excessive pressure and the need for revision.[17,18] If no pressure areas are present, the therapist increases the wearing time to 30-minute intervals. The therapist then increases the wearing time by adding 15 to 30 minutes until the maximum wearing period is reached.

An additional precaution when making a resting hand orthosis for a child who has moderately to severely increased tone is maintaining the integrity of the MCP joint of the thumb. The therapist directs pressure below the MCP joint of the thumb. Exner[15] cautions that distal force to the spastic thumb can result in hyperextension and dislocation of the MCP joint.

Wearing Schedule

The wearing schedule is determined on an individual basis, as are all other aspects of the intervention plan. In general, the more serious the threat of deformity the longer the orthosis is worn over 24 hours. If tone continues to increase at night, extend the wearing schedule unless it interferes with the child's sleep or presses against another part of the body. During the day, the orthosis is removed for periods of passive ranging, active movement, and opportunities for sensory experiences.

McClure and colleagues[26] provides a flow chart or algorithm for making clinical decisions regarding wearing schedules. They describe the biologic basis for limitations in joint ROM and for increasing ROM. This information is especially applicable with existing contractures. According to the authors, "the primary basis for using [orthoses] to increase ROM is that by holding the joint at or near its end-range over time, therapeutic tensile stress is applied to the restricted periarticular connective tissues (PCTs) and muscles. This tensile stress induces remodeling of the tissues to a new, longer length, which allows increased ROM."[26] McClure and colleagues[26] defined remodeling as "a biological phenomenon that occurs over long periods of time rather than a mechanically induced change that occurs within minutes."

The child benefits from participating in occupations immediately after removal of the resting hand orthosis to capitalize on increased hand expansion and elongation of tight muscles. If developing or improving functional hand skills is a primary goal, the orthosis is removed more frequently or for longer periods of time.

Instructions for Orthotic Application

Applying the child's orthosis correctly is important. Caregivers should understand the purpose of the orthosis, precautions, risks of incorrect usage, and how to reach the therapist with questions or concerns.

PROCEDURE   for Fabrication of a Dorsal Wrist Immobilization Orthosis

When selecting thermoplastic material for the wrist immobilization orthosis, use highly conforming material. For children who have wrist flexor spasticity, use rigid material. For smaller children, use ¹⁄₁₂-inch thick thermoplastic material. Whereas for larger children, use ⅛-inch thick material.

1. Position the child's hand palm down on a piece of paper. Make an outline of the child's hand from the finger tips to the forearm. The wrist is neutral with respect to radial and ulnar deviation. The fingers are in a natural resting position (not flat) and slightly abducted. Draw an outline of the fingers, hand, and forearm to the elbow.

2. While the child's hand is still on the paper, mark A at the MCP joints of the index finger, and mark B at the MCP joint of the little finger. Mark a C for the first web space. Mark a D for the ulnar border of the hand between the distal palmar crease and the wrist crease. Mark two-thirds the length of the forearm on each side with an X. Place another X on each side of the pattern about 1 inch outside and parallel to the two previous X markings for the approximate width of the orthosis. These markings are to accommodate for the side of the forearm trough.

3. Remove the child's hand from the pattern. Draw a line connecting the A and B markings of the MCP joints. Now, draw a new line 1 inch proximal to this line. This should match the child's distal palmar crease and marks the distal edge of the orthosis. Make sure that this line is angled towards the ulnar side of the hand.

4. Draw a kidney bean shape over the palmar area of the hand, leaving at least 1¼-inch border on each side and from the distal edge. This kidney bean shape matches with the first web space marked C on the radial side, and mark D on the ulnar side of the hand. This kidney bean shaped area will be cut out. Redraw all borders of the orthosis pattern and cut it out.

5. Trace the pattern onto the sheet of thermoplastic material.

6. Heat the thermoplastic material.

7. Cut the pattern out of the thermoplastic material. Carefully cut out the kidney bean shaped opening in the palm. Reheat the thermoplastic material until fully activated.

8. Mold the orthosis onto the child's hand. To fit the orthosis on the child, have the child's elbow rest on a pad on the table with the forearm in a pronated position.

9. Slip the child's four fingers through the distal cut out, and pull the material over the dorsum of the hand and wrist. Make sure to stop midway over the back of the hand, halfway down the length of the MPs.

10. Fold over the dorsal material at the level of the wrist to provide extra support for extension.

11. Flare the material away from a prominent ulnar styloid and at the proximal edge of the forearm. Make other adjustments to the orthosis as needed.

12. Position the child's wrist in extension as the material cools and hardens. Use your thumb to mold the palmar arch. Make sure the wrist remains correctly positioned as the thermoplastic material hardens.

13. Cut the Velcro hook adhesive into two 2-inch oval shaped pieces for the proximal edge of the orthosis. Heat the adhesive with a heat gun to encourage adherence before putting the Velcro pieces on the orthosis. If the material has a coating, use a solvent on the thermoplastic material or scratch the surface to remove some of the nonstick coating to increase adherence of the Velcro pieces.

14. The Velcro loop strap is placed at the proximal border of the orthosis. Depending on the child's size, it can be either a 1 inch or 2 inch wide strap. The strap should secure the orthosis snugly to the forearm.

15. Check the final fit of the orthosis. Make sure the orthosis is dorsally based and does not cover the volar surface of the forearm or wrist. Check the edges to ensure they are not impinging on the skin, or pressing on the bony prominences. Smooth all edges and round all corners.

Evaluation of the Orthosis

The self-evaluation described in Chapter 9 is used to evaluate the finished orthosis. The orthotic fit is reviewed at regular intervals. The orthosis' effectiveness in accomplishing stated goals and outcomes is reevaluated on an ongoing basis.

Dorsal Wrist Immobilization Orthosis

A dorsal based wrist immobilization orthosis offers excellent wrist support while allowing the palmar surface of the hand to be free for sensory input and play. Remember that children gain information from the world through exploration with their hands and fingers. Even while crawling, the dorsal based wrist immobilization orthosis supports the wrist in extension for weight-bearing. Using an appropriate thermoplastic material and slightly altering the pattern make weight-bearing easier while wearing the orthosis. Blocking the entire palmar surface in a weight-bearing orthosis may not be appropriate for all children. During crawling and weight-bearing activities, ensure that the child's fingers are not hyper flexed, but rather extended.

Instructions for Fabricating a Dorsal Wrist Immobilization Orthosis

The steps for fabricating a dorsal wrist immobilization orthosis can be found in the following procedure (Figure 16-18).

Soft Thumb Orthosis

A soft thumb orthosis with a thumb loop is often used with children who have mild spasticity or increased tone. The orthosis positions the thumb out of the palm. The material used for the wrist band and thumb loop is made from Neoprene. The strap forming the thumb loop is wide enough to support the thumb but not so wide that it buckles or wrinkles in the thumb web space. The strap forming the wrist band is wide enough to secure the thumb loop, remain in place on the wrist, and distribute pressure. The wrist band strap length is long enough to form an adequate overlap to secure the Velcro.

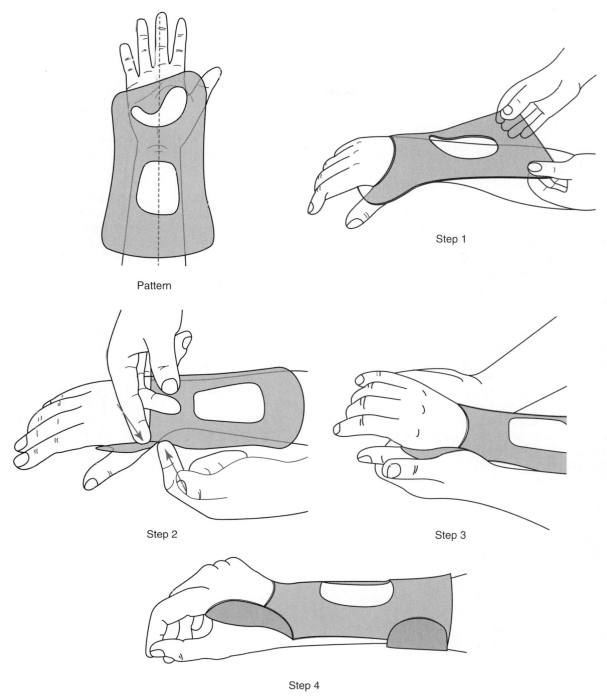

Pattern

Step 1

Step 2

Step 3

Step 4

Figure 16-18 Instructions for dorsal wrist cock-up orthosis. (Courtesy of Orfit Industries.)

Determine the specific dimensions by placing strap material on the child's arm and hand to measure lengths and widths to determine the desired angle of pull. Steps to fabricate a soft thumb orthosis can be found in the following procedure.

Rotation Strap

The rotation strap facilitates forearm supination or pronation, and it can be used to facilitate or augment shoulder rotation. The rotation strap is always coupled with a thumb or wrist orthosis. If used for shoulder motion, the strap must attach either to a therapeutic garment or strapping system at the trunk. A rotation strap is appropriate for children with

flexor tone that pulls the forearm into pronation or shoulder internal rotation. The strap can also be used for positioning the forearm after surgeries.

To make the strap, use colorful soft Velfoam, Beta Pile, or Neoprene. To augment a weaker movement, use Neoprene because it is more elastic. Strap width varies from ¾ inch for infants to 1½ to 2 inches for older children and adolescents. Wider straps have greater elasticity than narrower straps. The length of the strap is approximately 3 to 4 times the length of the forearm (for forearm rotation) or three times the length of the arm for shoulder rotation (Figure 16-20).

PROCEDURE | for Fabrication of a Soft Thumb Orthosis

To make the pattern, the wrist band overlaps on the volar side of the wrist. The length of the thumb loop is the distance from the proximal edge of the wrist band, around the thumb, and back around to the point of origin.

The materials and tools needed for fabrication of the soft thumb orthosis include:

- Neoprene
- Hook-and-loop Velcro
- Needle and thread and/or Neoprene tape
- Tape measure
- Scissors or roller cutter
- Straight edge ruler

1. Measure the child's thumb IP circumference with accuracy to the 1/16 inch. This measurement is used to create the pattern. When measuring an infant or toddler, it may be simplest to knot one end of a piece thread, wrap the thread snugly—not tightly—around the child's IP, and mark where the thread and knot intersect. Then straighten the thread and align it to a ruler's edge to obtain an accurate circumference measure.

2. Trace or photocopy of the palm side of the child's hand with fingers and thumb outstretched. If tracing, mark points on the outline to indicate the four corners of the palm where the palm intersects the wrist and the index and little fingers. Mark the two points where the line of the thumb IP intersects the outline of the thumb. As accurately as possible, draw a line for the distal palmar crease on the hand tracing.

3. From the photocopy or tracing determine the following measurements:

   - Measurement A: From the web space just below the distal palmar crease to the edge of the palm. Add 1 to 2 inches to this measurement.
   - Measurement B: Half the distance of the web space from the thumb IP to the index finger MCP.
   - Measurement C: Half of the thumb IP circumference. Add 1/16 inch if using 1.5 mm Neoprene. Add 1/8 inch is using 3.0 mm Neoprene.
   - Measurement D: Thumb IP to proximal edge of the thumb MCP joint.
   - Measurement E: Distance along the wrist crease from the ulnar to radial side of the wrist. Add 1 to 2 inches to this measurement.

4. Create the pattern using measurements A through E. Cut out the pattern, and trace it onto the Neoprene. Next cut the pattern from the Neoprene using either the scissors or roller cutter. Trace and cut a second pattern from the Neoprene. (*Note:* If the Neoprene has back and front sides, cut out mirror images.)

5. To assemble the orthosis, abut the two pieces of Neoprene side D to side D. Sew this seam by machine using a wide zigzag stitch. You may alternatively apply Neoprene tape or sew these two pieces together by hand. If sewing by hand, follow the directions for sewing by hand in #6.

6. Tape or sew by hand side B to side B. Neoprene heat-sensitive tape can be used to bond the two pieces together, because the thickness makes it difficult to sew together. If sewing by hand, use a single thread and embed the knot in the foam rubber within the seam. Use a running stitch to sew fabric to the fabric on the outside of the orthosis. Turn the orthosis inside out, pierce the needle through, and use a running stitch to sew fabric to fabric. This method avoids compressing the Neoprene at the joint, and thereby does not reduce the strength of the abutted joint. Using a single strand of thread reduces the possibility of creating irritation along the web of the child's hand.

7. Adjust volar and dorsal portions of the orthosis to achieve desired amount of thumb abduction and cut excess accordingly (dorsal portion overlaps volar portion by 1 inch for hook-and-loop closure).

8. Sew hook-and-loop fastener onto thumb sleeve, loop side down on dorsal portion, and hook side up on volar portion. The fit should be snug but not constricting.

9. Attach hook-and-loop Velcro to each end of the wrist band that is designed to overlap on the volar side of the forearm. To form the thumb loop, attach one end of the thumb loop to the dorsal portion of the wrist band. Then attach the loop Velcro to the free end of the thumb loop, and hook Velcro to the dorsal portion of the wrist band (partially covering the origin of the thumb loop).

10. The thumb loop is directed up across the web space, around the thenar eminence, and pulled diagonally to attach to the dorsal portion of the wrist band. The amount of tension on the thumb loop and the attachment location of the free end to the wrist band influence the amount of radial and palmar abduction of the thumb. If the wrist band does not fit snugly, the orthosis shifts distally on the wrist, thus reducing the amount of tension on the thumb loop. The wrist band must avoid circulatory restrictions (Figure 16-19).

Instructions for a Rotation Strap

Construction of a forearm rotation strap is simple. If cutting from a Neoprene bolt, use a roller cutter against a plastic ruler for accuracy. Before attaching the distal Velcro hook strip, trim the distal corners of the strap in a "V" to reduce bulk where the strap attaches to the hand or thumb orthosis. The proximal Velcro hook does not need to be sewn.

To apply the strap, attach to the hand thumb orthosis on the dorsal surface if promoting wrist extension. Likewise, attach to the palm side if promoting wrist flexion. Attaching the strap on the palm side and pulling through the web space may add unnecessary bulk to the orthosis and reduce hand function. Do not attach the strap ulnarly from the midline of the hand, because it promotes ulnar deviation. The strap is always attached near the thumb. To fabricate the

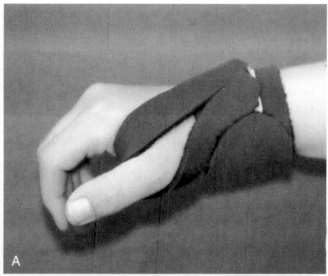

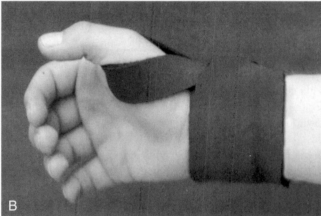

Figure 16-19 A, Radial view soft thumb orthosis with loop. **B,** Volar view soft thumb orthosis with loop. (Courtesy of Orfit Industries.)

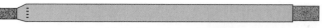

Figure 16-20 Forearm rotation strap.

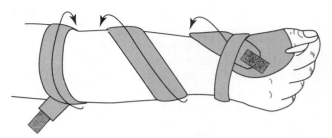

Figure 16-21 Pronation strapping.

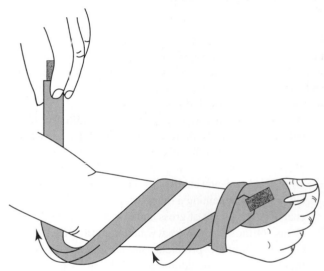

Figure 16-22 Supination strapping.

orthosis, position the child in a comfortable end range of desired rotation.

For a rotation strap that promotes supination, wrap the strap from the thumb side to ulnar side while spiraling up the forearm (Figure 16-21). Likewise, for an orthosis that promotes pronation, wrap the strap from the thumb side to the radial side while spiraling up the forearm (Figure 16-22).

Attach the strap to itself above the elbow with Velcro hook. You can assist in blocking elbow flexion if the strap is wrapped behind the elbow joint before securing it. This is a great addition to a thumb or hand-based orthosis. The strap can sometimes provide enough assistance with wrist extension to promote weight-bearing on the palm.

Anti-Swan Neck Orthosis

The goal of an anti-swan neck orthosis (Figure 16-23) is to prevent hyperextension or swan neck deformity of the PIP joint of the finger.

Fabrication of an Anti-Swan Neck Orthosis

The steps for fabricating an anti-swan neck orthosis can be found in the following procedure.

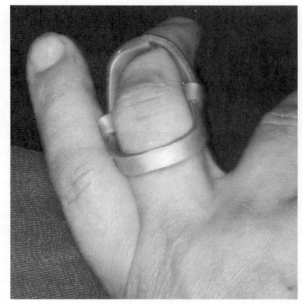

Figure 16-23 Anti- swan neck orthosis. (Courtesy of Orfit Industries.)

PROCEDURE	for Fabrication of an Anti-Swan Neck Orthosis

The orthosis is fabricated from thin strips of ½-inch coated thermoplastic material.

1. Position the child's finger in PIP joint flexion. Construct a thermoplastic oval shape over the proximal phalanx and middle phalanx. Overlap the ends, and let harden.
2. Place another strip of thermoplastic material directly under the PIP joint so that it overlaps onto the oval. Let harden. Carefully remove both strips and bond together with the use of a heat gun. Immediately dip into cold water to facilitate the bond and prevent over stretching of the material.
3. Ease the orthosis over the finger while it is flexed. The orthosis should allow for full finger flexion, but prevent hyperextension or "swanning" of the PIP joint.

Commercial Orthoses

Sometimes the most cost-effective option for orthotic provision is a commercial orthosis. Therapists select a product and measure for correct sizing. The following companies specialize in prefabricated pediatric orthoses:

1. Bamboo Brace (elbow extension orthosis) (http://professionaltherapies.com/PT-Bamboo-Brace-Adwords.aspx): The Bamboo Brace is a flexible pediatric arm brace (orthosis) placed around the elbow joint for children with CP and other developmental challenges. The Bamboo Brace assists children in maintaining a more extended elbow position to enable development of gross and fine motor skills.
2. Benik Orthoses (http://www.benik.com/): Benik sells custom Neoprene products, such as elbow wrist and thumb supports for adults and children. Measurement instructions are available online.
3. Comfy Splints (http://www.comfysplints.com/): These are prefabricated orthoses designed by occupational therapists and physicians. Their easy adjustability at multiple joints allows them to be used for many indications and deformities. They feature multi-layers for softness and new dri*release*® with FRESHGUARD® terrycloth covers. They are available in sizes for infants to large adults. The company sells a large selection of immobilization and mobilization orthoses.
4. The Joe Cool Company (http://www.joecoolco.com/): The Joe Cool thumb abduction orthosis maintains thumb abduction with minimal interference to grasp and sensation. Joe Cool thumb abduction orthoses are made of soft, flexible Neoprene and have an adjustable hook-and-loop closure system. They are latex-free and can be hand washed.
5. McKie Splints, LLC (www.mckiesplints.com): Dissatisfied with the bulkiness of commercially made thumb abduction orthoses for the 0 to 3 population, Ann McKie, an occupational therapist designed and patented the McKie thumb orthosis. Made from 1.5 mm Velcro-receptive Neoprene, the orthosis dynamically draws the thumb into opposition. The Velcro strap attaches at the head of the thumb MP to block hyperextension at the MCP joint. McKie Splints manufactures latex-free Neoprene thumb orthoses, supinator straps, and custom wrist-hand orthoses. All products are sized for premature infants, infants, children, teens, and adults and are available in a variety of colors. Low temperature thermoplastic stays are available on custom orthoses.

Evidence for Orthotic Intervention for Children

Table 16-3 summarizes evidence addressing the effectiveness of orthoses for children with a variety of diagnoses.

Summary

This chapter addressed the use of several types of orthoses for the management of children with a variety of conditions. Orthotic designs for a child differ from many of the adult designs. In addition to the dynamics of development, children differ from adults in the types of environments in which they live, learn, work, and play. Published case reports and research studies are needed to determine the effectiveness of the pediatric orthotic designs and optimal wearing schedules. Such outcomes will allow therapists to make decisions based on clinical reasoning and evidence.

Review Questions

1. How is orthotic intervention different with the pediatric population as compared to the adult population?
2. How would you prepare the room and the child to increase the probability of a successful orthotic fabrication session?
3. What factors should be considered when determining a wearing schedule for any pediatric orthosis?
4. What are the differences among the Bamboo Brace, Benik, Comfy Splints, Joe Cool, and McKie Splints commercial orthoses?
5. Name the pros and cons of using a soft orthoses versus thermoplastic material when providing an orthosis for a child?
6. What methods are appropriate for providing instructions to parents, teachers, and other caregivers to maximize correct application and usage of an orthosis?

Table 16-3   Evidence Based Practice for Pediatric Orthotic Intervention

AUTHORS/CITATION	DESIGN	NUMBER OF PARTICIPANTS	DESCRIPTION	RESULTS	LIMITATIONS
Banskota AK, Bijukachhe B, Rajbhandary T, et al: Radial club hand deformity—the continuing challenges and controversies, *Kathmandu Univ Med J* 3(1):30-34, 2005.	Retrospective study	Twenty-seven children with radial clubhand	Twenty-seven patient cases were evaluated retrospectively. Twenty-nine hands were treated conservatively with stretching, casting, splinting, and exercises. Six hands were treated surgically for wrist centralization.	Post-surgery, the six cases had a more stable but stiff wrist, and dexterity and hand function were compromised.	Small sample size, retrospective study, and no formal outcome measures evaluated
Ten Berge SR, Boonstra AM, Dijkstra1 PU, et al: A systematic evaluation of the effect of thumb opponens splints on hand function in children with unilateral spastic cerebral palsy, *Clin Rehabil* 26(4):362-371, 2012.	Randomized clinical trial	Seven children with hemiplegic CP	Children's performance on individualized ADLs were measured using goal-attainment and visual analog scaling first over a 1 month period under no splint condition, then for 2 months using the Neoprene thumb splint for at least 4 hours daily, and then for 1 month without the splint.	The Neoprene thumb splint improved ADL function in six of the children with lasting effects (1 month after the splint was removed) in four of the children.	Small sample size; missing data due to illness in the children and a requirement by parents for daily measures; selected ADL goals may not have been equal in difficulty; and unable to blind parents to splint on, splint off conditions
Burtner P, Poole J, Torres T, et al: Effect of wrist hand splints on grip, pinch, manual dexterity and muscle activation in children with spastic hemiplegia: a preliminary study, *J Hand Ther* 21:36-42, 2008.	Randomized clinical trial	Ten children with CP and five children without CP as controls	All children were fitted with custom-made static and dynamic spiral wrist orthoses (which allowed 30 degrees of wrist motion). The children with CP were fitted on their spastic hand, and the children without CP received two splints for each hand. During the second session, children wore the splints and performed grip strength testing, lateral pinch testing, and a pegboard test. Electrodes placed on eight muscle sites recorded activity levels during these activities. Children with CP demonstrated less wrist muscle activity with the static orthosis. Children demonstrated increased shoulder muscle activity during grip with the static orthosis and without. All children with CP demonstrated less grip and pinch measures than children without CP and were slower on dexterity tasks.	Children with CP demonstrated increased grip strength and dexterity while wearing dynamic spiral orthoses and increased pinch strength without an orthosis. Children without CP demonstrated no differences.	Small sample size and one time measurements only (Need follow-up long-term study on efficacy of dynamic spiral wrist orthosis.)

Continued

Table 16-3 Evidence Based Practice for Pediatric Orthotic Intervention—cont'd

AUTHORS/ CITATION	DESIGN	NUMBER OF PARTICIPANTS	DESCRIPTION	RESULTS	LIMITATIONS
Case-Smith J, DeLuca SC, Stevenson R, et al: Multicenter randomized controlled trial of pediatric constraint-induced movement therapy: 6-month follow-up, *Am J Occup Ther* 66:15-23, 2012.	Randomized clinical trial	Eighteen children with unilateral CP	Children were randomly assigned either 3 or 6 hours per day of CIMT for 21 days and wore a cast on the affected extremity.	Children were assessed at 1 week, 1 month, and 6 months with the following assessments: Assisted Hand Assessment and the Quality of Upper Extremity Skills Test, and parents completed the Motor Activity Skills log pre- and post-treatment. The procedures included casting the noninvolved hand, intensive structure motor learning, and individualized activities and objects to motivate each child.	Small sample size, and starting points and activities were not equivalent from the start (Predetermined activities, 24-hour per day casting, and the use of more natural settings may provide better information in future studies. However, 3 hours per day of cast use was enough to show positive results, but 6 hours per day did not significantly show increased results of hand function.)
Elliott CM, Reid SL, Alderson JA, et al: Lycra arm splints in conjunction with goal-directed training can improve movement in children with cerebral palsy, *Neurorehabilitation* 21(1):47-54, 2011.	Randomized clinical trial	Sixteen children with CP	Children were either given a lycra arm splint to wear continuously for 3 months or part of a control group. Three-dimensional (3D) upper limb kinematics was used to assess four functional tasks at baseline, on initial lycra 1 splint application, 3 months after lycra1 splint wear, and immediately after splint removal. Movement substructures of the motion of the wrist joint center were analyzed.	A significant difference was observed between baseline and 3 months of lycra 1 splint wear in the movement substructures; movement time, percentage of time, and distance in primary movement, jerk index, normalized jerk, and percentage of jerk in primary and secondary movements. The magnitude of changes in normalized jerk and the percentage of jerk in the primary movement from baseline to 3 months were greatest in children with dystonic hypertonia.	Small sample size
Kanellopoulos AD, Mavrogenis AF, Mitdiokapa EA, et al: Long lasting benefits following the combination of static night upper extremity splinting with botulinum toxin A injections in cerebral palsy children, *Eur J Rehabil Med* 49(4):501-506, 2009.	Randomized clinical trial	Twenty children with upper extremity spasticity	Twenty children received an injection of Botox. Ten were given a nighttime static orthosis. The Quality of Upper Extremity Skills test was used at baseline, 2 months, and 6 months post injection.	At 2 months, results were improved for the splinted group but not significant. At 6 months, results were statistically significant for the splinted group, showing improved function and reduced spasticity.	Small sample size, and no long-term follow up reported

Citation	Study Type	Sample	Methods	Results	Limitations
Plint A, Perry J, Correll R, et al: A randomized, controlled, controlled trial of removable splinting versus casting for wrist buckle fractures in children, Pediatrics117:691, 2006.	Randomized clinical trial	Eighty-seven children, 6-to 15-years-old with wrist buckle fracture	Children were randomly assigned to be casted or use a removable splint. Measures in ADL function using a modified ASK were taken at days 7, 14, 20, and 28.	Splinted children were independent earlier with their ADLs. No readjustments to the splint were needed in this group. The casted children by contrast had less independence, particularly with bathing and showering. Five children returned for recasting. Pain measures in both groups were equal. No refractures occurred in either group.	
Postans N, Wright P, Bromwich W, et al: The combined effect of dynamic splinting and neuromuscular electrical stimulation in reducing wrist and elbow contractures in six children with cerebral palsy, Prosthet Orthot Int 34(1):10-19, 2010.	Longitudinal single participant	Six children, ages 7 to 16 with fixed contractures	Children were encouraged to wear a dynamic orthosis for 1 hour daily over their contracted wrist or elbow with torque set at 0.0 for 12 weeks; the 12-week treatment phase combined daily, 1-hour torques set to provide tension to the contracted joint and NMES applied to wrist or elbow extensors for ½ hour of the treatment period; during the 12-week follow-up neither the orthosis nor NMES was applied. Assessment tools included the PEDI, the AS K, the Melbourne assessment, and manual and electric goniometers.	Increased PROM but no changes in active ROM in two children with elbow contractures, and increased active ROM in one child with wrist flexion contracture. No significant changes in function were measured.	Small sample size, possible noncompliance, examiners failed to address limits in supination that effected function, and limits in the developmental and functional tests to measure small changes
Shiozawa R, Uchiyama S, Sugimoto Y, et al: Comparison of splinting versus nonsplinting in the treatment of pediatric trigger finger, J Hand Surg 37(6):1211-1216, 2012.	Retrospective study	Twenty-four children with 47 affected fingers: 4 index, 28 middle, 11 ring, and 4 little	Twenty-four fingers treated with a static orthosis were compared to 23 fingers treated without orthosis.	Proportion of fingers requiring surgery in the group with orthoses was significantly lower than in the group without orthoses.	Small sample size

ADL, Activity of daily living; ASK, ***; CIMT, constraint induced movement therapy; CP, cerebral palsy; NMES, ***; PEDI, ***; PROM, passive range of motion; ROM, range of motion.

References

1. Abzug JM, Kozin SH: Current concepts: neonatal brachial plexus palsy, *Orthopaedics* 33(6):431–437, 2010.
2. Alexander R, Boehme R, Cupps B: *Normal development of functional motor skills: the first year of life*, ed 1, Tucson, AZ, 1993, Therapy Skill Builders pp 71–157.
3. American Occupational Therapy Association. (2008): Occupational therapy practice framework: domain and process, ed 2, *Am J Occup Ther* 62:625–683, 2008.
4. Armstrong J: Splinting the pediatric patient. In Fess EE, Gettle K, Philips C, Janson R, editors: *Hand and Upper Extremity Splinting: Principles and Methods*, ed 2, St. Louis, 2005, Mosby.
5. Banskota AK, Bijukachhe B, Rajbhandary T, et al.: Radial club hand deformity—the continuing challenges and controversies, *Kathmandu Univ Med J* 3(1):30–34, 2005.
6. Bell E, Graham HK: A new material for splinting neonatal limb deformities, *J of Ped Ortho* 15(5), 1995.
7. Beresford MW: Juvenile idiopathic arthritis: new insights into classification, measures of outcome, and pharmacotherapy, *Pediatr Drugs* 13(3):161–173, 2011.
8. Ten Berge SR, Boonstra AM, Dijkstra PU, et al.: A systematic evaluation of the effect of thumb opponens splints on hand function in children with unilateral spastic cerebral palsy, *Clin Rehabil* 26(4):362–371, 2012.
9. Boehme R: *Improving upper body control: an approach to assessment and treatment of tonal dysfunction*, Tucson, AZ, 1988, Therapy Skill Builders pp 86–118.
10. Colangelo C, Gorga D: *Occupational therapy practice guidelines for cerebral palsy*, ed 3, Bethesda, MD, 2004, American Occupational Therapy Association.
11. Collins LF: Splinting survey results, *OT Practice* 42–44, 1996.
12. de Boer IG, Peeters AJ, Rondays HK, et al.: The usage of functional wrist orthoses in patients with rheumatoid arthritis, *Disabil Rehabil* 30(4):286–295, 2008.
13. Duff SV, Charles J: Enhancing prehension in infants and children: Fostering neuromotor strategies, *Phys and Occup Ther Ped* 24:129–172, 2004.
14. Erhardt R: *Developmental hand dysfunction theory: assessment and treatment*, Tucson, AZ, 1994, Therapy Skill Builders.
15. Exner CE: Development of hand skills. In Case-Smith J, editor: *Occupational Therapy for Children*, ed 5, St. Louis, 2005, Mosby.
16. Granhaug KB: Splinting the upper extremity of a child. In Henderson A, Pehoski C, editors: *Hand function in the child: foundations for remediation*, ed 2, St Louis, 2006, Mosby, pp 401–432.
17. Hill SG: Current trends in upper extremity splinting. In Boehme R, editor: *Improving Upper Body Control*, Tucson, 1988, Therapy Skill Builders, pp 131–164.
18. Hogan L, Uditsky T: *Pediatric splinting: selection, fabrication, and clinical application of upper extremity splints*, San Antonio, TX, 1998, Therapy Skill Builders.
19. Howle J: *Neuro-developmental treatment approach theoretical foundations and principals of clinical practice*, Laguna Beach, CA, 2002, Neuro-Developmental Treatment Association, pp 85–88.
20. Jobe MT: Congenital Anomalies of the Hand. In Canale ST, Beaty JH, editors: *Campbell's operative orthopaedics*, ed 11, Philadelphia, PA, 2008, Elsevier, pp 4367–4461.
21. Kahn P: Juvenile idiopathic arthritis—current and future therapies, *Bull NYU Hosp Jt Dis* 67(3):291–302, 2009.
22. Kanellopoulos AD, Mavrogenis AF, Mitdiokapa EA, et al.: Long lasting benefits following the combination of static night upper extremity splinting with botulinum toxin A injections in cerebral palsy children, *Eur JRehabil Med* 49(4):501–506, 2009.
23. Lutz CS, Kozin SH: Congenital differences in the hand and upper extremity. In Burke SL, Higgins J, McClinton MA, et al.: *Hand and upper extremity rehabilitation: a practical guide*, ed 3, St Louis, 2006, Elsevier Churchill Livingstone, pp 659–688.
24. Manske PR, Goldfarb CA: Congenital failure of formation of the upper limb, *Hand Clin* 25(2):157–170, 2009.
25. McKie A: *Effectiveness of a neoprene hand splint on grasp in young children with cerebral palsy*, Master's Thesis, 1998, University of Wisconsin.
26. McClure PW, Blackburn LG, Dusold C: The use of splints in the treatment of joint stiffness: Biological rationale and an algorithm for making clinical decisions, *Physical Therapy* 74(12):1101–1110, 1994.
27. Ruchelsman DE, Pettrone S, Price AE, et al.: Brachial plexus birth palsy: an overview of early treatment considerations, *Bull NYU Hosp Jt Dis* 67(1):83–89, 2009.
28. Shiozawa R, Uchiyama S, Sugimoto Y, et al.: Comparison of splinting versus nonsplinting in the treatment of pediatric trigger finger, *J Hand Surg* 37(6):1211–1216, 2012.
29. Stern EB, Callinan N, Hank M, Lewis EJ, Schousboe JT, Ytterberg SR: Neoprene splinting: Dermatological issues, *Am J of Occup Ther* 52(7):573–578, 1998.
30. Snook J: Spasticity reduction splint, *Am J of Occup Ther* 33(10), 1979.
31. Tonkin MA: Failure of differentiation part i. syndactyly, *Hand Clin* 25(2):171–193, 2009.
32. Ty JM, James MA: Failure of differentiation: Part II (arthrogryposis, camptodactyly, clinodactyly, madelung deformity, trigger finger, and trigger thumb, *Hand Clin* 25(2):195–213, 2009.

APPENDIX 16-1 CASE STUDIES

CASE STUDY 16-1*

Read the following scenario, and answer the questions based on information in this chapter.

Ben is a 10-year-old boy who has cerebral palsy (CP) and is moderately mentally challenged. His family includes parents, a younger sister, and an older brother. Both parents work outside the home. There is supportive extended family, and the parents have been actively involved in programming decisions. Ben is in an educational program that includes special education, physical and occupational therapy, and speech and language therapy for augmentative communication. He has moderate to severely increased muscle tone in all four extremities with reduced tone in his trunk. Tone in the extremities remains increased at night and tends to increase further during the day when he is excited, upset, or exerting effort. Ben's functional use of his upper extremities is limited because of both increased tone and delayed development.

You have been Ben's therapist for the past 2 years. Among team goals are increasing opportunities to play; improving his ability to indicate choices in the classroom, at home, and for purposes of communication by eye or hand pointing; and increasing his active participation in dressing and eating. Specific objectives include increasing speed and accuracy of reach of the right upper extremity, improving functional gross grasp and release of the right hand, and facilitating any active movement of the left upper extremity. You selected neurodevelopmental treatment and biomechanical frames of reference to guide your intervention.

Orthotic intervention has not been part of his program to date. Over the past year, however, you have noted a decrease in the amount of wrist and finger extension bilaterally with more loss on the left side. You find that there is increased resistance to passive movement of his hands and arms when assisting Ben in functional activities. Ben's left hand is frequently tightly fisted with the thumb in the palm. His right hand is often loosely fisted, and although he can actively extend his fingers the right thumb remains in the palm. You are concerned about maintaining passive range of motion (PROM) but are hesitant to encumber his hands with orthoses that might interfere with development of grasp and release on the right side.

You are modifying Ben's intervention program to address increased tightness in the upper extremities. Which of the following options would you select, and why?

1. Option A: Increase the frequency of PROM and active range of motion (AROM) activities for both upper extremities and fabricate bilateral thermoplastic material thumb orthoses.
2. Option B: Fabricate resting hand orthoses for both hands and a thermoplastic material thumb orthosis for the right hand. Recommend wearing both resting hand orthoses at night and the left orthosis periodically during the day (depending on status of range of motion [ROM]). Recommend wearing the right thumb orthosis during functional grasp activities.
3. Option C: Fabricate resting hand orthoses for both upper extremities. Recommend that they be worn at night and during the day except during scheduled activities involving reach, grasp, and release.
4. Option D: Fabricate resting hand orthoses for both upper extremities. Because you are unsure if the orthoses would be put on correctly at home, recommend that they be worn only during the day at school. Both orthoses will be removed during scheduled activities involving reach, grasp, and release.

*See Appendix A for the answer key.

CASE STUDY 16-2*

Read the following scenario, and answer the question based on information in this chapter.

Mia is a 3-year-old girl with left hemiparesis resulting from an intracranial hemorrhage secondary to prematurity. She has full PROM and AROM in her left upper extremity, but there is mild to moderate increased tone. She has a fairly well controlled reach with the left arm, but her hand tends to close before reaching the object she is trying to grasp. Her thumb is usually adducted into her palm, which makes manipulation of objects difficult.

   Mia releases objects with her left hand, but this is slow, and she frequently flexes her left wrist by pressing on it with her right hand to assist with finger extension. Which of the following orthotic interventions would you consider as a component to her overall intervention program?

1. Option A: Fabricate a resting hand orthosis for the left upper extremity.
2. Option B: Fabricate a standard wrist extension orthosis for the left wrist.
3. Option C: Order or fabricate a Neoprene thumb abduction orthosis for the left hand and consider adding a C bar made from elastomer.

*See Appendix A for the answer key.

APPENDIX 16-2   LABORATORY EXERCISES

Laboratory Exercise 16-1* Recognizing Problems in Orthotic Fabrication No. 1

What problems in orthotic fabrication are present in the following picture?

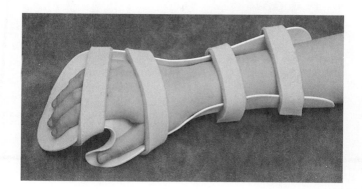

*See Appendix A for the answer key.

Laboratory Exercise 16-2* Recognizing Problems in Orthotic Fabrication No. 2

What problems in orthotic fabrication are present in the following picture?

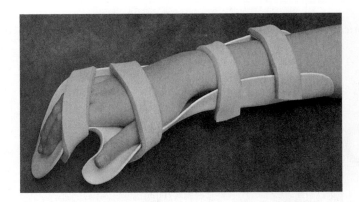

*See Appendix A for the answer key.

Topics Related to Orthosis

CHAPTER 17

Lower Extremity Orthotics

Christopher Robinson
Stefania Fatone
*Brittany Stryker**

Key Terms
biomechanical principles
normal gait
orthotic design principles
orthotic terminology
clinical considerations
pathologic gait

Chapter Objectives
1. Recognize the meaning of basic terminology used in lower extremity (LE) orthotic prescriptions.
2. Outline the role of the occupational therapist (OT) in the LE orthotic intervention program.
3. Recognize the importance of an interdisciplinary team approach to LE orthotic provision.
4. Describe the general purposes and basic functions of LE orthoses.
5. Describe the biomechanical principles of LE orthoses.
6. Describe the basic design principles of LE orthoses.
7. Describe various components and materials commonly used in the fabrication of LE orthoses.
8. Identify the basic components of normal and pathological gait.
9. Recognize commonly prescribed LE orthoses.

The International Organization for Standardization (ISO 8549-1:1989) defines an orthosis as an externally applied device used to modify the structural and functional characteristics of the neuromuscular and skeletal systems.[4] Orthoses are categorized based on the anatomic segments

and joints encompassed (ISO 8549-3:1989)[4] with standard abbreviations for lower extremity (LE) orthoses listed in Table 17-1. Consistency in terminology ensures effective communication within the rehabilitation team.

Evidence of orthotic applications has been found as early as 2750 BC[2] where excavation sites have uncovered mummies with various orthoses still intact. Wars and battles have always dramatically increased the number of people in need of assistive devices. However, it was the polio epidemics of the 1950s and the introduction of thermoplastics in the 1970s that spurred increased interest and development in the field of orthotics in the United States.[6] Today, continued advancements in technology promotes the development of new orthotic designs, materials, and components.

Role of the Occupational Therapist

In upper extremity orthotic practice, occupational therapists (OTs) typically provide comprehensive management including the design, fabrication, fitting, and functional training of the client with the orthosis. With increased emphasis on interdisciplinary care, OTs are increasingly engaged in the care of clients who use LE orthoses. However, in these cases, certified orthotists (COs) are responsible for the design, fabrication and fit of the LE orthoses, often working in concert with physical therapists in the provision of training in their use. OTs collaborate to ensure that LE orthoses are designed to facilitate successful occupational performance at each stage in the rehabilitation process. Common concerns addressed by OTs include acting as a client advocate, donning and doffing the orthosis, education regarding skin inspection for clients with insensate limbs, and integration of the orthosis into everyday use.

LE orthoses address specific biomechanical goals, such as providing knee stability during ambulation. In that case,

---

*With previous contributions from Deanna Fish, MS, CPO, Michael Lohman, MEd, OTR/L, CO, Dulcey Lima, OTR/L, CO, and Karyn Kessler OTR/L.

Table 17-1	Standard Abbreviations for Lower Limb Orthoses
ABBREVIATION	**NAME**
FO	Foot orthosis
AFO	Ankle-foot orthosis
KO	Knee orthosis
KAFO	Knee-ankle-foot orthosis
HO	Hip orthosis
HKAFO	Hip-knee-ankle-foot orthosis

From Condie D: International Organization for Standardization (ISO) terminology. In Hsu J, Michael J, Fisk J: *American Academy of Orthopaedic Surgeons' atlas of orthoses and assistive devices,* Philadelphia, 2008, Mosby, pp. 3-7.

Box 17-1	Clinical Objectives of Lower Extremity Orthotic Treatment

- Relieve pain
- Manage deformities
- Prevent excessive range of joint motion
- Increase the range of joint motion
- Compensate for abnormalities of segment length and shape
- Manage abnormal neuromuscular function (e.g., weakness or hyperactivity)
- Protect tissues
- Promote healing
- Provide other effects (e.g., placebo, warmth, postural feedback)

From Condie D: International Organization for Standardization (ISO) terminology. In Hsu J, Michael J, Fisk J: *American Academy of Orthopaedic Surgeons' atlas of orthoses and assistive devices,* Philadelphia, 2008, Mosby, pp. 3-7.

it may require the OT to help the client learn how to perform mobility tasks with a locked knee. It is the OT's role to anticipate performance issues that may occur when wearing LE orthoses and collaborate with the orthotist to ensure that these issues are considered during the design and fabrication processes. The potential of a LE orthosis to address biomechanical and gait impairments is irrelevant if it is rejected, because it is too difficult to don or doff or impedes activities of daily living (ADLs).

With pediatric clients, LE orthoses affect occupational performance differently from adults. LE orthoses may focus for example on the development of balance and equilibrium as a foundation for skill development and motor milestone acquisition. A LE orthosis designed to hold the hips in relatively extended and abducted position may provide a stable base of support to facilitate independent eating, playing, or writing skills but also impede crawling and transitional movements unless it is designed to avoid such problems.

An OT involved as part of the clinical team making decisions about LE orthotic management must have a working knowledge of terminology and basic biomechanical and **orthotic design principles** pertaining to LE orthoses. This chapter provides a basic understanding of LE orthotics but is not intended to be definitive or comprehensive in nature. Those with an interest in developing further expertise in this area should invest in additional training and reference texts, such as the *American Academy of Orthopedic Surgeons' Atlas of Orthoses and Assistive Devices.*[17]

Interdisciplinary Approach

Although this chapter focuses primarily on the roles of the OT and the CO, all members of the interdisciplinary team contribute the expertise needed to facilitate a client's progression through a comprehensive rehabilitation program involving LE orthoses. The suggestion to provide a LE orthosis can come from any member of the interdisciplinary team with effective collaboration required to ensure the best possible clinical outcome. Consideration must be given to the client's sensory, motor, and occupational performance. Skin integrity and sensation influences the choice of material for interface components. The client's strength is considered in relation to the weight and forces required to use the orthosis. Fine motor strength and coordination also influence the design of the strapping system. ADLs are considered with regards to donning and doffing of the device. The client's physical and cognitive capabilities are also considered for successful use of the device.

Upper extremity orthoses made by OTs are typically fabricated from low-temperature thermoplastic materials and are intended for interim use with a typical life span of 3 to 6 months. The properties of low-temperature thermoplastic materials are described in Chapter 3 of this text. Limitations in material properties, such as lack of sufficient rigidity, preclude use of low-temperature thermoplastics in most LE orthotic applications. Orthotists must access a much wider variety of materials in order to successfully fabricate LE orthoses that may be worn for months or even years while being able to withstand forces such as weight-bearing activity. With the proper tools and skills, LE orthoses can be adapted to address the client's changing clinical presentation as they progress through rehabilitation.

Orthotic Design Principles

General Concepts

When providing a client with LE orthoses, all involved must have a fundamental understanding of key biomechanical principles, clinical assessment, orthotic components, and material science to develop an orthotic intervention plan. Box 17-1 details the goals commonly addressed by LE orthoses. This intervention plan is created with input from the entire interdisciplinary team in order to ensure that it provides the client with the best possible outcome.

Biomechanical Principles

The orthotist's foundation for clinical decision making is based upon three fundamental **biomechanical principles:** three-point force systems, total contact, and kinaesthetic reminders. Although each of these principles may be used individually, they are often used in combination to achieve the best possible clinical outcome. These principles are summarized below in the context of LE applications.

Three-Point Force Systems

A three-point force system (Figure 17-1) is used to change the alignment of a joint through the application of two forces working in opposition to a counterforce (or fulcrum). The counterforce is positioned on the convex side of the joint deviation, close to the joint requiring the angular change. The opposite two forces are positioned proximally and distally to the counterforce, on the side of the joint concavity. The greater the linear distance between opposing forces, the less force is required to achieve/maintain the angular correction.

Total Contact

Total contact is utilized to distribute forces from the orthosis more evenly over the client's body. The equation

$$Pressure = Force/Area$$

demonstrates that for the same force, an increasing area results in a relative decrease in pressure. It is important that pressures are kept at reasonable magnitudes, otherwise the client is placed at risk for the development of skin breakdown. Breakdown could result in the inability to use the orthosis or infection if soft tissues are damaged and become a portal for bacteria. Some clinical presentations require relatively higher magnitudes of force from the orthosis to achieve biomechanical goals. The application of higher magnitudes of force requires increasing the surface area over which forces are applied, ensuring that tolerable and safe pressures are experienced by the soft tissues.

Kinaesthetic Reminder

A kinaesthetic reminder does not rely on the mechanical properties of an orthosis to achieve the intended function, but rather the sensation of wearing an orthosis. The sensation of being in physical contact with the orthosis may in some cases be sufficient to cue the client to alter movement patterns in a beneficial manner. For example, a child diagnosed with Down syndrome may present with excessive ankle dorsiflexion during the stance phase of gait (typically referred to as "crouch" gait) and can be provided a supramellolar orthosis (SMO), which has elastic straps that circumferentially wrap just proximal to the malleoli. Although the elastic straps do not have the material properties required to mechanically limit excessive dorsiflexion and forward progression of the child's tibia during gait, the sensation of the strap across the tibial crest cues the child to volitionally limit movements of the ankle joint.

Clinical Assessment for Lower Extremity Orthotic Management

The ultimate design of any orthosis should explicitly address the intervention goals identified for each individual client. Clinical objectives of orthotic treatment as identified by ISO 8551:2003 are listed in Box 17-1. Fabricating an orthosis without specific intervention goals identified will likely result in a less than optimal clinical outcome and decreased client acceptance of the orthosis. Making the client part of the clinical decision process is important because a single clinical presentation can be managed in many different ways. Defining appropriate orthotic intervention goals requires a thorough clinical assessment (Box 17-2). Physical examination includes both LEs to fully understand the client's current and potential function. LE orthoses may have intervention goals other than improving gait. Gait constitutes a large part of what LE orthoses address or compromise by their use. Hence, it is important to understand gait when dealing with LE orthoses. An overview of both normal and pathological gait biomechanics is discussed.

Having a strong working knowledge of the major joints and structures that contribute to LE movement and how to assess them enables informed clinical decisions. The key joints and structures contributing to lower limb movement are the oblique midtarsal (Chopart), subtalar, ankle, knee and hip joints (Figure 17-2). When in contact with the ground, these joints work in concert to facilitate efficient movement patterns. When a single joint is deficient in strength or motion to perform a functional task, adjacent joint segments are often affected as well. For example,

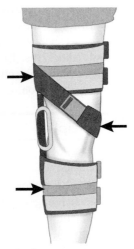

Figure 17-1 Three-point force system to correct genu valgum. Pictured is a three-point force system applied in the coronal plane to effect an angular change at the knee joint (i.e., resistance to genu valgum).

normal walking requires a person to have approximately 10 degrees of ankle dorsiflexion in order to allow the body to progress forward over the stance limb.[38] With a client who presents with a fixed plantar flexion contracture of 5 degrees at the ankle, tibial advancement is hindered. As a result, adjacent joints, including the oblique midtarsal joint and knee may exhibit excessive motion so as to allow the tibia to continue to advance in the sagittal plane. The midtarsal joints may dorsiflex, and the knee may hyperextend getting progressively worse over time as the client's body mass continues to progress forward with each step. This example only describes movement in a single plane. An orthosis aimed at addressing these impairments also accounts for coronal and transverse plane movements and the interplay that occurs between the joints, muscle groups, and motor control strategies needed to facilitate movement.

Once the orthotist has identified the specific joints, segments, and movements to address with the orthosis, the decision is made to control the joint directly or indirectly.[1] Direct control requires that the orthosis physically surrounds the segment or joint selected. Indirect control occurs when the orthosis attempts to modify the external forces acting on a joint beyond its physical boundaries. For example, an orthosis can address weak knee extensors utilizing either direct or indirect control. The direct approach would involve fabricating an orthosis that physically surrounds the knee joint (e.g., a knee orthosis or knee-ankle-foot orthosis). Hinges that lock when the knee is fully extended, act to stabilize the knee. An indirect approach would utilize an orthosis that encapsulates the foot, ankle, and calf musculature but terminates distal to the knee (i.e., an ankle-foot orthosis [AFO]). The AFO would rigidly hold the ankle joint in a fixed position, eliminating the ability of the tibia to advance over the foot during the stance phase of walking. Limiting ankle dorsiflexion in this way encourages the knee to remain extended during walking and standing without having an orthosis that physically surrounds the knee.

A helpful tool in the orthotic clinical decision making process is the technical analysis form (TAF).[26] The TAF allows orthotists to identify specific motion constraints to impart at each joint and in each plane. Classifications for joint motion constraints are shown in Table 17-2.

Box 17-2   Assessment for Lower Extremity Orthotic Intervention

- Personal history (i.e., initial presentation of disease, trauma or problem, course of disease to date, and so on)
- Medical background (i.e., current medications, previous interventions, and so on)
- Comorbid conditions that affect orthotic management (e.g., diabetes, neurological impairment, hand dysfunction, and so on)
- Current and previous orthotic use
- Current exercise/therapy program
- Individual goals and expectations
- Daily activity level (current and anticipated)
- Sitting and standing posture and balance
- Description of body size and habitus (e.g., weight, height, and so on)
- Skin integrity
- Presence of edema
- Areas of pain/discomfort
- Neurologic profile
- Sensation (i.e., light pressure, deep touch)
- Proprioception
- Range of available joint motion(s)
- Spasticity/tone
- Muscle strength
- Cognitive abilities (e.g., follow through with education and instructions regarding the orthosis)
- Static and dynamic alignment of joints
- Transfers and self-care tasks
- Observational gait assessment
- Functional testing to identify specific functional challenges (impact of condition on current functional status)

Data from Fish D, Kosta C, et al: Functional Walking: An EPIC Approach. Oregon Orthotic System Course Manual, 1997; Magee D: *Orthopedic physical assessment*, Philadelphia, PA, 1987, WB Saunders Company; Lustal H: The orthotic prescription. In Hsu J, Michael J, Fisk J: *American Academy of Orthopaedic Surgeons' atlas of orthoses and assistive devices*, Philadelphia PA, 2008, Mosby Elsevier, pp. 9-14.

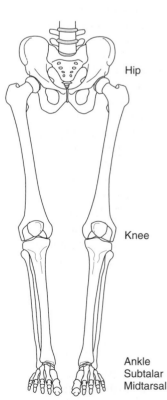

Figure 17-2 Key joints and structures contributing to lower limb movement.

Table 17-2	Control Options for Modification of Joint Motion by an Orthosis
TERMINOLOGY	**DESCRIPTION**
Free	Permit unencumbered motion in a plane or direction (e.g., free motion about the knee would allow flexion and extension of the knee through the full arc of motion).
Stop	To limit motion in a particular direction or plane (e.g., a plantar flexion stop mechanically blocks plantar flexion of the ankle but does not impede dorsiflexion).
Hold	To limit motion of a joint in both directions of a single plane of motion (e.g., a rigid orthosis preventing any motion at the ankle joint would be considered a hold).
Hold-variable	To limit motion of a joint in both directions of a single plane of motion without the joint being fixed (e.g., an orthosis made from a thin strut of flexible plastic posterior to the ankle can limit both plantar flexion and dorsiflexion without completely blocking all movement).
Assist	To encourage or facilitate motion in a specific direction for a plane of motion. Note assisting a motion will resist the opposing motion (e.g., a dorsiflexion-assist joint assists dorsiflexion movement while resisting plantar flexion movement).

Among other decisions, the orthotist decides whether to provide a prefabricated or custom fabricated orthosis. Prefabricated devices are also referred to as *custom-fit* because they still require a skilled orthotist to adjust and modify the device to ensure that it achieves the desired intervention goals. Custom-fit orthoses are beneficial in that they are potentially less costly than a custom fabricated device, and they allow for immediate fitting so long as the desired orthosis is in inventory. The dilemma with custom-fit orthoses is that they are designed for a broad range of individuals and typically available in limited sizes that may not match the anatomy of particular client. The severity of the pathology being treated may necessitate the use of a custom orthosis. For example, triplanar deformities often require a custom intervention because the affected segments lack the normal anatomical shape/alignment required to fit a prefabricated intervention. Custom fabricated orthoses require additional time and skill, but they offer an intervention that is customized, allowing the orthotist to choose the most optimal combination of materials and components to address a particular client's needs. The criteria that is most important to the selection of a custom-fit versus a custom fabricated intervention is the anatomical shape of the limb segments and the number of planes of motion.

Orthotic Components

Once the orthotist selects the motion controls to be incorporated into an orthosis, appropriate orthotic components are selected. Four categories of components are: interface components, articulating components, structural components, and cosmetic components (ISO 13404:2005).[4]

- Interface components: Interface components are defined by ISO as those components that are in direct contact with the orthosis user, are responsible for transmitting the forces required for function, and help hold the orthosis in place on the body. Examples include shells, pads, straps and, when used with an orthosis that encompass the feet, shoes.
- Articulating components: Articulating components are defined by ISO as components used to allow or control the motion of anatomical joints. Articulating components are further defined by the joint that they are intended to control, the permissible motion of the joint in the final orthosis, the form of articulation (i.e., either by motion between parts, as in a hinge, or deformation of a part of the joint). These components control the axis of rotation (i.e., monocentric or polycentric) and the type of motion control, which is described in Table 17-2.
- Structural components: As defined by ISO, structural components are those that connect the interface and articulating components, acting to maintain the alignment of the orthosis (e.g., metal uprights and plastic shells).
- Cosmetic components: Cosmetic components are the means of providing shape, color, and texture to orthoses. Examples may include fillers, covers, sleeves, and patterns or pictures embedded into plastic shells.

When selecting orthotic components, the orthotist considers the client's height, weight, and activity level to ensure that the components are robust enough to function optimally and be durable without being excessively heavy or bulky. Articulating components are available in a variety of configurations and can influence joint motion in many ways. The simplest configuration is a single axis joint that features a locking mechanism to create a hold in a specific plane. Orthoses may also feature relatively dynamic joints designed to impose an external torque across a joint. For example, a client who presents with a knee flexion contracture of 20 degrees may benefit from low load, long duration stretching if the interdisciplinary team feels that they have the potential to improve muscle length and range of motion. The orthotist may fit a device that utilizes a spring-loaded articulation to apply an external extension torque at the knee, with the ultimate goal of increasing knee range of motion over time. This dynamic joint enables clients to continue to gain the benefits of stretching, while being able to remove the orthosis for skin hygiene and comfort in contrast to serial casts that must remain in place 24 hours per day.

Regardless of joint design, alignment of anatomical and mechanical joint axes is important. If the axes do not coincide, undesirable forces (both shear and compressive) and moments (i.e., torques) are generated as joints move through their range.[8] Appropriate alignment of joint axes has consequences not only for the soft tissue at the interface, but also the integrity of the joint. However, there are occasions where joints are intentionally misaligned to create a desired outcome. For example, a posterior offset knee joint used in a knee-ankle-foot orthosis places the mechanical knee axis posterior to the client's anatomical knee axis in the sagittal plane but parallel in all other planes. The objective of this alignment is to position the client's weight line anterior to the mechanical joint thus creating an external extension moment (or torque) across the knee during stance phase. This facilitates knee stability without having to lock the mechanical knee joint entirely.

Materials Science

Once the orthotist chooses the specific components to be included in the orthosis, selection of the appropriate materials to create the structural components of the device occurs. Orthotists fabricate the vast majority of orthoses from thermoplastics, thermosets, metals/alloys, and foam interface materials. Within the realm of LE orthotics, metal or alloy systems were prominent until the 1970s when high-temperature thermoplastic materials and vacuum forming techniques were introduced into clinical practice. Although metal orthoses are still used (often by long-time users), thermoplastic systems have become the standard so long as there are no contraindications to their use, such as an allergy to the thermoplastic, heat sensitivity from total contact, or uncontrolled fluctuating edema.

High-temperature thermoplastics are typically used in the fabrication of LE orthoses, because they have greater strength and fatigue resistance when compared to the low-temperature thermoplastic materials typically used in the fabrication of upper extremity orthoses. High-temperature thermoplastic materials become malleable at temperatures above 80º C (180º F) and must therefore be shaped over a heat-resistant model of the client's limb. Thermoplastic materials are relatively inexpensive and available in a wide variety of strengths and thicknesses. They are popular because they can be heated multiple times and remolded, allowing for alterations to the contours of an orthosis in order to accommodate any changes in limb shape and volume. The most common high-temperature thermoplastic materials utilized in LE orthoses are polypropylene, copolymer, and polyethylene. Polypropylene is a strong but notch sensitive plastic that is typically used where rigidity is required, especially in clients who have higher weight or activity levels. Copolymer is also a relatively strong thermoplastic material but typically lacks the rigidity of polypropylene of the same thickness, often being used in instances where some flexibility is desired. Polyethylene is a flexible plastic that is well-suited to applications where weight is not necessarily borne through the material. Polypropylene and copolymer offer adequate tensile and bending strength for LE applications in pediatric and adult clients so long as the resultant orthosis is fabricated with appropriate thickness.

Thermoset materials used in LE orthoses generally consist of fiber-reinforced, laminated resins with layers of natural or synthetic fibers. Thermosets are comprised of three principle materials: resin, matrix, and promoter. The resin is in a liquid form until it is combined with a promoter. The promoter converts the liquid into a solid material. While in its liquid state, the resin is poured over the matrix and is allowed to set or cure until the material hardens. To manufacture a laminated orthosis, the orthotist relies on a positive model of the client's limb due to the exothermic reaction that occurs during curing. The material properties of the finished orthosis are more reliant on the type and orientation of the matrix materials than the chosen resin or hardener, which serves to bind the layers of matrix together. Common resins utilized in orthotic practice include: polyester, acrylic, and epoxy, while common matrices include nylon, carbon and glass fiber. Adding fibers and orienting them in an optimal manner increases the maximum strength and stiffness of the thermoset. Thermosets have the potential to provide relatively lightweight and stronger orthoses in contrast to thermoplastics but are potentially more costly. Once cured, thermosets cannot be reheated or reformed, although they can be sanded and trimmed; therefore they are best used with client's who are stable with regards to fluid volume.

Where durability is critical, orthoses can be fabricated primarily from metal and alloys. Metals and alloys are also used in thermoplastic or thermoset orthoses as many orthotic joints, rivets, screws, and chafes are manufactured from alloys. The most common metals/alloys used in the manufacture of LE orthoses are aluminum, stainless steel, and titanium. All of these materials can be treated and manufactured to create different properties. Aluminum and stainless steel are used more commonly in clinical practice as they are easier to work with from a fabrication standpoint and less expensive than titanium alloy.

Interface materials are the final consideration in the manufacture of orthoses. Orthotists use a wide array of natural and synthetic materials to create an interface between the client and the orthosis. The simplest interface is the application of a sock; a cotton or wool sock allows the skin to breath while wicking sweat and oils from the LE. Interface components may also be lined with materials designed to increase wearing comfort. Nylon, Neoprene, and thermoplastic foams can be attached to the inner surface of the interface component during the manufacturing process or as needed at follow-up assessments. For example, clients with peripheral neuropathy are at high risk of ulceration on the plantar surface of their feet. The orthotist may elect to line the plantar interface component of an orthosis with a foam such as plastazote, which is similar in durometer to soft tissue. With pressure, this material yields over areas of bony prominence and helps redistribute pressure over the plantar surface of the foot.

Gait Biomechanics

Observational Gait Analysis

As already mentioned, prescription criteria for LE orthoses are based on a thorough assessment of the client, including evaluation of gait where appropriate. Ideally, observational gait analysis (OGA) is performed with the client wearing minimal and/or snug fitting clothing. This allows the observer to relate the function of the lower limbs to the stability of the upper torso. Walking is observed with the client barefoot and then while wearing any existing orthoses or ambulation aids. Observation of gait is facilitated by use of video recordings that can be replayed and/or played in slow motion.

Normal Gait

Normal gait is characterized by smooth, rhythmic patterns of motion that require relatively little effort. Normal gait is often described in terms of a gait cycle, which is defined as initial contact of one foot to the next initial contact of the same foot (Figure 17-3). The gait cycle is partitioned into stance and swing phases, with stance phase including periods of double and single limb support. Stance phase is further divided into more specific functional subphases: loading response, mid-stance, terminal stance, and pre-swing; whereas swing phase can be divided into initial swing, mid-swing, and terminal swing.[38] Gard and Fatone[12] described the following important functions associated with normal walking: gait initiation and termination, balance and upright posture, stability of the stance leg, execution of the stepping motion, forward progression, shock absorption, and energy conservation. These functions are further detailed later.

Two-thirds of the body mass is carried above the hips when standing. Being top-heavy in this way challenges stability with active intervention required to maintain balance of the head, arms, and trunk over the legs and pelvis. Abdominal and pelvic muscular effort is reduced by holding the trunk vertical and positioned over the legs. During standing, static balance is achieved by positioning the body's center of gravity (weight line) within the base of support created by the perimeter of the feet. If the center of gravity moves outside the base of support, the person falls over.

However, during walking, the center of gravity does not need to be positioned directly over the base of support. The person walking maintains a dynamic equilibrium in which the motion of the body mass plays a role in maintaining an upright posture and balanced state. The dynamics associated with forward momentum of an able-bodied person enables body configurations to be assumed during gait for which static balance would not be possible.

Walking requires that a person successfully accelerate the body forward from a standing position, and stop walking while maintaining an upright, balanced state.[12] In able-bodied people, steady-state walking speed is achieved within two to three steps. During standing and walking, the stance leg must have the ability to support the weight of the body, especially during single support when the body progresses forward over the supporting leg while the contralateral leg is swinging forward. This requires a combination of adequate muscular strength and appropriate leg positioning. During walking, the body appears to increase stability of the lower limb joints through careful control of the ground reaction force (GRF) vector, reducing joint moments (i.e., torques) and muscle forces. The GRF is the reaction to the force exerted by the body on the ground.

Weight transfer onto the leading leg during gait is rapid and fairly abrupt. Weight transfer creates the challenge of accepting fast moving body weight in a manner that both absorbs the shock of floor contact and creates a stable limb over which the body can advance.[38] Normal ambulation is characterized by knee flexion during loading response, which serves to provide shock absorption by decreasing leg stiffness.[13]

Normal walking requires the ability to advance the leg from behind to in front of the body so as to execute the stepping motion in a smooth, efficient manner that does not disrupt forward progression. To accomplish this objective, the leg must be sufficiently shortened so that it does not contact the ground during swing, and it must then be rapidly

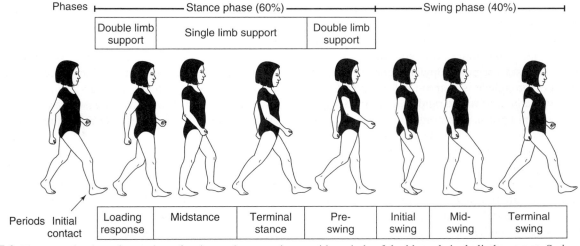

Figure 17-3 The normal gait cycle consists of swing and stance phases with periods of double and single limb support. Swing and stance phases are further subdivided into seven functional subphases.

lengthened as it moves in front of the body in preparation for initial contact and stance phase.

Able-bodied walking is characterized by symmetry with the stance and swing phases of one leg nearly equal in duration to those of the other, providing an even, rhythmic pattern. Stance phase duration during freely-selected able-bodied gait is about 62% of the gait cycle, with swing phase comprising about 38%, and double-support phases lasting approximately 12%. Phase durations are modified with faster or slower walking speeds.[31] The stepping rate (i.e., cadence) is influenced significantly by the swing leg: walking speed is difficult to change without the ability to control swing phase duration.

Able-bodied adults generally adopt a freely-selected walking speed of about 1.3 to 1.4 m/s, and are able to comfortably walk across a range of speeds from about 0.8 to 1.8 m/s.[24] Walking speed is determined by both step length and step rate. As the limb prepares for initial contact, the swing leg hip is flexed and the knee extended so as to move the foot to a position in front of the body, allowing for an adequate step length. Inability to flex the hip or extend the knee sufficiently results in short step lengths and slows forward progression. Faster walking speeds tend to be accompanied by greater pelvic rotation,[35] which serves to further increase step length. Rate of stepping relies on the ability to transfer body weight to the leading leg and swing the trailing leg forward without hindering forward progression.

Knee flexion is the primary mechanism by which the leg is effectively shortened for swing phase ground clearance of the foot. Knee flexion during swing phase converts the leg into a double (i.e., compound) pendulum, enabling the leg to swing forward with less effort and energy. Effort required to rotate the leg is reduced by knee flexion as it brings the foot and shank masses closer to the hip joint's axis of rotation. This also enables the leg to swing forward in shorter time than if the leg were fully extended.[23]

Able-bodied people utilize mechanisms to conserve mechanical energy and preserve forward momentum of the body, enabling forward progression with only relatively small additions of metabolic energy from step to step. Perry and Burnfield[38] suggested that three rocker mechanisms (heel, ankle, and forefoot) serve to facilitate forward progression, while Gard and Childress[11] proposed that these three rocker mechanisms can be integrated during walking to create a single, smooth "roll-over shape." Regardless of how it is defined, an altered foot rocker mechanism disrupts forward momentum of the body and decreases walking speed.[9]

During double support, body weight is rapidly transferred to the leading leg so that the trailing leg can be lifted and advanced in front of the body. Weight transfer must occur quickly and efficiently so that the knee of the trailing leg can begin flexing in preparation for swing phase and the leg can begin accelerating forward. Knee flexion and ankle plantar flexion in the trailing leg during double support phase serve to lengthen the leg. This allows the trailing leg to maintain contact with the ground and provide stability while facilitating transfer of load to the leading leg. Serving as a mobile link between the two legs, the pelvis facilitates smooth transmission of body weight from one leg to the other and provides shock absorption.[10] Rapid flexion of the hip in late stance accelerates the leg forward, and further knee flexion occurs passively. Inhibition of knee flexion at the end of stance phase or delay in knee flexion initiation reduces acceleration of the trailing leg, prolonging double support phase and slowing forward progression of the body.

Cushioning of impact forces generated during normal walking are achieved through the physical properties of biological tissues, footwear and walking surfaces,[20] and through actions of the lower limb and pelvis, such as stance phase knee flexion and coronal plane pelvic motion (i.e., pelvic obliquity).[10,13,38,43] The motions that occur during loading response provide shock absorption. At initial contact, ankle plantar flexion and knee flexion serve to lessen the impact of floor contact.[32,37,41] Increasing knee flexion in early stance decreases the stiffness of the leg and diminishes transmission of mechanical shock to the head.[15,20,27]

Able-bodied walking is characterized by remarkable efficiency, which seems to be accomplished by two primary means: managing the GRFs in such a manner that the internal muscle moments (i.e., torques) about joints are reduced, and by conserving mechanical energy associated with moving the segment masses of the body. Able-bodied people are able to capitalize on these energy conserving mechanisms, reducing the amount of metabolic energy that must be added from step to step. Recordings of muscle activity during walking show that for much of stance phase muscles are largely silent, indicating that little effort is required to maintain stability and advance the body forward.[38] Muscles appear to be used primarily to accelerate and decelerate the head, arms, trunk, and lower limb segments, with significant reliance on momentum of the body masses that enable muscles to be turned off in mid-stance and mid-swing. Perry and Burnfield[38] suggested that sufficient gait velocity is required to preserve the advantages of momentum and reduce demand on muscles.

Pathologic Gait

A **pathologic gait** pattern often develops secondary to neuromuscular deficits, joint instabilities, pain, disease processes, congenital impairments, and many other conditions. Excessive or insufficient joint motion can lead to exaggerated, inhibited, or compensatory movements of the body throughout the gait cycle.[38] As a result, the normal walking speed of the individual is often diminished. Clinical training in OGA ensures the identification of all pathologic gait deviations in need of LE orthotic intervention. Gait deviations are considered as either primary and directly caused by the pathology, or secondary compensatory maneuvers. When a primary deviation is identified, the observer looks for secondary gait deviations. Where a secondary gait deviation is observed, the observer looks elsewhere for the primary problem. It is important to realize that correction of the primary deviation will resolve the secondary deviation, but not vice versa. Deviations can occur in combination with each other (e.g., stiff knee gait coupled with hip hiking) and the magnitude of deviations in any individual subject may vary with severity of the pathology. Commonly observed primary gait deviations include drop foot, tone-induced equinovarus, knee hyperextension, knee instability, genu varum, genu valgum, and stiff knee gait. Commonly observed secondary or compensatory gait deviations include increased step width, vaulting, steppage gait, circumduction, hip hiking, and lateral, anterior, and posterior trunk lean. These gait deviations are described in more detail in the following sections.

Primary Deviations

Primary gait deviations may be due to the impairment or may also be caused by orthotic interventions acting appropriately or inappropriately (e.g., due to worn out orthotic components). Examples of primary gait deviations include drop foot (insufficient dorsiflexion during swing as a result of dorsiflexor muscle weakness) and tone-induced equinovarus (excessive plantar flexion during swing as a result of calf muscle spasticity or hypertonicity). A worn out plantar flexion stop or dorsiflexion assist spring on an ankle-foot orthosis can also create problems with the ankle alignment needed for swing phase ground clearance of the limb. When dorsiflexion of the ankle is compromised in any of these ways, not only will the toes drag on the ground during swing phase but initial contact with the ground during loading response will occur with the toes or forefoot rather than the heel. In response to these problems, clients will, if possible, adopt secondary gait deviations that provide ground clearance of the plantar flexed foot during swing phase, such as exaggerated hip and knee flexion (i.e., steppage gait) or hip circumduction. However, without the assistance of a LE orthosis, it is very difficult to compensate for the inappropriate initial contact. Disruption of the heel rocker in this manner compromises forward progression and slows walking.[34]

Secondary Deviations

Secondary (compensatory) gait deviations are a functional response to an impairment or orthotic intervention that disrupts the ability to walk. However, while secondary deviations facilitate walking, they can often be in and of themselves inefficient and energy expensive. Examples of common secondary gait deviations include vaulting, circumduction, and hip hiking. Each of these deviations compensate for a limb that is functionally too long during swing phase or cannot be shortened at the appropriate time (e.g., where knee motion is reduced due to a locked knee orthosis (KO) or hypertonicity/spasticity of the knee extensors; where there is a limb length discrepancy; where the dorsiflexor muscles are weak and the toe drags during swing). Vaulting involves exaggerated plantar flexion of the contralateral (uninvolved) ankle during mid-stance. By rising up on the stance limb, extra ground clearance is created for the swing limb in which

hip and knee flexion or ankle dorsiflexion are compromised. When circumducting, the impaired limb follows a laterally curved path during swing rather than swinging straight forward; less knee flexion is therefore needed for the foot to clear the ground during swing. Hip hiking involves elevation of the pelvis (and consequently the hip) on the impaired side in the coronal plane during swing. Hip hiking raises the leg more than it otherwise would be. While these deviations help ensure that the swing limb clears the ground during swing phase, they require larger displacement of segment masses, which increases muscular effort and energy expenditure and diminishes conservation of mechanical energies.

These energetic issues are even worse when trunk deviations (such as, lateral, anterior, or posterior trunk lean) are used to compensate for lower limb impairments, such as weak hip abductors, weak knee flexors, and weak hip extensors, respectively. Weakness of these muscles compromises stance phase stability at the respective joint. By shifting the trunk center of mass during stance on the impaired/weakened limb, the moments (or torques) that the weakened muscles must counteract to maintain upright stability are reduced. Moving the trunk laterally over the stance limb reduces the internal hip abductor moment needed from the muscle to maintain a level pelvis during single limb stance. Similarly, moving the trunk anteriorly over the stance limb increases the external knee extensor moment acting to stabilize the knee during single limb stance.

Some pathologic motions are more difficult to compensate for in a functional manner. Knee hyperextension is such a condition (Figure 17-4). This occurs as the knee moves in a backward direction during mid-stance (i.e., opposite to the direction of walking), often secondary to weakness of the quadriceps and/or calf muscle groups. Without hyperextension, the person experiences uncontrolled knee flexion and collapse. Unfortunately, on-going knee hyperextension results in increasing knee deformity and pain, and disrupting the efficiency of gait because the LE is forced backward as the body mass is attempting to move forward over the stance limb.

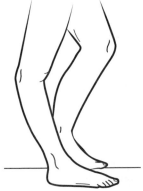

Figure 17-4 Knee hyperextension (genu recurvatum) is a progressive stance phase deformity. The knee moves posteriorly upon weight-bearing, serving to disrupt forward momentum and functionally shortening the limb during loading response.

Foot Orthoses

General Description

The most common LE orthoses are foot orthoses (FOs), not only because they form the basis of many of the more proximal LE orthoses, but because they are prescribed for an extremely broad range of pathologies from mild to severe. FOs are those devices that encompass all or part of the foot but terminate distal to the ankle joint.[4] A variety of FO designs are shown in Figure 17-5. They may extend the length of the foot, or terminate at the toe sulcus or proximal to the metatarsal heads. FOs benefit the foot primarily in stance and are held in position against the foot by shoes.[30] FOs may be used to treat foot instability or deformity caused by muscle weakness and/or imbalance, structural malalignment, and loss of structural integrity due to ligamentous laxity or rupture. FOs may also address more proximal disorders because the foot is the base of support for the entire body during standing and walking. Alignment of the foot can affect plantar pressure distribution, center of pressure progression, and moments occurring at proximal joints by altering the orientation of the GRF vector with respect to joint axes.

Shoes are an integral part of LE orthosis function because they form the base upon which almost all LE orthoses must work. Footwear must be spacious enough to accommodate the orthosis (e.g., they may be a half size larger or have removable inserts). To appropriately support the orthosis, it is helpful for the shoe to be of stable construction, including

a heel counter and a non-skid sole. For dysvascular feet at high risk of pressure ulcers, shoes should be made of soft materials, constructed without seams and provide extra depth to ensure the toe box does not place pressure on the dorsum of the foot. Velcro closures with longer openings can facilitate donning.

Most FOs are biplanar by design, addressing joint deviations and providing support in the sagittal (e.g., mid-foot depression) and coronal planes (e.g., hind-foot varus or valgus). More involved FO designs, such as the University of California Biomechanics Laboratory (UCBL), offer triplanar support with added control for transverse plane deviations (e.g., forefoot abduction or adduction).

Michael[29] identified three broad categories of FOs: accommodative or soft FOs, intermediate or semirigid FOs, and corrective or rigid FOs (see Figure 17-5). Soft FOs are made from soft or flexible materials, such as closed and open cell foams. Soft FOs accommodate and protect rigidly deformed or dysvascular feet. These orthoses attempt to increase the weight-bearing surface area, redistribute the plantar pressures, and decrease the forces applied to the tissues at risk for ulceration and breakdown. Semirigid FOs are made by layering different density foam materials. The composition of the layers dictate the degree of support and biomechanical control. Semirigid FOs include many prefabricated, commercially available FOs. Accommodative and semirigid devices are fabricated by molding foam directly to the plantar surface of the foot or by using crush boxes (blocks of foam whereby an impression of the foot is made by crushing the foam beneath the foot and subsequently filling the indentation with plaster to create a positive model of the foot used to vacuum-form the FO). Rigid FOs correct flexible deformities, especially those that include hind foot varus or valgus. The orthosis must be rigid to contour to the calcaneus (heel) and provide control of hind foot alignment and motion, especially during weight-bearing activities. Rigid orthoses are generally made from high-temperature thermoplastic materials and require a heat resistant positive model of the foot.

Clinical Considerations for the Occupational Therapist

When wearing FOs it is recommended that OTs educate clients with insensate feet about visual skin inspection. Education is important to ensure skin integrity and prevent skin breakdown. Handheld skin inspection mirrors are indicated for clients with reduced LE range of motion to ensure comprehensive inspection of the plantar surface of the foot. Checking the skin's color and temperature is essential for clients with major vascular issues and neuropathy. The OT plays an important role in educating the client for regular skin inspection and implications to overall health. Communicating any concerns to the interdisciplinary team is helpful to develop a long term care plan and to voice concerns to family members or care takers.

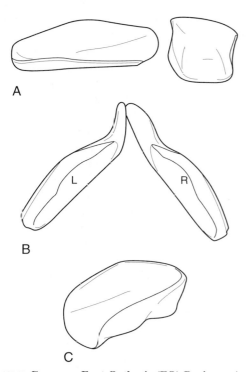

Figure 17-5 Common Foot Orthosis (FO) Designs. A, Accommodative or soft FO. **B,** Intermediate or semirigid FO. **C,** Corrective or rigid triplanar FO. (Courtesy of University of California Biomechanics Laboratory.)

Ankle-Foot Orthoses

General Description

AFOs are devices that encompass the ankle and the whole or part of the foot (Figure 17-6).[4] AFOs primarily provide ankle motion control in the presence of various foot and ankle pathologies. AFOs may also provide some control of subtalar motion. Some AFOs and SMOs have trimlines that terminate immediately proximal to the ankle. The more common AFO design includes a proximal trimline that terminates 20 mm distal to the neck of fibula. The trimline provides the longest possible lever arm for ankle motion control, particularly with spasticity of the calf muscle. Depending on the lever arm, an AFO not only controls the ankle directly, but also influences the knee (and perhaps the hip) indirectly by altering the moments acting about it.[4] AFOs are usually prescribed for clients who have muscle weakness controlling ankle-foot position, who have muscle hypertonicity or spasticity, or who have conditions resulting in pain or instability due to a loss of integrity of the structures of the lower leg, ankle, and foot.

AFOs may be made of metal, plastic, or a hybrid of metal and plastic. In most AFO designs, an anterior opening allows for donning and doffing. The anterior closure (calf strap)

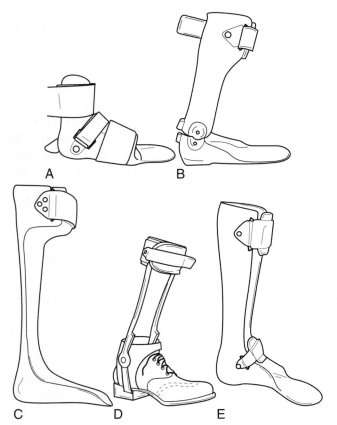

Figure 17-6 Various Ankle-Foot Orthosis (AFO) Designs. A, Supramalleolar orthosis (SMO). **B,** Articulated AFO with posterior plantar flexion stop and full-length foot plate. **C,** Posterior leaf spring AFO. **D,** Double-upright design with medial T-strap and dorsiflexion-assist ankle joints. **E,** Solid ankle AFO with instep strap.

secures the orthosis to the limb. The closure mechanism varies depending on the manual dexterity of the client. Most AFO designs incorporate a foot plate to control the foot and ankle, an articulated or non-articulated ankle (depending on the desired motion control), and a calf section to provide mechanical leverage for ankle and knee control. Metal AFO designs are attached externally to a shoe or incorporated into a foot plate that fits within the shoe. Thermoplastic material and thermoset AFO designs use a molded foot plate to improve midtarsal and subtalar joint control. This AFO improves aesthetics and allows different shoes to be worn. A common heel height when changing shoes is needed to maintain the desired ankle-foot and tibia-to-vertical alignment. In a thermoplastic AFO, the degree of ankle motion control is determined by material selection, trimline placement around the ankle, conformity, and articulation configuration. The function imparted by an AFO relies largely upon the degree of resistance provided to rotation about the ankle.[42] One function common to many AFOs is the support of the foot at an appropriate angle for clearance of the ground during swing. Clearance is usually accomplished by limiting plantar flexion range.

AFOs are either articulated or non-articulated. Non-articulated AFOs are used to rigidly encase the ankle joint (usually leaving only an anterior opening for donning and doffing), limiting ankle motion in the coronal and sagittal planes. Non-articulated AFOs are used when the ankle requires complete immobilization in order to reduce pain and/or ensure stability. However, a posterior leaf spring AFO is an example of a non-articulated AFO that permits dorsiflexion motion but provides resistance to plantar flexion. By virtue of its trimlines around the ankle joint, the posterior leaf spring orthosis is more flexible in one direction than the other, permitting dorsiflexion through bending of the plastic. Articulated AFOs allow ankle motion in the desired plane and direction by incorporating orthotic ankle joints and motion control devices (mechanical stops). Orthotic ankle joint components are configured to provide motion within a specific range, limit motion in a particular direction (e.g., a plantar flexion stop), and/or assist motion in a particular direction (e.g., dorsiflexion assist joints) (see Table 17-2).

An AFO is designated as a floor-reaction AFO if it is designed specifically to act indirectly at the knee. Manipulating ankle-foot alignment alters moments at the knee. Any AFO that affects ankle-foot alignment has an indirect affect at the more proximal joints. Creating an external knee extension moment during stance provides knee stability when it is absent or compromised. This moment is achieved with or without articulation at the ankle joint. An external knee extension moment is created during the stance phase by either a rigid AFO set in slight plantar flexion or an articulated AFO with a dorsiflexion stop.

Clinical Considerations for the Occupational Therapist

Similar issues apply for AFOs as for FOs with people who have insensate feet. The need for education regarding visual skin inspection exists. AFOs may be needed when the client is in a critical recovery or rehabilitation period, as in the case of cerebrovascular accident (CVA). OTs assist in making this process acceptable to the client by educating them on what to expect from the AFO. Educating clients on how the orthosis works, what muscles it may be assisting, and why it has to be constructed, is vital to acceptance of the orthosis, orthotic use, and recovery. Certain AFO design options positively or negatively influence occupational performance tasks. For example, a rigid ankle design provides appropriate biomechanical alignment and joint correction. The rigid design completely restricts ankle range of motion. The ankle movement restriction results in difficulty with activities, such as operating an automobile gas pedal, kneeling, bending at the waist, using stairs, or rising from a chair. Helping clients learn adaptive techniques to perform such activities while wearing the orthosis is important.

Knee Orthoses

General Description

KOs are generally prefabricated or custom fit to encompass the knee, and they act in the coronal and sagittal planes (Figure 17-7). As classified by the American Academy of Orthopaedic Surgeons (AAOS), the KO function falls into three categories: prophylactic, rehabilitative, and functional.[46] Prophylactic KOs prevent or reduce the severity of injury for otherwise healthy able-bodied persons involved in high-impact or contact sports. In these circumstances, KOs act kinesthetically to remind the wearer of a recent injury. Rehabilitative KOs are prescribed after a surgical procedure to limit knee range of motion while soft-tissue structures (e.g., reconstructed ligaments) heal. Functional KOs provide on-going mechanical stability to the chronically unstable or reconstructed knee joint or alter knee

moments and unload knee joint compartments affected by osteoarthritis.

Fit, joint alignment, and suspension are critical factors in the effectiveness of KOs. Given the cylindrical shape of the limb, mitigating distal migration of the orthosis can be challenging. If the orthosis is not maintained in proper position, joint alignment is sacrificed. Often a discrepancy is created between the anatomic and mechanical joint axes. Single-axis and polycentric joint designs refer to the pivoting motion of mechanical knee joints. A single-axis joint functions as a single hinged action. Polycentric joints produce a shifting axis to mimic the functional motion of the anatomical knee. Size, weight, function, and durability are important factors in selection. Specially designed straps, supracondylar pads, or inner sleeves prevent distal slipping of the orthosis during ADLs. The client must properly don and do periodic checks of the alignment of the orthosis throughout the day.

Clinical Considerations for the Occupational Therapist

People receiving functional KOs to prevent further osteoarthritic knee deformity may also experience upper extremity degenerative changes that limit hand function. Although most KO designs use Velcro closure systems, deciding between medial or lateral placement of closures is critical to enhance available functional dexterity. Closures that include a wider chafe opening allow the client with impaired hand function to feed Velcro straps through the opening with less difficulty.

Wherever possible, KOs are generally designed to provide total contact and are worn directly against the skin. Donning/doffing procedures are reviewed with the client to ensure that an effective dressing routine is established. For older adult clients, the sequencing of how to cinch straps is important to prevent migration of the orthosis and skin breakdown.

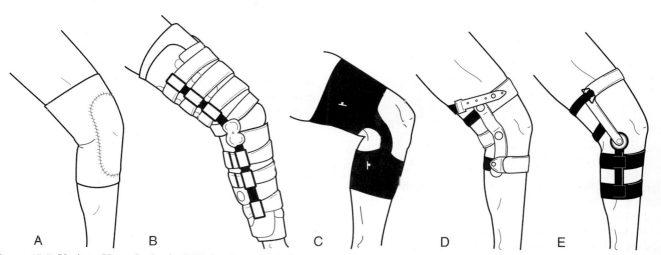

Figure 17-7 Various Knee Orthosis (KO) Designs. A, Soft Neoprene knee sleeve. **B,** Postoperative KO controls flexion and extension range of motion with adjustable joints. **C,** Prophylactic KO with lateral joint. **D,** Rehabilitative design to control knee hyperextension. **E,** Custom KO to stabilize injured knee.

Knee-Ankle-Foot Orthoses

General Description

Knee-ankle-foot orthoses (KAFOs) encompass the knee, ankle, and whole or part of the foot.[4] KAFOs include an AFO component and therefore incorporate some of the same concepts described previously. Compared to AFOs, KAFOs extend proximally, bridging the knee and containing the thigh tissues. KAFOs allow for coronal and sagittal plane control of the knee. Transverse plane control is determined distally by the AFO foot plate design. Skeletal knee alignment is achieved by applying corrective forces through the soft-tissue structures of the thigh. Therefore, a well-molded and fitted thigh shell is an important component of the orthotic design. Excessive gapping reduces the mechanical effect of the design and reduces potential stability and function. Most KAFOs are custom made from measurements or casts and are fabricated from metal and leather, thermoplastic, laminates, or combinations of these materials. Material selection is generally based on height, weight, activity level, and functional requirements (Figure 17-8).

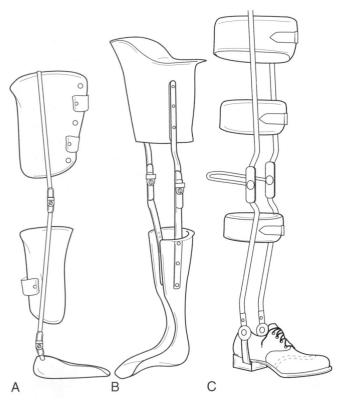

Figure 17-8 Various Knee-Ankle-Foot Orthosis (KAFO) Designs. A, Thermoplastic KAFO with molded foot plate, articulated ankle, long anterior tibial shell, drop locks, and circumferential thigh shell. **B,** Thermoplastic KAFO with molded foot plate, solid ankle, drop locks, and quadrilateral thigh shell for weight support. **C,** Double-upright KAFO attached to shoe with articulated ankle, posterior calf band, bail lock knee, and two posterior thigh bands.

The most proximal component of the KAFO is the thigh section. Posterior shells with anterior straps, anterior shells with posterior straps, and full circumferential shells are common thigh designs. Thigh shells are fabricated of rigid or flexible material. The thigh shell may be designed to "unweight" or "unload" the lower limb by providing a shelf for the ischium to sit on in combination with soft-tissue containment of the thigh tissues (see Figure 17-8, *B*). The principle impairments addressed by KAFOs are weakness of the muscles controlling the knee (and perhaps the hip and ankle), upper motor neuron lesions resulting in LE hypertonicity (spasticity), or loss of structural integrity of the hip or knee. KAFOs improve stability and functional mobility for clients with significant genu valgum, genu varum, genu recurvatum, or knee flexion instability.[7]

Similar to KOs, orthotic knee joints may be single-axis or polycentric. There are four basic knee control options available in KAFOs (Figure 17-9):

1. Free motion joints
2. Posterior offset joints (see Figure 17-9, *A*)
3. Joints with a manual lock (see Figure 17-9, *B* to *D*)
4. Stance control joints (see Figure 17-9, *E*)

Free motion joints provide support in the coronal plane while allowing sagittal plane motion. A mechanical block limits movement of the knee into an abnormal extension range. A locked knee KAFO provides support in the sagittal and coronal planes. The lock may be manually disengaged for sitting. Common locking mechanisms include the drop lock and bail or lever lock designs.[5] Drop locks are designed to fall into place over the mechanical hinge when the client stands. These locks must be manually lifted before engaging in any activity that requires knee flexion (e.g., sitting). Bail or lever locks are designed to snap into place, locking the knee once it is extended. The joints must be unlocked before sitting and can sometimes be disengaged by bumping the posterior lever mechanism on the seat of a chair. Although a locked KAFO is able to reliably provide stability in stance, it does not allow for flexion of the knee in swing, resulting in a functionally longer limb. The longer limb leads to secondary gait maneuvers, such as vaulting, hip hiking, and circumduction to ensure clearance of the ground by the foot during swing phase.[21,47] Walking with a locked knee results in a slower, more asymmetrical gait and increases the energy expenditure of walking.[16,18,25,39,44]

Posterior offset knee joints allow swing phase knee flexion and rely on geometric alignment to ensure stability of the knee in stance. The posterior offset knee joint assumes that in a normally aligned knee, the vertical GRF vector is oriented through the knee joint during limb loading. The alignment ensures stability with little muscular effort. By positioning the mechanical knee joint axis posterior to the anatomical knee joint axis in the sagittal plane, the vertical GRF vector is positioned anterior to the mechanical joint during the first part of stance. This alignment creates an external extensor moment (torque) and ensures that the mechanical joint is stable during weight-bearing. Consequently stability of the anatomical knee joint is assured. However, stability provided in this manner can be unreliable, especially over uneven terrain and slopes. Posterior offset knee joints should only be used when the client has:

- Adequate muscular control around the hip
- Proprioception at the knee
- Good balance

Such criteria ensures stumble recovery if geometric stability of the knee not be achieved.

Stance control knee joints employ various mechanisms to lock the knee in stance and automatically unlock in swing. Stance control knee joints include cable control, a position dependent pendulum, and microprocessors.[7] Depending on the mechanism, these joints are used with KOs and KAFOs. Stance control joints allow for a more normal gait pattern because the knee is not required to be locked during stance and swing to prevent stance phase knee flexion. Some of these joints offer a triphasic mode of operation: automatic lock/unlock, always unlocked, and always locked. Different modes are selected for different activities (e.g., the automatic mode for walking, unlock for sitting, and lock for standing or added security when walking over uneven terrain). The ideal candidate for stance control knee joints presents with isolated unilateral quadriceps weakness, a relatively sound contralateral side, minimal contractures, minimal spasticity, and reasonable hip musculature.[36]

Genu recurvatum is a common condition for KAFO application. Specifically, knee joint laxity allows the anatomic knee center to move posteriorly during weight-bearing. Genu recurvatum is usually an acquired deformity that develops secondary to weakness of the quadriceps or posterior calf muscles. The client compensates by maintaining the knee posteriorly and shifting the body weight anteriorly through hip flexion and anterior trunk lean. The compensations effectively place the body weight in front of the knee joint to prevent collapse and falling. Genu recurvatum may also develop secondary to a plantar flexion contracture at the ankle pulling the tibia backwards, forcing the knee posteriorly during loading response and disrupting forward progression during stance. Load-bearing stresses cause permanent damage to the posterior capsule and soft-tissue structures. Such deformity continues to progress over time. The potential for the development of a severe deformity with permanent damage to the knee necessitates prompt attention.

The objective of a KAFO varies for clients with genu recurvatum (see Figure 17-4). In some orthotic designs, complete sagittal plane correction is the goal as long as there is a mechanical means of providing stance stability to prevent collapse into knee flexion when weakness is noted. For other clients, partial correction reduces the deforming forces to the knee and limits progression of the deformity.

Clinical Considerations for Occupational Therapist

Using a KAFO that locks the knee in extension is a significant issue with regards to occupational performance. Unfortunately locking of the knee during walking was once unavoidable for clients who required knee stability and were at risk of falling because of quadriceps weakness. To some extent, locked knees are ameliorated with the availability of stance-control orthotic knee joints. However, some clients still use locked knee KAFOs. Then the OT considers the manual dexterity required to engage and disengage the locking mechanism safely. Additionally, a locking knee interferes with activities, such as rising from a chair, toileting, getting in and out of a car or confined space, and so on. Helping clients learn adaptive techniques for how to perform these activities with an immobile knee plays a major role in the successful occupational performance while wearing the KAFO. KAFOs in general have a number of straps and can be awkward to don and doff. This likewise will deserve the attention of an OT.

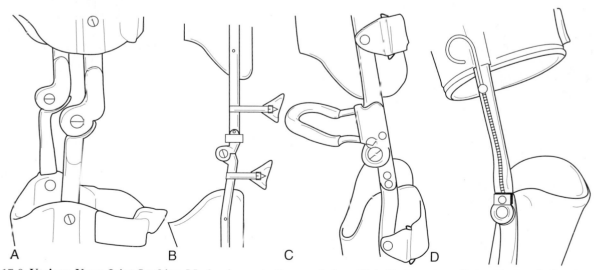

Figure 17-9 Various Knee Joint Locking Mechanisms. A, Free posterior offset. **B,** Posterior offset with drop locks. **C,** Bail lock. **D,** Trigger lock.

Hip Orthoses

General Description

Hip orthoses (HOs) are devices that encompass either unilaterally or bilaterally the hip(s), consisting of a pelvic section, mechanical hip joint(s), and thigh cuff(s). Occasionally, a shoulder strap is used to assist with suspension of the orthosis. HOs are primarily prescribed for problems associated with the femoral head or acetabulum where there is a need to control range of motion, alignment, and dislocation. However, the hip is a universal ball-and-socket joint with motion in all three planes. While many orthoses control abduction/adduction and flexion/extension reasonably well, controlling internal/external rotation is difficult.

HOs are used to treat congenital, dysplastic, traumatic, or degenerative hip conditions (Figure 17-10, *A* to *C*), or after postoperative hip procedures (see Figure 17-10, *D*).[14] Pediatric and adult populations require different orthotic approaches. Pediatric HOs for congenital hip disorders are typically designed to maintain good joint alignment during bone growth. Dysplastic joints present with varying degrees of severity. In the beginning of the disease process, occlusion of blood supply to the head of the femur promotes necrosis. Although revascularization eventually occurs, the bony contouring of the femoral head does not develop normally. Continued weight-bearing stresses increase deformation of the hip joint and can result in permanent disability. Maintaining maximum joint congruency and controlling forces through the hip joints using a variety of HO designs (see Figure 17-10) promotes normal development of the head of femur and acetabulum. As with most HOs, this type of orthotic treatment is temporary.

HOs for adults usually address the effects of joint deterioration. Clients with degenerative conditions are usually placed in HOs that limit range of motion to support and control compromised muscles, prevent dislocation following primary or revision surgery, and decrease pain. In adults who have had a hip replacement surgery, the HO is designed to provide different alignment options as the client progresses through the rehabilitation process. Usually, the hip joint is aligned to maintain 10 to 20 degrees of abduction and allows 0 to 70 degrees of flexion where there is risk of posterior dislocation following surgery.[22] When there is risk of anterior dislocation postoperatively, hip motion is blocked at 40 degrees extension and 70 degrees flexion. Flexion and extension ranges are limited to prevent dislocation while allowing the client sufficient motion to sit and walk. Internal and external rotation control is limited to some degree by "grasping" the soft tissue of the thigh. Proper fitting, adjustment, and donning of the orthosis are critical to maximizing function and benefit. Postoperatively, the HO is usually worn at all times for 3 to 6 months to allow the soft tissue to heal and to serve as a kinesthetic reminder to maintain proper positioning during ADLs. Although recurrent hip dislocation after surgical repair is rare, occasionally on-going external support may be required for complicated procedures, revisions, or poor surgical outcomes.

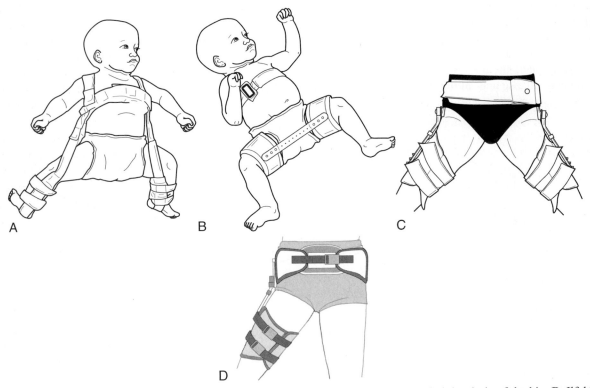

Figure 17-10 Various Hip Orthosis (HO) Designs. A, Pavlik harness used to manage congenital dysplasia of the hip. **B,** Ilfeld orthosis used to manage congenital dysplasia of the hip. **C,** Bilateral hip abduction orthoses with pelvic band. **D,** Postoperative hip abduction orthosis.

Children with spasticity of the hip muscles may develop hip instability and pain, requiring surgical release of the hip adductors, flexors, and internal rotators or more complicated bony osteotomies of the pelvis or femur. HOs used postoperatively in these cases ensure the hips are maintained in an appropriate position for healing while still allowing some small amount of motion to facilitate function. Additionally, HOs are usually equipped with two sets of liners that can be washed daily to eliminate odor and improve hygiene. When the HO is no longer used 24 hours per day to protect the surgical correction, it transitions to a functional orthosis during the day or a positioning orthosis at night.

Clinical Considerations for the Occupational Therapist

After total hip surgery and while wearing an HO, both adult and pediatric clients require training in self-care activities, such as dressing, bathing, toileting, and hygiene. An OT is essential in assisting a client to maintain hip precautions while donning the orthosis. An OT educates the client in the use of adaptive equipment (e.g., a reacher, sock-aid, long handled bath sponge, long handled shoe horn, and raised toilet seat) and may reduce excessive hip motion during hygiene and self-care.

Hip-Knee-Ankle-Foot Orthoses

General Considerations

Hip-knee-ankle-foot orthoses (HKAFOs) encompass all three major lower limb joints and build upon the basic concepts already outlined for KAFOs. HKAFOs provide varying levels of mechanical control (Figure 17-11). Most simply, a unilateral KAFO is attached to a pelvic band with a single axis joint to control rotational alignment of the limb during swing (see Figure 17-11, B). This alignment allows proper positioning of the limb for stance. Bilateral mechanical hip joints and a pelvic/trunk section are used to provide additional control and stability for paraplegic standing and ambulation. HKAFOs may be used for neurologic conditions resulting in severe muscle weakness (see Figure 17-11, A and C). The hip or pelvic section consists of a narrow band, or it may completely enclose the pelvis and trunk with a spinal orthosis attached to the LE orthoses. The amount of bracing of the trunk segment depends on the functional abilities, control, and upper body strength of the client. Hip and knee joints may be locked in extension during standing and walking, and the knees usually are locked.

Standing frames, such as the Parapodium and Swivel Walker,[40] are bilateral HKAFOs mounted to a base plate. These devices are designed to provide support for hands-free standing or limited mobility by swiveling, wherein shifting weight laterally by rocking or rotating the trunk unweights one limb and causes the orthosis to swivel forward on the weight-bearing side. Swivel walkers are only used

effectively on smooth, flat surfaces and provide extremely slow ambulation. Children are prescribed standing frames because standing is believed to provide a stimulus for normal development of bones and bowel and bladder function. In adults, standing is believed to reduce osteoporosis and improve peripheral circulation.

Ambulation with bilateral HKAFOs requires a "swing through" gait pattern assisted by a walker or crutches. The HKAFO is used to lift the whole body from the ground and swing it forward. Variations in this pattern of ambulation are known as "swing-to" and "drag-to" gait. HKAFOs are used for daily activities and therapeutic intervention programs. High energy costs of these type of gaits may prohibit use of this orthosis for all ADLs, and wheelchair mobility may be a better option for some clients.[7,45]

More complex HKAFO designs facilitate a reciprocal gait pattern so that extension of one limb promotes flexion of the contralateral limb, and vice versa (see Figure 17-11, D). These Reciprocating gait orthoses (RGOs) employ a linkage between the hip joints either by interlinked cables or a posterior, pivoting metal bar. RGOs are used in pediatric and adult populations, primarily for clients with flail bilateral lower limb involvement. Good upper extremity strength and adequate trunk control are prerequisites for RGOs because the main propulsive forces for this form of ambulation come from the arms via crutches or similar assistive devices. Reciprocal gait is more cosmetic and stable than swing through gait. However, a greater level of training is required to ensure effective ambulation and the complexity of orthotic design increases the need for maintenance. Although RGOs are used effectively by children with growth and body mass increases, it becomes more energy efficient to use a wheelchair than to ambulate with an RGO. Hence the use of RGOs is lower among adults.[7]

HKAFOs are commonly prescribed for clients with spina bifida or spinal cord injury, or for any client presenting with a flail lower limb and limited hip control. Individual height, weight, strength, endurance, motivation, physical assistance requirements, donning abilities, and psychosocial situations are evaluated with regard to the potential success of the orthotic program. Upright weight-bearing is believed to improve cardiopulmonary function, bowel and bladder function, circulation, and bone density.[19,28,33] Children benefit from the social interaction with their peers and can alternate with wheelchair mobility as needed. Almost all adult clients with traumatic spinal cord injury retain the desire to walk as a primary goal throughout their rehabilitation program.

Clinical Considerations for the Occupational Therapist

HKAFO systems require much higher levels of energy expenditure, upper extremity strength, and endurance than many clients are able to maintain on a regular basis. Although it may be apparent to members of the interdisciplinary rehabilitation team that the client achieves higher

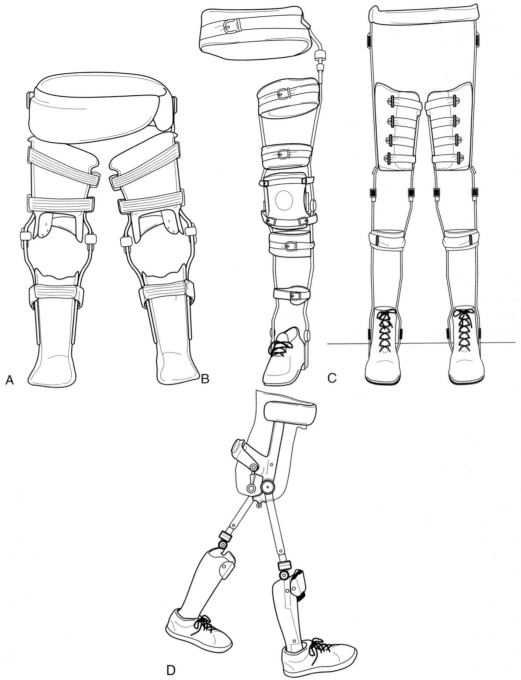

Figure 17-11 Various Hip-Knee-Ankle-Foot Orthosis (HKAFO) Designs. A, Bilateral thermoplastic HKAFOs. **B,** Unilateral double-upright HKAFO. **C,** Bilateral double-upright HKAFOs. **D,** Reciprocating gait orthosis (RGO).

levels of functional independence when using a wheelchair for mobility, the client may prefer to focus on ambulation as a primary goal. Adding a pelvic component, hip joint, knee joint, or ankle control to an orthosis increases the difficulty of dressing and undressing. Difficulty with dressing tasks is magnified when the client is at work or school, and it will require loose-fitting clothing and adaptive strategies for donning and doffing clothing. In addition, the OT provides consultation for proper seating for toileting, desk work, and transportation.

Summary

An interdisciplinary approach is important for all aspects of rehabilitation care including LE orthotic management. The OT should confer with the CO in the development of the LE orthotic prescription to ensure that the orthosis addresses the client's occupational goals. Such goals include but not limited to the ability to don/doff the orthosis successfully and integrate of the LE orthosis into ADLs. LE orthoses address a large number of issues from pain management to mobility.

Regardless of the goals it is important that the health care team have a working knowledge of the biomechanical principles necessary to achieve the intervention goals. LE orthotic management is unique when compared to the upper extremity in that it often requires more robust designs and materials due to the magnitude of the forces associated with weight-bearing activity and ambulation. Sound understanding of normal gait is important when assessing a client with mobility deficiencies. Knowing whether a gait deviation is primary or secondary (compensatory) is important to determine the ultimate design of the orthotic intervention. Once the specific biomechanical deficiencies are identified, the practitioner has a wide variety of orthotic designs available to address client's specific needs from relatively simple FOs to the reciprocating gait orthosis, which spans all major joints associated with LE function.

Review Questions

1. What health care professional provides custom orthotic services to persons with LE impairments?
2. What are four clinical objectives of a LE orthosis?
3. What are the major joints that contribute to lower limb function?
4. What are the three key biomechanical principles of LE orthotic management?
5. What are the basic differences between low-temperature and high-temperature thermoplastic materials?
6. What are the seven subphases of gait?
7. What is the main distinction between a primary and secondary gait deviation?
8. What is the role of the OT in the development of the orthotic intervention program?
9. What skin inspection techniques are taught to the person with insensate feet?
10. What are two control options for the ankle joint of an articulated AFO?
11. What are two design parameters that can be integrated into a KO to prevent migration and to ensure proper alignment of the anatomical and mechanical joint axes?
12. What are the four main types of knee joints used in KAFOs?
13. What type of training would a person wearing a postoperative HO require?
14. What clinical presentation would most benefit from a RGO?

References

1. Bowker P: The biomechanics of orthoses. In Bowker P, Condie D, Bader D, et al.: *Biomechanical basis of orthotic management*, Oxford, 1993, Butterworth-Heinemann.
2. Bunch W, Keagy R: *Principles of orthotic treatment*, St Louis, 1976, Mosby.
3. Condie D: International Organization for Standardization (ISO) terminology. In Hsu J, Michael J, Fisk J, editors: *American Academy of Orthopaedic Surgeons atlas of orthoses and assistive devices*, Philadelphia, 2008, Mosby, pp 3–7.
4. Condie E, Campbell J, et al.: *Report of a consensus conference on the orthotic management of stroke patients*, Copenhagen, Denmark, 2004, International Society for Prosthetics and Orthotics.
5. Dibello T, Kelley C, et al.: Orthoses for persons with postpolio sequelae. In Hsu J, Michael J, Fisk J, editors: *American Academy of Orthopaedic Surgeons atlas of orthoses and assistive devices*, Philadelphia, 2008, Mosby, pp 335–341.
6. Fatone S, Orthotics: In Akay M, editor: *Wiley encyclopedia of biomedical engineering*, Hoboken, NJ, 2006, John Wiley & Sons, Inc.
7. Fatone S: A review of the literature pertaining to KAFOs and HKAFOs for ambulation, *J Prosthet Orthot* 18(3):137–168, 2006.
8. Fatone S, Hansen AH: A model to predict the effect of ankle joint misalignment on calf band movement in ankle-foot orthoses, *Prosthet Orthot Int* 31(1):76–87, 2007.
9. Fish D, Kosta C: Walking impediments and gait inefficiencies in the CVA patient, *J Prosthet Orthot* 11(2):33–37, 1999.
10. Gard S, Childress D: The effect of pelvic list on the vertical displacement of the trunk during normal walking, *Gait Posture* 5(3):233–238, 1997.
11. Gard S, Childress D: What determines the vertical displacement of the body during normal walking? *J Prosthet Orthot* 13(3):64–67, 2001.
12. Gard S, Fatone S: Biomechanics of lower limb function and gait. In Condie E, Campbell J, Martina J, editors: *Report of a consensus conference on the orthotic management of stroke patients*, Copenhagen, Denmark, 2004, International Society for Prosthetics and Orthotics, pp 55–63.
13. Gard SA, Childress DS: The influence of stance-phase knee flexion on the vertical displacement of the trunk during normal walking, *Arch Phys Med Rehabil* 80(1):26–32, 1999.
14. Goldberg B, Hsu J: *Atlas of orthoses and assistive devices*, St Louis, 1997, Mosby.
15. Greene P, McMahon T: Reflex stiffness of man's anti-gravity muscles during kneebends while carrying extra weights, *J Biomech* 12(12):881–891, 1979.
16. Hanada E, Kerrigan DC: Energy consumption during level walking with arm and knee immobilized, *Arch Phys Med Rehabil* 82(9):1251–1254, 2001.
17. Hsu J, Michael J, Fisk J: *American Academy of Orthopedic Surgeons' atlas of orthoses and assistive devices*, Philadelphia, PA, 2008, Mosby Elsevier.
18. Kaufman KR, Irby SE, et al.: Energy-efficient knee-ankle foot orthosis: a case study, *J Prosthet Orthot* 8(3):79, 1996.
19. Kraft G, Lehmann J: Orthotics, *Phys Med Rehabil Clin N Am* 3(1):1–241, 1992.
20. Lafortune M, Lake M: Human pendulum approach to simulate and quantify locomotor impact loading, *J Biomech* 28(9):1111–1114, 1995.
21. Lage KJ, White SC, Yack HJ: The effects of unilateral knee immobilization on lower extremity gait mechanics, *Med Sci Sports Exerc* 27(1):8–14, 1995.
22. Lima D: Orthoses in Total Joint Replacement. In Hsu J, Michael J, Fisk J, editors: *American Academy of Orthopedic Surgeons' atlas of orthoses and assistive devices*, Philadelphia, PA, 2008, Mosby Elsevier, pp 335–341.
23. Maillardet F: The swing phase of locomotion, *Imeche* 6(3):67–75, 1977.
24. Margaria R: Biomechanics of human locomotion. In Margaria R, editor: *Biomechanics and energetics of muscular exercise*, Oxford, 1976, Oxford University Press, pp 67–144.

25. Mattsson E, Brostrom LA: The increase in energy cost of walking with an immobilized knee or an unstable ankle, *Scand J Rehabil Med* 22(1):51–53, 1990.

26. McCollough 3rd NC, Fryer CM, Glancy J: A new approach to patient analysis for orthotic prescription—part I: the lower extremity, *Artif Limbs* 14(2):68–80, 1970.

27. McMahon TA, Valiant G, Frederick EC: Groucho running, *J Appl Physiol* 62(6):2326–2337, 1987.

28. Merritt JL, Yoshida MK: Knee-ankle-foot orthoses: indications and practical applications of long leg braces, *Physical Medicine and Rehabilitation: State of the Art Reviews* 14(3):239–422, 2000.

29. Michael J: Lower limb orthoses. In Goldberg B, Hsu J, editors: *American Academy of Orthopaedic Surgeons' atlas of orthoses and assistive devices*, St Louis, 1997, Mosby.

30. Mojica M: Foot Orthoses. In Hsu J, Michael J, Fisk J, editors: *American Academy of Orthopaedic Surgeons' atlas of orthoses and assistive devices*, Philadelphia, PA, 2008, Mosby Elsevier, pp 335–341.

31. Murray MP, Kory RC, Clarkson BH, et al.: Comparison of free and fast speed walking patterns of normal men, *Am J Phys Med* 45(1):8–24, 1966.

32. Nack J, Phillips R: Shock absorption, *Clin Pod Med Surg* 7(2):391–397, 1990.

33. Nene A: Paraplegic locomotion: a review, *Spinal Cord* 34(9):507–524, 1996.

34. Nolan KJ, Yarossi M: Preservation of the first rocker is related to increases in gait speed in individuals with hemiplegia and AFO, *Clinical Biomechanics* 26(6):655–660, 2011.

35. Nottrodt J, Charteris J, et al.: The effects of speed on pelvic oscillations in the horizontal plane during level walking, *J Hum Mov Studies* 8(1):27–40, 1982.

36. Otto JP: The stance control orthosis: has its time finally come? *The O&P Edge*. (website) http://www.oandp.com/articles/2008-03_02.asp Accessed March 15, 2014.

37. Perry J: Kinesiology of lower extremity bracing, *Clinical Orthopedics* 102:18–31, 1974.

38. Perry J, Burnfield J: *Gait analysis: normal and pathological function*, Thorofare, NJ, 2010, Slack Inc.

39. Ralston H: Effects of immobilization of various body segments on the energy cost of human locomotion, *Ergonomics* 8(Suppl):53–60, 1965.

40. Rose GK, Henshaw JT: A swivel walker for paraplegics: medical and technical considerations, *Biomed Eng* 7(9-2):420–425, 1972.

41. Snyder RD, Powers CM, Fontaine C, et al.: The effect of five prosthetic feet on the gait and loading of the sound limb in dysvascular below-knee amputees, *J Rehabil Res Devel* 32(4):309–315, 1995.

42. Stills ML: Thermoformed ankle-foot orthoses, *Orthotics Prosthetics* 29(4):41–51, 1975.

43. Sutherland D, Kaufman K, et al.: Kinematics of normal human walking. In Rose J, Gamble J, editors: *Human walking*, Baltimore, MD, 1994, Williams & Wilkins, pp 23–44.

44. Waters RL, Campbell J, Thomas L, et al.: Energy costs of walking in lower-extremity plaster casts, *J Bone Joint Surg Am* 64(6):896–899, 1982.

45. Waters RL, Mulroy S: The energy expenditure of normal and pathologic gait, *Gait Posture* 9(3):207–231, 1999.

46. Wolters B: Knee orthoses for sports-related disorders. In Hsu J, Michael J, Fisk J, editors: *American Academy of Orthopaedic Surgeons' atlas of orthoses and assistive devices*, Philadelphia, PA, 2008, Mosby Elsevier, pp 335–341.

47. Zissimopoulos A, Fatone S, Gard SA: Biomechanical and energetic effects of a stance-control orthotic knee joint, *J Rehabil Res Dev* 44(4):503–514, 2007.

APPENDIX 17-1   CASE STUDIES

CASE STUDY 17-1*

Read the following scenario, and answer the questions based on information in this chapter.

A 67-year-old male sustained an acute cerebrovascular accident (CVA) to the right hemisphere of his brain and now presents with left sided hemiparesis. The client complains of difficulty ambulating, standing for long periods of time, and performing his activities of daily living (ADLs). During ambulation the client's left lower extremity (LE) presents with paralytic equinus during swing phase, lateral forefoot initial contact, and asymmetrical step lengths.

1. What are some of the potential roles an occupational therapist (OT) may play in the intervention of this client?
2. What intervention goals can be addressed for this client using a LE orthosis?
3. What biomechanical principles might be implemented in the design of this client's LE orthosis?
4. What type of LE orthosis might this client benefit from?

*See Appendix A for the answer key for Case Study 17-1.

CASE STUDY 17-2

A 62-year-old male client has a diagnosis of type II diabetes mellitus and associated peripheral neuropathy. The client complains of callousing on the plantar aspect of metatarsophalangeal (MTP) joints and tightness wearing the Oxford style shoes he typically wears. On clinical exam the client presents with clawed toes, atrophy of the intrinsic muscles of the foot, and depressed medial longitudinal arches during weight-bearing. Results from a monofilament assessment of the plantar aspect of the foot confirmed peripheral neuropathy. LE strength and active range of motion are within normal limits at all major joints. The client receives bilateral, custom fabricated, full-length accommodative foot orthoses (FOs) manufactured from multi-durometer foams and extra-depth footwear to accommodate the claw toe deformity. The multi-durometer foam construction allows for distribution of forces throughout the plantar aspect of the foot, which reduces peak plantar pressures and minimizes the risk of plantar ulceration. The extra depth footwear allows for needed adjustments of volumetric changes of the foot and accommodates the thickness of multidurometer FOs.

1. How might neuropathy negatively impact this client?
2. What benefits do extra-depth footwear have?
3. Why was the client provided accommodative instead of corrective foot orthoses?

CASE STUDY 17-3

A 62-year-old male client is 2 weeks post right total knee arthroplasty. During the surgery, he sustained an iatrogenic peroneal nerve lesion at the level of the fibular head. He complains of difficulty walking and is dragging his toe. The client is otherwise healthy and has no edema. On clinical exam, the client presents within functional limits for bilateral passive range of motion at the midfoot, ankle, subtalar, hip, and knee joints. A manual muscle test reveals he has 0/5 dorsiflexion and eversion. He has sensory loss over the dorsal aspect of the foot and lateral compartment of the leg. While ambulating, the client exhibits secondary compensations with hip hiking during the swing phase on the affected limb and initial contact with the lateral forefoot. The client receives a custom thermoplastic ankle-foot orthosis (AFO) with a flexible ankle trimline fabricated from ⁵⁄₃₂-inch (4 mm) copolymer (similar to Figure 17-5, *C*). Resistance to plantar flexion from the AFO coupled with the full-length foot plate provides the client with improved swing phase clearance. The foot plate eliminates the need for compensatory hip hiking and encourages a normal heel strike at initial contact. A flexible ankle trimline allows the tibia to progress forward during stance, and the thermoplastic design allows for a lightweight orthosis that can be readily changed from shoe to shoe with equal heel heights.

1. Why does the client present with both dorsiflexion and eversion weakness?
2. How would the client's gait be affected if he were provided a solid ankle AFO instead of the orthosis described above?

CASE STUDY 17-4

A 54-year-old female client has right lateral compartment osteoarthritis with associated genu valgum. The client complains of knee pain during weight-bearing activity that increases proportionately with activity level. Clinical evaluation reveals bilateral genu valgum and palpable swelling over the lateral joint line of the right knee. The client receives a functional knee orthosis (KO) to unload the lateral joint compartment of the right knee. The KO's three-point force system (acting through straps in the coronal plane) applies medially directed forces at the proximal and distal aspects. The KO's laterally directed force at the medial femoral condyle results in unloading of the lateral compartment of the knee joint. Polycentric knee joints are utilized to match the natural movements of the knee. Composite construction of the articulating and structural components ensures that the orthosis is structurally sound yet lightweight.

1. Why are polycentric articulations most appropriate when providing a knee orthosis?
2. What is the primary biomechanical objective for the provided orthosis?

CASE STUDY 17-5

A 47-year-old client has paralytic post-polio syndrome. The client complains of severe left knee pain while walking. The client was diagnosed with acute polio at 3 years of age and has noted increased symptoms of weakness with age. Clinical examination reveals that she has a 15 degree plantar flexion contracture and 30 degrees of knee hyperextension during loading response. There is laxity of the right knee in the sagittal plane and palpable swelling throughout the popliteal fossa. Sensation, vascular function, and proprioception are within normal limits. With ambulation the client exhibits secondary hip hiking during swing, initial contact with the forefoot, and severe hyperextension during stance. The client receives a thermoplastic knee-ankle-foot orthosis (KAFO) with posterior offset knee joints, solid ankle, and metatarsal length foot plate. The thermoplastic KAFO design accommodates the client's plantar flexion and knee hyperextension. The design allows the weight line to pass anterior to the anatomical knee and posterior offset knee joints. The posterior offset knee joints create a knee extension moment at both joints throughout stance phase. The KAFO serves to limit additional knee hyperextension and increases stability. The three-quarter length foot plate facilitates heel off in pre-swing, allowing the transition to swing phase.

1. How is the sensation and proprioception affected in a client with paralytic post-polio syndrome?
2. How would your recommendation change if the client presented with a 10 degree knee flexion contracture instead of knee hyperextension?

CASE STUDY 17-6

A 62-year-old client is seen in the post anesthesia recovery unit after a total hip arthroplasty revision. The client has a history of hip joint subluxation. The physician would like the hip to be maintained in a flexed and abducted position. The client has normal anatomy and a thin dressing placed at the incision anterior to the greater trochanter. The client receives a prefabricated hip orthosis (HO) with an adjustable range of motion joint. This articulation enables the orthotist to set the hip joint to a fixed abduction angle while allowing some flexion for ADLs. The orthotic alignment is intended to encourage proper healing of the soft tissues surrounding the hip prosthesis. Although the HO provides mechanical control of the hip joint, it is imperative that the OT reinforce hip joint precautions and facilitate the integration of the orthosis into ADLs.

1. Why would the physician request a flexed and abducted alignment?
2. What activities might the patient have difficulty achieving given the motion limitations the hip abduction orthosis is set to?

CASE STUDY 17-7

A 6-year-old child diagnosed with a low thoracic myelomeningocele lesion presents with absent sensation and motor function of bilateral LEs. The intervention goal is an orthosis that facilities static standing and the ability to ambulate in as normal manner as possible. The child has access to both pediatric physical therapists and OTs at school and has excellent upper limb strength and dexterity. The child is provided a custom reciprocating gait orthosis (RGO) because it facilitates static standing and step-over-step ambulation. In order to take advantage of this orthosis, it is imperative that the child have access to therapists to develop the skills needed to successfully integrate the orthosis into ADLs and have the requisite training to utilize crutches or other assistive devices necessary to successfully ambulate with the orthosis.

1. Why couldn't this client be provided ankle foot orthoses instead of the relatively cumbersome RGO?
2. What advantage does the RGO have over a hip knee ankle foot orthosis (HKAFO) with locked hips, knees and fixed ankles?

CHAPTER 18

Upper Extremity Prosthetics

Kris M. Vacek

Key Terms

biofeedback machine
body-powered prosthesis
componentry
contralateral limb
electrodes
externally-powered prosthesis
grip force
harness
hook rubbers
myoelectric prosthesis
nerve entrapment
overuse syndrome
phantom pain
phantom sensation
residual limb
socket

Chapter Objectives

1. Differentiate between various levels of upper extremity amputation as it relates to function.
2. Describe the various causes of an upper extremity amputation.
3. Differentiate the roles of the prosthetic team members.
4. Explain the unique role of the occupational therapist as a team member in upper extremity prosthetic rehabilitation.
5. Identify the characteristics of various upper extremity prosthetic devices.
6. Identify advantages and disadvantages of various upper extremity prosthetic devices.
7. Describe the phases of rehabilitation from an occupational therapy (OT) perspective.
8. Provide examples for OT intervention.
9. Discuss common psychological and social aspects of clients with amputations.
10. Discuss strategies for marketing upper extremity prosthetics specialty area to the wider community

Ray is a 52-year-old male who works in a meat processing plant. Ray's right, dominant hand was caught in a meat grinder. The surgeon who was scheduled to perform the right hand amputation called the Department of Occupational Therapy to have a therapist quickly consult on the best level of amputation for function. After the amputation, Ray was seen by an occupational therapist for pre-prosthetic training.

Orthotics and prosthetics are closely interrelated fields. This chapter serves as a resource for those therapists who serve this historically underserved population. There are approximately 2 million US people who are living with a limb loss.[37] Approximately 185,000 amputations occur in the United States each year.[37] The incidence of upper extremity amputation is lower than the incidence of lower extremity amputation (1:4 ratio).[4]

Approximately 50% of individuals with amputations are fitted with prostheses.[36] Of the 50% fitted with prostheses, only half actually wear the device. Experts cite numerous reasons for this trend.[46] Fit and prosthetic training appear to be the most salient factors that affect prosthetic wear.[10] Prostheses are often heavy and awkward to use. If the fit is not tolerable, or if the potential wearer has not been properly trained to use the device, the prosthesis may end up on the closet shelf. The purpose of an upper limb prosthesis depends on the client's goals. However, most prostheses assist in restoring body image and cosmesis and replace as much function of the limb as possible.[50] In conjunction with the health care team, the role of the prosthetist is to provide well-fitting prosthetic devices. It is the role of the occupational therapist to assist individuals to become independent users of their devices.

Unfortunately, only a small number of health care providers have extensive knowledge of the rehabilitation of the person with an upper extremity amputation. Typically therapists may encounter few individuals with upper extremity amputations. Thus, it is difficult to remain abreast of the current prosthetic trends and technologic developments that affect how therapists promote the maximal level of independence for clients with upper extremity amputations. However, occupational therapists can make a substantial difference in the lives of individuals with amputations if they possess knowledge of the various factors that impact the life of a person with an amputation.

Therapists who treat persons with orthotic needs will naturally be called upon to provide services to persons with upper extremity amputations. Thus, it is important for therapists to know to how access the information needed to provide occupational therapy (OT) to individuals with upper extremity amputations.

This chapter addresses the following content:
- Reasons for amputations
- General knowledge of upper extremity amputations and their impact on function
- Roles of team members
- Various prosthetic options and components
- Goals for OT intervention throughout the prosthetic rehabilitation process
- Psychological and social issues of clients with amputations
- Upper extremity prostheses for children
- Marketing strategies to increase prosthetic referrals

Causes of Upper Extremity Amputations

The causes of upper extremity amputations differ from lower extremity amputations. Lower extremity amputations are largely a result of vascular disease. The majority of upper extremity amputations result from trauma (69%) and a majority of these are due to war causalities[19,21] with other causes attributed to disease (27%) or congenital malformation (4%).[19] It is estimated that the number of individuals living with limb loss will more than double by 2050. This is largely due to the rise of vascular disorders.[19,52]

Amputation Levels and the Impact on Function and Satisfaction

Figure 18-1 provides an outline of the various amputation levels, along with their abbreviations. Older terminology included above elbow (AE) and below elbow (BE). It is believed this newer terminology is more appropriate. Newer terminology cites the anatomical level of amputation. For example, AE is called *transhumeral,* and BE is called *transradial* or *transradial-ulnar.* The level of amputation directly impacts function.

With levels of amputation, there is an inverse relationship between the amputation level and function. The more distal the amputation, the greater the functional ability of the extremity remains. Consequently, less is demanded of the prosthesis with increasingly distal amputations.[28] For

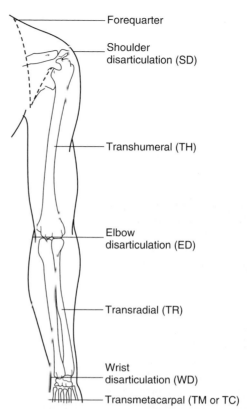

Figure 18-1 Levels of upper extremity amputation.

example, an individual who has an amputation at the midhumeral level may be functionally able to use shoulder internal and external rotation along with other shoulder motions. However, the individual lacks the functional motions of elbow flexion/extension and forearm supination/pronation, causing functional limitations. Regardless of level, prostheses in essence help compensate for the lost motions, but limitations remain. For example, when an individual with a midhumeral amputation wants to receive money from a cashier, more effort is required because of the functional limitations in motion. Compare this to someone whose limb loss is at the transradial level where often times some forearm motion is retained, allowing greater functional capacity of the upper extremity. More specifically, positioning and locking the elbow in flexion is necessary. Next, the person manually rotates the terminal device (TD) to the palm-up position with the sound side. Finally, the person is ready to perform the act of receiving the money. Conversely, an individual with an amputation at the wrist level is functionally able to pronate and supinate, flex and extend the elbow, and retain full shoulder function in the completion of activities of daily living (ADLs). The ability to pronate and supinate serves as a substantial advantage. Supination and pronation enables the person with the amputation to turn the prosthetic hand palm up as if to receive money from a cashier without the substitution movements of shoulder external rotation.

Whether or not an individual chooses to wear a prosthesis, the level of amputation directly may impact satisfaction. In a survey conducted in 2006, 93% of 109 respondents with an upper extremity amputation reported owning a prosthesis, whereas 12% of those respondents reported they did not wear it regularly.[4] A majority of those surveyed reported satisfaction with their prosthesis, but one-third reported dissatisfaction with it.[4] Contributing factors to dissatisfaction specifically include socket fit, comfort level, appearance, weight, and ease of use. Additionally, one-fourth of those surveyed received therapy, and the average number of visits was 25. Twenty percent of those who did not receive therapy reported cost as the leading factor preventing them from receiving the services they needed.[4]

The Team Members

The team treating clients with amputations must have knowledge in upper extremity prosthetics in order to facilitate success. The key team members consist of the client with the amputation, the prosthetist, and the therapist. Other important members include the surgeon, case manager, psychologist, and the insurer/reimbursement source. A team approach combines expertise and experience, creating a synergy of professionalism, with team members working together and promoting the maximal level of independence for the individual. The primary goal of therapy is to provide the individual with the proper tools and techniques to regain independence; however, OT is only one dimension of the entire process. The best results in upper extremity rehabilitation include interdisciplinary teamwork.[9]

The Client

The most important member of the team is the person with the amputation. Throughout the assessment and intervention process, several key factors of the client are considered including specific abilities, characteristics, or beliefs.[3] Factors such as the level of amputation, musculature, skin condition, range of motion, ability to learn, motivation, and values all contribute to the degree of participation in occupations.

The client's goals, desires, and needs establish the foundation for which the team develops the intervention plan. Clients' priorities for rehabilitation vary. It is important to ensure that clients are realistic with their expectations and are well educated on the prosthetic options available to them. Education can come from both the prosthetist and occupational therapist. The prosthetist discusses the various prosthetic options available, whereas the occupational therapist discusses the functional aspects of each device. This process is important because it helps the key team members formulate the individual intervention plan necessary for successful prosthetic delivery and use.[35] For example, an individual with a transhumeral amputation who works full-time in a factory and desires to return to work will have varying needs from an individual with a transradial amputation who is a home maker. The type of prosthesis selected differs, depending on a precise analysis of the client's desire to participate in meaningful occupations.[3]

The Prosthetist

Orthotics and prosthetics are closely interrelated fields. Forty-one percent of American Board for Certification (ABC) certified practitioners hold credentials in both orthotics and prosthetics, and fewer practitioners specialize in upper extremity prosthetic fabrication.[2] Since the incidence of upper extremity amputations is less than lower extremity amputations, it is important for the prosthetist to have a background in fabricating and fitting upper extremity prostheses. Prosthetists have knowledge of the technology and prosthetic **componentry** available. Technology for upper extremity prosthetics has significantly evolved since 1976 due to research and development in related technology, such as cell phones, computers, and video games.[13] Prosthetists are experts when it comes to fit and fabrication. Upon prosthetic delivery, prosthetists introduce, educate, and orient the clients about the controls and functions, all of which should be reinforced by the occupational therapist. In an ideal setting, prosthetists and therapists collaborate throughout the entire intervention process from assessment of prosthetic needs to return to occupational performance.

The Occupational Therapist

Unfortunately, only a small number of therapists have extensive knowledge of the rehabilitation of the person with an upper extremity amputation. In many practice settings, therapists rarely treat clients with upper extremity amputations. Thus, it is difficult to remain abreast of the current prosthetic and technologic developments. Such advances affect how therapists promote the maximal level of independence for these clients. However, occupational therapists can make a substantial difference in individuals with amputations when they possess knowledge of prosthetic intervention.

Occupational therapists' expertise is function. Therapists typically work with clients throughout the entire prosthetic rehabilitation process. Each phase of recovery presents its own challenges and demands. Without proper therapy, the benefits of prosthetic use may be limited. For example, the therapist may see the client immediately following surgery to address postsurgical issues, including pain, edema, wound healing, and shaping of the residual limb. The occupational therapist plays an important role as the client explores the various prosthetic devices. Finally, the therapist provides prosthetic rehabilitation upon delivery of the prosthesis and assists the client achievement of occupational performance.

The therapist reinforces and builds on residual movement, developing functional applications of the prosthesis to address the distinct ADL (e.g., brushing teeth) and instrumental ADL (e.g., driving) of each individual.[48] The therapist is responsible for ensuring that the client knows how to clean and maintain the prosthesis. In addition, the therapist provides opportunities for the client to practice using the prosthesis in specific daily activities. The therapist focuses on bilateral activities. Often, after amputation the individual

Table 18-1 Advantages and Disadvantages of Prosthetic Options

PROSTHETIC OPTION	ADVANTAGES	DISADVANTAGES
No prosthesis	Maintain full proprioception and sensation	Limited functional ability Difficult to perform bimanual tasks
Passive prosthesis	Light weight Minimal (if any) harnessing No cables; low maintenance	Prosthesis has no prehension abilities Difficult to perform bimanual tasks
Body-powered prosthesis	Heavy-duty construction and function Reduced maintenance cost Proprioception	Restrictive/uncomfortable harness Poor cosmesis Restrictive functional work area Limited grip force
Externally-powered prosthesis	Unlimited work area Function cosmetic restoration Increased grip force Harness system reduced or absent Increased comfort More modern, high-tech appeal Interchangeable components Development of technology to provide for individual custom fabrication	Battery maintenance Increased weight Susceptible to damage from moisture Increased cost

becomes successful in performing some ADLs unilaterally. Thus, therapy must begin early in the rehabilitation process to facilitate use of the prosthesis in bilateral activities.

Initial prosthetic training begins with a reorientation to the prosthesis and basic open-and-close control. Training then includes controlled grasp, such as opening the close control in small increments to grasp small items and then more fully to grasp larger items. Training emphasizes grasping objects of varied texture and density to be handled. Sessions incorporate work on prehension and timing of release. Functional and appropriate tasks are encouraged and require the client to use the prosthesis for gross and fine motor activities. Training also emphasizes tasks to achieve all of these components in a variety of planes.[30,39] With the combined efforts of the team members, the appropriate prosthetic components are chosen so that the individual can achieve goals through therapy, practice, and education.

Prosthetic Options

A prosthetic device cannot mechanically duplicate the amount of function, reliability, and cosmesis that the human upper extremity naturally provides. However, prostheses can improve functional abilities. In order to provide the appropriate prosthesis, a fundamental understanding of the components is necessary. Health care providers must continually stay abreast of prosthetic developments.

Generally, four categories of prosthetic options are available for the person with an upper extremity amputation. The options include (1) no prosthesis; (2) a passive (semi-active), cosmetic prosthesis; (3) a cable-driven body-powered prosthesis; and (4) an externally-powered, electrically-controlled prosthesis with either myoelectric sensors or specialized switches. Table 18-1 outlines the pros and cons of each prosthetic option.

No Prosthesis

Wearing no prosthesis is one approach, and for some individuals it is the best option. For example, an individual may not be able to tolerate the prosthesis for reasons such as residual limb hypersensitivity, soft tissue adhesions, and excessive scarring.[8] Reasons documented in literature for prosthetic rejection include limited usefulness, weight, and residual limb and socket discomfort.[34,51] Individuals choosing not to wear prostheses may find advantages and disadvantages with this option, which are found in Table 18-1.

Advantages of no prosthesis include increased proprioceptive and sensory input. Disadvantages include limited functional ability, bimanual task difficulty, and the potential for development of **overuse syndrome** and **nerve entrapment** in the **contralateral limb**.[42] Some individuals do not wear prostheses because (1) they do not know of their options, (2) they had a negative first prosthetic experience, (3) they lack funds, and (4) they are reluctant to undergo surgery for a prosthetic fit and reduction of hypersensitivity.[4]

Passive Prosthesis (Semi-Active)

A passive prosthesis option is common for individuals who have had amputation distal to the elbow in that they may maintain elbow flexion and extension and forearm pronation and supination. In this case, the obvious purpose is cosmetic. However, a passive prosthesis provides some degree of function. A passive prosthesis has many benefits, including its light weight, minimal (if any) harnessing, no cables, and low maintenance. Disadvantages include lack of prehensile abilities and difficulty in performing some bimanual tasks. Functionally, the digits of a passive prosthesis can be adjusted to assist with activities, such as carrying a purse or a document or operating the gearshift in an automobile.[33]

Body-Powered Prosthesis

The **body-powered prosthesis** is sturdy and allows for prehension. Body-powered upper limb prostheses are actuated by body motion, which generates tension in a cable. The cable courses from a shoulder harness through a housing to a prosthetic component, such as a hook or elbow. In other words, the active movements of the shoulder and arm cause the tension in the cable to open and close the hand or hand-like component (hook) as shown in Figure 18-2. Therapists help individuals with the amputation learn the names of the basic components, such as the figure-eight harness, cable, elbow unit, wrist unit, and TD.

Benefits of a body-powered prosthesis include its heavy-duty function and construction, decreased maintenance cost, and increased proprioceptive input. Disadvantages may include the restrictive uncomfortable harness, potential for nerve entrapment or compression, decreased cosmetic appearance, restricted functional work area (Figure 18-3), and limited **grip force** (see Table 18-1). Body-powered TDs generally weigh less than the externally-powered prostheses because they lack the heavy motors and circuitry placed within them to operate the myoelectric signals.

The Harness

The purpose of the **harness** is to suspend the prosthesis on the **residual limb.** It transmits force from the body to the prosthesis for independent operation of the prosthetic components.[36] The body-powered prosthesis always requires harnessing. There are two primary types of harness: a figure-eight and a chest strap. The figure-eight harness passes over the shoulder, across the back, and under the contralateral axilla. "The ring lies flat in the back, inferior to C7 and just to the sound side of the center of the spine."[46]

The standard figure-eight shoulder harness for the upper extremity has an axilla loop on the sound side that is commonly uncomfortable and can cause numbness and nerve damage.[15] The chest strap offers an alternative method of harnessing. It travels across the back, under the contralateral axilla, and across the chest. It is important that the harness, either figure-eight or chest strap, be tight enough to activate the TD without excessive effort and loose enough

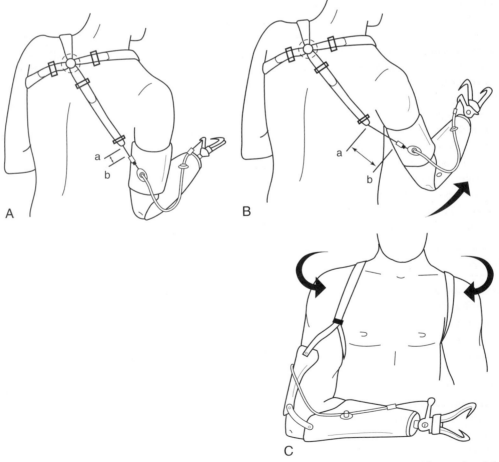

Figure 18-2 Body motions used to transmit force to terminal device (TD). **A,** Glenohumeral flexion. **B,** Bi-scapular abduction. **C,** Scapular adduction/retraction.

to be comfortable and allow freedom of movement of both arms and shoulders.

Long-term wear and inappropriate fit may cause discomfort or physical damage. The harness has been found to limit the functional work envelope, which is the space in front of the person who is able to use the prosthesis successfully for functional tasks. Harness systems limit successful prehension when the TD is outside the functional work area. With the body-powered prosthesis, function is limited above the head, behind the back, and near the ground, primarily because of the restricting harness (see Figure 18-3). The prosthesis functions as a result of the ability to move in these planes.

Discomfort and neurologic and musculoskeletal disorders can result from inefficient harness design[14] and long-term wear. After years of wearing a harness, the axilla of the sound side experiences increased force and pressure to operate the prosthesis repetitively throughout the day. This can result in neurologic damage. A strong case can be made for providing a myoelectric or externally-powered prosthesis that either eliminates or reduces the harnessing. This prevents the risk of long-term nerve damage on the sound side.

The prosthetist is responsible for fabrication of the harness, and the therapist occasionally may make minor adjustments to improve function. Sometimes several harness options are attempted to find the type of system that best fits the amputee. It is often a trial-and-error process. Another important factor is the awareness of the increased workload in the remaining arm, which may produce symptoms ranging from minor aches to serious conditions, such as nerve entrapment and overuse syndrome.[26]

The Socket

The **socket** is the part of the prosthesis that intimately fits over the individual's residual limb. It is the connection between the prosthesis and the individual's body. The socket is fabricated from an exact mold of the residual limb, and it is fabricated from various types of laminate or thermoplastic material. Development of high-temperature rigid plastic materials has made it possible to have total contact on the skin and allow decreased weight and increased durability. The use of carbon graphite and the introduction of flexible thermoplastics are more comfortable, lighter, and durable and have made soft sockets with windows possible. The prosthetist makes modifications over bony prominences and areas susceptible to torque and shear forces.[5] Typically, three to four sockets will be fabricated before the final one is delivered.

Intimate socket fit provides a stable foundation of support necessary to transfer forces from the TD. It provides evenly distributed pressure on the residual limb, which prevents skin breakdown or pressure sores. In the last decade, a multitude of design innovations have been incorporated, which have resulted in developing better comfort, suspension, stability, and range of motion. The new fitting techniques and socket designs appear to be more efficient for force of transmission and motion capture and more functionally consistent than traditional sockets.[1] Occasionally, the prosthetist instructs the individual to wear the socket before all components are attached. This increases wearing tolerance and facilitates reshaping of the residual limb.

As the person with the amputation ages, physical and physiologic changes occur. The person may experience

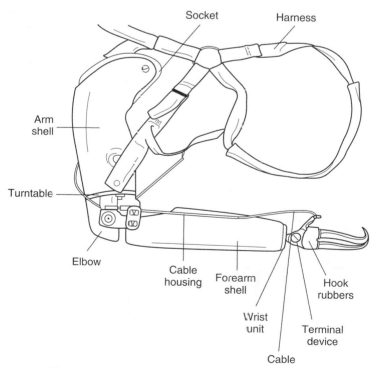

Figure 18-3 Components of a body-powered prosthesis.

weight loss or gain or muscle bulk increase or decrease. These changes have an impact on the size and condition of the residual limb, and the socket may no longer fit as it should. A new socket must be fabricated to fit the exact shape of the residual limb when changes occur. When a new socket is fabricated, it replaces the poorly fitting one in the individual's current prosthesis. An entirely new prosthesis is not needed because the socket is removable and replaceable. This saves on cost. The wearer of a body-powered prosthesis may benefit from using a second sheath or sock made of either a fabric or a gel-like substance to manage poor skin integrity, prevent breakdown, absorb moisture, or provide padding.

The Cable

The harness allows placement of the cable, which is the transmitting force that operates the prosthesis. Body-powered prostheses are operated by body motion that generates tension in the cable. The cable is routed from the harness through a housing to the TD or elbow.[14] The primary movement to operate the prosthesis is glenohumeral flexion. As the individual flexes the humerus, the TD opens. As the individual returns the humerus to neutral, the hook rubbers cause the TD to close. When the individual wishes to open the TD closer to the body, biscapular abduction is used, and adduction or retraction of the scapula allows the TD to close (Figure 18-4). The following quotation from a client with an upper extremity amputation highlights the importance of the cable system for functional tasks:

> *The rubber bands on my hooks regulate tension I put on objects. To force the hook open, I first lock the elbow in the desired position. Then I proceed to bring my shoulder forward, putting tension on the cables. After I have grasped the desired object, I bring my shoulder back to the original position.*[17]

Cables need periodic replacement when they fray or break. Cable replacement is generally the most common repair needed for the body-powered prosthesis wearer.[17] The occupational therapist and the client should know how to replace an old cable with a new one. The process is fairly simple, involving removal of the old cable and reattachment of the new cable to the TD and the harness. It is beneficial for the client to have two or three spare cables at home so that replacement is convenient.

Terminal Device

The TD is the hand component and appears in the form of a hand or a hook. Most body-powered prosthetic hands open and close in a three-point prehension pattern. The prosthetic hooks open and close in a lateral or tip pinch prehension pattern, depending on positioning of the TD. In addition, a variety of TDs are available for certain recreational activities, such as bowling, skiing, baseball, golfing, and volleyball (Figure 18-5).[41] Therapists should be familiar with TD options, because they will most likely introduce the person with the amputation to the available options and provide education in their use.

Generally, the initial goals of the prosthetist are to fit the person who has had an amputation with a standard prosthesis. The person with the amputation then requires time to adjust and become an independent user of the prosthetic device. This individual may not be visiting the prosthetist for some time but is interested in completing a specific activity. Sometimes the occupational therapist can fabricate a tool of thermoplastic or other material that can be attached to the TD to serve a specific function. At other times, collaboration with the prosthetist may be necessary to obtain a specific TD or a sophisticated adaptation.

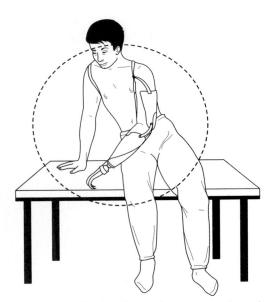

Figure 18-4 Functional work area (body-powered prosthesis).

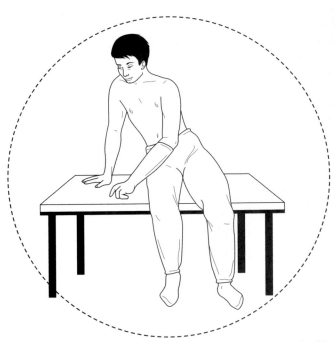

Figure 18-5 Functional work area (externally-powered prosthesis).

Some individuals benefit from two TD options. Typically, an individual has some form of a hand and a hook, which are interchangeable. For example, the client uses the handlike TD for basic ADL and uses the hooklike TD for more challenging activities such as quilting or changing a tire. Every TD has its pros and cons. Differences exist between the hand and hook TDs (Table 18-2). The handlike TD seems to be more cosmetically pleasing. However, digits 3, 4, and 5 are nonfunctional, often impairing function and providing increased bulk. The hooklike TD allows for successful fine motor prehension, is less bulky, and is more durable. However, it may be less cosmetically appealing than the handlike TD.

Grip Strength of Body-Powered Terminal Device

The body-powered grip can vary from 5 to 20 pounds, depending on the number of hook rubbers used. **Hook rubbers** are similar to thick, wide rubber bands providing resistance to the grip of the TD. Each rubber band provides 1 pound of grip force, consequently increasing the amount of pressure placed in the axilla on the contralateral side.

The Glove

The glove is the cosmetic covering of the handlike TD. Gloves are made of either latex or silicone substances and are removable and replaceable. Differences exist between the two types of glove. Latex gloves are sturdy and come in 10 to 15 shades of color. Individuals are matched to the shade that corresponds to their skin tone. Latex gloves easily absorb stains that do not wash off. However, latex gloves are more durable than silicone gloves.

A silicone glove is custom fabricated to match the individual in terms of shape, size, and coloring. It is difficult to differentiate between a silicone glove and a human hand by sight. Such a glove is truly a work of art. Silicone gloves are more costly and fragile than latex gloves. It is more difficult to permanently stain a silicone glove. However, they tear easily. Persons who have had an amputation generally request the silicone glove because of its lifelike appearance. Because silicone gloves are more expensive, funding for a silicone glove is difficult to obtain.

Externally-Powered Prosthesis

The **externally-powered prosthesis** is another prosthetic option. The externally-powered prosthesis is also called a **myoelectric prosthesis** because it operates from the electromyographic (EMG) signal transmitted from the muscles of the residual limb. An externally-powered prosthesis has several differences from the body-powered prosthesis, which are outlined in Table 18-1. Beneficial characteristics of a myoelectric prosthesis include an unlimited work area (see Figure 18-3), functional cosmetic restoration, increased grip force, elimination of harnessing, increased comfort, interchangeable componentry, and individualized custom fabrication. Thus, myoelectric control is most commonly used when possible.[16] Disadvantages of a myoelectric prosthesis include increased weight, increased cost, increased maintenance, and increased risk for damage. The therapist must have a general understanding of the components, such as the socket, electrodes, battery, glove, and TD as seen in Figure 18-5.

The externally-powered prosthesis comprises various components, as shown in Figure 18-6. The components include a socket, a forearm shell, electrodes, battery, glove, and TD.

The Harness

Most myoelectric prosthetic devices do not require a harness. Occasionally, a harness system is required if it is difficult to fit and maintain contact between the electrodes and the muscle signal or if the socket is loose because of weight loss or other factors. Because the harness system is either eliminated or reduced, the functional work area is expanded to include the areas above the head, behind the back, and near the ground compared with the body-powered prosthesis.

Externally-Powered Prosthetic Socket

The externally-powered prosthetic socket is unique in that it has **electrodes** that detect the EMG signals of the muscle. The electrodes are mounted directly in the walls of the flexible socket. The EMG signal stimulates the motor in the prosthesis to produce a desired motion. Prosthetics for clients with upper extremity amputations have dramatically

Table 18-2	Advantages and Disadvantages of the Hand and Hook Terminal Devices	
TERMINAL DEVICE	**ADVANTAGES**	**DISADVANTAGES**
Hand	Cosmetically appealing	Digits 3, 4, and 5 are nonfunctional Tendency to impair fine motor manipulation
Hook	Superior fine motor prehension Less bulky Durable	Cosmetically unappealing

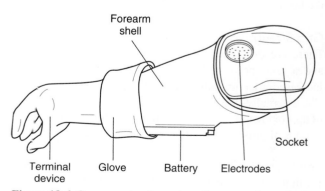

Figure 18-6 Components of an externally-powered prosthesis.

changed over the past several years. The main changes have occurred in components, socket fabrication, fitting techniques, suspension systems, and sources of power and electronic controls.[23]

There are a variety of electrodes available. Some are more sensitive than others in detecting the muscle EMG and controlling the movement of the TD. Through the collaborative effort of the team, the best-suited electrodes are determined. Single- or dual-site control systems are available. A single-site system is used if the client cannot differentiate and isolate control of two separate and opposing muscles for electrode sites. This may be beneficial for persons who are cognitively unable to control the dual site system, such as with pediatrics. For example, the TD would remain in the closed position when the individual's muscles are relaxed and open when the muscle contracts. Thus, if the individual wanted to grasp an object he or she would contract the muscle to open the TD, position it around the desired object, and relax. Upon relaxation, the TD automatically closes and remains closed until the next muscle contraction.

Commonly, a dual-site control system is preferred over a single-site system. The dual-site control system is activated by two separate muscle contractions. For example, the individual with a transradial amputation will most likely contract the wrist extensor muscle group to open the TD and the wrist flexor muscle group to close the TD. The TD has the ability to remain in any position as long as the muscle signals are absent. For example, the same individual can open the TD with contraction of the wrist extensors. Once the muscles are relaxed, the TD will stay open as if to shake the hand of a friend. As soon as the wrist flexors are contracted, the TD will close. With this system, a sheath or sock cannot be worn because it would interrupt the connection between the muscle and the electrode. As a precaution, it is important to remember that the externally-powered TD has a grip strength greater than that of the normal individual.

Externally-powered TDs have a greater opening range, allowing for the ability to grasp objects of larger size. The externally-powered prosthesis provides the ability to use prehension capabilities in all planes. This contributes to the expansion of the functional work area to include space above the head, behind the back, and near the ground.

Grip Strength of Externally-Powered Terminal Device

There are differences between an externally-powered TD and a body-powered TD. An externally-powered TD has increased grip strength compared to the body-powered TD. The externally-powered TD generally provides grip strength of approximately 20 to 30 pounds, compared with the 5 to 20 pounds of grip strength of the body-powered TD.

The Battery

Lithium-polymer battery technology advancements have improved the ease of externally-powered prostheses. The lithium-polymer batteries are 80% lighter, 70% smaller, and offer 30% more storage capacity than nickel-cadmium batteries.[11]

Prosthetic Rehabilitation

The educational background of occupational therapists includes motor control, motor learning, and movement as they relate to the upper extremity function required for occupational performance. Education in the psychological and social adjustment to disability is also the occupational therapist's area of expertise. The sooner therapy is initiated, the faster the client will be prepared for prosthetic fitting and the chances of engaging in bimanual activities will increase. Many long lasting deficits are prevented with early intervention from therapy.

Phases of Rehabilitation

Prosthetic rehabilitation is categorized into nine phases of evaluation and intervention (Box 18-1). Each phase contains specific items to evaluate along with typical areas to address.[22] The phases are:
1. Preoperative
2. Amputation surgery and dressing
3. Acute postsurgical
4. Pre-prosthetic
5. Prosthetic prescription and fabrication
6. Prosthetic training
7. Community integration
8. Vocational rehabilitation
9. Follow up

Preoperative Phase

Ideally, the assessment and intervention process begins before the amputation. The health care team forms a plan and educates the client on what to expect after surgery and during rehabilitation. Therapists assure realistic expectations and outline the typical rehabilitation process. Phantom pain and phantom sensation are explained, because they are common occurrences for individuals post amputation. The preoperative phase is a good time to assess hand dominance and determine the need for adaptive equipment. Adaptive equipment is provided on an as-needed basis only, because clients will eventually use their prostheses with daily activities, and adaptive equipment may interfere with the transition to prosthetic use.[22]

Amputation Surgery and Dressing Phase

Surgeons determine residual limb length prior to and during the surgery. Myoplastic closure of the wound is completed, ensuring soft tissue coverage of any distal bone. A rigid dressing or removable rigid dressing can assist in controlling pain.[22]

1. Preoperative phase
   - Team formulates a plan
   - Educate client on expectations
   - Provide adaptive equipment
2. Amputation surgery and dressing phase
   - Surgery
   - Determine length of residual limb
   - Wound care
   - Dressing wound
   - Pain control
3. Acute postsurgical phase
   - Pain control
   - Range of motion
   - Wound healing
   - Contracture prevention
   - Emotional support
   - Address phantom sensation/pain
4. Pre-prosthetic phase
   - Limb shrinkage and shaping
   - Increase muscle strength
   - Foster sense of control
   - Realistic expectations
5. Prosthetic prescription and fabrication phase
   - Prosthetic options considered
   - Prosthesis is delivered
6. Prosthetic training phase
   - Prosthetic fitting and training
   - Desensitization of residual limb
   - Unilateral independence
   - Educate client on prosthesis controls, etc.
7. Community integration phase
8. Vocational rehabilitation phase
9. Follow up phase
   - Purposeful activities
   - Participation in meaningful activities and occupations
   - Bilateral activities

Acute Postsurgical Phase

The goals after surgery for the team are pain control, maintenance of range of motion, and wound healing. Postsurgical therapy often incorporates wound care and contracture prevention. Emotional support to the client is essential. Discussions about phantom sensation and phantom pain continue.[22]

Wound Healing and Contracture Prevention

In addition, therapists assist persons to adjust to the amputation in many ways. Postsurgical goals include early motion, wound healing, scar management, desensitization, pain management, edema reduction, limb shrinkage/shaping and unilateral independence (change in hand dominance). Many interventions for motion, wound healing, scar management, desensitization, and pain management are the same interventions as used with other diagnoses. Interventions for edema reduction, limb shrinkage/shaping and change in hand dominance are more specific to this population.

Phantom Pain and Phantom Sensation

Clients with amputations often experience phantom sensation and phantom pain. The role of the health care team is to prepare clients and assure them that these phantom sensations and pain are to be expected and are normal.[20] **Phantom sensation** occurs when the individual feels as if the nonexistent limb is still present. The amputated extremity may feel exactly like the original limb in terms of shape, size, position, and ability to move. Rings or watches that were previously worn may be part of the sensation. Phantom sensation is described as a pins-and-needles or tingling sensation. Phantom sensation diminishes over time.

Phantom pain is different from phantom sensation. The phenomenon of phantom pain is not completely understood. It is common for an individual to experience pain in the phantom limb early on after amputation and have it fade over time. It is reported that 80% of individuals with an amputation experience phantom pain.[4]

Intervention related to phantom sensation and phantom pain is implemented as soon as possible. One study surveyed 65 individuals with upper amputations about phantom pain. Results suggested the best intervention for phantom pain was active participation in functional activity.[49] Other interventions include gentle massage, prosthetic wear, and transcutaneous electric nerve stimulation (TENS). As therapists, we are well equipped to work with clients to optimize the functional use of the extremity with an amputation.[20]

Pre-Prosthetic Phase

The primary goals during the pre-prosthetic phase are to shape the residual limb, increase muscle strength, and restore the person's sense of control over what is happening.[22]

Limb Shrinkage and Shaping

Limb shrinkage and shaping is addressed for this population. Custom compression garments are available for the client. Edema can be controlled through wrapping the residual limb in a diagonal design, so as not to compromise circulation. Compression garments or wraps should be worn as much as possible to ensure proper shaping of the residual limb. Compression has a direct impact on residual limb shrinkage and shaping. Elevation and retrograde massage are useful alternatives to decrease edema. It is important for the therapist to reinforce the importance of edema management because it has a direct impact on socket fit and comfort. The reduction of edema is a prerequisite for prosthetic fitting.[20]

Time during the pre-prosthetic phase is crucial for reinforcement of realistic expectations. Individuals with amputations may be under the assumption that they will perform all activities at the same level of independence they had prior to the amputation. This assumption needs to be discussed. Therapists explain that the prosthetic device will not replace the arm. Rather, it is an assistive tool used to stabilize, support, and hold objects during bimanual activities.

Prosthetic Prescription and Fabrication Phase

The prosthetic prescription and fabrication phase is the time when the team comes to consensus on the type of prosthesis that will best meet the client's needs and condition.[22] The pre-prosthetic period begins when the individual with the amputation begins exploration of prosthetic devices. The phase concludes upon prosthetic delivery.

Prosthetic Training Phase

During the prosthetic training phase, individuals frequently visit the prosthetist for fittings and modifications of the socket. Clients also see therapists for rehabilitation services. Individuals receiving body-powered prostheses move much quicker through the fabrication and rehabilitation process because electrodes are not required and muscle sites and signals do not need to be identified. Therapy continues to address any lingering issues from the acute postsurgical phase. Additional goals of therapy during this phase include preparation of the individual to tolerate wearing the prosthesis and using it independently for daily activities. Specifics include electrode training; desensitizing the residual limb to pressure, pain, and weight; maintaining range of motion; eliminating contractures; and unilateral independence.[22]

Electrode Training

If individuals receive an externally-powered prosthesis, the best muscle sites are identified and trained to operate the prosthetic features. Finding the sites and training the muscles for electrode placement are primarily the responsibility of the therapist. During this phase, therapists provide extensive training using biofeedback to teach individuals to contract the identified muscle or muscles on command. The therapist facilitates the improvement of muscle site control and focuses on isolated muscle contraction, strength, and endurance. Special **biofeedback machines** are available from prosthetists. It is important for clients to practice muscle contractions in a variety of positions, including lying, standing, and sitting. Practicing muscle contractions in different positions with the extremity in various planes enhances maximal success after delivery of the prosthesis.

Once electrode sites are established, the prosthetist is informed of the exact and most appropriate electrode location for the individual to obtain the most function. Locating and training for electrode sites is often a lengthy, rigorous, and trial-and-error process. Once the socket and electrode sites are sufficient to work the prosthesis, the prosthesis is ready for final fabrication. There may be a period of time after the pre-prosthetic phase when the individual is discharged from therapy with a home program until the prosthesis is delivered and therapy can resume.

Desensitizing the Residual Limb to Pressure, Pain, and Weight

Clients may experience disappointment when the prosthesis is delivered and they are unable to use it as they imagined. It is the duty of the health care team to inform individuals of the advantages and disadvantages of the various prosthetic components to provide a realistic picture of rehabilitation. Clients are usually surprised when they realize that the prosthesis is hard, cold, heavy, and not an exact replacement for the hand. With establishment of realistic expectations and acceptance, use of the device greatly improves.[6]

Clients commonly experience residual limb sensitivity. Therapists intervene by teaching and implementing the following desensitization techniques: wrapping, massage, weight-bearing, and pain management. Desensitization and pain management are additional components of therapy. Therapists provide modalities for pain and educate clients to manage their pain independently. Each client presents with different complaints, and the treatment is individualized.

In some instances, prosthetists provide clients with sockets to wear as precursors to full-time prosthetic wear. Sockets reshape the residual limb and allow clients to experience how the devices feel. Weights can be added to the distal ends of sockets for increasing tolerance to the weight of the devices.

Unilateral Independence

Unilateral independence involves using environmental adaptations and one-handed techniques. It may be necessary to teach clients to switch hand dominance if the dominant hand was amputated. Generally, therapists work to promote the maximal level of independence for the individual. Adaptive equipment is often used. For clients with amputations, it may promote better prosthetic success if therapists do not issue adaptive equipment until after prosthetic training, because clients may become efficient with the adaptive equipment and may not be motivated to learn to use the prosthesis.

Orientation and Control Training

Upon prosthetic delivery, the prosthetist educates clients about the prosthesis and its components. Therapists reorient clients to their prostheses. Prostheses are complex devices, and they cannot be mastered in one therapy session. Clients will not be independent with the prosthetic usage unless there is a complete understanding of all of the components.

Client orientation includes education on donning, doffing, operating switches and batteries, and caring for the prosthesis. Therapists ensure that prosthetic fit and function are adequate. Therapy includes evaluation of independence with prosthetic donning and doffing. Clients must be able to properly care for their prosthesis so as to prevent damage and maximize its potential.

Community Integration, Vocational Rehabilitation, and Follow-Up Phases

The final three phases of community integration, vocational rehabilitation, and follow up[22] are comprised of purposeful activities and participation in meaningful occupation-based activities.[3] These phases are intensive. Clients visits to other members of the team decrease, and therapists act as liaisons to the teams. These final phases are progressive and evolve as clients' skills develop. During this time, clients learn to operate the controls of their prostheses and practice until they become proficient. Depending on the prosthetic features, clients practice tasks, such as opening and closing the TD, elevating and lowering the elbow, and rotating the wrist on command. Practicing such activities is graded (e.g., controlling the TD to open in three, four, or five separate steps).

Purposeful Activity

With purposeful activity, clients learn how to operate prostheses by engaging in repetitive tasks to facilitate eventual functional use and endurance. Purposeful activity includes using the prostheses to grasp and release objects of various sizes, textures, and weights in different planes and positions. Objects above the head can be difficult to grasp because individuals must relax the wrist extensors and contract the flexors while the hand is elevated. Overhead grasp is difficult to accomplish because of the prosthetic weight. Examples of other activities practiced during this stage include holding and placing a tomato on a counter without crushing it or playing a card game with the cards held by the TD.

Bilateral activities are also a focus in therapy. Often, after amputation individuals become successful in performing some ADLs unilaterally. Thus, therapy must begin early in the rehabilitation process to facilitate use of the prosthesis in bilateral activities. Training includes controlled grasp, such as opening in small increments to grasp small items and then more fully to grasp larger items. Training emphasizes grasping objects of varied textures and density. Sessions incorporate work on prehension and timing of release. Functional and appropriate tasks are encouraged and require clients to use their prostheses for gross and fine motor activities in various planes.

Occupational-Based Activity

Occupational-based activity involves engaging the client in occupations that match clients' goals. Clients practice skills related to their lifestyle and interests. Training may include grooming and hygiene, meal preparation, dressing, child care, return to work activities, or other meaningful tasks. Tasks may also include preparation for return to employment or recreation.

The primary focus of therapy should include bilateral activities for occupational performance. Box 18-2 lists examples of bilateral tasks.[34] Individuals with amputations usually do not realize the functional benefits of their prostheses until they experience success with bilateral tasks. Bilateral task training may be difficult for some clients, who became proficient with one-handed techniques early in rehabilitation.

As stated earlier, clients are active participant in the rehabilitation process. Therapists design home programs for clients. The programs are continually updated as individuals progress to greater function and independence. Scheduling

---

Box 18-2   Examples of Bilateral Activities

- Insert a garbage bag into a trash receptacle
- Dry dishes with a towel
- Use cell phone
- Butter bread
- Put toothpaste on a toothbrush
- Lace and tie shoes
- Take a bill from a wallet
- Fold a letter and seal envelope
- Use power tools
- Crack eggs and separate the yolks from the whites
- Fold laundry
- Wash dishes in a sink
- Remove lids from jars
- Manage zippers or buttons
- Peel oranges
- Rake and bag leaves
- Peel and cut vegetables/fruits
- Cut meat
- Sewing on buttons
- Thread needles
- Use screw drivers
- Drive a vehicle
- Play sports or card games

---

periodic follow-up visits with the client to review progress and prosthesis function is important. Often therapy will be reinitiated when clients find new skills they need or desire to learn. Therapists are resources for clients, enabling them to achieve maximal function and independence for participation in meaningful activities during the course of a lifetime.

Psychological and Social Issues of Clients with Amputations

At any of the rehabilitation stages, psychological and social issues may arise, and it is important to make appropriate referrals to specialists as necessary. In 2002, Davidson stated "amputees volunteer that they have far more difficulty dealing with their social worlds than with their physical worlds."[20] Common issues can center around relationships with family, friends, co-workers, and significant others. Specific issues may include post-traumatic stress, body image concerns, loss of sense of wholeness, social isolation, decreased sexual activity, and depression.[43] One of the most common secondary conditions associated with limb loss is depressed mood.[4]

Family Dynamics

The dynamics of the family may be altered when a family member loses a limb. Significant others or direct family members of the injured person experience a series of losses and adjustments. Family members may fear that the individual is suffering and at risk of dying. Fear and anxiety may become overwhelming at times. Family members may worry about how the individual will adjust to his or her changed body. Issues about intimacy and dependency are common concerns. The therapist should encourage a reconnection between the person who has sustained an amputation and his or her partner.[31,32]

Impact on Rehabilitation

The rehabilitation team should become knowledgeable about the individual's response to the injury. Psychosocial aspects include change in self-image and body image, acceptance of the residual limb, and feeling comfortable in society as a person with an amputation. Some clients may be medically prepared to begin rehabilitation, but they are not psychologically ready. Health providers should not label the client as uncooperative and unmotivated. Rather, they should facilitate and reinforce good communication among the client and health care team. The client should be an active partner to establish rehabilitation goals.

Counseling People Who Have Amputations

According to Price and Fisher,[40] issues addressed during counseling sessions include depression, distress, sleeplessness, anxiety, changed body image, effects on relationships and intimacy, and feelings of anger and resentment. According to Kohl,[31,32] complaints of emotional distress in the early stages of rehabilitation seemed to be most apparent from 6 to 24 months after surgery.

Upper Extremity Prosthetic Intervention for Children

Early gross motor movements in children (such as prone and sitting) emerge between 4 and 6 months.[18] These movements directly involve the use of hands in order to balance, support, and stabilize the trunk. As a result, fitting children with prostheses is considered necessary in order to maintain and preserve normal development.[45] Exner[24] stated that "[t]he development of visual perception and eye-hand coordination skills in conjunction with cognitive and social development allow the child to engage in increasingly complex activities."

Early Fitting

According to Hanson and Mandacina,[27] "The single most important advantage of early fitting is the immediate acceptance of the prosthetic arm by the child." The most beneficial age range to receive a prosthesis is from 2 months to 2 years.[25,44,47] Children fitted with prostheses at a young age and who wear their prostheses regularly will demonstrate spontaneous use in daily activities.

Children fitted at later ages are less spontaneous and more inclined to use the prosthesis passively.[6,12,27] In addition, because hand skills develop gradually, children should be fitted early so that the prosthesis becomes naturally integrated with bilateral activities. While wearing their prostheses, children must practice activities that require crossing midline, hand position in space, grasping, bilateral tasks, and bringing hands to midline.[29] Table 18-3 suggests types of prostheses, goals, assessments, and interventions for children of different age groups.

Family Involvement

Acceptance of the prosthesis involves the family. The family should be involved in donning and doffing the prosthesis, playing with the child while the prosthesis is on, and developing wearing schedules. The family should be educated about the importance and advantages of early and consistent prosthetic use. Furthermore, children who have myoelectric prostheses require substantial one-to-one training and attention.[7]

Marketing Strategies and Recommendations

To specialize in upper extremity prosthetic rehabilitation, therapists must be motivated and persistent, just as in any area of practice. There are many avenues for gathering basic information on upper extremity prosthetics, such as journals, books, agencies, other therapists, and the Internet (see Appendix D). Important information from these resources augment basic prosthetic knowledge. Therapists should establish relationships with prosthetists that specialize in upper extremity prosthetics. Because the number of upper extremity amputations is generally low, it may be difficult for therapists to work full time in this area, unless they are willing to travel regionally or nationally. Some companies employ therapists who cover a designated region and provide prosthetic rehabilitation exclusively. If travel is not an option, therapists can network with prosthetic providers to be the primary referral for prosthetic rehabilitation in a geographic area. Typically, therapists who take this route work in an outpatient upper extremity rehabilitation facility.

Spending a week with a prosthetist to learn about the process of reimbursement, fabrication, and orientation to various prosthetic options is valuable. The reimbursement process can take much time, depending on the source of reimbursement and the insurance company's specific benefits regarding prostheses. It is important to remain focused on clients and to serve as advocates for individuals with the amputation. Phone calls and letters from health care professionals may expedite approval of prosthetic devices. Therapy can proceed without approval for the prosthetic devices in order to accomplish goals from the pre-prosthetic phase.

In addition, it is important to locate area case managers and physicians who work with this population. Case managers and physicians assist in establishing a referral base. It has been the experience of the author that physicians, prosthetists, and case managers are happy to know that therapists exist who want to work in upper extremity prosthetic rehabilitation. They are also often happy to refer clients. Upper extremity prosthetics is a rewarding field.

Table 18-3 Suggestions for Age Appropriate Prostheses, Goals, Assessment, and Interventions

AGE	TYPE OF PROSTHESIS	GOALS	ASSESSMENTS	INTERVENTION
2 months to 18 months	Passive fitting suspension socket with no harnessing	Weight bearing in sitting and standing Crawling and pulling to stand Rolling front to back Stabilizing toys Bilateral activities	PUFI Southhampton Hand test	No different than reaching all appropriate developmental milestones Gross motor skills using the prosthesis Fine motor skills with unaffected upper extremity
12 months to 24 months	Cookie Crusher myoelectric prosthesis (system discontinued at age 4)	Using prosthesis as an assist Discovering that the device opens and closes Opening hand upon request Placing toys in the myoelectric hand	Carrying large balls Weight bearing on the prosthesis while playing Stabilizing the body while completing table top activities Holding objects Riding toys	Typical screening assessments for age range

PUFI, Prosthetic Upper Extremity Function Index; *UNB*, University of New Brunswick.
Data from Shaperman J, Landsberger SE, Setoguchi Y: Early upper limb prosthesis fitting: when and what do we fit, *J Prosthet Orthot* 15(1):11-17, 2003; Stocker D, Caldwell R, Wedderburn Z: Review of infant fittings at the Institute of Biomedical Engineering: 13 years of service, *ACPOC News* 2:1-5, 1996.

SELF-QUIZ 18-1*

Answer the following questions.

1. The term *above elbow (AE) amputation* is now called:
   a. Transfemoral
   b. Transhumeral
   c. Transradial
   d. Transtibial
2. The term *below elbow (BE) amputation* is now called:
   a. Transfemoral
   b. Transhumeral
   c. Transradial
   d. Transtibial
3. The primary cause for an upper extremity amputation is:
   a. Congenital malformation
   b. Disease
   c. Trauma
   d. Vascular disorders
4. Which prosthetic option allows individuals to maintain grasp and release within an unlimited work area with full range of motion of the proximal upper extremity?
   a. Body-powered prosthesis
   b. Externally-powered prosthesis
   c. No prosthesis
   d. Passive prosthesis
5. Which prosthesis allows individuals to maintain proprioception for grasp and release?
   a. Body-powered prosthesis
   b. Externally-powered prosthesis
   c. No prosthesis
   d. Passive prosthesis

6. Which prosthetic option typically allows for increased grip/pinch strength?
   a. Body-powered prosthesis
   b. Externally-powered prosthesis
   c. No prosthesis
   d. Passive prosthesis
7. Often times therapists establish electrode sites and provide electrode training for externally-powered prostheses. In which phase of the rehabilitation process does this typically occur?
   a. Acute postsurgical
   b. Preoperative
   c. Pre-prosthetic
   d. Prosthetic training
8. A therapist receives an order to evaluate and treat an individual with a transhumeral amputation. The prosthetist indicates the client received the prosthesis one week ago. Rank in order the steps of the therapy intervention:
   Step 1: _____
   Step 2: _____
   Step 3: _____
   a. Purposeful activity
   b. Occupation-based activity
   c. Orientation and control training
9. In which phase of post-prosthetic training does the client learn to operate the controls of the prosthesis and practice until proficient?
   a. Purposeful activity
   b. Occupation-based activity
   c. Orientation and control training
10. Which secondary condition is most commonly associated with limb loss?
    a. Depressed mood
    b. Isolation
    c. Loss of sense of self
    d. Post-traumatic stress disorder

*See Appendix A for the answer key.

Review Questions

1. What is the relationship between the level of amputation and functional ability? List three reasons for prosthetic dissatisfaction.
2. What are the primary causes for upper extremity amputation?
3. Clarify the specific roles of the client, prosthetist, and occupational therapist when treating a person with an amputation?
4. What are the four prosthesis options available for people with upper extremity amputations?
5. How would you explain in lay terms the advantages and disadvantages of passive, body-powered, and externally-powered prostheses?
6. What is one therapy goal for each phase of prosthetic rehabilitation? What is one specific intervention for each phase?
7. What are the psychosocial impacts of an amputation that may arise?

References

1. Alley RD: *Advancement of upper extremity prosthetic interface and frame design*, From "MEC '02 The Next Generation," Proceedings of the 2002 MyoElectric Controls/Powered Prosthetics Symposium Fredericton New Brunswick, Canada, August 21-23, 2002, Copyright University of New Brunswick (website) http://dukespace.lib.duke.edu/dspace/bitstream/handle/10161/2684/r_alley_paper01.pdf?sequence=3. Accessed March 16, 2014.
2. American Board for Certification in Orthotics: Prosthetics & Pedorthics, Inc. Annual report [Brochure], 2011. Available for download at www.abcop.org.
3. American Occupational Therapy Association (AOTA): Occupational therapy practice framework: domain and process, *Amer J Occup Ther* 68(Suppl):S1-S48, 2014.
4. Amputee Coalition of America: *People with amputation speak out* (website) http://www.amputee-coalition.org/people-speak-out/index.html. Accessed March 16, 2014.
5. Andrews KL, Bouvette KA: Anatomy for fitting of prosthetics and orthotics, *Physical Medicine and Rehabilitation* 10(3):489–507, 1996.
6. Atkins DJ: Prosthetic Training. In Smith D, Michael J, Bowker J, editors: *Atlas of amputations and limb deficiencies: surgical, prosthetic, and rehabilitation principles*, Rosemont, IL, 2004, American Academy of Orthopaedic Surgeons, pp 275–284.

7. Atkins DJ: Pediatric prosthetics: a collection of considerations, *In Motion* 7(2):7–17. 1997.

8. Atkins DJ, Meier RH: *Comprehensive management of the upper-limb amputee*, New York, 1989, Springer-Verlag.

9. Baumgartner R, Bota P: Upper extremity amputation and prosthetics, *Medicine Orthotic Technology* 1:5–51, 1992.

10. Bennett JB, Alexander CB: Amputation levels and surgical techniques. In Atkins DJ, Meier RH, editors: *Comprehensive management of the upper-limb amputee*, New York, 1989, Springer-Verlag, pp 28–38.

11. Billock JN: Clinical evaluation and assessment principles in orthotics and prosthetics, *J Prosthet Orthot* 8(2):41–44, 2003.

12. Bowers R: Facing congenital differences, *First Step Magazine* 4:23–26, 2003.

13. Bowker JH, Pitham CH: The history of amputation surgery and prosthetics. In Smith D, Michael J, Bowker J, editors: *Atlas of amputations and limb deficiencies: surgical, prosthetic, and rehabilitation principles*, Rosemont, IL, 2004, American Academy of Orthopaedic Surgeons, pp 3–19.

14. Carlson LE, Veatch BD, Frey DD: Efficiency of prosthetic cable and housing, *J Prosthet Orthot* 7(3):96–99, 1995.

15. Collier M, LeBlanc M: Axilla bypass ring for shoulder harnesses for upper-limb prostheses, *J Prosthet Orthot* 8(2):130–131, 1996.

16. Corbett EA, Perreault EJ, Kuiken TA: Comparison of electromyography and force as interfaces for prosthetic control, *J Rehabil Res Dev* 48(6):629–642, 2011.

17. Crane V: Amputee adjusts, *Probe Magazine* 4:10–14, 1979.

18. Cronin A, Mandich MB: *Human development and performance throughout the lifespan*, New York, 2005, Thomson/Delmar Learning. 139–164.

19. Dillingham TR, Pezzin LE, MacKenzie EJ: Limb amputation and limb deficiency: epidemiology and recent trends in the United States, *South Med J* 95(8):875–883, 2002.

20. Davidson JH, Jones LE, Cornet J, et al.: Management of the multiple limb amputee, *Disabil Rehabil* 24(13):688–699, 2002.

21. Dougherty PJ: Wartime amputee care. In Smith D, Michael J, Bowker J, editors: *Atlas of amputations and limb deficiencies: surgical, prosthetic, and rehabilitation principles*, Rosemont, IL, 2004, American Academy of Orthopaedic Surgeons, pp 77–100.

22. Esquenazi A, DiGiacomo R: Rehabilitation after amputation, *J Am Podiatr Med Assoc* 91(1):13–22, 2001.

23. Esquinazi A, Meier R, Sears H: *The state of upper limb prosthetics*, Presentation at Orlando, FL, 2002, National Prosthetic and Orthotic Conference.

24. Exner CE: Development of hand functions. In Pratt PN, Allen AS, editors: *Occupational therapy for children*, ed 2, St Louis, 1989, Mosby, pp 235–259.

25. Fisher A: Initial fitting of the congenital below-elbow amputee: are we fitting early enough? *Inter-Clinic Information Bulletin* 15:7–10, 1976.

26. Jones LE, Davidson JH: Save the arm: a study of problems in the remaining arm of unilateral upper limb amputees, *Prosthet Orthot Int* 23(1):55–58, 1999.

27. Hanson WJ, Mandacina S: Microprocessor technology opens the door to success, *The O&P Edge* 5:36–38, 2003.

28. Hartigan BJ, Sarrafian SK: ***. In Smith D, Michael J, Bowker J, editors: *Atlas of amputations and limb deficiencies: surgical, prosthetic, and rehabilitation principles*, Rosemont, IL, 2004, American Academy of Orthopaedic Surgeons, pp 101–115.

29. Hubbard S, Bush G, Kurtz I, et al.: Myoelectric prostheses for the limb deficient child, *Physical Medicine Rehabilitation Clinical North America* 2:847–866, 1991.

30. Keenan DD: Myoelectric prosthesis protocol, *American Occupational Therapy Association Physical Disabilities Newsletter* 18(1):1–4, 1995.

31. Kohl SJ: Emotional coping with amputation. In Krueger DW, editor: *Rehabilitation psychology: a comprehensive textbook*, New York, 1984, Aspen, pp 272–281.

32. Kohl SJ: The process of psychological adaptation to traumatic limb loss. In Krueger DW, editor: *Emotional rehabilitation of physical trauma and disability*, ***, 1984, Spectrum Publications, pp 113–119.

33. Law HT: Engineering of upper limb prostheses, *Orthop Clin North Am* 12(4):929–951, 1981.

34. McFarland LV, Hubbard Winkler SL, et al.: Unilateral upper-limb loss: satisfaction and prosthetic-device use in veterans and servicemembers from Vietnam and OIF/OEF conflicts, *J Rehabil Res Dev* 47(4):299–316, 2010.

35. Miguelez JM. Critical factors in electrically powered upper-extremity prosthetics, *American Academy of Orthotics and Prosthetics* 14(1):36–38, 2002.

36. Muilenburg AL, LeBlanc MA: Body-powered upper limb components. In Atkins DJ, Meier RH, editors: *Comprehensive management of the upper-limb amputee*, New York, 1989, Springer-Verlag.

37. National Limb Loss Information Center: *Fact sheet—amputation statistics by cause:* limb loss in the United States. (website) http://www.amputee-coalition.org/fact_sheets/amp_stats_cause.html. Accessed March 16, 2014.

38. National Center for Health Statistics, N.D. [need full ref]

39. Patterson DB, McMillan PM, Rodriguez RP: Acceptance rate of myoelectric prosthesis, *Journal of the Association of Children's Prosthetic-Orthotic Clinics* 25(3):73–76, 1991.

40. Price EM, Fisher K: How does counseling help people with amputation, *J Prosthet Orthot* 14(2):102–106, 2002.

41. Radocy B: Upper-extremity prosthetics: considerations and designs for sports and recreation, *Clinical Prosthetics and Orthotics* 11(3):131–153, 1987.

42. Reddy MP: Nerve entrapment syndromes in the upper extremity contralateral to amputation, *Arch Phys Med Rehabil* 65(1):24–26, 1984.

43. Saradjian A, Thompson AR, Datta D: The experience of men using an upper limb prosthesis following amputation: positive coping and minimizing feeling different, *Disabil Rehabil* 30(11):871–883, 2008.

44. Scotland TD, Galway HR: A long-term review in children with congenital and acquired upper limb deficiency, *J Bone Joint Surg Br* 65(3):346–349, 1986.

45. Shaperman J, Landsberger SE, Setoguchi Y: Early upper limb prosthesis fitting: when and what do we fit, *J Prosthet Orthot* 15(1):11–17, 2003.

46. Shurr DG, Cook TM: *Prosthetics and orthotics*, Norwalk, CT, 1990, Appleton & Lange.

47. Stark G: Upper-extremity limb fitting, *In Motion* 12(4):47–52, 2001.

48. Toren S: Upper extremity, *First Step Magazine* 3:7–9, 2002.

49. Vacek KM: *Phantom pain and phantom sensation, Research Platform Presentation*, Kansas City, MO, June 2001, Amputee Coalition of Americas National Conference.

50. Williams 3rd TW: Progress on stabilizing and controlling powered upper-limb prostheses, *J Rehabil Res Dev* 48(6):ix–xix, 2011.

51. Wright TW, Hagen AD, Wood MB: Prosthetic usage in major upper extremity amputations, *J Hand Surg Am* 20(4):619–622, 1995.

52. Ziegler-Graham K, MacKenzie EJ, Ephraim PL, et al.: Estimating the prevalence of limb loss in the United States: 2005 to 2050, *Arch Phys Med Rehabil* 89(3):422–429, 2008.

CHAPTER 19

Ethical Issues Related to Orthotic Provision

Amy Marie Haddad

Key Terms

autonomy
beneficence
care-based ethics
duty
ethics
justice
morality
nonmaleficence
Occupational Therapy Code of Ethics and Ethics Standards
principles
self-determination
values
virtue

Chapter Objectives

1. Compare and contrast the various sources of moral guidance.
2. Define three traditional approaches to applied ethics: principle, care-based, and virtue.
3. Apply one of the traditional approaches to ethics to a complex case to reach a morally justifiable resolution.

Health care is fraught with ethical issues, including questions about whether to tell clients that you believe they are receiving inadequate care, how to deal with impaired or incompetent colleagues, or how to fairly distribute scarce and valuable resources. As one of the health professions, occupational therapy cannot help being involved in ethical problems and their resolutions. In fact, occupational therapists often find themselves caught between two moral goods. First is the desire to assist the client to function better with independence. The second moral good is the client's right to self-determination that may lead to non-adherence with agreed upon therapy and less than satisfactory outcomes.

The purpose of this chapter is to define applied ethics and its application to occupational therapy practice with a specific emphasis on the special types of problems encountered in orthotic provision. Sources of moral guidance and values are explored, along with three traditional approaches to ethics. The three approaches (principles, care-based ethics, and virtue) are applied to complex clinical situations involving orthotic provision in the later sections of this chapter. Resources to assist in the resolution of ethical problems are noted.

Ethics and Health Care

Ethics itself is hardly a new area of study. Its application to the practical problems of health care is a relative newcomer, beginning approximately in the late 1960s with questions about research on human subjects, vital organ transplantation, and hemodialysis.[9] What was needed at that time was a detailed study of professional ethics aimed at establishing standards of conduct and moral behavior. The need for the guidance that ethics provides continues to the present day.

Normative ethics is that level of ethical inquiry that asks "…whether there are any general principles or norms describing the characteristics that make actions right or wrong."[12] The results of applied ethics have direct bearing on practice and immediate consequences for action and policy.

In recent years, this definition of normative or applied ethics has expanded. Now it includes concerns about relationships and the particular experiences of those who are ill or injured, as opposed to abstract universal approaches. These types of concerns fall under the heading of care-based reasoning. Thus, a complete definition of normative ethics encompasses an examination of principles and virtues. It also includes what we should nurture and sustain as human beings to achieve the most of what is best in human life. The focus of this chapter is on the moral life in occupational therapy, particularly in the area of orthotic provision. To arrive at a clearer understanding of ethics, it is helpful to have a baseline of key terms. Three terms underlie the discussion in this chapter: ethics, morality, and values.

Ethics

Ethics is the exploration of moral duty, principles, human character or virtue, and human relationships. In effect, ethics involves the study of right and wrong, good and evil, moral conduct on an individual and societal basis, rules, promises, principles, and obligations. Taken together, these constitute the important concerns of ethics.

From this broad definition of ethics, it might appear that all human interactions on some level involve ethics. Although this is true, it is important to be able to sort out and differentiate the ethical issues central to the question at hand from those that are merely the underpinning or backdrop for daily experience. A simple guide to determining whether a situation involves ethics involves answering the following three questions[4]:

* Is there more than one morally plausible resolution?
* Is there no clear-cut best resolution?
* Is there direct reference to the welfare or dignity of others?

If the answer to any of these questions is yes, the situation in question involves ethics.

Morality

Human behavior or actions that are judged as either good or evil fall in the domain of **morality.** Although ethics can be thought of as the more formal and prescriptive of the two, many ethicists use the words *morality* and *ethics* synonymously. When we make a judgment about a person's conduct, saying "That action is bad or wrong," we are actually including a judgment about the act itself, the values attached to the action, and accountability for the action. If a therapist were to tell a lie, the very word we use to describe the action (lie) indicates that the action is wrong or at least opposed to the action of telling the truth. For example, suppose a client asked a therapist if she has any prior experience in fabricating a particular type of orthosis. Although the therapist has never made the specified orthosis before, she tells the client that she has made it on several occasions.

We can claim that the action is wrong only if we explore the values that support the worth or goodness of truth telling and why it is important to tell the truth. Telling the truth demonstrates respect for the other person and allows individuals to make decisions with accurate information. If we found while exploring the "liar's" action that he or she was completely unaware that lying was wrong or bad, we might excuse the person from moral wrongdoing because he or she did not know any better. When a person is unaware of the rightness or wrongness of actions, we consider him or her amoral.

Although it is difficult to believe that individuals would be unaware of the moral rules of the society in which they live, there are those who because of age or mental defect do not understand the moral implications of their actions. Persons who normally fall into this category are children, the mentally ill, or persons with severe cognitive disabilities. On the other hand, persons who know the difference between right and wrong conduct and yet choose to do the wrong thing are considered immoral and accountable for their actions.

Values

In the brief discussion of morality, it is clear that **values** are an important part of ethics. Values are the internal motivators for our actions. When individuals value something, they invest themselves psychologically and spiritually. They also attach emotions (positive or negative) and importance to persons, places, objects, actions, ideals, or goals that seem to be most relevant to or intimate with the self. Basic values and a value system are developed during childhood. Of course, early established values can be changed under great spiritual or emotional distress.

Values can also be changed when it becomes apparent that an old value does not effectively resolve a present dilemma and a new, more attractive and applicable, value does. A conflict of values is often the genesis for an ethical problem in clinical practice. Regardless of the origin of a value, the resulting personal and professional values can profoundly affect the ethical decisions occupational therapists make. For example, a first-year occupational therapy student used to think older adults over age 85 should not receive any type of orthotic intervention because it was too costly and life expectancy was probably minimal. However, after graduating with an occupational therapy degree and interacting with older adults in the clinical setting the new therapist now values the lives of older adults and has resolved the ageism bias.

Sources of Moral Guidance

The basic definitions of ethics, morality, and values set a foundation to separate ethical concerns from other types of problems and issues an occupational therapist faces in practice. Once it is clear that a situation or problem involves ethics, the next question is where you should look to determine what is right or morally correct. Are morals grounded in one's own opinion? Or that of significant others? In the law and regulations that govern professional practice? In the opinions of one's professional group or association? In the religious or philosophical beliefs of the individual or institution?

This section explores alternative sources of moral guidance. What is important is not to focus on determining what the right thing to do is, but to reflect on the various sources of moral authority that have particular impact on your professional practice and personal decision making. One should consider how these sources of authority shape one's behavior and character.

Family and Peers

One of the primary sources of support and guidance for moral decision making are peers and family members. In two separate national studies (one of registered nurses and the other of pharmacists) the majority of respondents stated that they would first turn to their spouse for moral advice or counsel, followed by a peer.[7,8] Setting aside concerns about breaches of confidentiality and privacy, seeking the advice of someone who is close and trusted is not too surprising, and it is likely that occupational therapists would respond in the same way their colleagues in nursing and pharmacy did.

Individuals who know us well and share the same perspectives and values are logically the first-line resource for most health professionals faced with a moral problem. However, even though it is understandable why an occupational therapist might turn to a peer for ethical advice, there is no reason to believe that the peer will be able to provide justifiable resolutions to the problem. In other words, peers and significant others may be sympathetic but they are not necessarily in the best position to sort through the complicated ethical issues encountered in practice.

Furthermore, significant others and peers would probably not be considered the source of moral authority, even if they were skilled in analyzing ethical problems. We must look further than the individuals who make up our families and our colleagues for moral guidance. For example, a therapist is faced with an ethical decision—whether or not to fabricate orthoses for a person who was burned over 90% of her body. Instead of the therapist asking his wife about the decision, the therapist could network with professional peers who are members of the hospital's ethics committee.

Laws and Regulations

At times it is difficult to distinguish between the law and ethics. Former Chief Justice of the Supreme Court, Earl Warren, described the relationship between the law and ethics as follows:

> *In civilized life, Law floats in a sea of Ethics. Each is indispensable to civilization. Without Law, we should be at the mercy of the least scrupulous; without Ethics, Law could not exist. Without ethical consciousness in most people, lawlessness would be rampant. Yet, without Law, civilization could not exist, for there are always people who, in the conflict of human interest, ignore their responsibility to their fellowman.[13]*

Thus, there is a delicate and changeable relationship between ethics and law. Laws and specific regulations that govern health care practice order our professional and institutional relationships. In an ideal world, the law would embody our ethical commitments. Yet, sometimes the law and ethics diverge.

It is possible that an occupational therapist could conclude that he or she should engage in civil disobedience to violate the law or public policy to do what is ethical. Of course, this sort of decision to disobey a law or regulation should not be taken lightly. If ethics sometimes requires civil disobedience, it implies that what is ethical is not determined solely by public policy or law. Therefore, this reasoning argues, the law is not a sufficient source of authority for determining proper ethical conduct for an occupational therapist.

Professional Codes of Ethics

Health professionals recognize that the question of what is moral has to do with professional ethics. Occupational therapists might turn to a professional code of ethics as a source of moral guidance. For American occupational therapists, this would be the current **Occupational Therapy Code of Ethics and Ethics Standards** of the American Occupational Therapy Association (AOTA).[1]

An occupational therapist faced with an ethical problem could turn to the Occupational Therapy Code of Ethics and Ethics Standards to see what guidance it offers regarding the specific issues at stake. Often the Code provides direction and assistance. "Health care professions specify and enforce obligations for their members, thereby seeking to ensure that persons who enter into relationships with these professionals will find them competent and trustworthy."[2] Most health care professions codify these rules of conduct into a formal code of ethics.

The purpose of professional codes is to set minimal expectations of those who practice within their respective profession. Professional codes can be aspirational in nature in that they set more than minimal expectations for members of the profession. The Occupational Therapy Code of Ethics and Ethics Standards[1] states that the code "is a guide to professional conduct when ethical issues arise. Ethical decision making is a process that includes awareness of how the outcome will impact occupational therapy clients in all spheres. Applications of Code of Ethics Standards Principles are considered situation-specific, and where a conflict exists, occupational therapy personnel will pursue responsible efforts for resolution." One limitation of codes is that they tend to oversimplify moral responsibilities.

The occupational therapist is obligated to abide by the tenets of the Code. It is possible that occupational therapists may believe that if they fulfill the requirements of the Code, they have done all they have to do, morally speaking. However, would an occupational therapist's conduct always be correct just because it conforms to the Occupational Therapy Code of Ethics and Ethics Standards?

Another limitation of codes of ethics is that the perspectives of the recipients of health care may be absent. What might the public proclaim as the fundamental obligations of occupational therapists if given the chance?

Finally, how do we account for changes in professional codes? Although the first version of the AOTA Code of Ethics was approved in 1977, it has already undergone several revisions. Each time the Occupational Therapy Code of Ethics and Ethics Standards changed, did the ethically correct behavior for occupational therapists really change—or only what AOTA members believed was the correct behavior? It seems that the foundation for ethics in occupational therapy is something more basic than current professional agreement based on these changes in the Code.

Religion

If an occupational therapist worked in a hospital or ambulatory care center sponsored by a religious organization, the institution's ethical code may be derived from religious beliefs and ethical commitments of the sponsoring group. For example, if the institution were Catholic and located in the United States, it would have to abide by the Ethical and Religious Directives for Catholic Health Care Services.[11] In addition, the occupational therapist may personally believe and hold to the beliefs and moral guidance of a religious tradition.

Should a religious tradition be considered a voice of moral authority? Religious traditions are a salient source of moral guidance on all-important matters of human life. Believers in a faith hold that a decision is right or morally correct because of divine authority. Thus, being a believer commits one to the ethical teachings of one's faith. Some argue that religion alone is the sufficient and ultimate justification for moral guidance. However, there is often plurality of beliefs regarding what is moral and good within a single faith tradition.

What if the religious beliefs of the institution and the occupational therapist differ? If there are differences in religious beliefs, whose beliefs should take precedence? For example, a female therapist receives an order to provide an orthosis for a male Hasidic Jew. The therapist recalls some information about the Hasidic Jewish culture. She thinks it may be inappropriate for her to touch this man's hand. The therapist is unsure what to do. She knows that this client needs her services and she is the only therapist in the clinic, but she also wishes to be culturally and religiously sensitive.

Because the moral authority for religious beliefs is by its very nature mutually exclusive, there would be no common language or set of ethical principles from which to engage in discussion. There is no common language because different people hold different religious beliefs. We would have to look for a view of ethics that is respectful and cognizant of religious beliefs but that exists outside individual belief systems in order to meet on common ground. In a pluralistic society, such as that encountered in the United States, secular ethical principles have great appeal because they are grounded on reason. Moreover, there is striking similarity among basic ethical principles and constructs held across diverse religious beliefs. This indicates that there is perhaps another, more basic source, of moral guidance. We now turn to three of these traditional approaches to secular ethics that allow us to talk across various faith traditions, cultures, and disciplines.

Classic Approaches to Ethics

One way of discussing morality is to observe that it involves obligations. The principles approach to ethics recognizes these obligations or duties and the universal nature of their application to moral decisions. Another way of viewing the moral life is through a more subjective lens with a concern for actual persons and their needs and relationships. **Care-based ethics** attempts to focus on the specific ethical issues that arise within the web of human relationships that nurture and sustain us as human beings.

Finally, we can view the moral life outside the moral problems encountered in clinical practice and instead focus on the character of the occupational therapist. When decisions have to be made in occupational therapy practice, it is often in a climate of stress and perhaps urgency. The best tools an occupational therapist can have for dealing with situations such as this are not those provided by principles or care-based reasoning but by a fixed habit of character or virtue. This provides a generally reliable response to ethical challenges. Virtue ethics takes the view that a person with a developed moral character knows when and what type of a decision needs to be made and has the perseverance to follow through. A brief description of each of these traditional approaches to ethics follows.

Principles Approach

Beauchamp and Childress[2] are the architects of the four principles approach to ethics. Although there are more than the four ethical principles selected by Beauchamp and Childress, these four principles do provide a comprehensive framework for ethical analysis. The four principles are as follows:
- Respect for **autonomy** (respecting the decision-making capacity of autonomous persons)
- **Nonmaleficence** (the **duty** not to harm)
- **Beneficence** (the duty to do good)
- **Justice** (a group of norms or rules that assist in the fair distribution of burdens and benefits)

Each of these **principles** has played a central role in health care. Respect for autonomy requires that we not only respect other human beings but that we have a regard for their **self-determination.** Autonomous adults have the right to make decisions about their lives without undue interference or coercion from others. Therapists must be aware of the autonomy of their clients. For example, a therapist may want to provide an orthosis for an older adult to slow deformity. The older adult may explicitly state that he or she does not wish to have the orthosis made.

Nonmaleficence is sometimes referred to as the most basic of all ethical principles in health care. Nonmaleficence is a perfect duty because it is always binding and forbids harm to others. For example, a physician may write a prescription for an orthosis that you know will cause a client harm. The therapist's duty of nonmaleficence guides the therapist to handle the situation for a different outcome.

Beneficence is an imperfect duty and one that is sometimes binding. Beneficence asserts that we should promote and do good for others. All of the occupational therapist's efforts are directed to the patient's good in the sense that interventions are directed to improving function and well-being. The very act of orthotic provision is a beneficent act because it is for the patient's welfare whether in the long or short term. In the relationship between health professionals and clients, the imperfect duty of beneficence takes on more weight and approximates the perfect duty of nonmaleficence.

Justice mediates the claims of self-interested individuals within communities. Distributive justice is of particular interest in health care because often there is not enough of a valuable resource for all those who need or want it, and decisions must be made about the fair distribution of such a resource. For example, a therapist knows that a client will benefit from an orthosis that is not covered by insurance. The therapist wishes to do good and refers the client to a pro bono clinic.

Generally speaking, principles are action guides to moral behavior. The principles approach responds most appropriately to the question of what is the morally correct thing to do. The principles are universally applicable (i.e., they apply to all people in all situations and provide a degree of impartiality to the decision-making process). Beauchamp and Childress emphasize that their four principles do not constitute a general ethical theory but provide a framework for identifying and reflecting on ethical problems.[2]

Principles must be specified to be of assistance in practical circumstances, especially when there is conflict between ethical principles. For example, a therapist is treating a client who is severely depressed and needs an orthosis to improve function. The client does not want the orthosis. The therapist must wrestle with the client's need for autonomy and the principles of beneficence and nonmaleficence. After specifying what autonomy, goods, and harms mean in the context of this case, the therapist could then turn to a more sophisticated level of reasoning to a moral decision; that is, ethical theory that prioritizes or balances the demands of the principles in conflict.

Care-Based Approach

Care-based reasoning emphasizes the particular and unique features of a situation. Care-based reasoning also emphasizes the moral relevance of such features as context, relationships, and power hidden in the more objective, universal view of the principles approach. A care-based approach to ethics recognizes that all persons are not situated so as to be independent decision makers of equal status. Many individuals (particularly clients) are disadvantaged, dependent, sometimes exploited, and often responsible for the care of others. All of these factors limit their ability to assert their rights in competition with the claims of others.

A care-based approach draws our attention to the actual persons involved in a case, and their needs, particular history, and connections. In addition, care-based theorists claim that a caring relationship is characterized by mutuality (recognition of the self in others) and transformation; that is, the relationship transforms or changes not only the recipient of care but the caregiver as well.[6,10] The recognition and protection of relationships are of prime importance to care-based ethics.

The following example demonstrates the ethical dilemma arising from a situation in which relationships, context, and power are intertwined. A therapist may wish to honor a child's goal to independently hold a crayon. To accomplish this goal, the therapist must provide the child with an orthosis. The child's parents are adamantly opposed to the child's wearing the orthosis because they wish to preserve the child's "normalcy" and do not want equipment that calls attention to the disability.

Virtue-Based Approach

Virtue is a morally good habit of one's nature. Virtue makes work, interactions, and all types of human exchanges good and makes individuals good. The distinction between a habit and action is important if one is to understand virtue, as human beings are constantly required to make choices between good and bad alternatives and to discern the right and reject the wrong. We need a constancy of mind or will to adhere to right principles. All of this calls for a foundation of solid virtues. Thus, we do the right thing or are inclined to do good as a matter of habit or character. Goodness is a part of who we are and is evident in how we act. An occupational therapist must have the virtues of compassion, wisdom, justice, temperance, and fortitude—to name a few essential virtues—to be deemed a good occupational therapist.

According to Aristotle, virtue means doing the right thing in relation to the right person, at the right time, and in the right manner. In other words, we should strive for moderation in all things, not going to excess or falling short of the Peter. For example, it is one thing to be courageous and another to take courage to the point of foolhardiness. If we exercise too little courage, we might be considered cowardly. Thus, to find the right balance is life's greatest good or *summum bonum* of the moral life. Virtue holds us fast to the right course. For example, a therapist's client tells her that her husband is abusing her and she is frightened to go home. The virtuous therapist makes the time to help this client and risks being reprimanded for low productivity units.

Application to Complex Cases

The three approaches to ethics provide different methods of analysis that highlight certain aspects of a case and minimize others. Each approach is applied to a different case dealing with occupational therapists involved in some aspect of orthotics. The first case highlights the ethical principles of nonmaleficence and beneficence and an additional principle, proportionality, that helps balance the two.

Case One: Harms and Benefits of Orthoses

Sarah, OTR/L, was somewhat surprised when she received an order for orthosis for a client from the oncology service in the large medical center in which she worked. The occupational therapy department did not receive many referrals from oncology. Sarah was concerned that the order might be inappropriate when she noted the age and primary diagnosis of the client, Sophie, who was dying of metastatic cancer of the breast. Sophie is 82 years old and is no longer a viable candidate for any type of treatment for cancer. She had undergone surgery several years before. Surgery was followed by radiation and chemotherapy. However, the cancer had returned and metastasized to her bones.

Sophie's husband died of cancer, and thus Sophie had first-hand knowledge of what dying could be like. She told her physician, "I saw how Frank died surrounded by tubes and equipment. That's not for me. I don't want to die in the hospital. I want my family and friends with me, and I don't want to be in pain." Recently, Sophie returned to the hospital for surgery to excise a tumor on her arm. Unfortunately, the tumor caused radial nerve compression that was not resolved by the surgery. The order Sarah received today was for a dynamic extension orthosis.

After Sarah finished reviewing the medical record, she walked down the hall to assess Sophie's condition. Sophie had fallen asleep in the chair in her room. As Sarah stood in the doorway and watched the slow rise and fall of Sophie's thin chest, she wondered if orthotic intervention made any sense in this case. What did Sophie stand to gain from the orthotic procedure? The dynamic extension orthosis was costly and inconvenient. A prefabricated orthosis would be less costly but may not offer the full function of a dynamic orthosis. How should Sarah weigh the potential benefits and harms of the two types of orthoses? How should Sarah weigh the potential benefits and harms of either orthosis against Sophie's overall prognosis?

There are at least two ethical questions raised by this case. The first is substantive: Is it ever appropriate to deliver care that offers little hope of benefit or is unduly burdensome to the client? The second is more procedural: What role should Sarah play in providing care to Sophie? Clearly, the two are linked but separate issues.

Sarah is obligated by the principles of nonmaleficence and beneficence to avoid harm and to provide good. This statement appears fairly straightforward. Yet, we know that certain clinical procedures (orthotic provision included) do cause harm in the form of inconvenience and cost. We justify this harm because of the potential benefit that will be realized. It is worthwhile, in other words, to bear some

inconvenience and higher cost in the present for greater function from stretching of soft tissue in the long term.

The principle of proportionality recognizes the need to balance the goods and harms of all types of clinical care. The risks of harm must be constantly weighed against possible benefit. We not only have a duty to avoid harm and do good but to weigh and balance possible benefits against possible harms to maximize benefits and minimize harms. Normally, the provision of a dynamic extension orthosis would be considered a moral good. If the orthosis does its job, the client will have greater flexibility and use of the wrist and hand, adding to the overall quality of life.

In this case, however, Sophie is already burdened with the pain and suffering of a terminal illness. It is unlikely that she will gain much benefit from any orthosis because there is little hope for an extended life span.

Competent clients have the right, according to autonomy, to make decisions about the benefit and burdens of intervention. This is especially important when a client nears the end of life. A death with dignity is sometimes defined as a death that is not "unduly burdened" by the clinical environment and medical technology to prolong life.[3] The intervention or technology in this case is not "life-sustaining" (e.g., a ventilator or artificial nutrition and hydration). However, it does have an impact on the quality of life Sophie will have until her death from other causes.

Clients are not obligated to undergo intervention that offers little hope of benefit or that involves excessive pain, expense, or other inconvenience. If the goals of intervention are not attainable (i.e., the use of particular therapy cannot or will not improve prognosis and recovery), the intervention need not be initiated or continued. The moral focus in this case is not on the type of disease or illness the client has, the state of medical science, or the type of intervention. In addition, questions of whether the intervention is customary, simple, inexpensive, or noninvasive are not the relevant ethical considerations. The true moral focus regarding any intervention, orthotic provision included, is the proportion between the benefit to the client and the burden involved. Furthermore, health care professionals are not mandated by law or morally obligated to render treatment that is deemed useless.

Sarah must first decide whether she considers an orthosis as plausible intervention. If the intervention is at least plausible, she has a duty to give Sophie the relevant information about the types of orthoses and their possible benefits and burdens. This should be done in a manner that Sophie understands so that she makes a decision about the intervention that is in keeping with her values and previously expressed wishes. If Sophie decides that the burdens of the intervention are disproportionate to the benefits, she is not obligated to undergo the orthotic procedure; nor is Sarah morally obligated to provide intervention that Sophie deems overly burdensome.

It should be noted that the physician ordered a specific orthosis for Sophie, and Sarah cannot ignore this additional obligation to a professional colleague. The physician has a right to expect that his orders will be carried out unless there is a good reason they should not be. Sarah should explain the outcome of her interaction with Sophie to the physician and work toward a mutually agreeable solution. Sarah could offer other methods of support to Sophie such as stretching exercises to improve the quality of her life for whatever time she has left.

The next case involves a situation in which the therapist is advised to deceive both the client and the third-party payer. The act of deception runs counter to the principle of respect for autonomy, and therefore requires justification. Another way to sort through the ethical issues and decide what ought to be done in this particular situation is through a care-based approach.

Case Two: Providing Less Than Optimal Services

The number of clients referred to the outpatient clinic of Centerview Medical Center seemed to increase every week. Peter, OTR/L, enjoyed the busy pace and the variety of clients he saw in the clinic. Peter was assigned a new client, Yongyue, a 28-year-old automobile manufacturing worker who sustained a severe crush injury of his hand on the job. Peter noted that there were orders to evaluate and begin intervention. As Peter read further in Yongyue's medical record, he saw that the physician specifically requested a certified hand therapist's (CHT's) services. Peter was not a CHT, so he approached his supervisor, Vivian, to discuss the problem. Peter explained that the physician's orders specified a CHT.

"How soon can Yongyue see the CHT?" Peter asked Vivian. "She's just too busy to take any new clients," Vivian responded. "I'll tell you what to do. I would hate to lose this case. It looks like it will take months of service to rehabilitate Yongyue. Why don't you just go ahead and provide services to him and have the CHT sign the notes? Who will know the difference?" Vivian then walked away.

Peter was left standing in the middle of the hallway with Yongyue's chart in his hand and a perplexed look on his face. Provide services to a client and have someone else sign off on them? On the face of it, that seemed very wrong to Peter. Yet he, too, would hate to lose this interesting case. He had briefly met Yongyue and instantly liked him. Would anyone really know the difference if he provided care to Yongyue or if the CHT did? Peter wondered what the right thing to do was. The application of a care-based approach includes the following[5]:

- Identifying the moral conflict within the specific context, considering the others who are involved in the conflict and how they are interrelated
- Feeling concern for relationships and individuals, and identifying oneself in relation to the individuals and problems involved

Generally speaking, if Peter took a care-based approach to resolving the ethical issues in the case, he would ask himself what it means to be "caring" within the context of this situation and its specific responsibilities. The moral conflict involves whether or not to provide services that are less than optimal to Yongyue; Peter is not a CHT. Could this be considered a "caring" action? The context of this case is a busy outpatient setting, perhaps too busy to handle the volume of clients and maintain quality. Because the physician specifically ordered that a CHT provide the care, the first logical alternative for Peter is to transfer Yongyue's care to a CHT. This is what Peter attempted to do and was told that the CHT caseload was backlogged.

If the beleaguered CHT at the Centerview Medical Center cannot see all of the clients who need her level of expertise, the clinic is obligated to either hire another CHT or to support and prepare another therapist who is already a member of the staff (such as Peter). After some time, this would allow Peter to become eligible to take the CHT certification examination. Both of these options are caring in several regards in that the special needs of all parties, including the overworked CHT, are considered.

The CHT would receive some assistance so that her work is more manageable, and probably less stressful, and clients would receive the level of care they deserve for their complex problems. However, these solutions are long term in nature and not immediately helpful to Peter. A caring, short-term solution could be to refer Yongyue to a CHT at another clinic or hospital. Alternatively, Peter could "trade" a patient with the CHT. In addition, Peter could work with the physician to see whether there is any room for negotiation about the requirement for the CHT. The latter option would be considered caring only if Peter truly believed he could deliver a quality of care approximating that of a CHT, perhaps under the indirect supervision of a CHT.

Vivian did not offer any of these alternative solutions to Peter's problem but suggested that Peter lie. Could a lie ever be considered a caring action? Perhaps, but in this situation we have to ask who the lie benefits? It appears that the clinic benefits because they won't lose reimbursement for billable service. Peter might also benefit to a limited extent because he would get to work with a client he likes and would learn from the experience of providing intervention to him.

Those who would be harmed are the physician and Yongyue. If either the physician or Yongyue found out that they had been deceived, how might they react? If Yongyue's care was insufficient, his function could be compromised. Of course, there are legal implications in the case, because what Vivian has suggested is fraud. However, there are moral implications as well.

Care-based ethics also focuses on the relationship of the individuals involved. Lies have a way of eroding relationships because they damage trust. If Peter chose to follow Vivian's recommendation, the entire time he was seeing Yongyue he would be doing so in a deceptive manner. It is important to understand that deception includes withholding information and outright falsehoods. In addition, Peter now knows that Vivian condones deception and this knowledge can hurt their relationship. Vivian did not demonstrate caring behavior to one of her subordinates but chose to place him in a moral dilemma in which he will be forced to oppose her recommendation to do the right thing.

Finally, because Peter "likes" Yongyue he may be more inclined to resist actions that are deceitful. Affection for clients makes it easier for us to recognize that they are fellow participants in life, facing the human condition. Another of the characteristics of care-based reasoning is mutuality; that is, empathizing with the other's position. If Peter were the client and had an injury similar to that sustained by Yongyue what sort of intervention would he want? As a client, would he accept the reasons for the deception Vivian has proposed? It is unlikely that any client would accept less than optimal care so that the clinic could make a profit.

In the next case, an occupational therapist wrestles with the conflicting obligations often encountered in clinical settings between clients and colleagues. Everyone makes a mistake at one time or another, but what if the mistake of a colleague has serious implications for a client's well-being? Should the therapist's primary loyalty always lie with the client?

Case Three: Covering for a Colleague

Justin, OTR/L, was filling in for a colleague and friend, Kara, who was absent from work with a bad case of the flu. Justin and Kara attended the same occupational therapy program, and after graduation both ended up working for the same health system in a large urban setting. Justin made it a habit to review the medical records, intervention plans, and progress reports of the clients he treated, even if he worked with them for only a day. He believed it was important to be familiar with their care and present status.

The first client on the schedule, Ben, was recovering from a flexor tendon injury, status post 2 weeks. The chart review indicated that Ben was a cooperative client. Justin began with an assessment of Ben's condition before proceeding with therapy. Justin immediately noticed that the tendon repair appeared to be ruptured. Justin began to question Ben about his activities. Ben reported doing his home exercise program as prescribed yesterday evening when he noted a significant sharp pain in his hand followed by the inability to bend his finger. "Should the therapist have told me to do those exercises like that?" Ben asked.

It appeared that Kara had not followed the protocol for flexor tendon injuries. Because she had given him a home exercise program with gripping exercises and put Ben through an inappropriate hand exercise regimen, the surgical repair was ruptured. Kara was responsible for the injury and the future pain and inconvenience that Ben would have to undergo having surgical repair of the injury a second time. Ben's question hung in the air as Justin thought about his obligations to a friend and colleague in contrast to his obligations to the client. This case raises numerous questions:

- Is this therapist simply inexperienced?

- How does one gauge the competence of a peer?
- How far does loyalty to peers extend?
- Is competency a matter of aesthetics?
- Are there sufficient safeguards in place to protect the public from incompetent providers?
- What are occupational therapy's obligations to society regarding the competence of its own practitioners and those in other fields?
- What does the public need to know?

It would be important to determine whether this was an isolated incident or a pattern in Kara's behavior. Overall competence is related to client good. Regardless of the reason for this particular act of incompetence, to remedy the incompetent behavior Justin must access the systems in place in the organization (such as Kara's supervisor or the risk management department). To report a friend and colleague, Justin must have the virtues of courage and perseverance. Justin's first obligation as a health care professional is to the best interests of clients.

Justin must also have the virtue of honesty. He has made an implied promise to clients to serve their best interests. In this case, that involves supplying information about what Justin suspects is the cause of Ben's injury. It is possible that Ben injured his hand himself, although he denies it. However, even if that is so Kara should not have engaged him in inappropriate active hand exercises.

Justin has a general moral obligation to tell the truth. He should not lie. Before Justin reveals the information about the ruptured tendon repair to Ben and the surgeon, who will need to know, he would first want to speak to Kara and confirm what actually happened. The morally virtuous occupational therapist is straightforward, thoughtful, and well-meaning. Given all of these virtues, Justin must make a decision (and quickly) as to how he will respond to Ben about his injury. He can be loyal to his peer and friend and still do the right thing, but he will need a strong moral character to act.

The Occupational Therapy Code of Ethics would support actions that maintain high-quality standards of care. In addition, balanced with this mandate of client benefit is Principle 7, which states, "Occupational therapy personnel shall treat colleagues and other professionals with respect, fairness, discretion, and integrity." Justin must make certain that Ben's welfare is protected, but he should do so in a way that minimizes harms to Kara.

Contribution of Ethics to Clinical Practice

In addition to the resources already enumerated to assist occupational therapists when making ethical decisions, there are resources within organizations or institutions. For example, policies and guidelines provide excellent support when they are thoughtfully written in keeping with the ethical norms provided herein and the values of the organization as a whole. Policies or guidelines should be available for commonly encountered ethical issues, such as informed consent, determination of decision-making ability, confidentiality, futility decisions, fair and safe distribution of staff and workload, and the role of surrogate decision makers.

Furthermore, personnel in specific areas of care (such as hand rehabilitation or burn care) could work together to establish mutually held values about the complex issues that comprise daily clinical experience. For example, what are the values regarding conflicts between religious values and those held by the institution regarding end-of-life intervention and pain management? Unless dedicated time is spent reflecting on issues such as these, it is likely that decisions will be made during highly emotional and urgent circumstances with less than satisfactory results.

Finally, another resource that is becoming more common is the institutional ethics committee. Occupational therapists should not only seek out the advice and support of ethics committees when problems seem beyond resolution; they should offer to serve on such committees, because their expertise and perspective are often missing from the committee's membership. Ethics committees offer the opportunity to discuss issues in a nonthreatening environment in a multidisciplinary manner. Although ethics committees do not make the decision for the individuals involved in an ethical problem, they do offer guidelines and affirm the values of the organization that form the parameters for decisions.

SELF-QUIZ 19-1*

In regard to the following questions, circle either true (T) or false (F).

1. T F By looking at the virtues of individuals, we are able to gauge their character.
2. T F Moral principles serve as action guides as we make ethical decisions.
3. T F Beneficence is a perfect duty.
4. T F Respect for autonomy obligates us to do good for others.
5. T F The principle of nonmaleficence requires that we avoid harming others at all times.
6. T F Care-based reasoning is concerned with the universal abstract aspects of the moral life.
7. T F Although not legally binding, professional codes of ethics set forth the highest standards of professions.
8. T F Ethics is an attempt to state what we should do, be, or care about to attain the most of what is best in human life.
9. T F Justice is concerned with the fair distribution of burdens and benefits in a community.
10. T F Proportionality requires that we balance the harms and goods in a situation and work to maximize the good.

*See Appendix A for the answer key.

Review Questions

1. How does one know if a situation involves ethics?
2. What is the difference among moral, amoral, and immoral behavior?
3. What are the basic differences between the three traditional approaches to ethics: principles, care-based, and virtue?
4. What are the four ethical principles that underlie the majority of interactions in health care?
5. What question does the principle approach to ethics best answer?
6. What does the principle of proportionality require us to do?
7. Can virtues be learned, practiced, and cultivated?
8. How does care-based ethics view the moral life?
9. How does virtue provide us with immediate responses to ethical challenges?
10. What are some of the limitations of professional codes of ethics?

References

1. American Occupational Therapy Association: *Occupational therapy code of ethics and ethics standards*, 2010 (website): http://www.aota.org/~/media/Corporate/Files/AboutOT/Ethics/Code%20and%20Ethics%20Standards%202010.ashx, Accessed March 16, 2014.
2. Beauchamp T, Childress J: *Principles of biomedical ethics*, ed 6, New York, 2009, Oxford University Press.
3. Catholic Health Association: *Caring for persons at the end of life*, St Louis, 1993, Catholic Health Association.
4. Chater R, Dockter D, Haddad A, et al.: Ethical decision making in pharmacy, *American Pharmacy NS* 33(4):73, 1993.
5. Fry ST, Killen AR, Robinson EM: Care-based reasoning, caring, and the ethic of care: a need for clarity, *J Clin Ethics* 7(1):41–47, 1996.
6. Gadow S: Body and self: a dialectic, *J Med Philos* 5(3):172–184, 1980.
7. Haddad AM: Ethical problems in nursing. In [editor], *Dissertation Abstracts International #AAG8818621*, Lincoln, NE, 1988, University of Nebraska at Lincoln.
8. Haddad AM: Ethical problems in pharmacy practice: a survey of difficulty and incidence, *Am J Pharm Educ* 55:1–6, 1991.

9. Jonsen AR: *The birth of bioethics*, New York, 1998, Oxford University Press.

10. Mayerhoff M: *On caring*, New York, 1971, Harper & Row.

11. United States Conference of Catholic Bishops: *Ethical and religious directives for catholic health care services*, ed 5, Washington, DC, 2009, US Conference of Catholic Bishops. Text also available at. http://www.usccb.org/about/doctrine/ethical-and-religious-directives.

12. Veatch RM, Haddad AM, English DC: *Case studies in biomedical ethics*, New York, 2010, Oxford University Press.

13. Warren E: Special address to the Lewis Marshall Award Dinner of the Jewish Theological Seminary of America, New York. Quote appears in: Bracker M, Warren favors profession to give advice on ethics, *New York Times* :1–2, 1962.

APPENDIX 19-1   CASE STUDY

CASE STUDY 19-1*

Read the following scenario, and answer the questions based on information in this chapter.

Valerie, OTR/L, is the clinical therapy manager at Francis Medical Center in a moderate-sized city with many referrals from the surrounding rural community. She spends approximately 25% of her time treating clients, on an inpatient and outpatient basis. The rest of her time is spent dealing with administrative responsibilities and management of the physical, occupational, and speech therapy staff and services.

Valerie has recently hired Sam, a new occupational therapy graduate, who is planning to take his occupational therapy board examination soon. Until Sam can take and pass his examination, Valerie decided she would review and co-sign Sam's documentation. Last week, Valerie was reviewing Sam's intervention plan and documentation for several outpatients with complex upper extremity injuries. One client with a chronic radial nerve injury was being seen too many times and had no orthotic provision to prevent contractures or to position for function. As a result, Valerie is concerned that Sam did not follow the usual diagnostic protocol to provide and monitor the orthosis every other week. She realizes that Sam needs more supervision and networking to improve his services for efficiency and efficacy.

Valerie knows that she does not have the flexibility or the time in her schedule to provide the mentoring Sam needs. There are no other qualified occupational therapists on staff because one recently retired and the other is on maternity leave. Although recruitment is in progress, no one has been hired to take the retired therapist's place. Thus, Valerie does not have another therapist to supervise and mentor Sam. What should Valerie do? Should she limit the type of client Sam sees so that he does not treat clients with complex injuries? However, how will Sam gain the experience he needs to adequately manage complex clients if he is not allowed to treat them? What are Valerie's responsibilities in this case?

1. Is there an ethical issue in the case? If so, list three questions pertinent to this position.
2. What is (are) the ethical problem(s) in the case? You may name them in terms of conflicts between principles or via a care-based or virtue approach.
3. Briefly describe four alternative actions Valerie could take to resolve the ethical problem(s) in the case. For each alternative, name the ethical principle that is upheld or threatened by the alternative.
4. Use the Occupational Therapy Code of Ethics and Ethics Standards to determine what principle(s) of the Code would be helpful to Valerie as she makes her decision. List the principle(s), and explain how it would be helpful.

*See Appendix A for the answer key.

Glossary

adherence   The extent that a client follows agreed-upon intervention without close supervision.

anterior elbow immobilization orthosis   Elbow immobilization orthosis positioned on the anterior aspect of the arm.

antideformity position   A position that includes the wrist in 30 to 40 degrees of extension, the thumb in 40 to 45 degrees of palmar abduction, the thumb interphalangeal (IP) joint in full extension, the metacarpophalangeals (MCPs) at 70 to 90 degrees of flexion, and the proximal interphalangeals (PIPs) and distal interphalangeals (DIPs) in full extension.

aponeurosis   A strong sheet of fibrous connective tissue that serves as a tendon to attach muscles to bone or as a fascia to bind muscles together.

area of force application   Area that force is supplied with an orthosis.

arthrogryposis   Severe contractures as a result of congenital limb deficits.

arteriovenous anastomosis   A blood vessel that connects directly to a venule without capillary intervention.

Assessment of Motor and Process Skills (AMPS)   A functional assessment that requires the client to perform an instrumental activity of daily living (IADL) and assesses motor and process skills.

autonomy   The capability of an adult to make decisions for himself or herself.

axonotmesis   An interruption of the axon with subsequent degeneration of the distal nerve segment.

beneficence   The duty to do good.

biofeedback machine   Equipment used to identify muscle signals and sites.

biomechanical   Considering the mechanical aspect of the body such as forces and muscle exertion.

biomechanical principles   Principles that include assessment of normal and pathologic gait patterns in a clinically observable evaluation.

biopsychosocial approach   Involving the interchange of biologic, psychological, and social factors.

body-powered prosthesis   Prosthesis activated and operated by body movements.

boutonnière deformity   A finger that postures with proximal interphalangeal (PIP) flexion and distal interphalangeal (DIP) hyperextension.

brachial plexus palsy   Paralysis or paresis of the brachial plexus a nerve plexus originating from the anterior braches including the last four cervical and first four thoracic spinal nerves. Plexus innervates the shoulder chest and arms.

buddy straps   Soft straps used to promote motion and support an injured digit to an adjacent digit.

camptodactyly   Permanent flexion of one or more of the interphalangeal finger joints usually caused by congenital factors.

Canadian Occupational Performance Measure (COPM)   A client-centered outcome measure used to assess self-care, productivity, and leisure.

care-based ethics   Focuses on the specific ethical issues that arise within the web of human relationships that nurture and sustain us as human beings.

carpal tunnel syndrome (CTS)   A common painful disorder of the wrist and hand induced by compression on the median nerve between the inelastic carpal ligament and other structures in the carpal tunnel.

central extensor tendon (CET)   This structure crosses the proximal interphalangeal (PIP) joint dorsally and is part of the PIP joint dorsal capsule.

cerebral palsy (CP)   A condition resulting in a non-progressive movement and postural disorder because of abnormal neural development or damage to the motor centers of the brain before, during or after birth.

circumferential   An orthosis that fits around the circumference of an extremity.

client-centered treatment   Treatment that focuses on meeting client goals as opposed to therapist-designed or protocol-driven goals.

client safety   Approach to client care that considers safety.

clinical reasoning   The in-depth deliberation and decision process that therapists apply in clinical practice involving several approaches towards thinking.

451

clinodactyly   A congenital condition resulting in permanent and abnormal lateral or medial flexion of one or more fingers.

collateral ligaments   Ligaments on each side of the joint that provide joint stability and restraint against deviation forces. The radial collateral ligament protects against ulnar deviation forces, and the ulnar collateral ligament protects against radial deviation forces.

complex regional pain syndrome (CRPS)   A chronic pain condition thought to be a result of impairment in the central or peripheral nerve systems.

componentry   The compilation of components toward assembling a prosthesis.

composite extension   Extension of all fingers together.

compression socks   Socks used to reduce swelling formation at an amputation site.

concomitant injury   Injury that occurs impacting two or more places simultaneously.

conduction   Transfers heat from one object to another. Heat is conducted from the higher-temperature object to the lower-temperature material.

congenital hand anomalies   Hand deformities found at birth

congenital trigger finger   Condition found at birth in which the finger is pulled into flexion.

constriction band syndrome   Treatment that focuses on meeting client goals as opposed to therapist-designed or protocol-driven goals

context   A variety of interrelated conditions within and surrounding the client that influence performance, including cultural, physical, social, personal, spiritual, temporal, and virtual aspects.

contracture   An abnormal, usually permanent, condition of a joint characterized by flexion and fixation and caused by atrophy and shortening of muscle fibers or by loss of the normal elasticity of the skin, such as that from the formation of extensive scar tissue over a joint.

contralateral limb   Limb on the opposite side to the referent.

convection   Transfers heat between a surface and a moving medium or agent.

creep   Response of soft tissue to prolonged stress. Can be with pain or inflammation or can be managed with controlled stress.

cumulative trauma disorder (CTD)   Musculoskeletal disorder resulting from repetitive motions (usually occupation) that develop over time. Symptoms include pain, inflammation, and function impairment.

degrees of freedom   The number of planes in which a joint axis(es) can move.

de Quervain tenosynovitis   The most commonly diagnosed wrist tendonitis that may be recognized by pain over the radial styloid, edema in the first dorsal compartment, and positive results from the Finkelstein test.

distal humerus   Fracture at the end of the humerus bone.

documentation   Professional writing in a formal medical record.

dorsal   Pertaining to the back or posterior.

double crush   Nerves that are compressed at more than one site.

dual site   The use of an externally powered prosthesis from two muscle sites.

Dupuytren contracture   A contracture characterized by the formation of finger flexion contractures with a thickened band of palmar fascia.

duty   An obligatory task, conduct, or function that arises from one's position.

dynamic orthosis   A mobilization orthosis that has a stable static base and an elastic mobilizing component.

ecchymosis   A subcutaneous hemorrhage marked by purple discoloration of the skin.

elbow arthroplasty   The resurfacing or replacement of the elbow joint.

elbow instability   Injury that results from a dislocation of the ulnohumeral joint and injury to the varus and valgus stabilizers of the elbow and to the radial head.

electrodes   Round or square metal used to read or "pick up" muscle signals.

end feel   Assessed by passively moving a joint to its maximal end range.

Erb palsy   Paralysis of the upper arm and shoulders but not hands caused by a lesion of the upper trunk of the brachial plexus or roots to the fifth and sixth cervical nerves.

Essex-Lopresti fracture   Fracture of the radial head along with dislocation of the distal radio-ulnar joint and accompanying issues with the interosseous membrane resulting from a fall from a height.

ethics   The exploration of moral duty, principles, human character or virtue, and human relationships involving the study of right and wrong, good and evil, and moral conduct on an individual and societal basis; rules, promises, principles, and obligations.

evidence-based practice   The process of reviewing a body of literature in order to select the most appropriate assessment or treatment for an individual client.

extensor lag   The joint can be passively extended but cannot be fully actively extended by the client.

externally-powered prosthesis   Prothesis operated by batteries.

finger loops   A method of applying dynamic force to a joint.

finger sprain   Stress or ligamentous injury to a joint. occurs in varying grades of severity.

flexion contracture   A joint that cannot be passively extended to neutral.

forearm trough   A component of the wrist immobilization orthosis that rests proximal to the wrist on one or more surfaces of the forearm. It provides counterforce leverage to support the weight of the forearm.

functional envelope   Area of work in front and around a person's hands.

functional position A position that includes the wrist in 20 to 30 degrees of extension, the thumb in 45 degrees of palmar abduction, the metacarpophalangeal (MCP) joints in 35 to 45 degrees of flexion, and all proximal interphalangeal (PIP) and distal interphalangeal (DIP) joints in slight flexion.

fusiform swelling Fullness at the proximal interphalangeal (PIP) joint and tapering proximally and distally. Often seen following finger PIP joint sprains.

grasp The result of holding an object against the rigid portion of the hand that the second and third digits provide. The flattening and cupping motions of the palm allow the hand to pick up and handle objects of various sizes.

grip force The amount of force given to a hand or a hook.

handling characteristics The properties of thermoplastic material when heated and softened.

hard end feel An abrupt hard stop to movement when bone contacts bone during PROM.

harness Strap system to suspend or hold a prosthesis.

heat gun An instrument used to make adjustments to thermoplastic materials.

Health Insurance Portability and Accountability Act (HIPPA) Health Insurrance Portability and Accountable Act regulates privacy standards that protects medical records and other health information.

hook rubbers Rubber bands used for hooks used to increase hook grip.

hypertonicity Being hypertonic or having excess tone.

hypoplasia Unfinished or under-development of an organ or part.

hypothenar bar A component of the wrist immobilization orthosis that palmarly supports the ulnar aspect of the transverse metacarpal arch.

immobilization Orthoses designed to immobilize primary or secondary joints.

integumentary system A system encompassing the integument (skin) and its derivatives.

intervention process Processes provided by therapists with intervention.

justice A group of norms or rules that assists in the fair distribution of burdens and benefits.

lamination Hard, permanent finish of prosthetic socket.

lateral bands Contributions from the intrinsic muscles that join dorsal to the proximal interphalangeal (PIP) joint axis. They displace volarly in a boutonnière deformity and dorsally in a swan neck deformity.

lateral epicondyle The tissue at the lower end of the humerus at the elbow joint.

mallet finger A finger that postures with distal interphalangeal (DIP) flexion.

McKie thumb orthosis A prefabricated Neoprene orthosis designed to position the thumb in opposition and in which a supinator strap may be added. The primary function is to provide biomechanically sound weight bearing, grasp, and manipulation of objects.

mechanical advantage The ratio of the output force developed by the muscles to the input force applied to the body structures the muscles move, especially the ratio of these forces associated with the body structures that act as levers.

mechanoreceptor Sensory nerve ending that responds to mechanical stimuli, such as touch, pressure, sound, and muscular contractions.

medial epicondyle The part of the humerus that gives attachment to the ulnar collateral ligament of the elbow joint, to the pronator teres, and to a common tendon of origin (the common flexor tendon) of some of the flexor muscles of the forearm.

median nerve One of the terminal branches of the brachial plexus, which extends along the radial parts of the forearm and the hand and supplies various muscles and the skin of these parts.

memory The ability of thermoplastic material to return to its preheated (original) shape and size when reheated.

metacarpal bar A component of the wrist immobilization orthosis that supports the transverse metacarpal arch dorsally or palmarly.

minimalist design A basic simplified orthotic design.

mobilization An orthosis designed to move or mobilize primary and secondary joints.

mobilization orthosis Orthosis designed to move or mobilize primary or secondary joints.

Monteggia fracture Dislocation of the proximal radioulnar joint along with a forearm fracture

morality Concerned with human behavior or actions that are judged as either good or evil.

myoelectric prosthesis The use of electronics to signal a muscle's electrical input.

Neoprene A soft orthotic material consisting of rubber with nylon lining on one side and pile material on the other, thus making the Velcro hook attachment quick. Neoprene retains warmth, has some degree of elasticity, and has contour for a snug fit.

nerve entrapment Pressure on a nerve.

neurapraxia A condition in which a nerve remains in place after a severe injury, although it no longer transmits impulses.

neurophysiologic Branch of physiology that addresses the nervous system.

neurotmesis A peripheral nerve injury in which laceration or traction completely disrupts the nerve.

nonmaleficence The duty not to harm.

normal gait Smooth, rhythmic patterns of motion requiring little effort involving a gait cycle from initial contact of one foot to the next initial contact of the same foot

oblique retinacular ligament (ORL) Also called the *ligament of Landsmeer*, this structure is determined to be tight if there is limitation of passive distal interphalangeal (DIP) flexion while the proximal interphalangeal (PIP) joint is extended.

occupational deprivation   A state wherein clients are unable to engage in chosen meaningful life occupations due to factors outside their control.

occupational disruption   A temporary and less severe condition than occupational deprivation that is also caused by an unexpected change in the ability to engage in meaningful activities.

occupational profile   The phase of the evaluation process that involves learning about a client from a contextual and performance viewpoint.

Occupational Therapy Code of Ethics and Ethics Standards   The professional code of ethics established by the American Occupational Therapy Association (AOTA). This code sets forth the minimal expectations for occupational therapists.

occupation-based orthotic intervention   A treatment approach that supports the goals of the treatment plan to promote the ability of clients to engage in meaningful and relevant life endeavors.

olecranon process   A proximal projection of the ulna that forms the tip of the elbow and fits into the olecranon fossa of the humerus when the forearm is extended at the proximal extremity of the ulna.

open reduction internal fixation (ORIF)   Two part surgical procedure for a broken bone including putting the bone back into place (reduction) followed by utilizing a means of internal fixation (screws, plates, rods, pins) to hold the bone.

orthotic intervention error   Treatment that focuses on meeting client goals as opposed to therapist-designed or protocol-driven goals

orthosis   A permanent device to replace or substitute for loss of muscle function.

orthosis   A temporary device that is part of a treatment program.

orthotic design principles   Principles that consider the interaction of anatomic and mechanical structures as well as functional considerations of orthotic components and materials.

orthotic terminology   Terminology derived from the anatomic area affected by the orthosis.

orthotic treatment objectives   Objectives that establish short- and long-term goals that enhance functional level with minimal orthotic intervention.

osteoarthritis (OA)   The most common form of arthritis, in which one or many joints undergo degenerative changes—including loss of articular cartilage and proliferation of bone spurs.

outrigger   A projection from the orthosis base that the therapist uses to position a mobilizing force.

overuse syndrome   Repetitive movements causing pain (usually contralateral limb).

pathologic gait   Abnormal gait which may develop from neuromuscular deficits, joint instabilities, pain, disease, or congenital impairment

performance characteristics   The properties of thermoplastic material after the material has cooled and hardened.

phantom pain   Burning, stabbing pain at the distal end of amputation.

phantom sensation   The feeling of presence of the nonexistent limb.

physical agent modality (PAM)   Modality that produces a biophysiologic response through the use of light, water, temperature, sound, electricity, or mechanical devices.

plaster bandage   Material used for casting

plasticity   The quality of being plastic or formative.

posterior elbow immobilization orthosis   A custommolded thermoplastic orthosis positioned in 80 to 90 degrees of flexion.

posterior interosseous nerve syndrome   A condition that includes weakness or paralysis of any muscles innervated by the posterior interosseous nerve and does not involve sensory loss.

preformed orthoses   Factory-produced orthoses premolded to a specific design.

prehension   The use of the hands and fingers to grasp or pick up objects.

pressure   Total force divided by the area of application.

principles   The universal nature of obligations and duties and their application to moral decisions.

pronator tunnel syndrome   The compression of the median nerve in the forearm between the two heads of the pronator teres muscle.

protocols   Written plans specifying the procedures for giving an examination, conducting research, or providing care for a particular condition.

radial   Pertaining to the radius or radial side of the forearm or hand.

radial club hand   A longitudinal deficiency of the radius associated with abnormal genetics resulting in missing or malformed radius and the small or missing thumb.

radial head   The disc-shaped portion of the radius closest to the elbow.

radial nerve   The largest branch of the brachial plexus, supplying the skin of the arm and forearm and their extensor muscles.

radial nerve injuries   Injuries commonly occurring from fractures of the humeral shaft, fractures and dislocation of the elbow, or compressions of the nerve.

radial tunnel syndrome   A condition in which a nerve in the forearm is compressed, causing elbow pain and weakness of the wrist or hand but without causing a loss of sensation.

reliability   The consistency of an assessment.

residual limb   The distal end portion of an amputation.

responsiveness   An assessment's sensitivity to measure differences in status.

rheumatoid arthritis (RA)   A chronic systemic disease that can affect the lungs, cardiovascular system, and eyes. Joint involvement resulting from inflammatory disease of the synovium is the primary clinical feature. The disease may range from mild to severe and can result in joint deformity and destruction of varying degrees.

scaphoid fracture   A break in the boat-shaped bone of the hand.

self-determination   The ability of the individual to freely choose his or her own actions.

sensory system modulation   The brain's ability to regulate and balance excitation and inhibition of sensory input.

serial casting   Casting used to gradually increase range of motion.

serial static orthosis   A type of mobilization orthosis that positions a joint near its elastic limits to overcome a loss in passive range of motion.

single site   The use of an externally-powered prosthesis from one muscle site.

socket   A hard material (resin and plastic) used to make temporary or permanent prostheses.

soft end feel   Soft compression of tissue felt when two body surfaces approximate each other

soft orthoses   Prefabricated or custom orthoses made from various soft materials.

spasticity   A form of muscular hypertonicity with increased resistance to stretch.

stages of healing   Refers to wound healing stages, such as the proliferative stage, which influence orthotic provision.

static progressive orthosis   An orthosis that uses nonelastic tension to provide a constant force.

stress   Any emotional, physical, social, economic, or other factor that requires a response or change.

stretch reflex   Reflex that is elicited through passive stretch used with orthotic fabrication for a person who has muscle done.

submaximum range   Placement of an orthosis 5-10 degrees below maximum passive range.

superficial agents   Heating agents or thermotherapy agents that penetrate the skin to a depth of 1 to 2 cm. They include moist hot packs, fluidotherapy, paraffin wax therapy, and cryotherapy.

suspension systems   Straps used to suspend or hold a prosthesis.

swan neck deformity   A finger that postures with proximal interphalangeal (PIP) hyperextension and distal interphalangeal (DIP) flexion.

syndactyly   Webbing between finger digits creating fusion of the digits.

task-oriented approach   Approach towards intervention that encourages hand usage with functional tasks

tendonitis   An inflammatory condition of a tendon, usually resulting from strain.

tenosynovitis   Inflammation of a tendon sheath caused by calcium deposits, repeated strain or trauma, high levels of blood cholesterol, rheumatoid arthritis, gout, or gonorrhea.

terminal device (TD)   Hand, hook, or tool used at the end of a prosthesis.

terminal extensor tendon   This delicate structure is formed by the uniting of the lateral bands and provides distal interphalangeal (DIP) extension.

thermoplastic material   Material that softens under heat and is capable of being molded into shape with pressure and then hardens upon cooling without undergoing a chemical change.

three-point pressure   A system consisting of three individual linear forces in which the middle force is directed in opposite direction to the other two forces.

torque   The effect a force has on rotational movement of a point. It can be calculated by multiplying the force by the length of the movement arm.

torque transmission   Orthoses that create motion of primary joints situated beyond the boundaries of the orthosis itself or that harness secondary "driver" joint(s) to create motion of primary joints that may be situated longitudinally or transversely to the driver joint(s).

transhumeral amputation   Amputation across the humerus bone.

transradial amputation   Amputation across the radius and ulna bones.

transverse retinacular ligament   This ligament helps prevent lateral band dorsal displacement and thereby contributes to the delicate balance of the extensor mechanism at the proximal interphalangeal (PIP) joint.

treatment protocol   Written plan specifying the procedures for treatment.

ulnar   Pertaining to the long medial bone of the forearm or ulnar side of the forearm or hand.

ulnar collateral ligament (UCL) injury   A common injury that can occur at the metacarpophalangeal (MCP) joint of the thumb. This is also known as *skier's thumb* or *gamekeeper's thumb.*

ulnar nerve   One of the termanl branches of the brachial plexus that supplies the muscles and skin on the ulnar side of the forearm and hand.

valgus   Deformed joint with the more distal of the bones deviating from the midline of the body.

validity   The extent to which an assessment measures what it is intended to measure.

values   The internal motivators for an individual's actions.

varus   Deformed joint which is bent inward with the angulation towards the midline of the body.

verbal analog scale (VeAS)   A scale used to determine a person's perception of pain intensity. The person is asked to rate pain on a scale from 0 to 10. (0 refers to no pain, and 10 refers to the worst pain ever experienced.)

virtue   A morally good habit of one's nature.

viscoelasticity   The skin's degree of viscosity and elasticity, which enables the skin to resist stress.

visual analog scale (ViAS)   A scale used to determine a person's perception of pain intensity. The person is asked to look at a 10-cm horizontal line. The left side of the line represents "no pain," and the right side represents "pain as bad as it could be." The person indicates pain level by marking a slash on the line, which represents the pain experienced.

volar   Also called *palmar,* this term pertains to the palm of the hand or the sole of the foot.

volar plate (VP) A fibrocartilaginous structure that prevents hyperextension of a joint.

Wallerian degeneration When a nerve is completely severed or the axon and myelin sheath are damaged, the segment of axon and the motor and sensory end receptors distal to the lesion suffer ischemia and begin to degenerate 3 to 5 days after the injury.

Wartenberg neuropathy Compression of the superficial radial nerve that usually includes numbness, tingling, and pain of the dorsoradial aspect of the forearm, wrist, and hand.

wearing schedules Planned schedules for donning and doffing orthoses.

working memory The short-term storage of information in the brain.

zones of the hand The division of the hand into distinct areas for ease of understanding literature, conversing with other health providers, and documenting pertinent information.

Answers to Self-Quizzes, Case Studies, and Laboratory Exercises

Chapter 1

Self-Quiz 1-1 Answers

1. b
2. c
3. a

Case Study 1-1 Answers

1. b
2. c
3. a

Chapter 2

Self-Quiz 2-1 Answers

1. The therapist should seek to learn about the culture of the client, either through personal interview with the individual or family or through reading. If the client speaks a language that you do not speak, ensure that a translator is present so that information is accurately transmitted between you and the client. Different cultures may have views about illness and disability that are different. They may also be of a different faith or have family obligations and responsibilities different from those you are accustomed to. Wearing a splint during certain ceremonies or religious events may not be acceptable to your client. Discuss the splint plan and appropriately explain the importance of compliance. If you learn that cultural difference may be a barrier to compliance, work with the client in an attempt to arrive at a workable solution.

2. The areas of occupation of play and education as well as developmentally appropriate activities of daily living (ADL) and instrumental activities of daily living (IADL) functions should be considered. Personal context factors such as age and gender will enter into color selection and the level of independence the child may have with splint donning/doffing and care. A younger child may need to have additional straps applied to prevent unwanted splint removal or shifting. An older child may be able to independently monitor a splinting schedule.

Case Study 2-1 Answers

1. Natasha's husband, who is her primary caretake, has accompanied her to treatment sessions. As an important part of her social context, and his role as caregiver, he is able to assist Natasha with accurate completion of the intake interview. To ensure that Natasha is empowered, and her family role as primary home and family caretaker is preserved to the extend possible within this traditional family, the therapist should first address questions to Natasha and verify responses with her husband only if needed.

2. Splint care sheet should be written in large, bold font. Instructions should be written in simple phrases and line drawings used as appropriate to illustrate splint and strap placement. Black-and-white or photocopied photos should be avoided because they may not provide high contrast. High-contrast color photos taken of the splint on Natasha's hand may assist with accurate placement but should not be used as the only pictorial representation. Splint care instructions must be reviewed with Natasha and her husband using the splint care sheet prior to issuing the device. Natasha should be asked to repeat instructions and precautions back to therapist with the assistance of her husband.

3. As with the splint care sheet, large font and line drawings can be used to assist with low vision. Instructions should be phrased simply and the order of the exercises should be clearly indicated. Line drawings can be effective, as can color photographs of Natasha's hand. Exercise instructions must be reviewed with Natasha and her

husband using the handout. Natasha should be asked to demonstrate the exercises and verbalize repetitions and frequency with the assistance of her husband prior to leaving the clinic.

Case Study 2-2 Answers

1. Graysen indicated that he is not satisfied with his ability to complete independent bill paying, use the computer to communicate with friends and family on social networking websites, or prepare his plate for independent eating. All of these areas scored poor in performance and satisfaction. Despite these issues being caused by limited hand function, they should be addressed during the first treatment sessions in order to enhance the quality of life for Graysen. Although these functions should return eventually as hand function improves, waiting for eventual hand movement, strength, and coordination will create an unnecessary lack of ability to complete meaningful life tasks. Computer use and social communication and bill paying are reported to be the most difficult and least satisfactory areas for Graysen.
2. A client-centered treatment model and a rehabilitative approach will expedite Graysen's return to function. The client-centered model focuses attention on his immediate concerns (bill paying, computer use and social communication, eating/plate preparation). The rehabilitative approach uses adaptations and modifications as treatment methods to enhance function.
3. The Canadian Occupational Performance Measure (COPM) was used to investigate the functional capabilities of the client within all areas of daily functioning. Issues were discovered within the patient's social, personal, and virtual contexts.

Chapter 4

Self-Quiz 4-1 Answers

Part I Answers
1. d
2. a
3. b
4. a
5. c

Part II Answers
1. distal palmar crease
2. proximal palmar crease
3. thenar crease
4. distal wrist crease
5. proximal wrist crease

Part III Answers
1. longitudinal arch
2. distal transverse arch
3. proximal transverse arch

Self-Quiz 4-2 Answers

1. F
2. F
3. T
4. T
5. F
6. T
7. F
8. T
9. T
10. F

Chapter 5

Self-Quiz 5-1 Answers

1. F
2. T
3. T
4. F
5. F
6. T
7. F
8. T
9. F
10. F
11. T
12. F
13. T
14. F

Chapter 6

Self-Quiz 6-1 Answers

1. F
2. T
3. T
4. T
5. F
6. T
7. F
8. F
9. F
10. T
11. T
12. F
13. F
14. T

Case Study 6-1 Answers

1. Steven has a radial nerve injury, which he sustained from falling asleep with his arm positioned over the top of a chair.

2. Never hesitate to call the physician's office. If the physician is not available, leave your question with the nurse.

3. The therapist should suggest an orthosis for radial nerve and research orthoses for that condition. He or she should review both textbooks and evidence-based practice articles, time permitting.

4. Steven should be educated about orthotic precautions, such as monitoring the orthosis for pressure sores, and about an orthotic-wearing schedule including removal for hygiene and exercise, so the orthotic provision is safe and effective.

5. As discussed, compliance can be a tricky issue because so many factors need to be considered for why a person is noncompliant. Is Steven's nonadherence related to a self-image problem with the orthosis or for some other reason that he has not stated? Refer to Box 6-3 for ideas of factors contributing to noncompliance. The therapist should provide open-ended questions to get Steven's perception about his noncompliance and what it would take for him to become compliant with orthotic wear. More specific education, including sharing of research evidence about the importance of orthotic wear with a radial nerve injury for regaining function, would be helpful. This education would also help Steven understand the slow process of nerve regeneration. Due to Steven's history of alcohol abuse leading to the development of the condition, he may need psychosocial support beyond the therapy clinic. Psychosocial support can be tactfully suggested by the therapist, and Steven can request a referral from his primary physician for intervention.

Case Study 6-2 Answers

1. Many areas were missing from the charting. Charting initially did not specify the extremity. It did not include client history of having de Quervain tenosynovitis or prior level of function. It did not mention prior treatment of receiving a prefabricated orthosis and did not specify where the reddened area was on the thumb. It provided an opinionated comment about client compliance. It would have been better to have provided factual information, such as a direct quote from Marie. The inclusion of normal measurements for range of motion, grip, and pinch strengths would make it easier for the reader to have a better understanding of deficits. It did not address the impact of the condition on doing work and home occupations. It did not address Marie's current level of pain. It should include the type of orthosis, position, and location. It should include a statement on fit, comfort, and function of the fabricated thumb immobilization orthosis. Goals are vague and not related to function. It would have been helpful to involve Marie with the goal setting, perhaps through administering the Canadian Occupational Performance Measure (COPM).

2. In every situation, questions using the interactive clinical reasoning approach will be different. The following are a few of many suggested questions:

- What questions do you have about wearing this fabricated orthosis? (This question may open up discussion, considering that Marie did not continue to wear the prefabricated orthosis due to developing some chafing on the volar surface of the thumb interphalangeal [IP] joint.)
- How will you go about following an orthotic schedule based on the home and work demands in your life? (This question may be helpful, considering Marie's history of noncompliance with the first orthosis.)
- What type of support do you need to help you with your orthosis and hand injury? (This question may help you better understand how Marie is coping with her condition.)

3. For this discussion, respect Marie's confidentiality by moving to a private area if in a large therapy room. You might assume that one reason Marie was noncompliant with the prefabricated orthosis was because it caused a reddened area on the thumb IP joint due to fitting improperly. However, you should tactfully question Marie for her reasons for noncompliance, which might be different from your assumption. Refer to Box 6-3 for ideas of factors that contribute to noncompliance and to Box 6-4 for ideas for open-ended questions to ask Marie. In any case, you should fabricate a well-fitted comfortable orthosis and monitor the fit carefully for potential pressure sores. Clear education about the reason for orthotic wear along with any evidence from research may help Marie's compliance. It will be important to check with Marie regularly about follow-through with the orthotic-wearing program. Consider making a phone call or emailing Marie to check on her level of compliance and to answer any questions.

4. Marie likely has worker's compensation insurance.

Chapter 7

Self-Quiz 7-1 Answers

1. T
2. T
3. F
4. T
5. T
6. F
7. F
8. T
9. F
10. F
11. F

Case Study 7-1 Answers

1. The two reasons are the following: (1) The prefabricated orthosis was not the best choice because it migrated up the forearm and did not fit properly, limiting finger and

thumb motions. (2) The orthosis was in the incorrect position of 20 degrees wrist extension and had not been readjusted to the correct position of neutral.

2. The wrist should be positioned as close to neutral as possible.

3. There are a variety of options for an orthotic-wearing schedule, but based on one study (Walker WC, Metzler M, Cifu DX, et al: Neutral wrist splinting in carpal tunnel syndrome: a comparison of night-only versus full-time wear instructions, *Arch Phys Med Rehabil* 81(4):424-429, 2000.) the person should wear the orthosis all the time with removal for exercise and hygiene.

4. The therapist should observe areas such as the ulnar styloid, the first web space, and the volar and dorsal aspects of the hand over the metacarpal bones for skin irritation. Beth should notify the therapist immediately if irritation occurs. In addition, Beth should be educated to not perform full finger flexion in the orthosis due to that motion causing increased pressure on the carpal tunnel.

5. In this case, trust was violated because Beth dutifully followed a wearing regimen for an orthosis that did not correctly fit and was exacerbating her condition. As McClure[42] suggests, providing research evidence specific to her situation might help her better understand the rationale for a custom-fabricated orthosis in a neutral position. Conservative management with using an orthosis may help because the condition was caught early,[26] and because after giving birth, carpal tunnel syndrome (CTS) symptoms may dissipate due to less fluid retention in the body and the client regaining hormonal balance.

Case Study 7-2 Answers

1. The therapist should use an orthosis to put Meggan's wrist in neutral to provide a low-load stretch.

2. The therapist should continue to use a serial orthosis to get Meggan's wrist into a functional wrist extension position.

3. This decision is made in collaboration with Meggan's physician based on her progress. Discontinuation of using an orthosis could occur when Meggan obtains more functional wrist extension, because wearing the orthosis too long will result in muscle weakness and/or joint stiffness. Once the orthosis is removed, the therapist will continue to work on obtaining increased active wrist extension and normal wrist motions for function.

Laboratory Exercise 7-2 Answers

Orthosis A

1. The wrist is positioned in extreme ulnar deviation. The wrist strap is placed incorrectly.

2. This extreme position stresses the wrist joint and possibly contributes to the development of other problems, such as wrist pain, pressure areas, and de Quervain tenosynovitis.

Orthosis B

1. The wrist is positioned in flexion instead of a functional hand position of extension. Positioning in wrist extension helps with digital flexion. If the wrist is flexed, the client loses functional grasp. The wrist strap is placed incorrectly.

Orthosis C

1. Metacarpophalangeal (MCP) flexion is inhibited because the orthotic metacarpal bar is too high. The wrist appears to be radially deviated. The wrist strap is placed incorrectly.

2. Potential development of skin irritation or pressure areas exists with digital flexion, and the person does not have a full functional grasp.

Chapter 8

Self-Quiz 8-1 Answers

1. T
2. F
3. T
4. F
5. T
6. T
7. F
8. F

Case Study 8-1 Answers

1. The hand is put in a hand-based thumb immobilization orthosis (MP radial and ulnar deviation restriction orthosis) with the carpometacarpal (CMC) joint in 40 degrees of palmar abduction and the metacarpophalangeal (MCP) joint in neutral to slight flexion and ulnar deviation.

2. To provide rest and protection during healing.

5. The orthosis is worn continuously for 4 to 5 weeks with removal for hygiene checks.

6. An option as suggested by Ford and colleagues[23] (Ford M, McKee P, Szilagyi M: A hybrid thermoplastic and neoprene thumb metacarpophalangeal joint orthosis, *J Hand Ther* 17(1):64-68, 2004.) is to fabricate a hybrid orthosis with a circumferential thermoplastic mold around the thumb covered by a Neoprene wrap. This orthosis will provide stability to the MCP joint and allow for functional movements during skiing.

Case Study 8-2 Answers

1. Based on Margaret's symptoms, the therapists should fabricate a hand-based orthosis. Because only the carpometacarpal (CMC) joint is involved, the orthosis designed by Colditz[14] (Colditz JC: The biomechanics of a thumb carpometacarpal immobilization splint: design

and fitting, *J Hand Ther* 13(3):228-235, 2000.)—which only immobilizes the CMC joint—would be appropriate.
2. To provide stability, and to control subluxation and pain.
3. Based on Colditz's[14] recommendations, Margaret should wear the orthosis continuously for 2 to 3 weeks (with removal for hygiene). After that time period, she should wear the orthosis during times when the thumb is irritated by activities.
4. Because of the wrist and thumb involvement, the therapist would consider fabricating a forearm-based thumb orthosis.
5.
6. The therapist should position the thumb metacarpophalangeal (MCP) joint in 30 degrees flexion and in palmar abduction as tolerated.

Laboratory Exercise 8-1 Answers

1. thumb post
2. metacarpal (palmar) bar
3. forearm trough

Laboratory Exercise 8-3 Answers

1. The two problems are the following: (1) The metacarpal bar is too high to allow full finger metacarpophalangeal (MCP) flexion and (2) the thumb interphalangeal (IP) joint flexion is limited because the material around the thumb extends too far distally.
2. An irritation might develop at the thumb IP joint (where the thumb opening is too high) and at the base of the index finger (where the metacarpal bar is too high). The orthosis limits full finger flexion.

Chapter 9

Case Study 9-1 Answers

1. b
2. c
3. b
4. b
5. b

Case Study 9-2 Answers

1. Diabetes mellitus is associated with Dupuytren disease.
2. Either a resting hand orthosis or a dorsal forearm-based static extension orthosis is appropriate to use after a Dupuytren contracture release.
3. The therapeutic position includes wrist in neutral or slight extension and metacarpophalangeals (MCPs), proximal interphalangeals (PIPs), and distal interphalangeals (DIPs) in full extension. The thumb does not need to be included in the orthosis.
4. Ken should wear his orthosis well after the wounds have completely healed. After healing, he should wear

the orthosis several weeks or months thereafter during the nighttime to provide stress and tension to counteract the scar contraction. (He may discontinue his resting hand orthosis in favor of individual finger orthoses.) The orthosis can be removed for hygiene, exercise, and activities of daily living (ADLs).
5. To accommodate for bandage thickness, the design of the orthosis should be wider. As bandage bulk is reduced, the orthosis should be modified to maintain as close to an ideal position as possible. Therefore, thermoplastic material that has memory will assist with the modification process. In addition, because this is a fairly long orthosis, a material with rigidity is helpful to adequately support the weight of the forearm, wrist, and hand.
6. Assuming no major complications in Ken's rehabilitation, he may require outpatient therapy. At a minimum, Ken should be seen for a home exercise program and monitored until the wound heals. The therapy may entail a minimum of one visit per week.
7. Ken may require assistance for any wound care and dressing changes initially. In addition, if he has difficulty with any one-handed techniques, he may require some assistance with ADLs or instrumental activities of daily living (IADLs) (particularly writing). Temporary accommodations may be required at work or when driving if the automobile has a manual transmission.

Laboratory Exercise 9-2 Answers

1. Thumb interphalangeal (IP) joint is flexed rather than extended, incorrect strap placement at distal forearm trough.
2. Radial deviation at the wrist; incorrect strap placement at distal forearm trough.
3. Poor wrist support; incorrect placement of straps at distal forearm trough.

Chapter 10

Self-Quiz 10-1 Answers

1. T
2. F
3. F
4. T
5. F
6. F
7. F
8. T
9. T
10. F

Case Study 10-1 Answers

1. Posterior elbow immobilization orthosis: Elbow in 120 degrees of flexion, forearm in neutral, and wrist in 15 degrees of extension.

2. Supine on a plinth, with the shoulder in 90 degrees of forward flexion, elbow in 120 degrees of flexion, forearm in neutral rotation, and wrist in neutral extension of 15 degrees.
3. Protect the olecranon, medial and lateral epicondyles, radial and ulnar heads, by padding the bony prominences and molding the orthosis over the padding.
4. The orthosis is worn at all times, and removed for protected range of motion exercises only in a protected environment.

Case Study 10–2 Answers

1. A commercial brace that can be blocked at 90 degrees of flexion and allow for active flexion from 90-degree position as tolerated.
2. To wear the brace at all times, and to perform the exercises within the brace. The brace will be adjusted in therapy every week to increase the flexion angle by 10 to 15 degrees.

Chapter 11

Self-Quiz 11-1 Answers

1. T
2. F
3. F
4. F
5. T

Case Study 11-1 Answers

1. The distal interphalangeal (DIP) joint of the right long finger.
2. All of the time except for skin care, during which time the joint needs to be supported in extension.
3. DIP gutter orthosis, dorsal-volar DIP orthosis, or stack orthosis.
4. Ryland is likely to need to wear his orthosis for 6 to 8 weeks.

Case Study 11-2 Answers

1. Darlene should have a dorsal proximal interphalangeal (PIP) orthosis, because the injury involved the volar plate.
2. The orthosis should cross the PIP joint in 20 to 30 degrees of flexion to protect the injured volar plate.
3. The index and long fingers should be buddy taped to support the injured long finger and maintain alignment. With injury to the radial collateral ligament, the middle phalanx would have a tendency to ulnarly deviate, and the buddy strap helps correct this tendency.
4. Teach Darlene how to use self-adherent compressive wrap to treat the edema. Consider building up the girth of her tennis racquet handle to minimize stress on her injured joint.

Case Study 11-3 Answers

1. Yes, Andrea would benefit from PIP hyperextension block orthoses to improve her active proximal interphalangeal (PIP) flexion.
2. You could fabricate trial thermoplastic orthoses for a few fingers and assess if they help.
3. Important client factors are Andrea's job dealing with the public and what she finds to be most cosmetically appealing. Orthoses will be needed for multiple fingers and will be used long term, and thus streamlined fit and durability are desired qualities. Orthosis adjustability may also be beneficial because PIP size may fluctuate from swelling related to her arthritis.
4. Andrea should wear her orthoses during the daytime only, because these are functional orthoses.

Laboratory Exercise 11-1 Answers

1. It blocks the proximal interphalangeal (PIP) joint.
2. It blocks the distal interphalangeal (DIP) joint.
3. It does not prevent the PIP from hyperextending, allowing the finger to still posture in a swan neck deformity.

Chapter 12

Self-Quiz 12-1 Answers

1. T
2. T
3. F
4. F
5. T
6. T

Chapter 13

Self-Quiz 13-1 Answers

1. T
2. T
3. F
4. F
5. F
6. T
7. T
8. F
9. F
10. T
11. T
12. F

Self-Quiz 13-2 Answers

1. B
2. F
3. A

4. G
5. D
6. E
7. C
8. H

Case Study 13-1 Answers

1. Activities that require grasp and pinch.
2. An elbow orthosis. Due to interosseous weakness, the hand should be monitored for a possible hand-based orthosis for ulnar nerve.
3. The elbow is flexed 30 to 45 degrees, and the wrist is in neutral to 20 degrees of extension.
4. There are a couple of options that the therapist may consider. The first option is lining the orthosis to make it more comfortable. Another option would be to consider the comfort benefits of a prefabricated elbow orthosis. Care must be taken, however, that the prefabricated orthosis correctly position his elbow in the appropriate amount of flexion.
5. Because symptoms are continuous, the therapist should suggest that Sally wear the orthosis all of the time.
6. Sally must become aware of activities that irritate her condition, such as sleeping with her elbow bent.

Case Study 13-2 Answers

1. b
2. a
3. b
4. b
5. b

Laboratory Exercise 13-1 Answers

S: "My pain has decreased."

O: Pt. reports that pain has decreased with resisted pronation from a score of 5 out of 10 to 2 out of 10. Manual muscle testing for the pronator quadratus, pronator teres, flexor carpi radialis, palmaris longus and flexor digitum superficialis, flexor pollicis longus, and flexor digitorium profundus to index and long fingers were all 4 (good). The long-arm orthosis was discontinued on [date] with physician order.

A: Pt. was receptive to continue doing ADLs and home exercise program. Pt. plans to modify work and home activities to decrease repetitive pronation and supination. Pt. has been instructed in a light strengthening program.

P: Occupational therapist will continue to monitor home exercise program.

Chapter 14

Case Study 14-1 Answers

1. d: A volar forearm-based hand immobilization orthosis that stretches and positions the wrist and the fingers in composite extension at or slightly greater than 5 degrees is most appropriate. Over time, the angle of wrist extension with the fingers in composite extension may be adjusted. Since Bertha also has edema, the orthosis facilitates edema reduction by keeping the hand upright and in a non-dependent position. A dorsal-based forearm platform with a volar hand component that positions the wrist and fingers in tolerable composite extension may position the hand in a desirable manner, but with Bertha's edema, donning the orthosis will be difficult. A volar finger spreader with volar forearm component is a viable alternative because it provides the added benefit of keeping the web spaces aerated. However, since Bertha reports pain with passive extension greater than 5 degrees, the position of maximum passive extension may increase the pain and compromise orthotic adherence. With Bertha's condition still in the acute stages of recovery, a rigid cast is not appropriate at this time. Finally, a volar cone orthosis is not appropriate because it may accentuate the edema and skin breakdown. In addition, placing the fingers in flexion over a cone and the wrist at submaximal stretch promotes contractures.

2. Prior to altering or discontinuing the orthosis, the therapist monitors how caregivers and the nursing staff apply the orthosis correctly. A common pitfall is when the straps are applied tightly creating chokepoints especially at the wrist. The therapist reinforces the importance of proper carry-over for the orthotic program to be successful. The therapist considers interventions to manage edema and evaluate other potential reasons for the swelling.

3. When a client has early signs of active control of hand movement, the therapist considers using orthoses to facilitate better hand control so that the client can engage in intensive, repetitive task practice. With the edema resolved, the appropriate orthosis is a Neoprene thumb-abduction and extension orthosis that extends to the forearm radially. The forearm component supports the wrist with emerging stability. Once the client is more capable of stabilizing the wrist during grip, the therapist may switch to a short opponens orthosis. Both Neoprene-based and short opponens orthoses restrict the thumb from assuming flexion-adduction. These orthoses prevent contracture formation and facilitate a greater repertoire of prehensile patterns. A finger spreader, a hard cone, and an inflatable orthosis are inappropriate substitutes because they only restrict hand use in a functional, task-oriented manner. If Bertha's spastic tone continues to pose problems with hand function, the therapist may provide a hand immobilization orthosis to provide wrist and hand flexor stretch during intervals of rest.

4. Using a Neoprene-based orthosis or a short opponens orthosis, family and caregivers encourage Bertha to her affected hand during activities, such as eating or drinking (e.g., holding a cup, picking up dense finger foods) and leisure (e.g., playing cards). The therapist considers active strategies and modalities to further develop strength and stability of grasp and maintain range of motion.

Chapter 15

Self-Quiz 15-1 Answers

1. T
2. F
3. F
4. T
5. F
6. T
7. F
8. F
9. T
10. F
11. T
12. T
13. T
14. T

Self-Quiz 15-2 Answers

1. A material that has high drapability and moldability is not a good choice for making antigravity orthoses. A material that has resistance to drape and memory is suitable. A slightly tacky orthotic material that lightly adheres to underlying stockinette may be helpful. Preshaping techniques assist in molding.
2. A positioning soft orthosis (such as, soft roll or palm protector) places the involved joints in submaximum extension. This position permits adequate skin hygiene.
3. An orthosis should not limit the use of uninvolved joints. An arthritis mitt orthosis immobilizes only the affected joints and positions the thumb in a resting position. The client can still use the fingers for functional activities at night.
4. Pad the outside of the orthosis.
5. The straps should be soft, wide foam straps that are cut a little long to adjust for edema. The orthotic design should be made wide enough to accommodate the edema.

Case Study 15-1 Answers

1. c
2. a and c
3. b, c, and d
4. d

Case Study 15-2 Answers

1. a and d
2. d
3. a
4. d
5. c

Laboratory Exercise 15-1 Answers

1. The orthosis blocks the wrist and thumb interphalangeal (IP) joint.
2. The figure-eight is not properly positioned to effectively prevent hyperextension of the thumb IP joint. The figure-eight orthosis should be rotated and placed on the finger to prevent IP hyperextension

Chapter 16

Laboratory Exercise 16-1 Answer

Two fabrication problems are present in this orthosis. First, the C bar does not fit into the web space of the thumb and provides inadequate positioning of the thumb between radial and palmar abduction. Second, the sides of the forearm trough are too high—resulting in bridging of the straps.

Laboratory Exercise 16-2 Answer

The straps are not keeping the wrist positioned in the orthosis. The distal forearm strap should be placed just proximal to the ulnar styloid, and a second strap should be added just distal to the ulnar styloid—preventing the flexor action of the wrist from lifting the wrist away from the orthosis's surface. The orthosis does not fit snugly into the thumb web space.

Laboratory Exercise 16-3 Answer

The orthosis does not fit snugly into the web space. In addition, the thumb trough is slightly too long and does not allow tactile contact of the tip of the thumb with an object being grasped.

Case Study 16-1 Answers

1. Option A would probably not be adequate to address concerns of losing range of motion (ROM) of the wrist and fingers. Once range is lost, it can be difficult (if not impossible) to regain. Therefore prevention is paramount. Relying on passive range of motion (PROM) may be disruptive to other activities and occupations during the day. The constant effects of moderately to severely increased tone will be difficult to overcome with activities alone. The thumb orthoses alone would not be adequate to address concerns with the wrist and finger flexors.
2. Option B would probably best meet Ben's needs at this time. Prolonged stretch to the wrist and finger flexors could occur at night. Active functional movement during play, z-care, communication, and school activities could be emphasized during his waking hours. Because the left upper extremity is tighter and less functional, it would also be prudent to wear the left resting orthosis on this hand periodically during the day. A thermoplastic thumb orthosis for the right hand would control some

of the increased tone in the hand but leave the wrist and fingers free for active and functional movement. ROM measurements would be required to determine optimal wearing schedules.

You will contact Ben's parents to discuss your recommendations for using the orthoses and the purpose of the orthoses and to get their input. Assuming they are in agreement, you arrange a meeting with his parents prior to the orthoses' going home. At this time, you will review the purpose of the orthoses, demonstrate how to apply the orthoses, and provide an opportunity for the parents to practice donning and doffing the orthoses. You will also give the parents written instructions, precautions, and your phone number. Photographs of the orthoses on Ben's hands will be included if needed.

3. Option C would be excessive use of resting hand orthoses at the present time. Ben should continue to experience active movement and sensory feedback as much as possible during the day, especially with the right hand.

4. Option D would unnecessarily restrict active use of the hands during the day while leaving the wrist and finger flexors shortened during the night and on weekends. This family is involved in Ben's programming, and you will address the issue of correct application at home by meeting with the parents as described in Option B. If you have questions regarding follow-through at home, you should obtain more information about the family's strengths and limitations, the parents' understanding of intervention, and family routines. You should then individualize your style of collaboration and provide instruction for that family.

Case Study 16-2 Answers

1. Option A, a resting hand orthosis, would not be appropriate because Mia has full passive range of motion (PROM) in the left wrist and hand. Elongation of wrist and finger flexors is desirable but could be accomplished through weight-bearing activities.

2. Option B, a standard wrist cock-up (immobilization) orthosis, would not adequately address the problem of thumb adduction into the palm. It is likely that positioning the thumb in opposition will have an inhibitory effect on the wrist and hand. If the wrist flexion continues to be a problem after the thumb is addressed, other orthotic or treatment options could be considered.

3. Option C, using a Neoprene thumb orthosis as part of an overall intervention plan, is the correct answer. The thumb can serve as a key point of control for the hand, and once positioned may have an overall inhibitory affect. Tone is probably not severe enough to start with a thermoplastic thumb orthosis, but Mia might need additional assistance in the form of an added C bar attached to the Neoprene thumb orthosis. If Neoprene does not adequately limit thumb adduction, a thermoplastic thumb orthosis could be considered.

Chapter 17

Case Study 17-1 Answers

1. The occupational therapist could assist with donning and doffing of the device, developing wear schedules based upon the client's needs and develop skills to integrate the device into activities of dialing living.

2. An optimally provided orthosis could address the client's concerns with mobility and ADL that require LE functionality.

3. Total contact, 3 point pressure systems and kinesthetic reminder could each play a role in this particular client. 3 point pressure systems could address the client's paralytic equinus in swing phase, total contact would distribute the pressure throughout a larger area of the limb and the sensation of wearing an orthosis could enhance proprioception.

4. This client would most benefit from a thermoplastic ankle foot orthosis (AFO). The AFO would enable a heel strike at initial contact, modulate forward progression of the tibia during stance phase and eliminate equinus positioning throughout swing phase.

Case Study 17-2 Answers

1. Neuropathy can negatively affect the sensory, motor and autonomic functions. Sensory deficits could result in diminished protective sensation making the client unaware of injury. Motor neuropathy can result in atrophy of the intrinsic muscles of the foot resulting in an imbalance of the muscles that facilitate locomotion and other weight bearing activities. Autonomic neuropathy can result in diminished function of the glands within the feet compromising skin integrity, which may compromise the soft tissue envelope increasing the risk of infection.

2. Extra-depth footwear have the ability to be adjusted to achieve an optimal fit to the client's foot be creating additional volume for deformities such as clawed does.

3. Accomodative foot orthoses create an interface for the diabetic foot that conforms to the client's present alignment ensuring pressure is distributed over the largest possible surface area. A corrective orthosis applies specific forces to achieve an alignment different from the patients in situ presentation which could potentially result in skin breakdown where forces are excessive.

Case Study 17-3 Answers

1. The common peroneal nerve bifurcates into the deep and superficial peroneal nerve which innervate the anterior and lateral compartments of the leg.

2. Swing phase functionality would be affected in a similar manner, but the solid ankle trimline would not allow for the client's tibia would be unable to progress forward

to 10 degrees of relative dorsiflexion at terminal stance forcing the patient to either take a shorter contralateral step or hyperextend the knee on the ipsilateral side to maintain step length symmetry.

Case Study 17-4 Answers

1. The anatomical knee joint is a polycentric joint. The application of a single axis joint would not accurately follow the knees axis of rotation as it moves through normal range-of-motion which could result in the orthosis migrating and placing less than optimal forces through the client's knee.
2. The 3 point pressure system is exemplified in the coronal plane to create an unloading of the client's osteoarthritic lateral compartment.

Case Study 17-5 Answers

1. Both sensation and proprioception are unaffected by paralytic post-polio syndrome as polio affects the anterior horn of the spinal cord resulting in only motor deficits.
2. The client should be provided a knee joint that locks as the posterior offset joint on the provided orthosis relies on maintaining the weight line anterior to the knee joint which cannot consistently be done with a client that does not achieve terminal extension.

Case Study 17-6 Answers

1. This position seats the prosthesis into the socket encouraging joint stability. Relative adduction or excessive hip flexion could encourage the prosthesis the shift out of the socket.
2. Sitting and transferring would be more difficult and require modifications to perform these tasks.

Case Study 17-7 Answers

1. A client with a thoracic level lesion would not have adequate volitional strength at the hips or knees to facilitate ambulation with just ankle foot orthoses.
2. Ambulation with the HKAFO would require a swing-through gait versus the much more natural reciprocating pattern that is enabled by the RGO.

Chapter 18

Self-Quiz 18-1 Answers

1. B
2. C
3. C
4. B
5. A
6. B

7. C
8. Step 1: C
Step 2: A
Step 3: B
9. A
10. A

Chapter 19

Self-Quiz 19-1 Answers

1. T
2. T
3. F
4. F
5. T
6. F
7. F
8. T
9. T
10. T

Case Study 19-1 Answers

1. The guide to determining whether a situation involves ethics includes answering the following three questions:
   * Is there more than one morally plausible resolution?
   * Is there no clear-cut best resolution?
   * Is there direct reference to the welfare or dignity of others?

   In this case, because Sam is inexperienced, one could expect that he would need supervision as he gains mastery over the techniques necessary to treat clients. Valerie has already noted that Sam needs more supervision. Thus, the welfare of clients is affected. Valerie realizes that the ideal solution would be for her to spend more time supervising Sam, but she does not believe this is possible because of her administrative duties. There is more than one morally plausible option in the case. Because the answer to two of the three criteria is "yes," the case does involve an ethical issue.

2. Clearly, the ethical principles of nonmaleficence and beneficence are involved. Valerie and Sam have an obligation to protect all clients from unnecessary harm and to do good for them within the constraints of available resources. There are not enough qualified staff members to supervise Sam. The lack of senior staff members could be considered a problem of justice. There is not enough of Valerie to go around. She is not capable of completing all of the tasks assigned to her, and thus she must make decisions about what takes priority.

   A fair and equitable work setting should have adequate personnel to do the job safely and effectively. The current shortage of staff could be due to chance (i.e., the unfortunate coincidence of a retirement and maternity leave). However, both of these events are predictable.

Thus, as the manager Valerie should have foreseen that there would be a problem and made advance plans for it. If Valerie is making a good-faith effort to recruit replacement staff, we would not hold her accountable for sustaining a work environment that is unsafe and short staffed. We could, however, hold her accountable for poor planning and the impact this has had on Sam's orientation and client care.

According to care-based reasoning, Valerie should consider what a caring work environment would look like for new employees and clients. It is true that novices do not become expert without experience, but how we provide experience makes a great deal of difference.

Finally, virtues that are required in this situation could include perseverance, compassion, courage, justice, and integrity. One of the alternatives available to Valerie is to reassign her administrative and management responsibilities to someone else, in that there is no one else in her institution who is an occupational therapist and can supervise direct client care. It would take courage to delegate administrative authority, because it would require relinquishing power. However, if client care holds a central position in the values of the organization, this is a plausible option.

3. The first alternative action is that Valerie could limit the type of clients Sam treats, selecting only those he can treat safely with minimal supervision. The principles that support this action are nonmaleficence and beneficence, in that clients would be protected. Sam would not receive the type of experience he would like, which might interfere with his autonomy, but client welfare would not be in jeopardy.

The second alternative action is that Valerie could maintain the status quo and continue with things the way they are, with minimal supervision. The principles of nonmaleficence and beneficence are threatened. It is possible that Sam would not commit any serious mistakes, but because of his inexperience it is clear that clients would not be getting the quality of care they need or deserve.

The third option is that Valerie could ask for release time from her administrative duties so that she could be free for direct client care. The principles of nonmaleficence, beneficence, and justice are supported by this action—in that client welfare is protected and Sam receives the type of supervision that he should have to become a competent clinician.

The fourth option is to hire an occupational therapist on a temporary basis for specific supervision of Sam and complex cases. This action may require greater expense, but it would allow Valerie to continue with her administrative duties (if those duties contribute to the benefit of clients), and Sam would receive the supervision he needs. Clients would be protected from harm and would benefit from the expertise of an experienced therapist.

4. The principles in the Code of Ethics that are helpful in this case include principle 4, which demands the maintenance of high standards of competence. There is a clear responsibility for all occupational therapists to maintain their own level of competence and to monitor that of peers. Depending on the reason for incompetence, various methods can be taken to resolve the problem, such as further education, increased staffing, workshops, drug and alcohol treatment programs, and so on. In this case, Sam is incompetent because he is inexperienced and needs more supervision. This is a state that is temporary and could be resolved with adequate supervision. Second, principle 1C strictly enjoins protecting clients from harm. Valerie should be guided by this principle above all others as she attempts to resolve the problem.

Web Resources and Vendors

Societies, Organizations, Education

American Academy of Orthopaedic Surgeons
http://www.aaos.org/
American Association for Hand Surgery
http://www.handsurgery.org/
American Hand Therapy Foundation
http://www.ahtf.org/
The American Occupational Therapy Association, Inc.
http://www.aota.org/
The American Occupational Therapy Foundation
http://www.aotf.org/
American Orthotic & Prosthetic Association
http://www.aopanet.org/
American Physical Therapy Association
http://www.apta.org/
American Society of Hand Therapists
http://www.asht.org/
American Society for Surgery of the Hand
http://www.assh.org/
Canadian Association of Occupational Therapists
http://www.caot.ca/
E-hand.com The Electronic Textbook of Hand Surgery
http://www.eatonhand.com/
Exploring Hand Therapy
http://www.exploringhandtherapy.com/
Hand Rehabilitation Foundation
http://www.handrehabfoundation.org/
Handsights (special interest group of hand therapists attending
the surgery meetings)
http://www.handsights.net/
Hand Therapy Certification Commission
http://www.htcc.org/
International Federation of Societies for Hand Therapy
http://www.ifsht.org/
Journal of Hand Therapy
http://journals.elsevierhealth.com/periodicals/hanthe
World Federation of Occupational Therapists
http://www.wfot.org/

Orthotic Materials and Accessories Suppliers

The following list is of course not exhaustive. Neither is the quality and/or service of products implied, and company contact information is subject to change.
AliMed 1-800-225-2610
http://www.alimed.com/
Bio Med Sciences, Inc. 1-800-25-SILON
http://www.silon.com/
Bioness, Inc. 1-800-211-9136
http://www.bionessinc.com
Chesapeake Medical Products, Inc. 1-888-560-2674
http://www.chesapeakemedical.com/
DeRoyal 1-800-deroyal
http://www.deroyal.com/
Human Factors Engineering 928-684-9606
http://www.splinting.com/
Kinex Medical Company 1-800-845-6364
http://www.kinexmedical.com/
Klarity Medical Products, Inc. 740-788-8107
http://www.klaritymedical.com/
North Coast Medical 1-800-821-9319
http://www.ncmedical.com/
Orfit Industries 1-888-ORFIT-US
http://www.orfit.com/
Patterson Medical 1-800-323-5547
http://www.pattersoncompanies.com/medical
Silver Ring Splint 1-800-311-7028
http://www.silverringsplint.com/
U.E. Tech 1-800-736-1894
http://www.uetech.com/
WFR Corporation 1-800-526-5247
http://www.reveals.com/

Resources for Upper Extremity Prosthetics

Amputee Coalition of America
    www.amputee-coalition.org
American Academy of Orthotists & Prosthetists
    www.oandp.org
American Orthotic & Prosthetic Association
    www.aopanet.org

American Amputee Foundation
    www.americanamputee.org
American Board for Certification in Orthotics, Prosthetics
    & Pedorthics
    www.abcop.org

Index

Note: Page numbers followed by "b", "f" and "t" indicate boxes, figures and tables respectively.